Handbook of Experimental Pharmacology

Volume 258

The *Handbook of Experimental Pharmacology* is one of the most authoritative and influential book series in pharmacology. It provides critical and comprehensive discussions of the most significant areas of pharmacological research, written by leading international authorities. Each volume in the series represents the most informative and contemporary account of its subject available, making it an unrivalled reference source.

HEP is indexed in PubMed and Scopus.

More information about this series at http://www.springer.com/series/164

Michael A. Nader • Yasmin L. Hurd
Editors

Substance Use Disorders

From Etiology to Treatment

Springer

Editors
Michael A. Nader
Wake Forest School of Medicine
Winston-Salem, NC, USA

Yasmin L. Hurd
Addiction Institute of Mount Sinai
Icahn School of Medicine at Mount Sinai
New York, NY, USA

ISSN 0171-2004 ISSN 1865-0325 (electronic)
Handbook of Experimental Pharmacology
ISBN 978-3-030-33678-3 ISBN 978-3-030-33679-0 (eBook)
https://doi.org/10.1007/978-3-030-33679-0

This Springer imprint is published by the registered company Springer Nature Switzerland AG.
The registered company address is: Gewerbestrasse 11, 6330 Cham, Switzerland

Preface

Drug abuse continues to be a major public health problem worldwide contributing to extensive morbidity and mortality that have tremendous economic and human costs. Many Western countries have seen a dramatic increase in the use of opioid drugs where, for example, in the USA the use of both prescription and illicit opioids have contributed to the death of over 300,000 people in the past decade (Center for Disease Control 2018). Many communities are now experiencing a new wave of cocaine and other stimulant use as well as the emergence of synthetic drugs. While much attention is given to illegal drugs, the two prominent legal substances, tobacco and alcohol, continue to exert the biggest threat to human health worldwide with an estimated 143.7 deaths per 100,000 people per year (Peacock et al. 2018). Another drug that now straddles the legal and illegal markets is cannabis where dramatic sociopolitical changes in many countries have led to the legalization of medicinal and recreational cannabis. The societal and health consequences of these policy changes are still unknown, but what is clear is that similar to other drugs, cannabis can lead to a pathological use disorder for which there are limited treatment options. Disturbingly, there are today still few available treatments for substance use disorders (SUDs). The growing use of drugs combined with the low-risk perception of the harm of these substances in society has raised significant alarm and brought renewed awareness of the critical need for advanced knowledge about the effects of these psychoactive drugs on the brain that can guide the development of much needed new treatment strategies to save lives.

The primary problem facing clinicians treating individuals with SUD is relapse (O'Brien and Anthony 2005). In fact, relapse rates have remained unchanged over the last 40 years (Dong et al. 2017). It has been noted (Humphreys and Bickel 2018) that there are common neuroadaptations across SUDs, but there are still significant gaps of knowledge about how these common neural pathways and circuits contribute to relapse vulnerability, as well as whether and how they recover during long-term abstinence. There is also a wide range of individual differences in behavioral and neurobiological responses to chronic drug abuse; these differences manifest themselves during recovery attempts, with some people having a greater ability to maintain abstinence than others. Clearly, more research is needed to understand these individual differences in attempts to develop a personalized treatment strategy for SUDs.

The goal of this volume is to describe innovative basic science and clinical research focused on various drugs of abuse given their critical impact in many communities today. The first three chapters provide overviews of research techniques: population-based research, molecular techniques, and small-molecule chemistry. The remaining chapters focus on (1) molecular mechanisms, (2) preclinical behavioral pharmacology, and (3) clinical pharmacology for opioids (mu and kappa receptor), stimulants (cocaine and amphetamines), marijuana, nicotine, alcohol, and newly emerging substances of abuse. Together, these chapters bridge preclinical and clinical behavioral pharmacology in expanding knowledge about the current state of the field.

Some highlights from this volume:

- Recent advances in developing novel opioid analgesics from an understanding of mu receptor structure and function, including the study of biased agonists;
- Drugs acting at mu opioid receptors, including abused opioids, can vary on a number of dimensions, including pharmacological efficacy, drug-receptor interactions, receptor selectivity, and pharmacokinetics; these differences impact the behavioral effects of drugs acting at mu opioid receptors;
- Individual differences are a hallmark of SUD. In fact, most people that try drugs do not become dependent on them. The neurobiological and genetic underpinnings of individual differences in vulnerability are discussed;
- In individuals with SUDs, epigenetic molecular adaptations (DNA modification to increase or decrease the probability of gene expression) underlie persistent drug-seeking behavior;
- Research on cannabinoids led to the discovery of the endogenous cannabinoid system. Studies are described showing the benefits, as well as harmful effects of this neurotransmitter system on human health;
- Clinical trials involving pharmacotherapies for cannabis use disorder highlight the importance of individual differences and the contribution of concurrent mental health conditions;
- Research is described involving nicotine's direct actions in the brain in regard to specific genes that mitigate the vulnerability to develop nicotine dependence, as well as the role that other constituents in nicotine and tobacco products have on maintaining dependence;
- Given the relapse rates with existing Food and Drug Administration (FDA)-approved medications for smoking cessation, novel pharmacotherapies are being developed through clinical trials that might hold additional promise;
- Alcohol use disorder (AUD) is prevalent in adolescents and adults; however the mechanisms mediating AUD may not be the same in these two populations. Preclinical models of adolescent vulnerability are described focusing on GABAergic and glutamatergic neurotransmission within regions/circuits that regulate cognitive function, emotion, and their integration;
- Three medications have been approved in the USA, by the FDA, and in other countries to treat patients with AUD: disulfiram, naltrexone (oral and long-acting), and acamprosate. Individual differences in treatment response continued

to push for the development of other medications that have shown efficacy in clinical trials;

- The use of synthetic drugs has soared. Epidemiology, chemistry, pharmacophysiology, clinical effects, laboratory detection, and clinical treatment are discussed for newly emerging drugs of abuse; the challenge to detect these drugs are of particular importance for hospital employees, medical examiners, and law enforcement personnel.

This volume reflects the culmination of significant efforts by many individuals who wrote, organized, and assembled these chapters. We would like to thank Dr. James E. Barrett, Editor-in-Chief of the *Handbook of Experimental Pharmacology* series, for inviting us to edit this volume and for his guidance throughout the process. We also would like to acknowledge the outstanding efforts of Susanne Dathe, Coral Zhou, Anand Ventakachalam, and Gerit Rother. Finally, we would like to thank the contributors to this volume. Their insight and vision should guide clinicians and researchers into innovative treatment strategies for substance use disorders.

Winston-Salem, NC, USA — Michael A. Nader
New York, NY, USA — Yasmin L. Hurd

References

Center for Disease Control. Drug overdose deaths in the United States, 1999–2017. NCHS Data Brief, No. 329, Nov 2018

Dong Y et al (2017) Circuit and synaptic plasticity mechanisms of drug relapse. J Neurosci 37:10867–10876

Humphreys K, Bickel WK (2018) Toward a neuroscience of long-term recovery from addiction. JAMA Psychiatry 75:875–876

O'Brien MS, Anthony JC (2005) Risk of becoming cocaine dependent: epidemiological estimates for the United States, 2000–2001. Neuropsychopharmacology 30:1006–1018

Peacock A, Leung J, Larney S, Colledge S, Hickman M, Rehm J, Giovino GA, West R, Hall W, Griffiths P, Ali R, Gowing L, Marsden J, Ferrari AJ, Grebely J, Farrell M, Degenhardt L (2018) Global statistics on alcohol, tobacco and illicit drug use: 2017 status report. Addiction 113:1905–1926

Contents

Methods for Population Research on Substance Use and Consequences 1
Mark Wolfson, Kimberly G. Wagoner, Eunyoung Y. Song, Melinda Pankratz, and Sunday Azagba

Translational Molecular Approaches in Substance Abuse Research 31
Sasha L. Fulton and Ian Maze

Small Molecule Neuropeptide S and Melanocortin 4 Receptor Ligands as Potential Treatments for Substance Use Disorders 61
Bruce Blough and Ojas Namjoshi

Emerging Insights into Mu Opioid Pharmacology 89
Gavril W. Pasternak, Steven R. Childers, and Ying-Xian Pan

Behavioral Pharmacology of Drugs Acting at Mu Opioid Receptors 127
Lisa R. Gerak, David R. Maguire, and Charles P. France

The Rise and Fall of Kappa-Opioid Receptors in Drug Abuse Research 147
Matthew L. Banks

Clinical Trials for Opioid Use Disorder 167
Esther Blessing, Sanya Virani, and John Rotrosen

Modelling Differential Vulnerability to Substance Use Disorder in Rodents: Neurobiological Mechanisms 203
Bianca Jupp, Jolyon A. Jones, and Jeffrey W. Dalley

Activity-Dependent Epigenetic Remodeling in Cocaine Use Disorder . . . 231
Alberto J. López, Cody A. Siciliano, and Erin S. Calipari

Molecular Mechanisms of Amphetamines 265
Maarten E. A. Reith and Margaret E. Gnegy

Clinical Trials for Stimulant Use Disorders: Addressing Heterogeneities That May Undermine Treatment Outcomes 299
Paul S. Regier, Kyle M. Kampman, and Anna Rose Childress

Molecular Mechanism and Cannabinoid Pharmacology 323
Lesley D. Schurman, Dai Lu, Debra A. Kendall, Allyn C. Howlett, and Aron H. Lichtman

Pharmacotherapies for Cannabis Use Disorders: Clinical Challenges and Promising Therapeutic Agents 355
Suzanne Nielsen, Pamela Sabioni, Linda Gowing, and Bernard Le Foll

Molecular Mechanisms Associated with Nicotine Pharmacology and Dependence 373
Christie D. Fowler, Jill R. Turner, and M. Imad Damaj

Randomized Clinical Trials Investigating Innovative Interventions for Smoking Cessation in the Last Decade 395
Marie N. S. Gendy, Christine Ibrahim, Matthew E. Sloan, and Bernard Le Foll

Adolescent Vulnerability to Alcohol Use Disorder: Neurophysiological Mechanisms from Preclinical Studies 421
Brian A. McCool and Molly M. McGinnis

Medication Development for Alcohol Use Disorder: A Focus on Clinical Studies 443
Lorenzo Leggio, Daniel E. Falk, Megan L. Ryan, Joanne Fertig, and Raye Z. Litten

Newly Emerging Drugs of Abuse 463
Kenichi Tamama and Michael J. Lynch

Methods for Population Research on Substance Use and Consequences

Mark Wolfson, Kimberly G. Wagoner, Eunyoung Y. Song, Melinda Pankratz, and Sunday Azagba

Contents

1 Introduction 2
2 Population Research on Substance Use and Consequences 3
2.1 Data Collection Methods 3
3 Measures 11
3.1 Measures of Own Use 11
3.2 Harming Others 15
4 Causal Factors and Correlates of Substance Use and Consequences 15
4.1 Individual Causal Factors and Correlates 16
4.2 Environmental Causal Factors and Correlates 17
5 Summary and Conclusion 20
5.1 Accumulation of Knowledge 20
5.2 Translation of Knowledge 21
5.3 Limitations 21
References 21

Abstract

This chapter reviews the array of methods used in contemporary research on population-level research on substance use and its consequences. We argue that there are critical questions that can best – or in some cases, only – be addressed at

M. Wolfson (✉)
Department of Social Medicine, Population, and Public Health, School of Medicine, University of California, Riverside, CA, USA
e-mail: mark.wolfson@medsch.ucr.edu

K. G. Wagoner · E. Y. Song · M. Pankratz
Department of Social Sciences and Health Policy, Wake Forest School of Medicine, Winston-Salem, NC, USA
e-mail: kwagoner@wakehealth.edu; esong@wakehealth.edu; mpankrat@wakehealth.edu

S. Azagba
Department of Family and Preventive Medicine, University of Utah, Salt Lake City, UT, USA
e-mail: Sunday.Azagba@utah.edu

M. A. Nader, Y. L. Hurd (eds.), *Substance Use Disorders*,
Handbook of Experimental Pharmacology 258, https://doi.org/10.1007/164_2019_319

the level of a population. We then describe the major categories of data collection methods used in population research, including surveys, ecological momentary assessment, administrative data, audit methods, and unobtrusive assessment of substance use. Two categories of measures are then discussed: measures of an individual's use of substances and related problems and measures of harm to others caused by one's use. We then review factors that may be considered causes or correlates of substance use and consequences, including both individual and environmental factors. We close with a few thoughts on the accumulation of knowledge and its translation to policy and practice.

Keywords
Alcohol · Drugs · Population health · Public health · Research · Tobacco

1 Introduction

This chapter reviews the array of methods used in contemporary research on population-level research on substance use and its consequences. These include methods that have been utilized for decades (such as population-based surveys and administrative data), as well as methods of more recent vintage (such as response-driven sampling and a variety of audit methods).

A useful starting point is to ask the question, "why is it important to examine substance use at the population level?" After all, there is an abundance of research on the dynamics of substance use in individuals and small, handpicked samples, as evidenced by many of the chapters in this volume. This research is extraordinarily useful for answering a number of key questions related to human drug-seeking, drug-taking, and physiological and psychological responses. However, there are also critical questions that can best – or in some cases, only – be addressed at the level of a population (we discuss alternative definitions of "populations," below). These include:

1. What is the incidence and prevalence of substance use in a population? Answering this question is not only important from a scientific standpoint but also important for informing public policy at local, state, national, and cross-national levels.
2. What are the relationships between population-level patterns of substance use and rates of negative consequences of use? From both scientific and policy standpoints, it is important to understand how rates of substance use translate into rates of problems.
3. What individual and environmental factors underlie rates of substance use and consequences in populations? Individual factors (as discussed below) may include age, race and ethnicity, gender, sexual identity, sexual orientation, socioeconomic status, genetic makeup, personality, beliefs and attitudes, and life experiences. Environmental or contextual factors may include the availability of drugs with abuse potential, neighborhood factors (e.g., housing, socioeconomic status, crime rates), the presence or absence of relevant policies, and enforcement practices, among others.

It is also important to define what we mean by *substance use*. We define substance use as the intentional consumption of psychoactive drugs, which conventionally include alcohol, tobacco, marijuana, illicit drugs (such as cocaine, hallucinogens, heroin), inhalants, and prescription drugs that are either not used as prescribed or used by someone for whom they were not prescribed. We define consequences of substance use to include individual or group changes in health, behavior, family situation, economic status, educational status, legal status, or other outcomes which may be attributed, at least in part, to use of one or more substances.

Finally, it is important to define what we mean by a "population." As in all areas of science, the definition of a population is the subject of contention and debate (see Krieger 2012 for a recent summary of the issues). We use here a conventional (and conservative) definition of a population as the "inhabitants of an area" (see Krieger 2012), although we briefly reference other definitions, such as a geographically dispersed aggregation of people who are united by some other characteristic or feature, such as sexual identity.

In the following sections of this chapter, we review methods for population research on substance use and its consequences, focusing on data collection methods (including surveys, ecological momentary assessment, administrative data, electronic health records, audits, and unobtrusive methods) for producing data on (1) substance use, (2) consequences of use, and (3) contexts of use and environmental factors. We follow this with a discussion of future directions in methods.

2 Population Research on Substance Use and Consequences

2.1 Data Collection Methods

Below we review methods for population research on substance use and its consequences, focusing on data collection methods, including surveys, ecological momentary assessment, administrative data, electronic health records, audits, and unobtrusive methods.

2.1.1 Surveys

Dating back at least to the 1970s, there is a long history of national surveys on substance use. For example, the National Survey on Drug Use and Health (originally known as the National Household Survey on Drug Abuse), sponsored by what is now known as the Substance Abuse and Mental Health Services Administration (SAMHSA), was first fielded in 1971. Monitoring the Future, which includes annual national surveys of high school students and periodic follow-up surveys of subsamples of these students, was launched in 1974 (Bachman et al. 2001).

Table 1 displays information on basic characteristics of major survey datasets that include extensive data on substance use.

This table does not include surveys that are no longer active, such as the Harvard College Alcohol Study, conducted in a sample of over 100 college campuses in 1993, 1997, 1999, and 2001 (Wechsler and Nelson 2008).

Table 1 Major survey datasets that include extensive data on alcohol, tobacco, and other drug use and consequences

	Sample				
Survey name	Age range	Other sample characteristics	Years	Sponsor	Website
National Survey on Drug Use and Health	Age 12 and up	Random sample of households. Repeated cross-sectional design. Face-to-face interviews	1971–present	Substance Abuse and Mental Health Services Administration	https://nsduhweb.rti.org/respweb/homepage.cfm
Monitoring the Future	8th, 10th, and 12th grade students (12th graders since 1975 and 8th and 10th graders since 1991)	School-based survey. Repeated cross-sectional design with a longitudinal follow-up component	1975–present	National Institute on Drug Abuse	http://www.monitoringthefuture.org/
Behavioral Risk Factor Surveillance System	Adults aged 18 years or older	Multimode (mail, landline phone, and cell phone) health survey. Repeated cross-sectional design. Fifty-one projects used a disproportionate stratified sample (DSS) design for their landline samples. Guam, Puerto Rico, and the US Virgin Islands used a simple random sample design	1984–present	Centers for Disease Control and Prevention	https://www.cdc.gov/brfss/
Youth Risk Behavior Surveillance System	Students in grades 9–12	Cross-sectional school-based survey	1975–present	Centers for Disease Control and Prevention	https://www.cdc.gov/healthyyouth/data/yrbs/index.htm
National Longitudinal Study of Adolescent to Adult Health	Sample of adolescents in grades 7–12 in the United States during the 1994–1995 school year	Periodic longitudinal follow-up survey. In-home interview	Wave 1: 1994–1995 Wave 2: 1996 Wave 3: 2001–2002 Wave 4: 2008 Wave 5: 2016–2018	National Institute of Child Health and Human Development	https://www.cpc.unc.edu/projects/addhealth/

National Health and Nutrition Examination Survey	Noninstitutionalized civilian resident population. Adults and children	Multistage, unequal probability and cluster sampling methods. Interviews and physical examinations	1971–present	Centers for Disease Control and Prevention	https://www.cdc.gov/nchs/nhanes/index.htm
National Health Interview Survey	Aged 65 or older	Cross-sectional household interview survey	1957–present	Centers for Disease Control and Prevention	https://www.cdc.gov/nchs/nhis/index.htm
Pregnancy Risk Assessment Monitoring System	A sample of women who have had a recent birth	Population-based sampling frame "follows back" a stratified sample of women several months postpartum, surveying them about their own and their infant's prenatal, birth, and postpartum behavior and experiences	1988–present	Centers for Disease Control and Prevention	https://www.cdc.gov/prams/index.htm
General Social Survey	Noninstitutionalized adults who speak either English or Spanish	Repeated cross-sectional interview survey	1972–present	The University of Chicago	http://gss.norc.org/
National Alcohol Survey	Individuals ages 18 and over	Periodic national survey	1964–present	Alcohol Research Group	http://arg.org/center/national-alcohol-surveys/
National Epidemiologic Survey on Alcohol and Related Conditions	Ages 18 and over	Face-to-face interviews. Periodic cross-sectional survey	Wave 1: 2001–2002 Wave 2: 2004–2005 Wave 3: 2012–2013	National Institute on Alcohol Abuse and Alcoholism	https://www.niaaa.nih.gov/research/nesarc-iii
National Adult Tobacco Survey	Noninstitutionalized adults ages 18 and over	Landline and cell phone survey	2009–present	Centers for Disease Control and Prevention	https://www.cdc.gov/tobacco/data_statistics/surveys/nats/index.htm

(continued)

Table 1 (continued)

Survey name	Sample		Years	Sponsor	Website
	Age range	Other sample characteristics			
National Youth Tobacco Survey	Middle school (grades 6–8) and high school (grades 9–12) students	School-based survey	2000–present	Centers for Disease Control and Prevention and Food and Drug Administration	https://www.cdc.gov/tobacco/data_statistics/surveys/nyts/index.htm
Population Assessment of Tobacco and Health	First wave of data collection included responses from over 32,000 adults and 13,000 youth	National longitudinal study of individuals ages 12 and over. In-person interviews	2013–present	National Institutes of Health and Food and Drug Administration	https://pathstudyinfo.nih.gov/UI/HomeMobile.aspx

The sponsoring agency or the organization that implements each of these surveys issues periodic reports on major findings from the surveys, usually related to prevalence of use of various substances, and changes in prevalence over time (e.g., Johnston et al. 2019; Mack et al. 2017). In addition, raw data (stripped of any personal identifiers) from these surveys are available to the research community. These datasets are widely used by researchers, who sometimes use them to contest the "official" findings (e.g., Borders 2018), as well as for a wide variety of studies examining such topics as the association of state recreational marijuana laws and adolescent marijuana use (Cerdá et al. 2017 using Monitoring the Future data), rankings of states on the prevalence of adolescent substance use (Moss et al. 2018 using National Survey on Drug Use and Health and Youth Risk Behavior Surveillance System data), and the relationship of initiation of e-cigarette use and smoking reduction and cessation (Berry et al. 2019 using Population Assessment of Tobacco and Health data).

In addition to these widely used national datasets, many states and local organizations (e.g., health departments) implement their own surveys to document more local conditions. In addition, researchers field their own, specially designed surveys, based on a need for a sample that is defined in different ways or that asks different questions than included in the existing national or state surveys. For example, a researcher may have an interest in alcohol use among LGBT youth (Newcomb et al. 2012), associations between the experience of racial discrimination and substance use (Gibbons et al. 2010), or ask about contexts or behaviors insufficiently addressed in standard surveys (e.g., adolescent alcohol and drug use at own home or someone else's (Egan et al. 2019)).

A fundamental question faced by organizations fielding surveys as well as individual researchers or research teams is how to draw a sample to be surveyed. A comprehensive review of sampling strategies for substance abuse research is beyond the scope of this chapter (see Gfroerer et al. 2017 for such a review). Major categories of these strategies include general population surveys (such as the National Survey on Drug Use and Health), student surveys (such as Monitoring the Future and the Youth Risk Behavior Survey), and "special population" surveys, such as surveys of individuals housed in prisons or jails (such as the National Inmate Survey; see Bronson et al. 2017; Gfroerer et al. 2017).

In addition to sampling strategy, survey mode is also an important decision. Surveys may be conducted by in-person interviews, telephone interviews, Internet surveys, and paper-and-pencil questionnaires, among others (Johnson and VanGeest 2017). Choice of mode involves consideration of important feasibility and coverage issues (e.g., some households will lack a landline phone or cell phone coverage; see Livingston et al. 2013). In addition, researchers need to consider the potential influence of survey mode on responses to questions, especially questions involving sensitive behaviors such as illicit or underage drug use and harms caused to others. There is evidence that modes of data collection that require direct interaction with another individual (such as in-person or telephone interviewer) are associated with lower rates of self-reported drug use (especially illicit drug use; see Johnson and VanGeest 2017) and one's own drug use resulting in harms to others. Alternatively, methods such as audio computer-assisted self-interviews (ACASI) appear to produce the highest rates of endorsement of substance use (McNeely et al. 2016).

The sampling approaches described above all have the potential of drawing what is known as a "probability sample" – that is, the likelihood of any individual being selected is known, which allows statistical inference to characterize the population as a whole. In addition, there are a variety of nonprobability samples that are used in research on substance use.

An approach known as respondent-driven sampling (RDS) is particularly useful for research on substance use. While probability sampling is the gold standard for ensuring generalizability of the sample to the larger population (Shadish et al. 2001), random selection is not feasible or efficient for many studies that focus on "hidden populations" with relatively rare behaviors (Heckathorn 1997). RDS is a non-probability, chain-referral approach to sampling in which participants recruit their peers, who often share some behaviors, from their own social networks. It provides a basis to calculate unbiased estimates of population parameters (Heckathorn 1997; Heckathorn et al. 2002). RDS relies on respondents (known as "seeds") who then recruit a limited number of subsequent respondents who are members of their social networks. RDS has been extensively used in research on people who inject drugs (McKnight et al. 2006) and other relatively rare or "hidden" populations, such as methamphetamine smokers (Kimani et al. 2014; see Leon et al. 2016 for an in-depth review of the theory and application of RDS).

Another approach to gathering data from populations that might not be adequately represented in standard probability samples is time-space sampling, which is a systematic approach to generating representative samples of populations defined by locations (Parsons et al. 2008). It has been used to gather data on the use of "club drugs" (e.g., MDMA, ketamine, GHB, cocaine, methamphetamine, and LSD) among young adults who frequent dance clubs (Ramo et al. 2010).

2.1.2 Ecological Momentary Assessment

While conventional surveys can be powerful tools for assessing substance use in populations, they are typically limited in their frequency, with many taking place annually. This makes assessment of alcohol and/or drug use in shorter time periods problematic, especially given the difficulties of accurate recall. In addition, it may be challenging in conventional surveys to accurately measure the settings in which alcohol and/or drug use takes place. An approach known as ecological momentary assessment (EMA) "is particularly suitable for studying substance use, because use is episodic and thought to be related to mood and context" (Shiffman 2009). EMA is a mobile health (mHealth) method that typically uses smartphones or other portable devices to collect data from individuals over short time periods (Linas et al. 2016).

2.1.3 Administrative Data

In addition to survey data, there are many administrative datasets – data routinely compiled by units of government or other organizations, such as hospitals and health systems – that are frequently used in research on substance use and consequences in populations (see Table 2).

Table 2 Major administrative datasets that include extensive data on alcohol, tobacco, and other drug use or consequences

Dataset name	Sample		Years	Sponsor	Website
	Age range	Other sample characteristics			
Treatment Episode Data Set	Aged 12 or older	Tracks annual admissions and discharges to public and private substance abuse treatment facilities receiving federal funding	1992–present	Substance Abuse and Mental Health Services Administration	https://wwwdasis.samhsa.gov/dasis2/teds.htm
Fatality Analysis Reporting System		Fatal injuries suffered in motor vehicle traffic crashes	1975–present	National Highway Traffic Safety Administration	https://www.nhtsa.gov/research-data/fatality-analysis-reporting-system-fars
Fatal injury data		Injury-related mortality data	1981–present	Centers for Disease Control and Prevention	https://www.cdc.gov/injury/wisqars/fatal.html
Public drug treatment and Medicaid systems		Drug treatment, deaths, hospitalization	1991–present	Centers for Medicare and Medicaid Services	https://www.medicaid.gov/medicaid/prescription-drugs/index.html
Health maintenance organization		Drug treatment		Health Maintenance Organization	
Social Security Administration		Social Security benefits		US Social Security Administration	https://www.ssa.gov/
Child welfare and public drug treatment system		Drug treatment		National Center on Substance Abuse and Child Welfare	https://ncsacw.samhsa.gov/default.aspx
Mental Health Systems		Mental health and drug and alcohol recovery services	1978–present	Mental Health Systems	https://www.mhsinc.org/
Uniform Crime Reporting Program		Law enforcement administration, operation, and management	1930–present	US Department of Justice, FBI	https://www.fbi.gov/services/cjis/ucr

For example, the Fatality Analysis Reporting System (FARS) has been extensively used to assess alcohol and other drug involvement in fatal motor vehicle crashes. It has been a central resource for research on the effects of state and national laws (e.g., the minimum legal drinking age, state "per se" laws, and administrative license revocation laws) on alcohol-involved fatal motor vehicle crashes (Voas et al. 2000; Fell et al. 2016). Other administrative databases that have been used extensively in population research on substance use include the Treatment Episode Data Set (TEDS), which tracks annual admissions and discharges to public and private substance abuse facilities. For example, TEDS has been used to estimate the percentage of individuals in need of substance abuse treatment who actually received it (the percentage was 8.3%; see Batts et al. 2014).

Finally, there has been substantial research using patients' electronic health records (EHRs) in recent years. These are records on patients that include information on medical diagnoses and treatments that are maintained by individual healthcare delivery organizations (Wu et al. 2016). For example, a number of researchers have used EHR to investigate the relationship between patients experiencing chronic pain and the development of opioid use disorder (Hser et al. 2017).

2.1.4 Audit Methods

An audit study is "a specific type of field experiment that permits researchers to examine difficult to detect behavior ... and decision-making in real-world scenarios" (Gaddis 2017).

The earliest audit studies focused on racial and gender discrimination in real-world settings, such as situations involving home rental or home buying (e.g., Wienk Ronald et al. 1979). Audit studies have been used in substance abuse research since the late 1980s. Examples include assessment of the willingness of retail outlets to sell or serve tobacco products, alcoholic beverages, or (in states where recreational use of marijuana is legal) cannabis products to underage individuals (e.g., DiFranza et al. 1987; Forster et al. 1996, 1997; Buller et al. 2016) or serve alcohol to intoxicated individuals (Toomey et al. 2016). With the rise of new products in alcohol and tobacco as well as the changing marijuana landscape, audits are not only conducted in these physical locations but are increasingly being conducted online as well (Williams et al. 2015). In addition to purchase attempts, audit studies often involve an assessment of the availability and marketing of a product, including the retail outlet density and proximity of retailers to specific locations, such as schools, daycares, and parks. These retail assessments may be conducted using a variety of methods. Data can be collected via paper-and-pencil forms or electronically using mobile technology like iPads or cellular phones. Sometimes, photographic documentation is needed so that a post-assessment content analysis of product advertising can be conducted, as analysis cannot reliably be completed during real-time data collection (i.e., while in the store) (Riffe et al. 2005). To do this, electronic devices or wearable imaging technology, such as glasses with built-in cameras, is needed (Cantrell et al. 2013; Widome et al. 2013; Wagoner et al. 2014, 2018). Wearable imaging technology allows advertisements to be photographically documented at timed increments, making this method more efficient and less obtrusive than taking photos with tablets or mobile phones.

2.1.5 Unobtrusive Assessment of Substance Use

In addition to the methods described above, there are emerging methods that do not involve direct interaction with individuals or retail environments. One example is what is sometimes referred to as "sewage" or "wastewater" epidemiology, which involves laboratory assessment of excreted drug residues in wastewater to monitor community-level use of drugs of abuse in near real time (Zuccato et al. 2008; Tillett 2008). A recent wastewater measure of cannabis consumption provided evidence that there was a substantial increase in marijuana consumption in Washington state following legalization (Burgard et al. 2019).

A second unobtrusive approach to population health research involves the analysis of social media data, using "big data" approaches (Kim et al. 2017). For example, researchers have examined Twitter posts about JUUL, a popular brand of e-cigarette, and documented that adolescents were following the company's official Twitter account and sharing the messages with others (Chu et al. 2018).

3 Measures

There is an extensive literature on measurement of substance use and its correlates and consequences (see, e.g., Grigsby et al. 2018), of which we can only touch the surface here. Below we present a brief overview of the assessment of an individual's own use, proxy reports on someone else's use, and harm caused to others. We then touch on a few critical points related to measurement of correlates of use and problems, emphasizing the importance of research looking at both endogenous (intraindividual) and exogenous (extra-individual) factors associated with use and problems.

3.1 Measures of Own Use

One of two methods is typically used to measure an individual's use of substances: self-reports or biological measures (sometimes these are both used in the same study). Self-reports, as the name suggests, involve an individual reporting on his or her own substance use behaviors. There is a substantial empirical literature on the reliability and validity of self-reports, as substance use, settings, and consequences may be sensitive topics, with self-reports subject to social desirability as well as recall issues common to self-reported behaviors. A variety of methods have been developed in response to concerns about both social desirability and inaccurate reporting. These include survey methods minimizing or eliminating direct interaction with research staff (e.g., ACASI, described above), triangulation with biological measures, "bogus pipeline" methods, and "randomized response" methods.

Biological measures (sometimes known as "biomarkers") involve the collection of specimens from individuals followed by lab testing to detect the presence and concentration of drugs with abuse potential. Biomarkers from urine, hair, oral fluid, blood, sweat, and breath have been used in substance abuse research (Fendrich et al. 2017; Peterson 2004; Dick 2017; Sharma et al. 2016).

3.1.1 Type of Substance

Researchers almost always find it useful to try to ascertain the type of substance being used. That said, there is considerable variation in the granularity that is sought. For example, a researcher may include survey questions simply on alcohol use, with alcohol including any type. Or they may be interested in the type of alcohol used (e.g., beer, wine, or distilled spirits). For example, some researchers have examined the relationship between the type of alcohol used and the probability of negative consequences (Maldonado-Molina et al. 2010). Some recent work has gone beyond assessing type of alcohol used to actually ascertaining the brand of alcohol, motivated in part by an interest in understanding the connections between alcohol marketing and underage and adult alcohol use (Padon et al. 2018; for similar research on tobacco, see Perks et al. 2018). Researchers studying cannabis use face a host of challenges due to wide variation in strains, which are associated with differences in the concentration of active substances (e.g., THC, CBD) and the presence of contaminants or adulterants (National Academies of Sciences, Engineering, and Medicine 2017). These challenges are often present when assessing the type of illicit drug being used (Napper et al. 2010).

3.1.2 Mode of Consumption

While national surveys often ask about the use of different categories of drugs, many drugs can be consumed in different ways, with important implications for use patterns, progression to addiction, and other consequences of use (Novak and Kral 2011). Examples of modes of consumption include injection, inhalation, and smoking. Even within any one of these categories, there may be important variations – for example, injection directly into a vein ("mainlining") or injection under the skin ("skin-popping"). A further complication is the use of clean needles or reusing needles when injection drugs. For example, a 2015 HIV outbreak in Indiana that stemmed from reuse of needles while injecting the opioid analgesic oxymorphone drew national attention (Conrad et al. 2015). Large increases in rates of acute hepatitis C infection over the past decade in the United States have been linked to injection of heroin and prescription opioid analgesics using contaminated needles (Zibbell et al. 2018). Efforts to identify the mode of consumption are reflected in recent research on heroin, methamphetamine, cocaine (Novak and Kral 2011), and marijuana use (Johnson et al. 2016).

3.1.3 Quantity and Frequency of Use

Quantity and frequency of drug use are typically assessed in research, given their association with impairment and downstream consequences (Grigsby et al. 2018). That said, assessing each of these features of substance use can pose a number of challenges. For example, the quantity of alcohol use is typically measured by asking questions about the number of drinks that a respondent has consumed during a given time period or drinking occasion. This is sometimes accompanied by definitions of a "standard drink": 12 fluid ounces of beer, 8–9 fluid ounces of malt liquor, 5 fluid ounces of wine, and 1.5 fluid ounces of distilled spirits (National Institute on Alcohol Abuse and Alcoholism 2019). However, individuals typically have little idea of the actual size of the drink they have consumed (Greenfield and Kerr 2008). There are continuing efforts to improve upon and standardize assessment of quantity, using particular sequences of questions that have been shown to elicit more accurate estimates of the quantity of alcohol consumed (such as the quantity-frequency instrument and the beverage-specific quantity-frequency instrument (see Greenfield and Kerr 2008; Nugawela et al. 2016; Vichitkunakorn et al. 2018)).

In the United States, there has been a long history of using a measure of "binge drinking" as a marker of a heavy drinking occasion (the National Institute on Alcohol Abuse and Alcoholism definition of binge drinking is four or more drinks for females and five or more drinks for males in a 2 h period; this level of consumption typically elevates blood alcohol levels to 0.08 g/dl (NIAAA 2015)). Recent research has demonstrated that use of an additional, higher threshold for "high-intensity drinking" – eight or more drinks for females and ten or more for males – is useful for identifying particularly risky drinking occasions (Patrick 2016; Cox et al. 2019).

The emergence of new tobacco products (e.g., e-cigarettes) presents unresolved challenges for measurement. As noted by Wong et al. (2019), the reliability and validity (as well as comparability across studies) of quantity measures such as the number of puffs, vaping episodes, cartridges, and quantity of e-liquid consumed has not been established and may make more or less sense depending on the particular features of the product (also see Cooper et al. 2016).

Similarly, a variety of methods have been used to assess the history or frequency of substance use (often using combined measures of quantity and frequency). This is motivated by researchers' interests in specifying, and understanding the consequences associated with, different patterns of substance use over time. As mentioned earlier, social desirability, as well as recall issues, can pose challenges to accurate measurement of use patterns over a period of time. One often-used method for increasing the accuracy of retrospective self-reports of substance use is the timeline followback method (TLFB; Robinson et al. 2014). The TLFB approach uses a calendar to assist individuals in providing retrospective estimates of their drinking over a specified time period, which can range from a week to 12 months preceding the time of the survey or interview. There are continuing debates about the optimal period of time to measure use using TLFB (e.g., 30-day versus 7-day periods; Hoeppner et al. 2010).

3.1.4 Setting

National surveys often ask questions about substance use without consideration of the context or setting of use. This may provide an incomplete and inadequate understanding of use, since (1) patterns of use may vary considerably across settings and (2) different settings may be associated with variation in the types and likelihood of consequences. An example of the former is cigarette smoking by young adults in public settings, such as bars, which tends to be more episodic than smoking in private settings, such as in homes (Guillory et al. 2017). An example of the latter is research on underage alcohol use in party settings. Alcohol use by young people at parties is associated with higher rates of negative consequences, including sexual assaults, subsequent drinking and driving, and violence, than drinking in many other settings (Wagoner et al. 2012). Moreover, heightened risk of negative consequences is associated with characteristics of parties, such as whether there is adult presence or supervision, the number of individuals at the party, and whether illicit drugs, such as marijuana, are also being used (Egan et al. 2019; Cox et al. 2019). In recognition of the importance of understanding setting, many studies now try to assess the setting or context in which substance use takes place and analyze the relationship of various settings to patterns of consumption and problems (Grüne et al. 2017; Dunbar et al. 2010; Padilla et al. 2015).

3.1.5 Source

Historically, up until about the 1990s, the source from which a substance with abuse potential was obtained was not an important focus of research. However, in the late 1980s and the 1990s, studies showing the ease with which youth could obtain cigarettes (DiFranza et al. 1987; Forster et al. 1997) and alcohol (Forster et al. 1995) from retail outlets led to an important focus on source that has continued to this day. For example, recent work has focused on the sources of opioid analgesics used without a prescription (Daniulaityte et al. 2014). Research on sources of drugs has the potential to inform effective prevention efforts, such as efforts to restrict youth access to tobacco and alcohol and efforts to reduce inappropriate prescribing of opioid analgesics (Forster and Wolfson 1998; Barglow 2018).

3.1.6 Problems Associated with Use

Problems stemming from substance use are, of course, a critical focus of research. It is important to document the prevalence and extent of such problems and to analyze relationships between patterns of use, individual characteristics, environmental characteristics, and the occurrence of problems.

Many substances have the potential for users to become addicted, so, appropriately, addiction or dependence is an important problem to be measured. If assessment takes place in an interview format, validated instruments commonly used to assess alcohol and drug misuse include the Substance Dependence Severity Scale, the Addiction Severity Index, the Comprehensive Addiction Severity Index for Adolescents, and DSM 5 SCID (see Grigsby et al. 2018 for a review). If an assessment is to be self-administered (e.g., a self-administered survey), validated brief instruments used to assess misuse include the CAGE, CRAFFT, Michigan Alcohol Screening Test (MAST), the Drug Abuse Screening Test (DAST), and the Alcohol Use Disorders Identification Test (AUDIT), among others (see Grigsby et al. 2018). Choices of the particular instrument to be used typically depend on the population being assessed, the logistics of assessment (e.g., interviewer- or self-administered), and the particular interests of the researchers.

The introduction of new products can present challenges for researchers. For example, efforts are ongoing to adapt existing, validated tools, such as the Fagerström Test for Nicotine Dependence (FTND) and the Nicotine Dependence Syndrome Scale (NDSS) for assessing dependence on e-cigarettes (González et al. 2017) and water pipe tobacco smoking (Myers et al. 2016).

Of course, researchers may be interested in a variety of consequences of substance use that may not be adequately assessed in existing tools, including particular health, educational, social, and legal outcomes. Administrative data sources are also an important tool for examining such outcomes. To cite just one example, the Fatality Analysis Reporting System has been a critical resource for understanding the nature, extent, and societal impact of alcohol-impaired driving (Fell et al. 2009).

3.2 Harming Others

An individual's use of substances can result in a variety of harms to others, ranging from minor annoyances to serious injury and death (Giesbrecht et al. 2010). This is another topic that, until recent years, has been underemphasized in population research on substance use and consequences (Rossow 2016). One line of research that has emerged is the examination of individuals providing substances to others, by way of sharing, gift, or sale. For example, Wolfson et al. (1997) found that more than two-thirds of adolescent smokers had provided tobacco to another adolescent in the previous 30 days, underscoring the importance of social as well as commercial availability of tobacco products.

More generally, in recent years, there has been a proliferation of efforts to assess the harms associated with alcohol and other drugs in college populations (Rhodes et al. 2009a, b) and a number of nation-states, including Australia (Laslett et al. 2014), New Zealand (Casswell et al. 2011), and the United States (Greenfield et al. 2009).

4 Causal Factors and Correlates of Substance Use and Consequences

Accurate and comprehensive description of patterns of use and consequences is critical. But in order to advance the development and implementation of effective prevention, harm reduction, and treatment strategies, population research must also identify causes or correlates of substance use and consequences. This, of course, is a broad topic and has been the focus of 1,000s of scientific articles and books. For the purposes of this chapter, we provide an overview of the kinds of variables that have been examined for the potential role they may play in understanding patterns of substance use and associated problems. We group these factors into two categories, (1) individual and (2) environmental, and, for each, provide some examples of the ways in which the factors have been conceptualized and measured in population research on substance use.

4.1 Individual Causal Factors and Correlates

In this section, we discuss individual-level factors – usually characteristics or attributes of individuals.

4.1.1 Sociodemographic Factors

Sociodemographic factors, including age, race and ethnicity, gender, and socioeconomic status, are typically assessed in population research on substance use and problems. This enables researchers to examine differences in the incidence and prevalence of use and the associations of use with problems across categories of age (e.g., young adolescents, older adolescents, young adults, and older adults), race and ethnicity, and gender. Of particular concern are disparities in exposure to prevention, harm reduction, and treatment by race, ethnicity, and income (e.g., Melnick 2011), as well as disproportionate legal sanctioning of African Americans for drug offenses (Mooney et al. 2018).

4.1.2 Sexual Orientation and Identity

Increasingly, research on substance use and problems includes assessment of sexual orientation and examination of differences in substance use and problems by this attribute (Kerr and Oglesby 2017; Rhodes et al. 2009a, b). Several studies suggest that LGBT populations are at higher risk for substance use and substance use disorders (Marshal et al. 2008; Azagba et al. 2019).

4.1.3 Personality and Attitudinal Factors

A wide variety of personality factors has been assessed and analyzed in population research on substance use and problems. For example, the five-factor model of personality (the factors are neuroticism, extraversion, openness to experience, agreeableness, and conscientiousness) has been applied in research on community samples (Terracciano et al. 2008). Other factors that have been extensively examined in population research on substance use include time attitudes, self-efficacy, and sensation seeking (McKay et al. 2016). Finally, favorable attitudes about specific substances have been found to predict later use of those substances (Guo et al. 2001).

4.1.4 Personality and Attitudinal Factors

Religiosity, as defined by religious beliefs and attendance at religious services, has been found to be negatively associated with substance use in a large number of studies (Edlund et al. 2010), although there is variation in this relationship by denomination (Michalak et al. 2007).

4.1.5 Mental Health

The co-occurrence of mental health problems and substance misuse has been a mainstay of population research. It is estimated that as many as half of individuals who experience a mental health episode will also experience substance misuse. Santucci (2012) suggests that the substantial overlap between mental health problems and substance abuse may involve some combination of four reasons: risk factors common to both disorders, substance use precipitating mental disorder, self-medication hypothesis, and the presence of either mental illness or SUD contributing to the development of the other.

4.2 Environmental Causal Factors and Correlates

In this section, we examine extra-individual or "environmental" factors that have been the subject of population research on substance use and problems. Many of these factors are of particular interest because they are potentially modifiable.

4.2.1 Situational Factors

Situational factors refer to characteristics of a particular drinking event. These may include the physical location, the social occasion, the day of the week and the time of day, and the presence of, and relationship to, other individuals participating in or observing the event (Jackson et al. 2016). Situational factors are usually measured by survey respondent self-reports, for example, using some variant of the TLFB method described earlier, or ecological momentary assessment (Freisthler et al. 2014).

4.2.2 Family Factors

As one might expect, parenting practices and family dynamics have been the focus of a considerable amount of research on substance use and problems among youth and young adults. For example, high family conflict and low family bonding have been found to increase the risk of initiation of illicit drugs as a child moves through adolescence into young adulthood (Guo et al. 2001). Parental use of drugs is also a risk factor for initiation by youth. Most often, scales of parenting practices and family dynamics are based on self-reports of youth. However, some studies incorporate direct parental reports, which are then linked with data on the child, into measurement of parenting style and family climate and functioning (Rusby et al. 2018). In recent years, researchers have examined how drinking with parents, parents hosting parties, and parents providing alcohol to their adolescents are associated with adolescents' drinking practices and alcohol-related problems (Foley et al. 2004; Reboussin et al. 2012; Cox et al. 2019).

4.2.3 Peer Networks

Having peers who use alcohol, drugs, and tobacco products is also associated with adolescent use (Trucco et al. 2011). This is most often assessed by asking questions about parental behavior on surveys or interviews. However, in some cases, researchers have used social network analysis (SNA) methods to directly ascertain alcohol, tobacco, and drug use within an individual's social networks. For example, Fujimoto and Valente (2012) used data on social networks from the national Add Health survey. The In-School Survey had students nominate their five best male and five best female friends from a school roster, who were also participants in the survey. Thus, the investigators were able to examine the characteristics of social networks and the association of these characteristics and a youth's position in the network with his or her substance use behaviors.

4.2.4 Availability of Substances

Availability of substances, to both youth and adults, has been extensively examined, using a variety of methods, in recent years. One dimension of this is availability in the home. Broman (2016) used subjective questions to assess this among youth: "Is alcohol easily available to you in your home?" "Are illegal drugs easily available to you in your home?"

Availability of drugs with abuse potential from commercial outlets is also an important focus of research. This can also be assessed using a measure of perceived availability, for example, youth perceptions of the availability of alcohol from bars, grocery stores, or package stores (Foley et al. 2004). But researchers have also used other, objective, measures to assess availability. One is the density or proximity of stores that sell alcohol, tobacco, or marijuana products (in states where medical and/or recreational marijuana can be legally sold) (Mair et al. 2015). In states that require licensing of such stores, density can be computed by geocoding the location of licensed outlets. In states that do not have such a licensing requirement, researchers may generate their own lists of outlets, using a combination of online business listing services (Lee et al. 2016) or physical inspection ("ground-truthing") (Feld et al. 2016). The Centers for Disease Control and Prevention have published a guide on methods for measuring alcohol outlet density (Centers for Disease Control and Prevention 2017).

Using audit methods described earlier in this chapter, researchers have assessed alcohol, tobacco, and marijuana outlets' propensity to sell or serve alcohol, tobacco, or marijuana products to youth, using the outcomes from these audits as a measure of availability (Forster et al. 1997). In addition, they have assessed retailer attitudes and practices (e.g., server or seller training) by conducting systematic observations or surveys of store owners or managers (Wolfson et al. 1996).

Availability of prescription drugs with abuse potential, such as prescription opioid analgesics, has become an important focus of research coinciding with the advent of the opioid crisis in the United States. Availability has been measured by calculating the number of prescriptions of a drug of interest (e.g., an opioid analgesic) divided by the population of a geopolitical unit (e.g., a state), as well as by the rate of high-dose prescribing (defined as a daily dose of 90 morphine milligram equivalents or higher) per capita (Schuchat et al. 2017). County-level data on rates of prescribing are published by many states, based on their prescription drug monitoring program. State-level and national data are published by the CDC (Schuchat et al. 2017).

4.2.5 Price

The price of legal and illicit drugs, which is sometimes considered to be an aspect of availability, is another "environmental" factor that has received substantial attention. Increasing the price of legal substances, often by way of tax increases, is a key tool in efforts to reduce use and harms from alcohol and tobacco use (Sharma et al. 2017). For both alcohol and tobacco research, there are debates about the best kind of data to use to measure price (Ruhm et al. 2012). Data can be person-level survey data (i.e., asking people the price they pay for products), aggregate data from secondary data sources available at the state or national level, or local retail "scanner" data from supermarkets (Adhikari et al. 2012). For illicit drugs, there is not a nationwide consistent and sustained source of reliable data on price, which creates challenges for researchers interested in this dimension of the environment for illicit drugs (Johnson and Golub 2007).

4.2.6 Marketing

Industry marketing, including advertising and promotions by manufacturers and retailers, is an important influence on alcohol and tobacco use, including initiation of use by individuals under the legal age to purchase and use these products (Tanski et al. 2015). With the advent of legal medical and recreational cannabis in some states, researchers have begun to document similar patterns for marijuana (D'Amico et al. 2018). Exposure to marketing is typically measured using self-reports in surveys, which can either be cued (by showing part of an ad but without brand information) or un-cued (simply asking individuals whether they have seen ads). While conventional television and magazine advertising has been most often assessed, recent work focused on marketing via channels involving the Internet (McClure et al. 2016). Recent work has also used EMA (described earlier) to measure exposure to marketing using real-time self-reports (Roberts et al. 2019).

4.2.7 Policy

Federal, state, and local public policy, as well as institutional policy (i.e., policy instituted by nongovernmental organizations, such as healthcare systems, alcohol and tobacco manufacturers and retailers, and social service organizations), are important topics for substance abuse research. There is now a considerable literature on methods for assessing and characterizing policy related to substance use and problems (e.g., see Wagenaar and Burris 2013). In some cases, there are existing databases that indicate which states or localities have a particular policy of interest. For example, NIAAA's Alcohol Policy Information System (APIS) contains extensive information about federal and state alcohol policies, as well as recreational cannabis policies. If an existing database is not used, researchers may rely on online federal, state, or local codes or statutes, although sometimes responsible officials (such as city clerks) are simply asked in surveys about the existence of particular policies (e.g., Forster et al. 1996). Often researchers are interested in assessing whether or not a policy achieved its intended impact; however, it is also important to investigate potential unintended consequences of policy (Wolfson and Hourigan 1997).

4.2.8 Enforcement Practices

Once policies are put in place, they may or may not be enforced. Moreover, there may be considerable variation across jurisdictions in the ways in which policies, such as the minimum legal drinking age, are enforced. Researchers have used both observational and survey methods to collect data on law enforcement agencies regarding their policies, priorities, and practices with respect to enforcement of laws related to illicit substance use, possession, and other behaviors, such as driving while impaired by alcohol or drugs (Montgomery et al. 2006; Bernat et al. 2014).

4.2.9 Community Characteristics

Researchers may have interests in more general features of communities and their relationship to substance use and related problems. These may include whether communities are rural or urban; the composition of the population with respect to race, ethnicity, and income; the presence of concentrated poverty; and the age distribution of a community, among others. The US Census and American Community Survey data are often used for studies exploring these questions. States, cities, or more granular units, such as census tracts, may be used as a unit of aggregation (see Song et al. 2009; Reboussin et al. 2010). There has also been a long-standing interest in exploring the relationship between social determinants of health and substance use and related problems; this interest has intensified with the now widespread attention to the opioid crisis and awareness that certain areas, such as rural communities and Appalachia, have been particularly hard hit (Dasgupta et al. 2018).

5 Summary and Conclusion

5.1 Accumulation of Knowledge

Population research on substance use and related problems has a long history as a vibrant, interdisciplinary field of inquiry. However, it is fair to ask how successful it has been in integrating and accumulating knowledge. One potential obstacle to knowledge accumulation and integration is the use of a multiplicity of measures, which can constitute an obstacle to the development of generalizable knowledge. Recently, federal funders of substance abuse research and others have examined the extent to which common or commensurate measures are used across research studies. One examination of the commonality of shared measurement, based on a sample of applications for funded grants involving human subjects research supported by the National Institute on Drug Abuse (NIDA) and the National Institute on Alcohol Abuse and Alcoholism (NIAAA), found that commonality of measures was generally low, although research on prevention and treatment had somewhat greater commonality than research involving epidemiology and services (Conway et al. 2014). This raises concerns about the generalizability of findings and the cumulative nature of research. A couple of different strategies have emerged in response to this concern. One response is intentional curating measures into compendia, whose use is subsequently promoted by funding agencies. A prominent example of this is NIDA's support for the development and promotion of the PhenX Toolkit (Hendershot et al. 2015; also see https://www.drugabuse.gov/researchers/research-resources/data-harmonization-projects). A second response to the problem of non-common measures is "data harmonization." This term describes efforts to combine data from different surveys or data sources, where questions may not be exactly the same or difference in methods (sometimes also referred to as "integrative data analysis"; Mun et al. 2015). In addition, in recent years, there has been a movement toward publishing more meta-analyses and systematic reviews (e.g., Hulme et al. 2018; Duke et al. 2018), which can promote accumulation and integration of knowledge.

5.2 Translation of Knowledge

A second important macro question is the extent to which research in a field of study gets translated into policy and practice. Some have argued that substance misuse research is not optimally aligned with the needs of treatment, harm reduction and prevention policymakers and practitioners. One potential, partial remedy that has been suggested is establishing a closer connection between policymakers, practitioners, and researchers in all stages of research – i.e., in the formulation of research problems, implementation of the research, and interpretation and dissemination of results (Dick 2017; Wolfson et al. 2017).

5.3 Limitations

In this chapter, we have attempted to survey a large, complex field within the relatively brief compass of a single chapter. Inevitably, the first limitation is that we were of necessity selective and may have neglected some areas of particular interest to readers. Specific limitations worth acknowledging are that we have for the most part drawn on literature based on research conducted in the United States. We also have mainly discussed observational research. However, throughout the chapter, we refer the reader to other volumes that explore the wide variety of research designs, including large-scale experiments (e.g., community trials and natural experiments), which can be powerful vehicles of knowledge generation in population research on substance use and related problems. Despite these shortcomings, we hope the reader will find some facts, references, or opinions of value in this chapter.

References

Adhikari BB, Zhen C, Kahende JW, Goetz J, Loomis B (2012) Price responsiveness of cigarette demand in US: retail scanner data (1994–2007). Econ Res Int 2012:1. https://doi.org/10.1155/2012/148702

Azagba S, Latham K, Shan L (2019) Cigarette smoking, e-cigarette use, and sexual identity among high school students in the USA. Eur J Pediatr 178:1–9

Bachman JG, Johnson LD, O'Malley PM (2001) The monitoring the future project after twenty-seven years: design and procedures. In: Monitoring the future occasional paper 54. Institute for Social Research, University of Michigan, Ann Arbor. http://monitoringthefuture.org/pubs/occpapers/occ54.pdf

Barglow P (2018) Commentary: the opioid overdose epidemic: evidence-based interventions. Am J Addict 27:605–607. https://doi.org/10.1111/ajad.12823

Batts K, Pemberton M, Bose J et al (2014) Comparing and evaluating substance use treatment utilization estimates from the National Survey on Drug Use and Health and other data sources. Center for Behavioral Health Statistics and Quality, Rockville

Bernat DH, Lenk KM, Nelson TF et al (2014) College law enforcement and security department responses to alcohol-related incidents: a National Study. Alcohol Clin Exp Res 38:2253–2259. https://doi.org/10.1111/acer.12490

Berry KM, Reynolds LM, Collins JM et al (2019) E-cigarette initiation and associated changes in smoking cessation and reduction: the population assessment of tobacco and health study, 2013–2015. Tob Control 28(1):42–49. https://doi.org/10.1136/tobaccocontrol-2017-054108

Borders TF (2018) Portraying a more complete picture of illicit drug use epidemiology and policy for rural America: a competing viewpoint to the CDC's *MMWR* report. J Rural Health 34:3–5. https://doi.org/10.1111/jrh.12289

Broman CL (2016) The availability of substances in adolescence: influences in emerging adulthood. J Child Adolesc Subst Abuse 25(5):487–495. https://doi.org/10.1080/1067828X.2015.1103346

Bronson J, Stroop J, Zimmer S et al (2017) Drug use, dependence, and abuse among state prisoners and jail inmates, 2007-2009. U.S. Department of Justice, Washington, DC. https://www.bjs.gov/content/pub/pdf/dudaspji0709.pdf

Buller DB, Woodall WG, Saltz R et al (2016) Pseudo-underage assessment of compliance with identification regulations at retail marijuana outlets in Colorado. J Stud Alcohol Drugs 77 (6):868–872. https://doi.org/10.15288/jsad.2016.77.868

Burgard DA, Williams J, Westerman D, Rushing R, Carpenter R, LaRock A, Sadetsky J, Clarke J, Fryhle H, Pellman M, Banta-Green CJ (2019) Using wastewater-based analysis to monitor the effects of legalized retail sales on Cannabis consumption in Washington State, USA. Addiction 114:1582. https://doi.org/10.1111/add.14641

Cantrell J, Kreslake JM, Ganz O et al (2013) Marketing little cigars and cigarillos: advertising, price, and associations with neighborhood demographics. Am J Public Health 103:1902–1909

Casswell S, Harding JF, You RQ et al (2011) Alcohol's harm to others: self-reports from a representative sample of New Zealanders. N Z Med J 124(1336):75–84

Centers for Disease Control and Prevention (2017) Guide for measuring alcohol outlet density. Centers for Disease Control and Prevention, U.S. Department of Health and Human Services, Atlanta

Cerdá M, Wall M, Feng T et al (2017) Association of state recreational marijuana laws with adolescent marijuana use. JAMA Pediatr 171(2):142–149. https://doi.org/10.1001/jamapediatrics.2016.3624

Chu K-H, Colditz JB, Primack BA, Shensa A, Allem J-P, Miller E et al (2018) JUUL: spreading online and offline. J Adolesc Health 63(5):582–586. https://doi.org/10.1016/j.jadohealth.2018.08.002

Conrad C, Bradley H, Broz D, Buddha S, Chapman E, Galang R et al (2015) Community outbreak of HIV infection linked to injection drug use of oxymorphone – Indiana, 2015. Morb Mortal Wkly Rep 64(16):443–444

Conway KP, Vullo GC, Kennedy AP et al (2014) Data compatibility in the addiction sciences: an examination of measure commonality. Drug Alcohol Depend 141:153–158. https://doi.org/10.1016/j.drugalcdep.2014.04.029

Cooper M, Harrell MB, Perry CL (2016) A qualitative approach to understanding real-world electronic cigarette use: implications for measurement and regulation. Prev Chronic Dis 13: E07. https://doi.org/10.5888/pcd13.150502

Cox MJ, Egan KL, Suerken CK, Reboussin BA, Song EY, Wagoner KG, Wolfson M (2019) Social and situational party characteristics associated with high-intensity alcohol use among youth and young adults. Alcohol Clin Exp Res 43:1957

D'Amico EJ, Rodriguez A, Tucker JS, Pedersen ER, Shih RA (2018) Planting the seed for marijuana use: changes in exposure to medical marijuana advertising and subsequent adolescent marijuana use, cognitions, and consequences over seven years. Drug Alcohol Depend 188:385–391. https://doi.org/10.1016/j.drugalcdep.2018.03.031

Daniulaityte R, Falck R, Carlson RG (2014) Sources of pharmaceutical opioids for non-medical use among young adults. J Psychoactive Drugs 46(3):198–207. https://doi.org/10.1080/02791072.2014.916833

Dasgupta N, Beletsky L, Ciccarone D (2018) Opioid crisis: no easy fix to its social and economic determinants. Am J Public Health 108(2):182–186. https://doi.org/10.2105/AJPH.2017.304187

Dick DM (2017) Rethinking the way we do research: the benefits of community-engaged, citizen science approaches and nontraditional collaborators. Alcohol Clin Exp Res 41:1849–1856. https://doi.org/10.1111/acer.13492

DiFranza JR, Norwood BD, Garner DW et al (1987) Legislative efforts to protect children from tobacco. JAMA 257(24):3387–3389. https://doi.org/10.1001/jama.1987.03390240093030

Duke AA, Smith KMZ, Oberleitner LMS, Westphal A, McKee SA (2018) Alcohol, drugs, and violence: a meta-meta-analysis. Psychol Violence 8(2):238–249. https://doi.org/10.1037/vio0000106

Dunbar MS, Scharf D, Kirchner T, Shiffman S (2010) Do smokers crave cigarettes in some smoking situations more than others? Situational correlates of craving when smoking. Nicotine Tob Res 12(3):226–234. https://doi.org/10.1093/ntr/ntp198

Edlund MJ, Harris KM, Koenig HG, Han X, Sullivan G, Mattox R, Tang L (2010) Religiosity and decreased risk of substance use disorders: is the effect mediated by social support or mental health status? Soc Psychiatry Psychiatr Epidemiol 45(8):827–836. https://doi.org/10.1007/s00127-009-0124-3

Egan KL, Suerken C, Debinski DV, Reboussin BA, Wagoner KG, Sutfin EL, Wolfson M (2019) More than just alcohol: marijuana and illicit drug use at parties attended by 15–20 year olds. Subst Use Misuse 54(2):297–306. https://doi.org/10.1080/10826084.2018.1517798

Feld AL, Johnson TO, Byerly KW, Ribisl KM (2016) How to conduct store observations of tobacco marketing and products. Prev Chronic Dis 13:150504. https://doi.org/10.5888/pcd13.150504

Fell JC, Tippetts AS, Voas RB (2009) Fatal traffic crashes involving drinking drivers: what have we learned? Ann Adv Automot Med 53:63–76

Fell JC, Scherer M, Thomas S et al (2016) Assessing the impact of twenty underage drinking Laws. J Stud Alcohol Drugs 77(2):249–260. https://doi.org/10.15288/jsad.2016.77.249

Fendrich M, Johnson TP, Becker J (2017) The use of biological measures in social research on drug misuse. In: VanGeest JB, Johnson TP, Alemagno SA (eds) Research methods in the study of substance abuse. Springer, New York, pp 285–314

Foley KL, Wolfson M, Altman D, DuRant DH (2004) Adult approval and adolescent alcohol use. J Adolesc Health 35(4):345.e17

Forster JL, Wolfson M (1998) Youth access to tobacco: policies and politics. Annu Rev Public Health 19:203–235

Forster JL, Murray D, Wolfson M, Wagenaar AC (1995) Commercial availability of alcohol to young people: results of alcohol purchase attempts. Prev Med 24:342–347

Forster JL, Komro KA, Wolfson M (1996) Survey of city ordinances and local enforcement regarding commercial availability of tobacco to minors in Minnesota (USA). Tob Control 5(1):46–51

Forster JL, Wolfson M, Murray DM et al (1997) Perceived and measured availability of tobacco to youth in fourteen Minnesota communities: the TPOP study. Am J Prev Med 13(3):167–174

Freisthler B, Lipperman-Kreda S, Bersamin M, Gruenewald PJ (2014) Tracking the when, where, and with whom of alcohol use: integrating ecological momentary assessment and geospatial data to examine risk for alcohol-related problems. Alcohol Res 36(1):29–38

Fujimoto K, Valente TW (2012) Social network influences on adolescent substance use: disentangling structural equivalence from cohesion. Soc Sci Med 74(12):1952–1960. https://doi.org/10.1016/j.socscimed.2012.02.009

Gaddis SM (2017) An introduction to audit studies in the social sciences. In: Gaddis SM (ed) Audit studies: behind the scenes with theory, method, and nuance. Springer, Cham, pp 2–38

Gfroerer J, Hughes A, Bose J et al (2017) Sampling strategies for substance abuse research. In: VanGeest JB et al (eds) Research methods in the study of substance abuse. Springer, New York, pp 65–80

Gibbons FX, Etcheverry PE, Stock ML et al (2010) Exploring the link between racial discrimination and substance use: what mediates? What buffers? J Pers Soc Psychol 99(5):785–801. https://doi.org/10.1037/a0019880

Giesbrecht N, Cukier S, Steeves D (2010) Collateral damage from alcohol: implications of 'second-hand effects of drinking' for populations and health priorities. Addiction 105(8):1323–1325

González Roz A, Secades Villa R, Weidberg S (2017) Evaluating nicotine dependence levels in E-cigarette users. Adicciones 29(2):136–138. https://doi.org/10.20882/adicciones.905

Greenfield TK, Kerr WC (2008) Alcohol measurement methodology in epidemiology: recent advances and opportunities. Addiction 103:1082–1099

Greenfield TK, Ye Y, Kerr WC et al (2009) Externalities from alcohol consumption in the 2005 US National Alcohol Survey: implications for policy. Int J Environ Res Public Health 6:3205–3224

Grigsby TJ, Sussman S, Chou CP et al (2018) Assessment of substance misuse. In: VanGeest JB, Johnson TP, Alemagno SA (eds) Research methods in the study of substance abuse. Springer, New York, pp 197–233

Grüne B, Piontek D, Sleczka P, Kraus L, Pogarell O (2017) Drinking location and drinking culture and their association with alcohol use among girls and boys in Europe. J Stud Alcohol Drugs 78(4):549–557. https://doi.org/10.15288/jsad.2017.78.549

Guillory J, Lisha N, Lee YO, Ling PM (2017) Phantom smoking among young adult bar patrons. Tob Control 26(2):153–157. https://doi.org/10.1136/tobaccocontrol-2015-052821

Guo J, Hawkins JD, Hill KG, Abbott RD (2001) Childhood and adolescent predictors of alcohol abuse and dependence in young adulthood. J Stud Alcohol 62(6):754–762

Heckathorn DD (1997) Respondent-driven sampling: a new approach to the study of hidden populations. Soc Probl 44(2):26. https://doi.org/10.2307/3096941

Heckathorn DD, Broadhead RS, Hughes JJ (2002) Extensions of respondent-driven sampling: a new approach to the study of injection drug users aged 18–25. AIDS Behav 6(1):13. https://doi.org/10.1023/A:1014528612685

Hendershot T, Pan H, Haines J et al (2015) Using the PhenX toolkit to add standard measures to a study. Curr Protoc Hum Genet 86:1.21.1–1.21.17. https://doi.org/10.1002/0471142905.hg0121s86

Hoeppner BB, Stout RL, Jackson KM, Barnett NP (2010) How good is fine-grained timeline follow-Back data? Comparing 30-day TLFB and repeated 7-day TLFB alcohol consumption reports on the person and daily level. Addict Behav 35(12):1138–1143. https://doi.org/10.1016/j.addbeh.2010.08.013

Hser YI, Mooney LJ, Saxon AJ et al (2017) Chronic pain among patients with opioid use disorder: results from electronic health records data. J Subst Abus Treat 77:26–30. https://doi.org/10.1016/j.jsat.2017.03.006

Hulme S, Bright D, Nielsen S (2018) The source and diversion of pharmaceutical drugs for non-medical use: a systematic review and meta-analysis. Drug Alcohol Depend 186:242–256. https://doi.org/10.1016/j.drugalcdep.2018.02.010

Jackson KM, Merrill JE, Barnett NP et al (2016) Contextual influences on early drinking: characteristics of drinking and nondrinking days. Psychol Addict Behav 30(5):566–577

Johnson BD, Golub A (2007) The potential for accurately measuring behavioral and economic dimensions of consumption, prices, and markets for illegal drugs. Drug Alcohol Depend 90(S1):S16–S26

Johnson TP, VanGeest JB (2017) Using surveys to study substance use behavior. In: VanGeest JB, Johnson TP, Almagno SA (eds) Research methods in the study of substance abuse. Springer, New York

Johnson RM, Brooks-Russell A, Ma MJ, Fairman B, Rickey L, Tolliver J, Levinson AH (2016) Usual modes of marijuana consumption among high school students in Colorado. J Stud Alcohol Drugs 77(4):580–588. https://doi.org/10.15288/jsad.2016.77.580

Johnston LD, Miech RA, O'Malley PM et al (2019) Monitoring the future national survey results on drug use, 1975–2018: overview, key findings on adolescent drug use. Institute for Social Research, The University of Michigan, Ann Arbor, p 119

Kerr DL, Oglesby WH (2017) LGBT populations and substance abuse research. In: VanGeest JA (ed) Research methods in the study of substance abuse. Springer, New York, pp 197–233

Kim SJ, Marsch LA, Hancock JT et al (2017) Scaling up research on drug abuse and addiction through social media big data. J Med Internet Res 19(10):e353. https://www.jmir.org/2017/10/e353. https://doi.org/10.2196/jmir.6426

Kimani SM, Watt MH, Merli MG et al (2014) Respondent driven sampling is an effective method for engaging methamphetamine users in HIV prevention research in South Africa. Drug Alcohol Depend 143:134–140

Krieger N (2012) Who and what is a "population"? Historical debates, current controversies, and implications for understanding "population health" and rectifying health inequities. Milbank Q 90(4):634–681. https://doi.org/10.1111/j.1468-0009.2012.00678.x

Laslett AM, Wilkinson C, Room R et al (2014) Alcohol's harm to others: an overview of Australian work and results so far. Australas Epidemiol 21(2):10

Lee JGL, D'Angelo H, Kuteh JD, Martin RJ (2016) Identification of vape shops in two North Carolina counties: an approach for states without retailer licensing. Int J Environ Res Public Health 13(11):1050. https://doi.org/10.3390/ijerph13111050

Leon L, Des Jarlais D, Jauffret-Roustide MJ, Le Strat Y (2016) Update on respondent-driven sampling: theory and practical considerations for studies of persons who inject drugs. Methodol Innov 9:205979911667287. https://doi.org/10.1177/2059799116672878

Linas B, Genz A, Westergaard RP et al (2016) Ecological momentary assessment of illicit drug use compared to biological and self-reported methods. JMIR Mhealth Uhealth 4(1):e27. https://doi.org/10.2196/mhealth.4470. https://mhealth.jmir.org/2016/1/e27

Livingston M, Dietze P, Ferris J et al (2013) Surveying alcohol and other drug use through telephone sampling: a comparison of landline and mobile phone samples. BMC Med Res Methodol 13(1):41. https://doi.org/10.1186/1471-2288-13-41

Mack KA, Jones CM, Ballesteros MF (2017) Illicit drug use, illicit drug use disorders, and drug overdose deaths in metropolitan and nonmetropolitan areas – United States. MMWR Surveill Summ 66(SS-19):1–12. https://doi.org/10.15585/mmwr.ss6619a1

Mair C, Freisthler B, Ponicki WR, Gaidus A (2015) The impacts of marijuana dispensary density and neighborhood ecology on marijuana abuse and dependence. Drug Alcohol Depend 154:111–116. https://doi.org/10.1016/j.drugalcdep.2015.06.019

Maldonado-Molina MM, Reingle JM, Tobler AL, Komro KA (2010) Effects of beverage-specific alcohol consumption on drinking behaviors among urban youth. J Drug Educ 40(3):265–280. https://doi.org/10.2190/DE.40.3.d

Marshal MP, Friedman MS, Stall R, King KM, Miles J, Gold MA, Bukstein OG, Morse JQ (2008) Sexual orientation and adolescent substance use: a meta-analysis and methodological review. Addiction 103(4):546–556. https://doi.org/10.1111/j.1360-0443.2008.02149.x

McClure AC, Tanski SE, Li Z, Jackson K, Morgenstern M, Li Z, Sargent JD (2016) Internet alcohol marketing and underage alcohol use. Pediatrics 137(2):e20152149. https://doi.org/10.1542/peds.2015-2149

McKay MT, Percy A, Cole JC, Worrell FC, Andretta JR (2016) The relationship between time attitudes profiles and self-efficacy, sensation seeking, and alcohol use: an exploratory study. Personal Individ Differ 97:203–209. https://doi.org/10.1016/j.paid.2016.03.060

McKnight C, Des Jarlais D, Bramson H et al (2006) Respondent-driven sampling in a study of drug users in New York City: notes from the field. J Urban Health 83:54

McNeely J, Strauss SM, Rotrosen J et al (2016) Validation of an audio computer-assisted self-interview (ACASI) version of the alcohol, smoking and substance involvement screening test (ASSIST) in primary care patients. Addiction 111(2):233–244. https://doi.org/10.1111/add.13165

Melnick G, Duncan A, Thompson A, Wexler HK, Chaple M, Cleland CM (2011) Racial disparities in substance abuse treatment and the ecological fallacy. J Ethn Subst Abuse 10(3):226–245. https://doi.org/10.1080/15332640.2011.600201

Michalak L, Trocki K, Bond J (2007) Religion and alcohol in the U.S. National Alcohol Survey: how important is religion for abstention and drinking? Drug Alcohol Depend 87(2–3):268–280. https://doi.org/10.1016/j.drugalcdep.2006.07.013

Montgomery J, Foley KL, Wolfson M (2006) Enforcing the minimum drinking age: state, local and agency characteristics associated with compliance checks and cops in shops programs. Addiction 101(2):223–231

Mooney AC, Giannella E, Glymour MM, Neilands TB, Morris MD, Tulsky J, Sudhinaraset M (2018) Racial/ethnic disparities in arrests for drug possession after California proposition 47, 2011–2016. Am J Public Health 108(8):987–993. https://doi.org/10.2105/AJPH.2018.304445

Moss JL, Liu B, Ahu L (2018) State prevalence and ranks of adolescent substance use: implications for cancer prevention. Prev Chronic Dis 15:170345. https://doi.org/10.5888/pcd15.170345

Mun EY, de la Torre J, Atkins DC et al (2015) Project INTEGRATE: an integrative study of brief alcohol interventions for college students. Psychol Addict Behav 29(1):34–48

Myers K, Ward KD, Maziak W (2016) Dependence measures based on hookah smokers' experiences and context are needed. Addiction 111:936–940. https://doi.org/10.1111/add.13287

Napper LE, Fisher DG, Johnson ME, Wood MM (2010) The reliability and validity of drug users' self reports of amphetamine use among primarily heroin and cocaine users. Addict Behav 35(4):350–354. https://doi.org/10.1016/j.addbeh.2009.12.006

National Academies of Sciences, Engineering, and Medicine (2017) The health effects of cannabis and cannabinoids: the current state of evidence and recommendations for research. The National Academies Press, Washington, DC. https://doi.org/10.17226/24625

National Institute on Alcohol Abuse and Alcoholism [NIAAA Website] (2015) Alcohol facts and statistics. http://pubs.niaaa.nih.gov/publications/AlcoholFacts&Stats/AlcoholFacts&Stats.pdf. Accessed 22 June 2019

National Institute on Alcohol Abuse and Alcoholism (2019) What is a standard drink? https://www.niaaa.nih.gov/alcohol-health/overview-alcohol-consumption/what-standard-drink. Accessed 22 June 2019

Newcomb ME, Heinz AJ, Mustanski B (2012) Examining risk and protective factors for alcohol use in lesbian, gay, bisexual, and transgender youth: a longitudinal multilevel analysis. J Stud Alcohol Drugs 73(5):783–793

Novak SP, Kral AH (2011) Comparing injection and non-injection routes of administration for heroin, methamphetamine, and cocaine users in the United States. J Addict Dis 30(3):248–257. https://doi.org/10.1080/10550887.2011.581989

Nugawela MD, Langley T, Szatkowski L, Lewis S (2016) Measuring alcohol consumption in population surveys: a review of international guidelines and comparison with surveys in England. Alcohol Alcohol 51(1):84–92. https://doi.org/10.1093/alcalc/agv073

Padilla M, Berg CJ, Schauer GL, Lang DL, Kegler MC (2015) Allowing cigarette or marijuana smoking in the home and car: prevalence and correlates in a young adult sample. Health Educ Res 30(1):179–191. https://doi.org/10.1093/her/cyu051

Padon AA, Rimal RN, Siegel M, DeJong W, Naimi TS, Jernigan DH (2018) Alcohol brand use of youth-appealing advertising and consumption by youth and adults. J Public Health Res 7(1):22–28. https://doi.org/10.4081/jphr.2018.1269

Parsons JT, Grov C, Kelly BC (2008) Comparing the effectiveness of two forms of time-space sampling to identify club drug-using young adults. J Drug Issues 38(4):1061–1081

Patrick ME (2016) A call for research on high-intensity alcohol use. Alcohol Clin Exp Res 40:256–259

Perks SN, Armour B, Agaku IT (2018) Cigarette brand preference and pro-tobacco advertising among middle and high school students – United States, 2012–2016. MMWR Morb Mortal Wkly Rep 67:119–124. https://doi.org/10.15585/mmwr.mm6704a3

Peterson K (2004) Biomarkers for alcohol use and abuse. Alcohol Res Health 28:1

Ramo DE, Grov C, Delucchi K et al (2010) Typology of club drug use among young adults recruited using time-space sampling. Drug Alcohol Depend 107(2–3):119–127. https://doi.org/10.1016/j.drugalcdep.2009.09.014

Reboussin BA, Preisser JS, Song E-Y, Wolfson M (2010) Geographic clustering of underage drinking and the influence of community characteristics. Drug Alcohol Depend 106(1):38–47. https://doi.org/10.1016/j.drugalcdep.2009.07.019

Reboussin BA, Song E, Wolfson M (2012) Social influences on the clustering of underage risky drinking and its consequences in communities. J Stud Alcohol Drugs 73(6):890–898

Rhodes SD, McCoy TP, Omli MR, Cohen GM, Wagoner KG, RH DR, Vissman AT, Wolfson M (2009a) The negative consequences of other students' drinking: inventory development and assessment of differences by student characteristics and risk behaviors. Int J Adolesc Med Health 21(4):519–529

Rhodes SD, McCoy TP, Wilkin AM, Wolfson M (2009b) Behavioral risk disparities in a random sample of self-identifying gay and non-gay male university students. J Homosex 56(8):1083–1100

Riffe D, Lacy S, Fico FG (2005) Analyzing media messages: using quantitative content analysis in research, 2nd edn. Lawrence Erlbaum, Mahwah

Roberts ME, Keller-Hamilton B, Hinton A, Browning CR, Slater MD, Xi W, Ferketich AK (2019) The magnitude and impact of tobacco marketing exposure in adolescents' day-to-day lives: an ecological momentary assessment (EMA) study. Addict Behav 88:144–149. https://doi.org/10.1016/j.addbeh.2018.08.035

Robinson SM, Sobell LC, Sobell MB, Leo GI (2014) Reliability of the timeline followback for cocaine, cannabis, and cigarette use. Psychol Addict Behav 28(1):154–162. https://doi.org/10.1037/a0030992

Rossow I (2016) How well do survey studies capture alcohol's harm to others? Subst Abuse 9(Suppl 2):99–106. https://doi.org/10.4137/SART.S23503

Ruhm CJ, Jones AS, McGeary KA, Kerr WC, Terza JV, Greenfield TK, Pandian RS (2012) What U.S. data should be used to measure the price elasticity of demand for alcohol? J Health Econ 31(6):851–862. https://doi.org/10.1016/j.jhealeco.2012.08.002

Rusby JC, Light JM, Crowley R, Westling E (2018) Influence of parent–youth relationship, parental monitoring, and parent substance use on adolescent substance use onset. J Fam Psychol 32(3):310–320. https://doi.org/10.1037/fam0000350

Santucci K (2012) Psychiatric disease and drug abuse. Curr Opin Pediatr 24(2):233–237. https://doi.org/10.1097/MOP.0b013e3283504fbf

Schuchat A, Houry D, Guy GP Jr (2017) New data on opioid use and prescribing in the United States. JAMA 318(5):425–426. https://doi.org/10.1001/jama.2017.8913

Shadish WR, Cook TD, Campbell DT (2001) Experimental and quasi-experimental designs for generalized causal inference. Houghton Mifflin, Boston

Sharma G, Oden N, VanVeldhuisen PC et al (2016) Hair analysis and its concordance with self-report for drug users presenting in emergency department. Drug Alcohol Depend 167:149–155. https://doi.org/10.1016/j.drugalcdep.2016.08.007. http://www.sciencedirect.com/science/article/pii/S0376871616302447

Sharma A, Sinha K, Vandenberg B (2017) Pricing as a means of controlling alcohol consumption. Br Med Bull 123(1):149–158. https://doi.org/10.1093/bmb/ldx020

Shiffman S (2009) Ecological momentary assessment (EMA) in studies of substance use. Psychol Assess 21(4):486–497. https://doi.org/10.1037/a0017074

Song E, Reboussin BA, Foley KL, Kaltenbach LA, Wagoner KG, Wolfson M (2009) Selected community characteristics and underage drinking. Subst Use Misuse 44(2):179–194. https://doi.org/10.1080/10826080802347594

Tanski SE, McClure AC, Li Z et al (2015) Cued recall of alcohol advertising on television and underage drinking behavior. JAMA Pediatr 169(3):264–271

Terracciano A, Löckenhoff CE, Crum RM, Bienvenu OJ, Costa PT Jr (2008) Five-factor model personality profiles of drug users. BMC Psychiatry 8:22. https://doi.org/10.1186/1471-244X-8-22

Tillett T (2008) Getting straight on what's flushed: "sewage epidemiology" measures community drug consumption. Environ Health Perspect 116(8):A351–A351

Toomey TL, Lenk KM, Nederhoff DM et al (2016) Can obviously intoxicated patrons still easily buy alcohol at on-premise establishments? Alcohol Clin Exp Res 40:616–622. https://doi.org/10.1111/acer.12985

Trucco EM, Colder CR, Wieczorek WF (2011) Vulnerability to peer influence: a moderated mediation study of early adolescent alcohol use initiation. Addict Behav 36(7):729–736. https://doi.org/10.1016/j.addbeh.2011.02.008

Vichitkunakorn P, Balthip K, Geater A, Assanangkornchai S (2018) Comparisons between context-specific and beverage-specific quantity frequency instruments to assess alcohol consumption indices: individual and sample level analysis. PLoS One 13(8):e0202756. https://doi.org/10.1371/journal.pone.0202756

Voas RB, Tippetts AS, Fell J (2000) The relationship of alcohol safety laws to drinking drivers in fatal crashes. Accid Anal Prev 32(4):483–492. https://doi.org/10.1016/S0001-4575(99)00063-9

Wagenaar AC, Burris S (eds) (2013) Public health law research: theory and methods. Jossey-Bass, San Francisco

Wagoner KG, Francisco VT, Sparks M, Wyrick D, Nichols T, Wolfson M (2012) A review of social host policies focused on underage drinking parties: suggestions for future research. J Drug Educ 42(1):99–117

Wagoner KG, Song EY, Egan KL, Sutfin EL, Reboussin BA, Spangler J, Wolfson M (2014) E-cigarette availability and promotion among retail outlets near college campuses in two southeastern states. Nicotine Tob Res 16:1150–1155

Wagoner KG, Song EY, King JL, Egan KL, Debinski B, Wolfson M, Spangler J, Sufin EL (2018) Availability and placement of electronic nicotine delivery systems at the point-of-sale. Nicotine Tob Res 20:1020–1024

Wagoner KG, Berman M, Rose SW, Song E, Ross JC, Klein EG, Kelley DE, King JL, Wolfson M, Sutfin EL (2019) Health claims made in vape shops: an observational study and content analysis. Tob Control. https://doi.org/10.1136/tobaccocontrol-2018-054537

Wechsler H, Nelson TF (2008) What we have learned from the Harvard School of Public Health College Alcohol Study: focusing attention on college student alcohol consumption and the environmental conditions that promote it. J Stud Alcohol Drugs 69(4):481–490

Widome R, Brock B, Noble P et al (2013) The relationship of neighborhood demographic characteristics to point-of-sale tobacco advertising and marketing. Ethn Health 18:136–151

Wienk Ronald E, Clifford ER, Simonson JC et al (1979) Measuring racial discrimination in American housing markets: the housing market practices survey. Department of Housing and Urban Development, Office of Policy Development and Research, Washington, D.C.

Williams RS, Derrick J, Ribisl KM (2015) Electronic cigarette sales to minors via the internet. JAMA Pediatr 169(3):e1563. https://doi.org/10.1001/jamapediatrics.2015.63

Wolfson M, Hourigan M (1997) Unintended consequences and professional ethics: criminalization of alcohol and tobacco use by youth and young adults. Addiction 92:1159–1164. https://doi.org/10.1111/j.1360-0443.1997.tb03675.x

Wolfson M, Toomey TL, Forster JL et al (1996) Alcohol outlet policies and practices concerning sales to underage people. Addiction 91(4):589–602

Wolfson M, Forster JL, Claxton AJ et al (1997) Adolescent smokers' provision of tobacco to other adolescents. Am J Public Health 87(4):649–651

Wolfson M, Wagoner KG, Rhodes SD et al (2017) Co-production of research questions and research evidence in public health: the study to prevent teen drinking parties. Biomed Res Int 2017:3639596. https://doi.org/10.1155/2017/3639596

Wong S-W, Lin H-C, Piper ME, Siddiqui A, Buu A (2019) Measuring characteristics of E-cigarette consumption among college students. J Am Coll Heal 67(4):338–347. https://doi.org/10.1080/07448481.2018.1481075

Wu LT, Brady KT, Spratt SE et al (2016) Using electronic health record data for substance use Screening, Brief Intervention, and Referral to Treatment among adults with type 2 diabetes: design of a National Drug Abuse Treatment Clinical Trials Network study. Contemp Clin Trials 46:30–38. https://doi.org/10.1016/j.cct.2015.11.009

Zibbell JE, Asher AK, Patel RC, Kupronis B, Iqbal K, Ward JW, Holtzman D (2018) Increases in acute hepatitis C virus infection related to a growing opioid epidemic and associated injection drug use, United States, 2004 to 2014. Am J Public Health 108(2):175–181. https://doi.org/10.2105/ajph.2017.304132

Zuccato E, Chiabrando C, Castiglioni S et al (2008) Estimating community drug abuse by wastewater analysis. Environ Health Perspect 116(8):1027–1032

Translational Molecular Approaches in Substance Abuse Research

Sasha L. Fulton and Ian Maze

Contents

1 Introduction 32
2 The Neurobiology of Substance Use Disorder 33
3 Substance Use Disorder Heritability 34
4 Genetic Components of SUD 35
4.1 Consideration of SUD Phenotypes in Human Clinical Populations 35
4.2 Genome-Wide Associations and Functional Validation Studies Reveal Genetic Susceptibility and Neurobiological Mechanisms of Substance Use Disorder 36
4.3 GWAS Identified a nAChR Subunit Risk Variant Associated with Nicotine Dependence 37
4.4 Molecular and Pharmacological Approaches Have Defined Roles for Genetic Polymorphisms in Substance Use Disorder Physiology 41
4.5 Animals: Behavioral Models of Substance Use Disorder 42
4.6 Use of Animal Models to Explore Genetic Polymorphisms Associated with Substance Use Disorder 43
4.7 Transcriptomics and Substance Use Disorder 45
4.8 Cell-Type Specificity: Single-Cell and FACS-Based Approaches 46
5 Epigenetic Components of SUD 47
5.1 Histone Modifications 47
5.2 DNA Methylation 51
5.3 Chromatin Structure 52

S. L. Fulton
Department of Neuroscience, Friedman Brain Institute, Icahn School of Medicine at Mount Sinai, New York, NY, USA

I. Maze (✉)
Department of Neuroscience, Friedman Brain Institute, Icahn School of Medicine at Mount Sinai, New York, NY, USA

Department of Pharmacological Sciences, Icahn School of Medicine at Mount Sinai, New York, NY, USA
e-mail: ian.maze@mssm.edu

M. A. Nader, Y. L. Hurd (eds.), *Substance Use Disorders*,
Handbook of Experimental Pharmacology 258, https://doi.org/10.1007/164_2019_259

6 Conclusions and Future Directions 53
References 54

Abstract

Excessive abuse of psychoactive substances is one of the leading contributors to morbidity and mortality worldwide. In this book chapter, we review translational research strategies that are applied in the pursuit of new and more effective therapeutics for substance use disorder (SUD). The complex, multidimensional nature of psychiatric disorders like SUD presents difficult challenges to investigators. While animal models are critical for outlining the mechanistic relationships between defined behaviors and genetic and/or molecular changes, the heterogeneous pathophysiology of brain diseases is uniquely human, necessitating the use of human studies and translational research schemes. Translational research describes a cross-species approach in which findings from human patient-based data can be used to guide molecular genetic investigations in preclinical animal models in order to delineate the mechanisms of reward circuitry changes in the addicted state. Results from animal studies can then inform clinical investigations toward the development of novel treatments for SUD. Here we describe the strategies that are used to identify and functionally validate genetic variants in the human genome which may contribute to increased risk for SUD, starting from early candidate gene approaches to more recent genome-wide association studies. We will next examine studies aimed at understanding how transcriptional and epigenetic dysregulation in SUD can persistently alter cellular function in the disease state. In our discussion, we then focus on examples from the literature illustrating molecular genetic methodologies that have been applied to studies of different substances of abuse – from alcohol and nicotine to stimulants and opioids – in order to exemplify how these approaches can both delineate the underlying molecular systems driving drug addiction and provide insights into the genetic basis of SUD.

Keywords

Epigenetics · Genetics · Molecular approaches · Substance use disorder · Translational research

1 Introduction

Excessive abuse of psychoactive substances is one of the leading contributors to morbidity and mortality worldwide, affecting a population of nearly half a billion (Degenhardt and Hall 2012). In the United States, 11.3% of Americans smoked cigarettes daily, 5.9% abused alcohol, and 2.9% had an illicit drug use disorder in the past year – an estimated 30.2 million people in total (Abuse and Administration 2016). Effective treatments for substance use disorder (SUD) are lacking, and recovery rates are often very low – for example, while 68% of US smokers stated they wanted to quit, only 7% have ceased using tobacco (Babb 2017). SUD is a chronic relapsing disease driven by neuroadaptations in the brain's reward circuitry. Persistent changes in these systems trigger compulsive drug-seeking behaviors despite negative consequences, though the precise mechanisms that underlie the progression from drug exposures to drug abuse are not well understood. Given the present shortage of treatment possibilities and prevention options, it is critical that new advances in translational research be leveraged and integrated with current methods in order to parse the neurobiological mechanisms underlying SUD.

In this book chapter, we review translational research strategies that are applied in the pursuit of new and more effective therapeutics for SUD. The complex, multidimensional nature of psychiatric disorders presents difficult challenges to investigators. While animal models are critical for outlining the mechanistic relationships between defined behaviors and genetic and/or molecular changes, the heterogeneous pathophysiology of brain diseases is uniquely human. Many of the cortical brain regions involved in psychiatric disorders have weak conservation with nonhuman species, including other primates (Konopka et al. 2012), necessitating the use of human studies and translational research schemes. Translational research describes a cross-species approach in which findings from human patient-based data can be used to guide molecular genetic investigations in preclinical animal models in order to delineate the mechanisms of reward circuitry changes in the addicted state. Results from animal studies in turn can inform clinical trials for the development of novel treatments for substance abuse.

In the following sections, we will begin by describing strategies that are used to identify and functionally validate genetic variants in the human genome which may contribute to increased risk for SUD, starting from early candidate gene approaches to more recent genome-wide association studies. We will next examine studies aimed at understanding how transcriptional and epigenetic dysregulation in SUD can persistently alter cellular function in the disease state. In our discussion, we then focus on examples from the literature illustrating molecular genetic methodologies that have been applied to studies of different substances of abuse – from alcohol and nicotine to stimulants and opioids – in order to exemplify how these approaches can both delineate the underlying molecular systems driving drug addiction and provide insights into the genetic basis of SUD. Our emphasis will be on developments that have markedly advanced our mechanistic understanding of SUD, as well as those that have identified novel biomarkers and promising new therapeutic targets for improved pharmacogenomics-based treatments.

2 The Neurobiology of Substance Use Disorder

SUD is a chronic relapsing disorder characterized by aberrant plasticity in reward and learning-related processing systems. The three major stages of SUD have been conceptualized in a heuristic framework that is defined by disturbances in three major neurocircuits (Koob and Volkow 2016). In the initial binge/intoxication stage, the acutely reinforcing use of psychoactive substances works through their primary sites of action to influence dopamine and opioid signaling in the basal ganglia, including the ventral tegmental area (VTA) and nucleus accumbens (NAc), which integrates dopaminergic and glutamatergic input from the midbrain and cortex to modulate emotion, motivation, reward, and goal-directed behavior (Nestler 2005; Lüscher and Malenka 2011). Maladaptations in these regions can cause drug use to escalate to compulsive use and dependence. During the withdrawal/negative affective stage, there is a marked increase in anxiety, depression, amotivational symptoms, and physiological states that involves a reduction in dopaminergic signaling and concomitant increases in stress-related neurotransmitters in the extended amygdala. Such negative withdrawal symptoms in turn precipitate craving and cognitive deficits in the preoccupation/anticipation stage, which recruits pre-frontal cortex and insular afferents back to the basal ganglia and amygdala, often leading to relapse (D'Souza 2015; Scofield et al. 2016). This recurring pattern can repeat in cycles and is associated with enormous medical, social, and occupational consequences. The ultimate aim of addiction research is to identify and characterize both the environmental and genetic molecular drivers of these functional alterations in reward circuitries in order to better leverage for targeted SUD therapeutics.

3 Substance Use Disorder Heritability

SUD is a highly complex, multifactorial psychiatric disorder driven by both genetic and environmental influences. Importantly, not all people who use addictive substances develop SUD; individual genetic differences influence susceptibility to the disease. Establishing evidence for heritable vulnerability to substance abuse across specific drug classes has emerged based on large-scale family-based genetic studies, including family pedigree analyses, adoption, and twin linkage studies (Uhl et al. 1995; Merikangas et al. 1998; Kendler et al. 2000). Early family-based studies examined risks for SUD in first-degree relatives of individuals with and without the disorder. For example, in a study of individuals with alcohol dependence and their siblings, it was found that, relative to controls, siblings of alcohol-dependent cases had increased rates of alcohol dependence themselves – up to 50% for men and 25% for women (Bierut et al. 1998). In a similar study surveying first-degree relatives of addicted individuals, an eightfold increase in risk was reported for developing SUD for a range of addictive substances (including opioids, cocaine, cannabis, and alcohol) (Merikangas et al. 1998), implicating familial influences as a non-specific risk factor for drug dependence. While these types of family studies revealed that SUD clusters in related individuals, pedigree-based designs cannot separate the specific contributions of genetics vs. environment to a given disease.

In adoption studies, concordance between offspring and biological parents indicates genetic influences on behavior, while similarity between offspring and adoptive parents suggests environmental influences. This type of research scheme is based on comparing the correlation between addiction status of offspring and the characteristics of both biological and adoptive parents. By isolating the influence of environmental exposures from potential genetic confounds on risks for addiction,

Cadoret et al. determined that alcohol dependence in biological parents predicted increased drug abuse in adopted individuals, which held across both males and females (Cadoret et al. 1986, 1996). Limitations of adoption studies include the fact that adoptive children and their biological parents are not necessarily a representative sample of the population as a whole; biological parents of adopted children are more likely to have higher rates of drug addiction, while adoptive parents are less likely. In addition, prenatal environmental influences, including drug exposure in utero, cannot be ruled out.

Classical twin studies, on the other hand, have used data from monozygotic (MZ) and dizygotic (DZ) twin pairs, raised together, in order to deconstruct roles of genetic vs. environmental influences on variation measured within a given phenotype. Twin studies yield insights into the mode of inheritance for a given disease state. A polygenic disease is determined by the combination of many genetic variants, all of which individually contribute to a small percentage of genetic vulnerability. When inherited together, however, these variants can drive expression of a disease phenotype. MZ/DZ twin concordance ratios provide some insights into this issue, since MZ twins share 100% of genetic variants, where DZ twins do not. A high MZ/DZ ratio for a disease (as in, e.g., schizophrenia) indicates that a disease may be polygenic. For SUD, the MZ/DZ twin concordance ratios hover between 2:1 for hallucinogens and 4:1 for cocaine, indicating moderate polygenic effects (Swan et al. 1997). Other factors that are not captured in twin studies include epigenetic modifications and stochastic DNA changes that may occur in one twin and not in the other. For alcohol, opioids, cocaine, and cannabis, multiple groups have reported that a genetic contribution to drug disorders constitutes increased risk ranging from 0.2–0.3 (for hallucinogens and cannabis) to around 0.6–0.8 (for opiates and cocaine) and varies depending on the specific substance examined (Tsuang et al. 2001; Agrawal and Lynskey 2008). Again, these studies indicate that some risk factors for SUD genetically segregate across different substances, while others are substance-specific (Goldman and Bergen 1998).

Although these early findings support a strong heritable component associated with vulnerability to SUD, these designs are not able to identify the specific genes that drive susceptibility to the disease. In order to classify the particular genes involved in SUD risk and progression, researchers within recent years utilize genome-wide sequencing methods and molecular profiling techniques, as discussed below.

4 Genetic Components of SUD

4.1 Consideration of SUD Phenotypes in Human Clinical Populations

A forward genetic approach begins with a phenotype of interest and aims to reveal genetic variants or genotypes that may contribute to that phenotype. Precise phenotypic definitions of case vs. control individuals (e.g., subjects exposed vs. unexposed to psychoactive substances) is a central issue in the analysis of complex traits and is an essential component of forward genetics. Quantitative phenotypes or endophenotypes may afford greater reliability and reproducibility compared to an overt addiction diagnosis by providing researchers with a more clinically or biologically homogenous case population. For example, for nicotine use, the Fagerstrom Test of Nicotine Dependence (FTND), a validated, expert-recommended, low-burden questionnaire of six items used to assess severity of physiological nicotine dependence symptoms among cigarette smokers (Breslau and Johnson 2000; Thorgeirsson et al. 2010), is the most widely used measure of nicotine dependence. Other examples of quantitative phenotypes for nicotine use include number of cigarettes per day and urine levels of nicotine metabolites or other equivalents, such as cotinine, which act as specific biomarkers of nicotine update and tobacco exposure (Scherer et al. 2007; Wang et al. 2011).

While quantitative phenotypes help researchers standardize domains of a diagnosed disease, endophenotypes define phenotypes that may emerge before a disease is clinically diagnosed. Endophenotypes are biological or psychological phenomena of a disorder that may be intermediates in the causal chain between genetic contributions to a disorder and diagnosable symptoms of a psychopathology. For SUD, examples include novelty seeking, reward sensitivity, and risk taking. When considering results from forward genetic approaches, careful consideration should be taken into how these measures map onto phenotypic outcomes of drug addiction (e.g., DSM-IV vs. DSM-V criteria or other validated and heritable outcome measures).

4.2 Genome-Wide Associations and Functional Validation Studies Reveal Genetic Susceptibility and Neurobiological Mechanisms of Substance Use Disorder

Given the high heritability of SUD, enormous efforts have been taken to resolve genetic variations that may cause vulnerability to the disease. In addition, it has been shown that treatment response is highly dependent on genetic variation in genes that regulate the synthesis, metabolism, and transport of major neurotransmitters involved in reward behaviors and drug use. Exploring the mechanisms of the strong link between treatment responsiveness and genetic profile may thereby improve the efficacy of pharmacotherapies for SUD (Heilig et al. 2011).

Genome-wide association studies (GWAS) measure and analyze DNA sequence variation across the entire genome to identify genetic risk factors for complex diseases. In large genetic association studies, several important factors determine the power of this approach to detect important risk variants. The number of subjects examined, number of genetic markers compared between subjects, the specificity and definition of case vs. control subjects, etc. are all critical to the impact of these studies. Ultimately, the goal of GWAS is to exploit such results to improve predictions about individuals and populations at higher risk for developing a given disease. From GWAS datasets, researchers can also establish which molecular systems are critical to disease susceptibility and progression. These data in turn can be used in the development of prevention and treatment strategies – including those based on tailoring specific treatments to individuals based upon genotype. Several classes of genes have been elucidated as being important to the genetic component of SUD through GWAS (Table 1). Overall, genes identified in GWAS as being related to SUD tend to cluster around components of drug mechanisms of action, as well as factors associated with neuroplasticity: gene components of extracellular proteins, cytoskeleton/cell adhesion, cell signaling, and gene expression regulation. In the next section, we will examine an example of a genetic risk variant for SUD identified with GWAS and the series of studies that applied molecular genetic techniques to validate and characterize this polymorphism in vitro and in animal models.

4.3 GWAS Identified a nAChR Subunit Risk Variant Associated with Nicotine Dependence

The first addiction GWAS reports focused on nicotine dependence (Bierut et al. 2006; Saccone et al. 2006). Comparing 1,050 cases defined by FTND scores for nicotine dependence vs. 879 controls, these studies identified significant associations for variants in a region on human chromosome 15 encoding the α3, α5, and β4 subunits of the nicotinic acetylcholine receptor (nAChR). Nicotine acts as a potent agonist for these nAChR ligand-gated ion channels, which are distributed in specific reward-related brain regions in varying combinations of subunits, each with diverse functional characteristics. The risk polymorphisms in these genes were found to increase probabilities for nicotine dependence (Bierut et al. 2006; Sherva et al. 2008). One of the identified variants, the non-synonymous SNP rs16969968 found in exon 5 of the α5 gene (α5SNP), causes an amino acid change (D398N). This SNP is fairly frequent in the general population, found in approximately 35% of Europeans and 50% of Middle Eastern populations (Saccone et al. 2006). In meta-analyses of human clinical populations, it has been associated with an increased risk for nicotine dependence, lung cancer, lower aversive experience to smoking, and increased cognitive enhancement after nicotine exposure (Saccone et al. 2006; Chen et al. 2015). Moreover, the haplotype carrying the rs16969968 risk allele has implications for cessation treatment success, with smokers at highest nicotine dependence risk being less likely to quit smoking overall but responding most effectively to pharmacologic treatments (Chen et al. 2015). These findings highlight the potential for personalized cessation treatments based upon genetic risk variants for nicotine dependence. However, the exact structural changes and resulting functional differences caused by this SNP could not be determined from simple genome associations. In the years following the discovery of this SNP, the connection between nicotine dependence and genetic variation at this locus has become the most widely replicated GWAS finding in the psychiatric disease literature, providing a particularly illustrative example of the variety of molecular genetic techniques that are applied to investigate genetic variants identified by human GWAS.

Table 1 Summary table of genetic loci identified at genome-wide statistical significance ($P < 5 \times 10^{-8}$) in GWAS of SUD-related phenotypes/biomarkers

Drug	Associated gene	Chromosome	SNP	Annotation	Phenotype/biomarker
Nicotine	*UGT2B10-UGT2A3*	4q13	rs115765562	Upstream	Cotinine glucuronidation (Patel et al. 2015)
			rs114612145	Downstream	Cotinine levels (Ware et al. 2016)
	PDE1C	7p14	rs215605	Intronic	CPD (Thorgeirsson et al. 2010), heavy vs. never (Wain et al. 2015)
	CHRNB3-CHRNA6	8p11	rs6474412	Upstream	CPD (Thorgeirsson et al. 2010)
			rs1451240	Upstream	Nicotine dependence (Rice et al. 2012)
	DBH	9q34	rs3025343	Intronic	Current vs. former (Furberg et al. 2010), current vs. former (Siedlinski et al. 2011), current vs. former (David et al. 2012), FTND score (Yang et al. 2015), heavy vs. never (Wain et al. 2015)
	BDNF	11p14	rs6265	Missense	Ever vs. never (Furberg et al. 2010), heavy vs. never (Wain et al. 2015)
	CHRNA5-CHRNA3-CHRNB4	15q25	rs16969968	Missense	Nicotine dependence (Bierut et al. 2006; Saccone et al. 2006), CPD (Furberg et al. 2010; Thorgeirsson et al. 2010; David et al. 2012), CPD, years of smoking, pack-years, current vs. former (Gabrielsen et al. 2013), CPD (Munafò et al. 2012), CPD (Richmond-Rakerd et al. 2016)
			rs1051730	Synonymous	CPD (Furberg et al. 2010; Thorgeirsson et al. 2010; David et al. 2012), heavy vs. light (Wain et al. 2015), adherence to NRT, NRT dose (Ware et al. 2015)
			rs2036527	Intergenic	CPD (David et al. 2012), Nicotine dependence (Broms et al. 2012), abstinence (Zhu et al. 2014)
			rs34684276	Intronic	Nicotine dependence (Hancock et al. 2015)
	EGLN2	19q13	rs3733829	Intronic	CPD (Furberg et al. 2010), CPD, exhaled CO (Bloom et al. 2013)
	CYP2A6-CYP2B6	19q13	rs4105144	Upstream	CPD (Thorgeirsson et al. 2010), CPD (Siedlinski et al. 2011), cotinine levels (Timofeeva et al. 2011)
			rs8102683	Upstream	CPD (Kumasaka et al. 2012)
			rs56113850	Intronic	NMR (Loukola et al. 2015)
	DNMT3B	20q11	rs910083	Intronic	Nicotine dependence (Hancock et al. 2015), heavy vs. never (Hancock et al. 2015; Wain et al. 2015)
	NOL4L	20q11	rs57342388	Intronic	Heavy vs. never (Wain et al. 2015), nicotine dependence (Hancock et al. 2015)

	CHRNA4	20q13	rs2273500	Splice acceptor	Nicotine dependence, heavy vs. never (Hancock et al. 2015)
Alcohol	*SERPINC1*	1q25	rs1799876	Intronic	Maximum drinks in 24-h period (Xu et al. 2015), weekly alcohol intake (Jorgenson et al. 2017)
	GCKR	2p23	rs780094	Intronic	Daily alcohol intake (Schumann et al. 2016)
			rs4665985	Downstream	Weekly alcohol intake, drinker vs. nondrinker (Jorgenson et al. 2017)
	SGOL1	3p24	rs11128951	Upstream	Drinker vs. nondrinker (Jorgenson et al. 2017)
	TF-SRPRB	3q22	rs1799899	Missense	CDT% (Kutalik et al. 2011)
			rs3811647	Intronic	Total transferrin (Kutalik et al. 2011)
			rs1534166	Intronic	CDT concentration (Kutalik et al. 2011)
	KLB	4p14	rs11940694	Intronic	Daily alcohol intake (Schumann et al. 2016)
			rs7686419	Upstream	Drinker vs. nondrinker, weekly alcohol intake (Jorgenson et al. 2017)
	ADH1B-ADH1C	4q23	rs1789891	Intronic	DSM-IV-defined cases vs. controls (Frank et al. 2012), DSM-IV-defined cases vs. controls (Way et al. 2015)
			rs1229984	Missense	Ever vs. never (Takeuchi et al. 2011), DSM-IV-defined cases vs. controls, maximum drinks in 24-h period (Bierut et al. 2012), DSM-IV-defined cases vs. controls (Park et al. 2013), DSM-IV symptom count (Gelernter et al. 2014a), maximum drinks in a 24-h period (Xu et al. 2015), DSM-IV-defined cases vs. controls (Way et al. 2015), weekly alcohol intake, drinker vs. nondrinker (Jorgenson et al. 2017)
			rs2066702	Missense	DSM-IV symptom count (Gelernter et al. 2014a) Maximum drinks in 24-h period (Xu et al. 2015)
			rs145452708	Intronic	Weekly alcohol intake (Clarke et al. 2017)
			rs141973904	Intronic	Alcohol use disorder identification test (AUDIT) score (Sanchez-Roige et al. 2019)
	AUTS2	7q11	rs6943555	Intronic	Average consumption (grams/day/kg body weight) (Schumann et al. 2011)
	ALDH2	12q24	rs2074356	Intronic	Average consumption (grams alcohol/day) (Baik et al. 2011)
			rs671	Missense	Ever vs. never (Takeuchi et al. 2011), DSM-IV-defined cases vs. controls (Park et al. 2013), past year drinkers vs. nondrinkers (Yang et al. 2013),

(continued)

Table 1 (continued)

Drug	Associated gene	Chromosome	SNP	Annotation	Phenotype/biomarker
					maximum drinks in a 24-h period, flush response, alcohol dependence (Quillen et al. 2014), drinker vs. nondrinker, weekly alcohol intake (Jorgenson et al. 2017)
			rs11066280	5′ untranslated	Past year drinkers vs. nondrinkers, daily alcohol intake (Yang et al. 2013)
Amphetamine	*CDH13*	16	rs3784943	Intronic	Positive subjective drug response to amphetamine (Hart et al. 2012)
Cocaine	*FAM53B*	10	rs2629540	Intronic	DSM-IV symptom count for cocaine dependence (Gelernter et al. 2014c)
Opioids[a]	*KCNG2*	18	rs62103177	Intronic	Opioid dependence (Gelernter et al. 2014b)
	KCNC1	11	rs60349741	UTR_3	Opioid dependence (Gelernter et al. 2014b)
	APBB2	4	rs114070671a	Intronic	Opioid dependence (Gelernter et al. 2014b)
	CNIH3	1	rs10799590	Intronic	Opioid-dependent daily injectors ($N = 1{,}167$) with opioid misusers who never progressed to daily injection (Nelson et al. 2014)

[a]Identified SNPs that have not been independently replicated

4.4 Molecular and Pharmacological Approaches Have Defined Roles for Genetic Polymorphisms in Substance Use Disorder Physiology

Candidate loci identified by GWAS provide valuable targets for mechanistic dissections in preclinical models. Once a genetic variant has been identified through GWAS, it is critical to determine if the polymorphism has an effect on the gene product's expression or function. Once a definitive effect is identified, researchers can then use molecular genetic and pharmacological approaches to determine its specific role in the drug's mechanism of action.

In vitro studies are those performed using molecules, cells, or organisms outside of their biological context and can be powerful tools for examining the ultimate effect of a SNP on a protein's structure and function before investigations in more complex animal models. In the case of the CHRNA5 polymorphism, early in vitro studies utilized HEK cells to validate the effects of the rs16969968:G > A SNP and found that the amino acid variant confers a partial loss of function to the nAChR by reducing Ca^{2+} influx after nicotine-mediated activation, implying that the variant receptor desensitizes more quickly vs. its wild-type counterpart (Saccone et al. 2006; Kuryatov et al. 2011). While these studies provided critical validation of CHRNA5's effect on receptor function, HEK cell lines are derived from human embryonic kidney cells grown in tissue culture and cannot recapitulate the cell-type-specific genetic architectures and proteomes of differentiated human neurons.

A more biologically relevant in vitro system has been made available with recent advances in induced pluripotent stem cells (hiPSCs), which have allowed researchers to create differentiated cell types with skin fibroblasts collected from a human patient. Differentiated cells from hiPSCs have the exact genome as the donor patient and thus can be utilized as a model cellular system. Recently, Deflorio et al. generated hiPSCs from individuals with and without polymorphisms in the nAChR α5 subunit and then differentiated them into midbrain dopaminergic (DA) neurons. By measuring the functional electrophysiological properties of wild-type (WT) vs. variant nAChRs expressed in these human DA neurons, the authors discovered that with this SNP, more nicotine and/or acetylcholine chloride is necessary to obtain the same downstream calcium influx in comparison to the wild-type receptor (Deflorio et al. 2016). Moving forward, this hiPSC system can be used in drug discovery approaches to further dissect dependence-related phenotypes and screen for compounds that interact specifically with human wild-type vs. polymorphic nAChRs (Collo et al. 2018). While in vitro studies are indispensable for probing the functional consequences of genetic variation identified in GWAS, they are performed in artificial systems isolated from the complexity of a biological context. Moreover, in disease modeling, the most valuable translational insights inform how a gene or gene variant impacts behavior. For this purpose, genetically engineered rodents are one of the most important means used to tease out functional roles for specific genes.

4.5 Animals: Behavioral Models of Substance Use Disorder

Animal models are critical for use in genetic manipulation experiments aimed at mechanistic investigation, which are currently impossible to perform in human subjects. Achieving face and construct validity for an animal model of psychiatric disease is one of the primary concerns when designing behavioral paradigms of SUD. However, the models for SUD described here are some of the most reproducible and useful for studying distinct aspects of the addiction cycle. Because the vast majority of animal studies for SUD have been conducted in rodents (i.e., mice and rats), we will focus on paradigms utilizing these species. It should be noted, however, that there are examples of investigations performed in nonhuman primates to analyze more complex behaviors, as well as research that has utilized more basic models, such as *Drosophila*, to examine conserved mechanisms of drug-taking behaviors (often with alcohol or cocaine). Drugs that have positive reinforcing effects in rodents and primates mirror closely with those that have high abuse potential in humans, including alcohol, cocaine, and heroin. Below, we will briefly describe a couple of the behavioral paradigms used to investigate SUD in rodents.

Conditioned Place Preference (CPP) The basic characteristics of this task involve the association of a particular environment with drug treatment, followed by the association of a different environment with the absence of said drug (i.e., the drug's vehicle). In a simple version of the CPP paradigm, animals are first exposed to two distinct environments, each of which is paired with either a drug or nondrug state – note that in these assays, the drug is often passively administered, which should be considered in the evaluation of studies utilizing CPP. During the testing phase, the animal is then given the choice to enter and explore both environments, with the time spent in either the drug-paired vs. vehicle-paired environments (e.g., the animal's place preference) used as an index of the reinforcing value of the drug. Animals will often spend more time in a drug-associated environment and will avoid environments paired with aversive states, such as drug withdrawal, which can be applied in a variation of CPP called conditioned place aversion.

Self-Administration (SA) The intravenous drug self-administration animal model is a powerful tool for investigating the addictive cycle of rewarding drugs. An intravenous catheter is implanted in the animal, such that upon completion of a task (often a lever press or nose poke), the drug of interest is delivered directly to the bloodstream. Intravenous cocaine and heroin self-administration in rodents thus recapitulates the voluntary pattern of behavior of the human addiction cycle, including preoccupation/anticipation, drug seeking, escalation of drug taking, withdrawal, extinction, and cue-induced seeking or relapse. Experimental manipulations that increase the rate of self-administration, such as administering a drug that counteracts the effects of the drug of abuse, may be interpreted as decreasing the reinforcing potency of the drug. Once an animal is tested with a particular experimental drug, additional pharmacological manipulations can be done with standard reference compounds, using the same animals to validate the effects.

These paradigms can be carried out to study the effects of acute (or short-term) vs. chronic (long-term) drug taking, with the desired behavioral or molecular readouts assessed immediately after drug taking or after extended periods of abstinence to mimic long-term adaptations that develop during withdrawal and/or relapse.

4.6 Use of Animal Models to Explore Genetic Polymorphisms Associated with Substance Use Disorder

In the case of nicotinic receptor variants identified in human GWAS studies, manipulation of these receptor subunit genes in rodents has greatly expanded our understanding of the neurobiology of nicotine addiction. One of the earliest genetic editing studies conducted for the *CHRNA5* risk variant was the generation of a Chrna5 subunit knockout (KO) mouse, in which the gene for Chrna5 was silenced or excised from the germline. A KO mouse can give researchers clues into the overall function of a gene of interest and the effects of disrupting its protein product. A series of these studies showed that mice lacking the α5 subunit escalate their nicotine self-administration at high doses in comparison to normal control mice (Fowler et al. 2011; Morel et al. 2014), while wild-type animals appear to titrate the amount of nicotine self-administered to maintain a consistent dosage. Several brain regions involved in nicotine dependence have been evaluated for potential changes in function after disruption of the *Chrna5* gene. Fowler et al. reported increased nicotine intake in mice with a null mutation in *Chrna5*. This effect was "rescued" in knockout mice by re-expressing wild-type α5 subunits in the medial habenula (MHb), a brain region associated with inhibition of rewarding signals during an aversive experience. Interestingly, knocking down the α5 subunit in the MHb did not change reinforcing effects of nicotine but did eliminate the MHb's inhibitory brake on nicotine taking at high doses, which would otherwise be aversive.

Such KO and rescue studies yield invaluable insights into the overall function of a gene of interest and the role that it might play in producing a given phenotype. However, they cannot precisely address the consequences of constitutive expression of a specific SNP throughout development. Until recently, the available toolbox of rat genetics lacked the ability to easily introduce site-directed, heritable mutations into the genome to create KO or knock in (KI) rats. To this end, programmable molecular gene-editing systems have been developed in progressively accessible iterations, including zinc finger nucleases (ZFNs), transcription activator-like effector nucleases (TALENs), and CRISPR (clustered regularly interspaced short palindromic repeat)-associated protein 9 (Cas9) RNA-guided engineered nucleases (RGENs) (Kim and Kim 2014). These gene-editing machineries can be injected into single-cell rat embryos to induce sequence-specific double-strand breaks and the subsequent insertion of a transgene through homologous recombination. Recently, researchers were able to utilize the ZFN system to KO the WT nCHR5 subunit and replace it with the rs16969968:G > A SNP in rat germline, creating animals constitutively expressing the variant form of this subunit during development (Forget et al.

2018). The authors then ran WT vs. KO vs. α5SNP rats through a self-administration paradigm in order to determine the differential effects of manipulating this gene on nicotine taking behavior. Unlike the WT animals, the nCHR5 KO rats did not acquire self-administration of nicotine at the dose used in this study, which is consistent with previous reports in mice showing that KO animals require higher doses of nicotine to develop a learned response – suggesting the nCHR5 subunit is important for sensitivity to nicotine. At high nicotine doses, however, KO mice do show increased nicotine taking over WT mice. Interestingly in this study, the α5SNP rats were able to acquire nicotine taking at the lower dose of nicotine similarly to the WT rats, but unlike the WT condition, the α5SNP did not reduce their nicotine intake at high doses and were willing to exert more energy to obtain a nicotine infusion. These results demonstrate how different the resulting phenotype can be when a gene is knocked out vs. when the same gene with disease-relevant mutations is edited in.

These gene-editing strategies can be used to gain even more specific control of transgene expression by using systems like Cre recombinase in order to create cell-type-specific or inducible expression of the editing molecule in a certain brain region or cell type of interest. Cre recombinase is a protein that recognizes and mediates site-specific recombination between loxP site sequences. This unique property can be harnessed by inserting these loxP sites around a transgene of interest. When Cre recombinase is expressed in a cell containing these loxP sites, researchers can elicit gene deletion, insertion, translocation, and inversion depending on the location and orientation of the sites. The Cre/loxP recombination system has become an ideal tool for genetic manipulation in mammalian cells and genetically modified animal models. For example, Morel et al. utilized a Cre recombinase approach in order to investigate the role of the mutant nCHR5 subunit specifically in dopaminergic neurons in the mouse ventral tegmental area (VTA) (Morel et al. 2014). In this paper, the authors utilized the Cre recombinase system to re-express the α5SNP version of the subunit under control of the dopamine transporter (DAT), which resulted in a partial loss of nicotine-evoked receptor function and yielded intermediate behavioral and electrophysiological phenotypes compared with those of the α5 KO mice, suggesting that the α5 subunit has a critical role in defining the sensitivity of the VTA DA system to nicotine through its effects on raising the threshold for dopaminergic release in this brain region.

Taken together, these functional validation studies have helped to form a more complete picture of nAChRs subunit genetic variants and their role in nicotine addiction. In the case of smoking cessation, there are now three FDA-approved medications in existence: *nicotine replacement therapy*; *varenicline* – a partial agonist of the α4β2 nicotine receptors that produces less effects on dopamine release in comparison to nicotine; and *bupropion, an atypical norepinephrine-dopamine reuptake inhibitor (NDRI) antidepressant and nicotinic receptor antagonist.* Emerging evidence suggests that stratifying patients based on *CHRNA5* genetic biomarkers may improve responsiveness to nicotine replacement therapy (Chen et al. 2015). For example, Chen et al. described two randomized cessation trials in which the efficacy of nicotine replacement therapy varied with rs16969968 genotype but not for varenicline treatment. This variant also contributes to increased risk for lung cancer and chronic obstructive pulmonary disease (Hung et al. 2008; Timofeeva et al. 2012), highlighting its association with heavier smoking and a lower likelihood of quitting. While there is equivocal evidence of an interaction between genotype and treatment efficacy, the *CHRNA5* SNP is a known biomarker for difficulty in quitting smoking, and genotyping can help to identify individuals with CHRNA5 high-risk alleles, as they typically have an increased need for pharmacological cessation aids (Chen et al. 2015).

Finally, the α5-containing nAChRs impacted by *CHRNA5* variation may represent an important target for medication development. Considering that *CHRNA5* risk variants result in hypofunction of α5 nAChRs, novel pharmacological agents that enhance the activity of a5 nAChRs may decrease nicotine use by restoring appropriate cholinergic signals that mediate the aversive properties of nicotine. Moving forward, advances in methodological approaches will allow studies to leverage our current knowledge of CHRNA5 and other variants in order to better characterize their downstream effects toward improved treatments.

4.7 Transcriptomics and Substance Use Disorder

Persistent changes in gene expression drive neuroplastic maladaptations in the reward circuitry that underlie craving, drug-seeking, and relapse during SUD progression (Lüscher and Malenka 2011). For this reason, researchers have sought to outline the coordinated alterations in transcriptional programs that may precipitate aberrant synaptic plasticity in these cells. Moreover, GWAS results can be integrated and overlaid with transcriptomic data to reveal where SNPS and CNVs might be associated with gene expression changes in key brain regions implicated in reward learning. Much of the early work interrogating gene expression in clinical SUD and in animal models of addiction utilized real-time polymerase chain reaction or in situ hybridization in a priori, hypothesis-driven approaches to measure amounts of candidate genes in controls vs. cases – studies that corroborated the idea of transcriptional dysregulation in the reward system (Nikoshkov et al. 2005; Bach et al. 2014). More recently, transcriptomic analysis of the full complement of mRNA in a given tissue with next-generation sequencing techniques, such as RNA-seq, has provided researchers with greater insights into the coordinated networks of gene expression changes that may underlie SUD progression (Wolf 2010; Robison and Nestler 2011; Egervari et al. 2017).

In order to illustrate how profiling studies can validate and extend our understanding of genetic association findings, we will use the example of the *OPRM1* gene, which encodes the human G-protein coupled mu opioid receptor (MOR). The MOR is responsible for mediating the rewarding effects of opioids. Numerous SNPs in the *ORPM*1 gene have been identified as associated with heroin addiction in candidate genome association studies (Nelson et al. 2014). Several years of work have used in vitro studies and mouse genetics to demonstrate that MOR represents the primary in vivo molecular target for both the most clinically useful (morphine) and most largely abused (heroin) opiates (Bond et al. 1998; Befort et al. 2001; Wang et al. 2001). MOR KO in mice abolishes both heroin and morphine CPP and self-administration (Becker et al. 2000; Contet et al. 2004). Targeted expression studies have shown that one of the most common SNPs in this locus, A118G, is a functional variant with deleterious effects on both mRNA and protein levels (Zhang et al. 2005). However, the transcriptional events downstream of reduced ORPM1 expression associated with this SNP were not well characterized. Sillivan et al. thus performed transcriptional microarray analyses on NAc from human patients dependent on heroin, a brain region involved in goal-directed behavior and reward processing (Sillivan et al. 2013), whereby they revealed evidence of dysregulated MOR signaling pathways in heroin abusers compared to controls. The authors then analyzed differentially expressed genes using pathway analyses and identified the ELK1 transcription factor as an important regulator of these genes. ELK1 is a known target of the ERK signaling pathway, which itself has been widely studied in cocaine-related dopaminergic signaling. Interestingly, ELK1 expression was found to also correlate with risk variants of ORPM1 in a dose-dependent manner, suggesting a link between ELK1-associated transcriptional programs and reduced expression of ORPM1. Furthermore, ELK1 expression correlates with the severity of heroin use in both human subjects and rat self-administration models of heroin abuse. ELK1 has also been implicated in the mechanisms of drug addiction to other substances besides heroin, including synthetic opioids, THC, and cocaine (Valjent et al. 2001). Several other studies have identified ELK1-regulated genes as being differentially expressed after drug exposures. For example, after ELK1 was identified in mechanistic and transcriptional studies of cocaine administration, Besnard et al. used a cell-penetrating peptide, named TAT-DEF-Elk-1 (TDE), to specifically inhibit ELK1 phosphorylation and the subsequent induction of plasticity-related genes. In doing so, they found that such inhibition reverses cocaine-induced increases in dendritic spine density and delays CPP for cocaine (Besnard et al. 2011). Together, these findings indicate ELK1 as a potential molecular target mediating cellular phenotypes in opioid addiction and highlight transcriptomics as a powerful tool in probing the mechanisms of SUD.

4.8 Cell-Type Specificity: Single-Cell and FACS-Based Approaches

The extreme cellular heterogeneity of the brain is maintained by transcriptional and epigenetic signatures that are unique to given cell types of interest. For this reason, detecting important differences in gene expression in bulk tissue preparations may be occluded by inclusion of many different heterogeneous profiles. In addition, several lines of research have demonstrated the importance of non-neuronal cells in the etiology of SUD, including astrocytes, microglia, oligodendrocytes, and neuroimmune cells (Knapp and Hauser 1996; Slezak et al. 2013). For example, it has been well documented that heroin users have deficits in white matter integrity and myelination, processes that are mediated by oligodendrocytes (Bora et al. 2012; Li et al. 2016). Advances in microfluidics and sequencing technology have made it feasible to analyze thousands of single-cell transcriptomes in a single experiment.

Single-cell RNA sequencing (scRNA-seq) platforms have been developed (Klein et al. 2015; Zheng et al. 2017), enabling the characterization of dozens of molecularly distinct CNS cell types from multiple regions. To investigate cell-type-specific transcription response to opioid administration, Avey et al. performed single-cell RNA sequencing (scRNA-seq) of mouse NAc following acute morphine treatments, where they identified unique morphine-dependent transcriptional responses in both oligodendrocytes and astrocytes (Avey et al. 2018). While not a model of addiction per se, these types of studies allow researchers to further narrow the biological response to abused substances. Further analyses using RNA-seq of FACS-purified oligodendrocytes revealed a large gene set regulated by morphine that were highly enriched for roles in oligodendrocyte maturation and myelination, including the unfolded protein response, confirming the hypothesis that aberrant oligodendrocyte function may contribute to white matter deficits in heroin addiction. These data demonstrate that single-cell and cell-type-specific techniques can illuminate mechanistic insights into the etiology of SUD and that, going forward, it will be critical that addiction studies take into consideration cell-type-specific contributions to SUD phenotypes.

5 Epigenetic Components of SUD

Over a decade of GWAS, studies have indicated that the majority of SNPs that contribute to risk for SUD reside in noncoding regions of DNA or the regulatory sequences that determine how a gene is expressed, termed gene regulatory elements (GREs). How and when these GREs are made available for transcription factor binding is determined by chromatin-based (so-called epigenetic) influences, such as posttranslational covalent modifications to DNA or histone proteins, which ultimately function to alter the accessibility of GREs and/or gene coding loci in order to allow trans-regulatory factors to bind and increase/decrease the probability of transcription events occurring at a given locus. Dynamic restructuring of nucleosome organization in order to allow for transcription machinery access to regulatory DNA sequences is the basis of epigenetic regulation of gene expression. In the following section, we will briefly turn our attention to epigenetic profiling and validation methods (see Fig. 1 for overview of methods) – with a focus on histone and DNA modifications – that are commonly used to reveal both the stable and dynamic properties of chromatin that modify the transcriptomes in SUD.

5.1 Histone Modifications

The basic unit of transcription (i.e., the nucleosome) is comprised of a protein/DNA complex composed of ~147 base pairs of double-stranded DNA wrapped around a core histone octamer containing two copies each of the histone proteins H2A, H2B, H3, and H4. Histones are small, highly alkaline proteins containing both globular domains and more flexible N- and C-terminal "tails" that can undergo

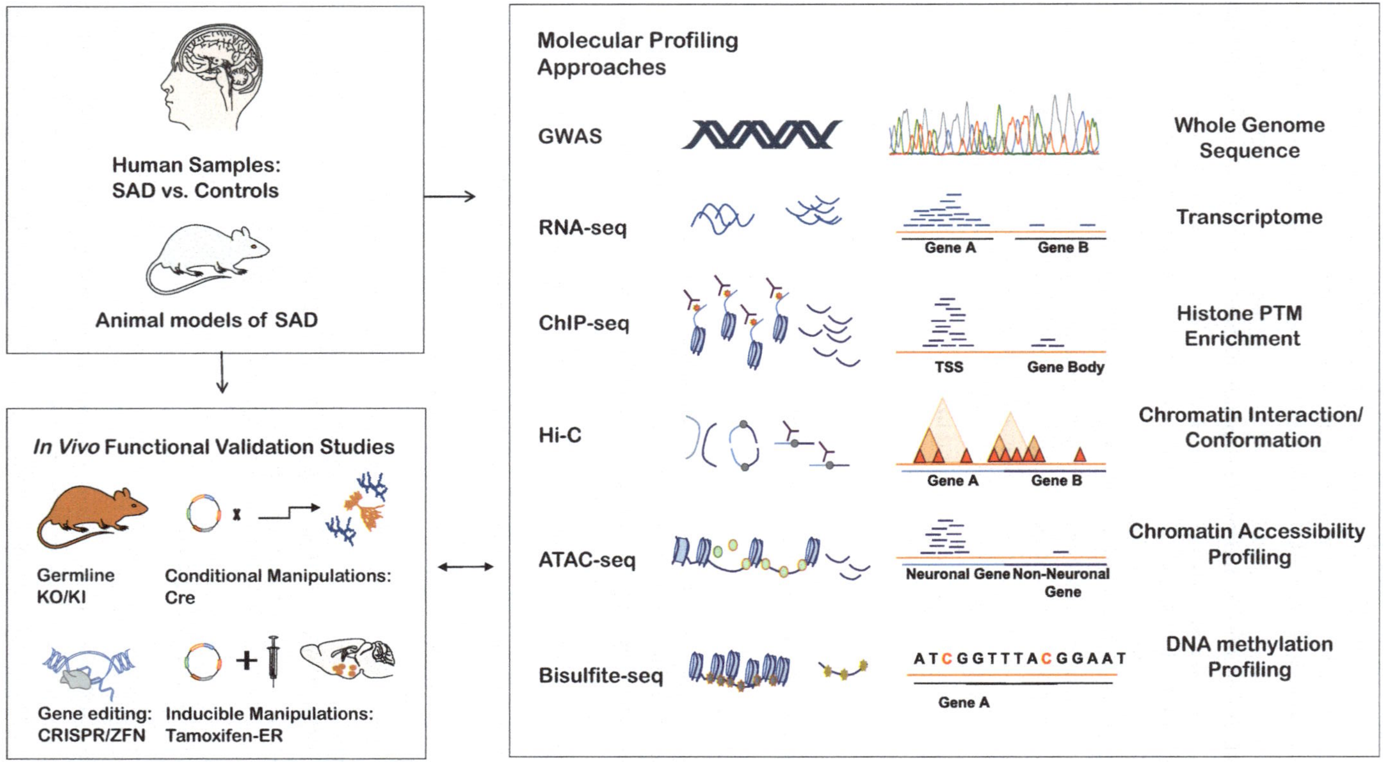

Fig. 1 Translational approaches for investigating SUD: Both clinical SUD human samples and preclinical animal models of SUD can be utilized in molecular disease profiling. *Molecular profiling approaches*: Alterations in chromatin following drug-related experience underlies the development of SUD. Measuring these changes can be achieved by using cell-tagging methods or isolation of distinct cell populations. (1) GWAS studies sequence entire genomes to find associations between genetic variants and disease phenotypes. (2) RNA-seq measures relative levels of transcripts. (3) ChIP-seq utilizes antibodies specific for

Fig. 1 (continued) histone PTMs and/or transcription factors, with associated DNA then being isolated to examine genomic enrichment. (4) Hi-C is used to discover contacts between proximal and distal genomic loci. (5) ATAC-seq uses the transposase Tn5 to cut and ligate specific adapters to open chromatin regions that can be used for downstream sequencing of chromatin accessibility. (6) Bisulfite-seq converts unmethylated cytosines into uracil, and DNA sequences are amplified to detect methylation profile. *In vivo functional validation studies*: Candidate target genes, modifications, or proteins identified in profiling studies can be manipulated in functional validation studies in rodent models using genetic approaches. (1) Germline mutations: knockout (KO) will remove a gene from all cells in an animal. Knock in (KI) will insert a transgene in all cells. (2) Conditional manipulations allow knockout/induction of transgene expression only when Cre recombinase is present. (3) Inducible manipulations allow induction of transgene expression only upon injection of a specific compound, such as tamoxifen. (4) Gene editing with CRISPR or zinc finger nucleases (ZFNs) will replace the endogenous version of a gene with a risk variant or other mutation

posttranslational modifications in order to alter their structure and change the nature of their interactions with neighboring DNA. These tails are heavily modified by the covalent addition of acetyl, methyl, phospho, ubiquitin, and other chemical groups that affect their charge and/or how they interact with DNA-binding proteins. These modifications are placed by specialized enzymes termed "writers" that have highly specific motifs that recognize a combination of DNA sequence/amino acid position/ histone modifications, and they are removed by equally specific "eraser" enzymes. Complex combinatorial "histone codes" are thus hypothesized to dictate which regions of DNA will be accessible to transcription factors, enhancers, silencers, and other regulatory factors. These histone marks provide a reversible, labile substrate for the aberrant neural plasticity observed in drug addiction. As SUD is expressed as an aberrant form of neural plasticity (Hyman et al. 2006), there has been much focus on examining potential epigenetic sources of gene regulation in drug addiction (LaPlant and Nestler 2011; Walker et al. 2015).

Over the past 10 years, many studies have demonstrated alterations in global, temporally defined histone modification states in the human and rodent brain in response to cocaine administration (Kumar et al. 2005; Maze et al. 2010; LaPlant and Nestler 2011). Similar phenomena have been observed for other drugs of abuse, including methamphetamine (Schmidt et al. 2012; Jayanthi et al. 2014) and morphine (Mashayekhi et al. 2012). Global levels of histone modifications can be evaluated using chromatin immunoprecipitation-sequencing (ChIP-seq) methods. ChIP-seq begins by cross-linking the DNA from a given cell population to all associated DNA-bound proteins and then using antibodies specific to a protein of interest to immunoprecipitate and sequence the stretches of DNA associated with that protein. These types of studies in animal models of SUD suggest that the presence of distinct histone modification marks at gene promoters (e.g., on H4 vs. H3) can encode the temporal progression of drug taking in the form of chromatin structural changes from acute to chronic exposures through relapse.

Manipulation of the enzymatic machineries responsible for depositing/removing these marks can yield insights into the regulatory mechanics of histone modification changes. For example, Maze et al. identified persistent decreases in levels of classical repressive H3 lysine methylation, as well as in the expression of the G9a K-methyl transferase, 24 h after cocaine administration, events that correlated with increased synaptic plasticity and the upregulation of a subset of plasticity-related genes (Maze et al. 2010). We subsequently used a series of regional-specific conditional manipulations of G9a in the mouse NAc to selectively knock down G9a in this brain region to directly determine its role in cocaine-induced neuronal plasticity and CPP behaviors. In doing so, we found that G9a downregulation increased dendritic spine plasticity of NAc neurons and enhanced preferences for cocaine, thereby establishing a crucial role for histone methylation in the long-term actions of cocaine (Maze et al. 2010). Interestingly, the example of G9a manipulation in animal models of cocaine taking also offers a demonstration of the complexities of interpreting different drug-related behavioral paradigms. Recently, it was shown that even though artificially reducing G9a in the NAc enhances cocaine CPP and overexpression reduces cocaine CPP, overexpression of G9a actually increased cocaine-seeking behavior in a different experimental paradigm, self-administration (Anderson et al. 2018). The authors also revealed the anxiogenic effect of G9a overexpression during the self-administration training, and overall these data highlight the importance of carefully defining the drug-related behavioral phenotype in question. These and many other studies have cemented a role of histone modifications in neural plasticity and SUD. However, many of the approaches used above measure and manipulate overall levels of a given histone modification across the genome but do not necessarily address the downstream effects of individual histone modification located at specific gene loci. Below, we discuss examples of new approaches that can be used to further examine the role of gene-specific deposition of histone modifications in the precipitation of molecular and behavioral effects caused by drug exposures.

Recent advances in gene targeting have allowed a more specific dissection of the role of histone modifications related to given phenotypes using engineered transcription factors, zinc finger proteins (ZFPs) (Snowden et al. 2002), and/or transcription activator-like effectors (TALEs) (Sanjana et al. 2012) that can be designed to recognize and bind to specific loci throughout the genome in order to deliver histone modifications directly to genes of interest in vivo. This gene-targeted approach makes it possible to directly examine the behavioral and biochemical consequences of *various* epigenetic marks in the context of drug exposures (Heller et al. 2014).

Recently, Heller et al. utilized this technique to investigate the role of a transcriptionally permissive modification, histone H3 lysine 9/14 acetylation (H3K9/14 ac), vs. a repressive mark, histone H3 lysine 9 dimethylation (H3K9me2), targeted specifically to the *Cdk5* locus in NAc, a gene implicated in reward-related behaviors in this brain region. In doing so, they demonstrated increased cocaine-induced locomotor behaviors, as well as resilience to social stress, following activation of *Cdk5* (Heller et al. 2016). Conversely, *Cdk5* repression by H3K9me2 was found to attenuate both cocaine-induced locomotor behaviors and conditioned place preference (Heller et al. 2016). These data are especially compelling given that previous work has identified different behavioral responses upon *Cdk5* overexpression vs. knockdown, demonstrating the importance of targeted epigenetic remodeling tools in studies of tunable molecular changes occurring in disease states.

5.2 DNA Methylation

Another important epigenetic modification that contributes to chromatin structure and accessibility is DNA methylation, which occurs when a methyl group is covalently added to a cytosine nucleotide (Jaenisch and Bird 2003). This modification is catalyzed by a family of enzymes called DNA methyltransferases (DNMTs). DNA methylation is often associated with targeted genomic silencing and closed heterochromatic genome regions. Methylation patterns are established and modified throughout development in tissue- and cell-type-specific configurations. In the past decade, accumulating evidence has implicated DNA methylation in learning, cognition, and neural plasticity in response to environmental cues, making it a key mechanism of interest in epigenetic regulation of SUD-related plasticity.

A range of studies have investigated levels of DNMTs in self-administration animal models of SUD, finding global changes in DNMT expression over temporally defined stages of self-administration. For example, immediately following the last session of cocaine taking, Dnmt3a was upregulated at an early time point of withdrawal (4 h after the last cocaine dose), followed by downregulation after 24 h (LaPlant et al. 2010). However, after 28 days of withdrawal following either cocaine IP injections or cocaine self-administration, Dnmt3a was upregulated in NAc, demonstrating long-lasting inductions of Dmnt3a expression and regulation of genes downstream of Dnmt3a activity. Furthermore, artificially manipulating levels of Dnmts – and/or associated methyl-binding proteins – via knockdown or overexpression in key reward-related brain regions have been found to affect addiction-related behaviors in rodent models. For example, MeCP2 is a reader protein for DNA methylation and is thought to act primarily as a transcriptional repressor through recruitment of histone deacetylases to methylated DNA (Bird 2002). MeCP2 is broadly implicated in addiction, as extended cocaine self-administration increases its expression in the dorsal striatum and other limbic regions, and genetic manipulations of (Im et al. 2010) MeCP2 levels alter addiction-related behaviors in rodents. Given that the machinery involved in placing and recognizing DNA methylation seems to be involved in the molecular changes related to addiction behaviors, efforts have been undertaken to use genome-wide approaches to examine genetic loci where DNA methylation is gained or lost during chronic exposures to psychoactive substances.

Recently, Kozlenkov et al. performed genome-wide bisulfite sequencing on orbitofrontal cortex (OFC) of heroin addicts who died of overdose. Importantly, this profiling study was performed on FACS-purified neuronal nuclei separated from glial cells, allowing the authors to determine cell-type-specific effects of heroin abuse on methylation (Kozlenkov et al. 2017). Using this approach, they identified hypermethylated regions in exons of synaptic plasticity genes enriched in glutamatergic, but not GABAergic, neuronal subtypes. Hypomethylated regions were preferentially found in promoter and enhancer regions of genes related to transcription factor activity and gene expression regulation. Altogether, these results concur with previous reports of reduced glutamatergic transmission in the frontal cortex observed in rodent models following drug exposures, and they highlight that DNA methylation changes in neurons are specific to targeted gene regions. These observations also suggest that DNA methylation may be recruited to different genic features or regulatory domains in the context of heroin use to influence aspects of transcription.

5.3 Chromatin Structure

Chromatin conformation is the ultimate determinant of DNA accessibility, which regulates gene expression. Histone modifications and DNA methylation converge on the regulation of chromatin structure. Both nicotine and cocaine induce global nucleosome repositioning, suggesting that chromatin accessibility represents an initial dynamic genome-wide alteration of the transcriptional landscape preceding more selective downstream transcriptional reprogramming, which characterizes cell- and tissue-specific responses to drugs of abuse (Brown et al. 2015). Advances in sequencing technology have led to new methods that allow chromatin accessibility to be analyzed using whole genome approaches, such as Hi-C, which allows for capture of the three-dimensional interactions between chromatin structure, and the *A*ssay for *T*ransposase-*A*ccessible *C*hromatin-Sequencing (ATAC-seq), which makes use of transposase enzymes to label and amplify open chromatin regions for subsequent sequencing. Egervari et al. recently used ATAC-seq in an integrated transcriptomic and epigenetic approach to investigate molecular changes in the striatum of human heroin abusers and rat SA models (Egervari et al. 2017). The authors performed microarray analyses and ATAC-seq on case vs. controls and identified striatal transcriptional dysregulation for genes related to glutamatergic neurotransmission. Moreover, at key striatal glutamatergic gene loci, both human heroin addicts and heroin SA rats displayed increased levels of a specific histone modification, H3K27ac that mapped precisely onto regions of increased chromatin accessibility, suggesting a mechanistic link between this mark and chromatin remodeling. Most interestingly, the authors found that by administering a pharmacological agent that specifically targets the enzymatic machinery that reads H3K27ac, JQ1 – an inhibitor of select bromodomain containing acetyl reader proteins – in a rodent SA model, they could alter cocaine- and fear-associated memories. This study demonstrates the power of translational approaches that combine chromatin-based genome-wide sequencing and targeted epigenetic investigations in human and rodent models.

6 Conclusions and Future Directions

Together, the studies described in this chapter exemplify the basic scheme of a translational research approach to investigating SUD mechanisms involving both genetic and epigenetic contributors to the disease. Extended focus should be given to promising new areas of genetic and epigenetic SUD research not reviewed here, such as miRNAs, alternative splicing mechanisms, exosome signaling, and immune-response pathologies. Moving forward, an emergent theme in SUD research will be the importance of integrating large-scale studies and genome-wide datasets across experimental modalities, drugs of abuse, and species of interest in order to optimize identification of important genes, pathways, and regulatory mechanisms in SUD. Toward this aim, it is critical that researchers continue to expand currently available large-scale datasets in the study of clinical and nonhuman models of SUD with methods like ATAC-seq and Hi-C to probe chromatin structures, Chip-seq and bisulfite sequencing to examine epigenetic modifications, screening for peripheral biomarkers, and improved GWAS designs to probe genetic vulnerability – strategies that have already been successfully applied in other diseases and neuropsychiatric disorders. In addition, future mechanistic investigations into gene targets using model systems should take into consideration environmental contributors to the molecular neurobiology of SUD – stress, enriched environment, and early life experiences (aberrant or otherwise). Given the vast diversity and heterogeneity of the neural systems involved, targeted approaches will need to pay special attention to the spatial specificity of manipulations using recently developed tools like FACS and the cell-type-specific expression of genetic constructs and gene-editing systems that allow for precise targeting of brain regions, circuits, and cell types of interest. Finer temporal specificity can also be achieved using inducible manipulations that allow researchers to turn on or off a transgene of interest at a specific time point in the development of addictive-like states to investigate risk factors that may precipitate SUD or during the addiction cycle to further delineate the progression of SUD (including withdrawal periods to examine long-term changes after drug use and/or during treatment). Together, these approaches promise to accelerate our understanding of SUD neurobiology and will aid in the search for more effective therapeutics for addiction.

Acknowledgments We thank the National Institutes of Health (DP1DA042078, R01MH116900, R21DA044767 to I.M.) for their gracious support of this work.

References

Abuse S, M. H. S. Administration (2016) 2015 National survey on drug use and health. Substance Abuse and Mental Health Services Administration, Rockville

Agrawal A, Lynskey MT (2008) Are there genetic influences on addiction: evidence from family, adoption and twin studies. Addiction 103:1069–1081

Anderson EM, Larson EB, Guzman D, Wissman AM, Neve RL et al (2018) Overexpression of the histone dimethyltransferase G9a in nucleus accumbens shell increases cocaine self-administration, stress-induced reinstatement, and anxiety. J Neurosci 38:803–813

Avey D, Sankararaman S, Yim AK, Barve R, Milbrandt J et al (2018) Single-cell RNA-seq uncovers a robust transcriptional response to morphine by glia. Cell Rep 24:3619–3629. e3614

Babb S (2017) Quitting smoking among adults—United States, 2000–2015. MMWR Morb Mortal Wkly Rep 65:1457–1464

Bach H, Arango V, Kassir SA, Tsaava T, Dwork AJ et al (2014) Alcoholics have more tryptophan hydroxylase 2 mRNA and protein in the dorsal and median raphe nuclei. Alcohol Clin Exp Res 38:1894–1901

Baik I, Cho NH, Kim SH, Han B-G, Shin C (2011) Genome-wide association studies identify genetic loci related to alcohol consumption in Korean men. Am J Clin Nutr 93:809–816

Becker A, Grecksch G, Brödemann R, Kraus J, Peters B et al (2000) Morphine self-administration in μ-opioid receptor-deficient mice. Naunyn Schmiedebergs Arch Pharmacol 361:584–589

Befort K, Filliol D, Décaillot FM, Gavériaux-Ruff C, Hoehe MR et al (2001) A single nucleotide polymorphic mutation in the human μ-opioid receptor severely impairs receptor signaling. J Biol Chem 276:3130–3137

Besnard A, Bouveyron N, Kappes V, Pascoli V, Pagès C et al (2011) Alterations of molecular and behavioral responses to cocaine by selective inhibition of Elk-1 phosphorylation. J Neurosci 31:14296–14307

Bierut LJ, Dinwiddie SH, Begleiter H, Crowe RR, Hesselbrock V et al (1998) Familial transmission of substance dependence: alcohol, marijuana, cocaine, and habitual smoking: a report from the Collaborative Study on the Genetics of Alcoholism. Arch Gen Psychiatry 55:982–988

Bierut LJ, Madden PA, Breslau N, Johnson EO, Hatsukami D et al (2006) Novel genes identified in a high-density genome wide association study for nicotine dependence. Hum Mol Genet 16:24–35

Bierut LJ, Goate AM, Breslau N, Johnson EO, Bertelsen S et al (2012) ADH1B is associated with alcohol dependence and alcohol consumption in populations of European and African ancestry. Mol Psychiatry 17:445

Bird A (2002) DNA methylation patterns and epigenetic memory. Genes Dev 16:6–21

Bloom AJ, Baker TB, Chen L-S, Breslau N, Hatsukami D et al (2013) Variants in two adjacent genes, EGLN2 and CYP2A6, influence smoking behavior related to disease risk via different mechanisms. Hum Mol Genet 23:555–561

Bond C, LaForge KS, Tian M, Melia D, Zhang S et al (1998) Single-nucleotide polymorphism in the human mu opioid receptor gene alters β-endorphin binding and activity: possible implications for opiate addiction. Proc Natl Acad Sci 95:9608–9613

Bora E, Yücel M, Fornito A, Pantelis C, Harrison BJ et al (2012) White matter microstructure in opiate addiction. Addict Biol 17:141–148

Breslau N, Johnson EO (2000) Predicting smoking cessation and major depression in nicotine-dependent smokers. Am J Public Health 90:1122

Broms U, Wedenoja J, Largeau MR, Korhonen T, Pitkäniemi J et al (2012) Analysis of detailed phenotype profiles reveals CHRNA5-CHRNA3-CHRNB4 gene cluster association with several nicotine dependence traits. Nicotine Tob Res 14:720–733

Brown AN, Vied C, Dennis JH, Bhide PG (2015) Nucleosome repositioning: a novel mechanism for nicotine-and cocaine-induced epigenetic changes. PLoS One 10:e0139103

Cadoret RJ, Troughton E, O'Gorman TW, Heywood E (1986) An adoption study of genetic and environmental factors in drug abuse. Arch Gen Psychiatry 43:1131–1136

Cadoret RJ, Yates WR, Troughton E, Woodworth G, Stewart MA (1996) An adoption study of drug abuse/dependency in females. Compr Psychiatry 37:88–94

Chen L-S, Hung RJ, Baker T, Horton A, Culverhouse R et al (2015) CHRNA5 risk variant predicts delayed smoking cessation and earlier lung cancer diagnosis—a meta-analysis. J Natl Cancer Inst 107:djv100

Clarke T-K, Adams MJ, Davies G, Howard DM, Hall LS et al (2017) Genome-wide association study of alcohol consumption and genetic overlap with other health-related traits in UK Biobank (N=112 117). Mol Psychiatry 22:1376

Collo G, Cavalleri L, Zoli M, Maskos U, Merlo Pich E (2018) Alpha6-containing nicotinic acetylcholine receptors mediate nicotine-induced structural plasticity in mouse and human iPSC-derived dopaminergic neurons. Front Pharmacol 9:572

Contet C, Kieffer BL, Befort K (2004) Mu opioid receptor: a gateway to drug addiction. Curr Opin Neurobiol 14:370–378

David S, Hamidovic A, Chen G, Bergen A, Wessel J et al (2012) Genome-wide meta-analyses of smoking behaviors in African Americans. Transl Psychiatry 2:e119

Deflorio C, Blanchard S, Carla Carisì M, Bohl D, Maskos U (2016) Human polymorphisms in nicotinic receptors: a functional analysis in iPS-derived dopaminergic neurons. FASEB J 31:828–839

Degenhardt L, Hall W (2012) Extent of illicit drug use and dependence, and their contribution to the global burden of disease. Lancet 379:55–70

D'Souza MS (2015) Glutamatergic transmission in drug reward: implications for drug addiction. Front Neurosci 9:404

Egervari G, Landry J, Callens J, Fullard JF, Roussos P et al (2017) Striatal H3K27 acetylation linked to glutamatergic gene dysregulation in human heroin abusers holds promise as therapeutic target. Biol Psychiatry 81:585–594

Forget B, Scholze P, Langa F, Morel C, Pons S et al (2018) A human polymorphism in CHRNA5 is linked to relapse to nicotine seeking in transgenic rats. Curr Biol 28:3244–3253. e3247
Fowler CD, Lu Q, Johnson PM, Marks MJ, Kenny PJ (2011) Habenular α5 nicotinic receptor subunit signalling controls nicotine intake. Nature 471:597
Frank J, Cichon S, Treutlein J, Ridinger M, Mattheisen M et al (2012) Genome-wide significant association between alcohol dependence and a variant in the ADH gene cluster. Addict Biol 17:171–180
Furberg H, Kim Y, Dackor J, Boerwinkle E, Franceschini N et al (2010) Genome-wide meta-analyses identify multiple loci associated with smoking behavior. Nat Genet 42:441
Gabrielsen ME, Romundstad P, Langhammer A, Krokan HE, Skorpen F (2013) Association between a 15q25 gene variant, nicotine-related habits, lung cancer and COPD among 56 307 individuals from the HUNT study in Norway. Eur J Hum Genet 21:1293
Gelernter J, Kranzler H, Sherva R, Almasy L, Koesterer R et al (2014a) Genome-wide association study of alcohol dependence: significant findings in African-and European-Americans including novel risk loci. Mol Psychiatry 19:41
Gelernter J, Kranzler HR, Sherva R, Koesterer R, Almasy L et al (2014b) Genome-wide association study of opioid dependence: multiple associations mapped to calcium and potassium pathways. Biol Psychiatry 76:66–74
Gelernter J, Sherva R, Koesterer R, Almasy L, Zhao H et al (2014c) Genome-wide association study of cocaine dependence and related traits: FAM53B identified as a risk gene. Mol Psychiatry 19:717
Goldman D, Bergen A (1998) General and specific inheritance of substance abuse and alcoholism. Arch Gen Psychiatry 55:964–965
Hancock D, Reginsson G, Gaddis N, Chen X, Saccone N et al (2015) Genome-wide meta-analysis reveals common splice site acceptor variant in CHRNA4 associated with nicotine dependence. Transl Psychiatry 5:e651
Hart AB, Engelhardt BE, Wardle MC, Sokoloff G, Stephens M et al (2012) Genome-wide association study of d-amphetamine response in healthy volunteers identifies putative associations, including cadherin 13 (CDH13). PLoS One 7:e42646
Heilig M, Goldman D, Berrettini W, O'brien CP (2011) Pharmacogenetic approaches to the treatment of alcohol addiction. Nat Rev Neurosci 12:670
Heller EA, Cates HM, Peña CJ, Sun H, Shao N et al (2014) Locus-specific epigenetic remodeling controls addiction-and depression-related behaviors. Nat Neurosci 17:1720
Heller EA, Hamilton PJ, Burek DD, Lombroso SI, Peña CJ et al (2016) Targeted epigenetic remodeling of the Cdk5 gene in nucleus accumbens regulates cocaine-and stress-evoked behavior. J Neurosci 36:4690–4697
Hung RJ, McKay JD, Gaborieau V, Boffetta P, Hashibe M et al (2008) A susceptibility locus for lung cancer maps to nicotinic acetylcholine receptor subunit genes on 15q25. Nature 452:633
Hyman SE, Malenka RC, Nestler EJ (2006) Neural mechanisms of addiction: the role of reward-related learning and memory. Annu Rev Neurosci 29:565–598
Im H-I, Hollander JA, Bali P, Kenny PJ (2010) MeCP2 controls BDNF expression and cocaine intake through homeostatic interactions with microRNA-212. Nat Neurosci 13:1120
Jaenisch R, Bird A (2003) Epigenetic regulation of gene expression: how the genome integrates intrinsic and environmental signals. Nat Genet 33:245
Jayanthi S, McCoy MT, Chen B, Britt JP, Kourrich S et al (2014) Methamphetamine downregulates striatal glutamate receptors via diverse epigenetic mechanisms. Biol Psychiatry 76:47–56
Jorgenson E, Thai KK, Hoffmann TJ, Sakoda LC, Kvale MN et al (2017) Genetic contributors to variation in alcohol consumption vary by race/ethnicity in a large multi-ethnic genome-wide association study. Mol Psychiatry 22:1359
Kendler KS, Karkowski LM, Neale MC, Prescott CA (2000) Illicit psychoactive substance use, heavy use, abuse, and dependence in a US population-based sample of male twins. Arch Gen Psychiatry 57:261–269

Kim H, Kim J-S (2014) A guide to genome engineering with programmable nucleases. Nat Rev Genet 15:321

Klein AM, Mazutis L, Akartuna I, Tallapragada N, Veres A et al (2015) Droplet barcoding for single-cell transcriptomics applied to embryonic stem cells. Cell 161:1187–1201

Knapp PE, Hauser KF (1996) μ-Opioid receptor activation enhances DNA synthesis in immature oligodendrocytes. Brain Res 743:341–345

Konopka G, Friedrich T, Davis-Turak J, Winden K, Oldham MC et al (2012) Human-specific transcriptional networks in the brain. Neuron 75:601–617

Koob GF, Volkow ND (2016) Neurobiology of addiction: a neurocircuitry analysis. Lancet Psychiatry 3:760–773

Kozlenkov A, Jaffe AE, Timashpolsky A, Apontes P, Rudchenko S et al (2017) DNA methylation profiling of human prefrontal cortex neurons in heroin users shows significant difference between genomic contexts of hyper-and hypomethylation and a younger epigenetic age. Genes 8:152

Kumar A, Choi K-H, Renthal W, Tsankova NM, Theobald DE et al (2005) Chromatin remodeling is a key mechanism underlying cocaine-induced plasticity in striatum. Neuron 48:303–314

Kumasaka N, Aoki M, Okada Y, Takahashi A, Ozaki K et al (2012) Haplotypes with copy number and single nucleotide polymorphisms in CYP2A6 locus are associated with smoking quantity in a Japanese population. PLoS One 7:e44507

Kuryatov A, Berrettini W, Lindstrom J (2011) Acetylcholine receptor (AChR) α5 subunit variant associated with risk for nicotine dependence and lung cancer reduces (α4β2) 2α5 AChR function. Mol Pharmacol 79:119–125

Kutalik Z, Benyamin B, Bergmann S, Mooser V, Waeber G et al (2011) Genome-wide association study identifies two loci strongly affecting transferrin glycosylation. Hum Mol Genet 20:3710–3717

LaPlant Q, Nestler EJ (2011) CRACKing the histone code: cocaine's effects on chromatin structure and function. Horm Behav 59:321–330

LaPlant Q, Vialou V, Covington HE III, Dumitriu D, Feng J et al (2010) Dnmt3a regulates emotional behavior and spine plasticity in the nucleus accumbens. Nat Neurosci 13:1137

Li W, Zhu J, Li Q, Ye J, Chen J et al (2016) Brain white matter integrity in heroin addicts during methadone maintenance treatment is related to relapse propensity. Brain Behav 6:e00436

Loukola A, Buchwald J, Gupta R, Palviainen T, Hällfors J et al (2015) A genome-wide association study of a biomarker of nicotine metabolism. PLoS Genet 11:e1005498

Lüscher C, Malenka RC (2011) Drug-evoked synaptic plasticity in addiction: from molecular changes to circuit remodeling. Neuron 69:650–663

Mashayekhi FJ, Rasti M, Rahvar M, Mokarram P, Namavar MR et al (2012) Expression levels of the BDNF gene and histone modifications around its promoters in the ventral tegmental area and locus ceruleus of rats during forced abstinence from morphine. Neurochem Res 37:1517–1523

Maze I, Covington HE, Dietz DM, LaPlant Q, Renthal W et al (2010) Essential role of the histone methyltransferase G9a in cocaine-induced plasticity. Science 327:213–216

Merikangas KR, Stolar M, Stevens DE, Goulet J, Preisig MA et al (1998) Familial transmission of substance use disorders. Arch Gen Psychiatry 55:973–979

Morel C, Fattore L, Pons S, Hay Y, Marti F et al (2014) Nicotine consumption is regulated by a human polymorphism in dopamine neurons. Mol Psychiatry 19:930

Munafò MR, Timofeeva MN, Morris RW, Prieto-Merino D, Sattar N et al (2012) Association between genetic variants on chromosome 15q25 locus and objective measures of tobacco exposure. J Natl Cancer Inst 104:740–748

Nelson EC, Lynskey MT, Heath AC, Wray N, Agrawal A et al (2014) Association of OPRD1 polymorphisms with heroin dependence in a large case-control series. Addict Biol 19:111–121

Nestler EJ (2005) Is there a common molecular pathway for addiction? Nat Neurosci 8:1445

Nikoshkov A, Hurd YL, Yakovleva T, Bazov I, Marinova Z et al (2005) Prodynorphin transcripts and proteins differentially expressed and regulated in the adult human brain. FASEB J 19:1543–1545

Park BL, Kim JW, Cheong HS, Kim LH, Lee BC et al (2013) Extended genetic effects of ADH cluster genes on the risk of alcohol dependence: from GWAS to replication. Hum Genet 132:657–668

Patel YM, Stram DO, Wilkens LR, Park S-SL, Henderson BE et al (2015) The contribution of common genetic variation to nicotine and cotinine glucuronidation in multiple ethnic/racial populations. Cancer Epidemiol Biomark Prev 24:119–127

Quillen EE, Chen XD, Almasy L, Yang F, He H et al (2014) ALDH2 is associated to alcohol dependence and is the major genetic determinant of "daily maximum drinks" in a GWAS study of an isolated rural Chinese sample. Am J Med Genet Part B: Neuropsychiatr Genet 165:103–110

Rice JP, Hartz SM, Agrawal A, Almasy L, Bennett S et al (2012) CHRNB3 is more strongly associated with Fagerström Test for Cigarette Dependence-based nicotine dependence than cigarettes per day: phenotype definition changes genome-wide association studies results. Addiction 107:2019–2028

Richmond-Rakerd LS, Otto JM, Slutske WS, Ehlers CL, Wilhelmsen KC et al (2016) A novel tobacco use phenotype suggests the 15q25 and 19q13 loci may be differentially associated with cigarettes per day and tobacco-related problems. Nicotine Tob Res 19:426–434

Robison AJ, Nestler EJ (2011) Transcriptional and epigenetic mechanisms of addiction. Nat Rev Neurosci 12:623

Saccone SF, Hinrichs AL, Saccone NL, Chase GA, Konvicka K et al (2006) Cholinergic nicotinic receptor genes implicated in a nicotine dependence association study targeting 348 candidate genes with 3713 SNPs. Hum Mol Genet 16:36–49

Sanchez-Roige S, Fontanillas P, Elson SL, a. R. Team, Gray JC et al (2019) Genome-wide association study of alcohol use disorder identification test (AUDIT) scores in 20 328 research participants of European ancestry. Addict Biol 24:121–131

Sanjana NE, Cong L, Zhou Y, Cunniff MM, Feng G et al (2012) A transcription activator-like effector toolbox for genome engineering. Nat Protoc 7:171

Scherer G, Engl J, Urban M, Gilch G, Janket D et al (2007) Relationship between machine-derived smoke yields and biomarkers in cigarette smokers in Germany. Regul Toxicol Pharmacol 47:171–183

Schmidt HD, Sangrey GR, Darnell SB, Schassburger RL, Cha JHJ et al (2012) Increased brain-derived neurotrophic factor (BDNF) expression in the ventral tegmental area during cocaine abstinence is associated with increased histone acetylation at BDNF exon I-containing promoters. J Neurochem 120:202–209

Schumann G, Coin LJ, Lourdusamy A, Charoen P, Berger KH et al (2011) Genome-wide association and genetic functional studies identify autism susceptibility candidate 2 gene (AUTS2) in the regulation of alcohol consumption. Proc Natl Acad Sci 108:7119–7124

Schumann G, Liu C, O'Reilly P, Gao H, Song P et al (2016) KLB is associated with alcohol drinking, and its gene product β-Klotho is necessary for FGF21 regulation of alcohol preference. Proc Natl Acad Sci 113:14372–14377

Scofield M, Heinsbroek J, Gipson C, Kupchik Y, Spencer S et al (2016) The nucleus accumbens: mechanisms of addiction across drug classes reflect the importance of glutamate homeostasis. Pharmacol Rev 68:816–871

Sherva R, Wilhelmsen K, Pomerleau CS, Chasse SA, Rice JP et al (2008) Association of a single nucleotide polymorphism in neuronal acetylcholine receptor subunit alpha 5 (CHRNA5) with smoking status and with 'pleasurable buzz'during early experimentation with smoking. Addiction 103:1544–1552

Siedlinski M, Cho MH, Bakke P, Gulsvik A, Lomas DA et al (2011) Genome-wide association study of smoking behaviours in patients with COPD. Thorax 66(10):894–902

Sillivan SE, Whittard JD, Jacobs MM, Ren Y, Mazloom AR et al (2013) ELK1 transcription factor linked to dysregulated striatal mu opioid receptor signaling network and OPRM1 polymorphism in human heroin abusers. Biol Psychiatry 74:511–519

Slezak M, Korostynski M, Gieryk A, Golda S, Dzbek J et al (2013) Astrocytes are a neural target of morphine action via glucocorticoid receptor-dependent signaling. Glia 61:623–635

Snowden AW, Gregory PD, Case CC, Pabo CO (2002) Gene-specific targeting of H3K9 methylation is sufficient for initiating repression in vivo. Curr Biol 12:2159–2166

Swan GE, Carmelli D, Cardon LR (1997) Heavy consumption of cigarettes, alcohol and coffee in male twins. J Stud Alcohol 58:182–190

Takeuchi F, Isono M, Nabika T, Katsuya T, Sugiyama T et al (2011) Confirmation of ALDH2 as a Major locus of drinking behavior and of its variants regulating multiple metabolic phenotypes in a Japanese population. Circ J 75:911–918

Thorgeirsson TE, Gudbjartsson DF, Surakka I, Vink JM, Amin N et al (2010) Sequence variants at CHRNB3–CHRNA6 and CYP2A6 affect smoking behavior. Nat Genet 42:448

Timofeeva MN, McKay JD, Davey SG, Johansson M, Byrnes GB et al (2011) Genetic polymorphisms in 15q25 and 19q13 loci, cotinine levels, and risk of lung cancer in EPIC. Cancer Epidemiol Biomark Prev 20:2250–2261

Timofeeva MN, Hung RJ, Rafnar T, Christiani DC, Field JK et al (2012) Influence of common genetic variation on lung cancer risk: meta-analysis of 14 900 cases and 29 485 controls. Hum Mol Genet 21:4980–4995

Tsuang MT, Bar JL, Harley RM, Lyons MJ (2001) The Harvard twin study of substance abuse: what we have learned. Harv Rev Psychiatry 9:267–279

Uhl G, Elmer G, Labuda M, Pickens R (1995) Genetic influences in drug abuse. In: Psychopharmacology: The fourth generation of progress. Raven Press, New York, pp 1793–1806

Valjent E, Pagès C, Rogard M, Besson MJ, Maldonado R et al (2001) Δ9-tetrahydrocannabinol-induced MAPK/ERK and Elk-1 activation in vivo depends on dopaminergic transmission. Eur J Neurosci 14:342–352

Wain LV, Shrine N, Miller S, Jackson VE, Ntalla I et al (2015) Novel insights into the genetics of smoking behaviour, lung function, and chronic obstructive pulmonary disease (UK BiLEVE): a genetic association study in UK Biobank. Lancet Respir Med 3:769–781

Walker DM, Cates HM, Heller EA, Nestler EJ (2015) Regulation of chromatin states by drugs of abuse. Curr Opin Neurobiol 30:112–121

Wang D, Quillan JM, Winans K, Lucas JL, Sadée W (2001) Single nucleotide polymorphisms in the human μ opioid receptor gene alter basal G protein coupling and calmodulin binding. J Biol Chem 276:34624–34630

Wang J, Liang Q, Mendes P, Sarkar M (2011) Is 24h nicotine equivalents a surrogate for smoke exposure based on its relationship with other biomarkers of exposure? Biomarkers 16:144–154

Ware JJ, Aveyard P, Broderick P, Houlston RS, Eisen T et al (2015) The association of rs1051730 genotype on adherence to and consumption of prescribed nicotine replacement therapy dose during a smoking cessation attempt. Drug Alcohol Depend 151:236–240

Ware JJ, Chen X, Vink J, Loukola A, Minica C et al (2016) Genome-wide meta-analysis of cotinine levels in cigarette smokers identifies locus at 4q13.2. Sci Rep 6:20092

Way M, McQuillin A, Saini J, Ruparelia K, Lydall GJ et al (2015) Genetic variants in or near ADH 1 B and ADH 1 C affect susceptibility to alcohol dependence in a British and Irish population. Addict Biol 20:594–604

Wolf ME (2010) The Bermuda Triangle of cocaine-induced neuroadaptations. Trends Neurosci 33:391–398

Xu K, Kranzler HR, Sherva R, Sartor CE, Almasy L et al (2015) Genomewide association study for maximum number of alcoholic drinks in European Americans and African Americans. Alcohol Clin Exp Res 39:1137–1147

Yang X, Lu X, Wang L, Chen S, Li J et al (2013) Common variants at 12q24 are associated with drinking behavior in Han Chinese. Am J Clin Nutr 97:545–551

Yang J, Wang S, Yang Z, Hodgkinson CA, Iarikova P et al (2015) The contribution of rare and common variants in 30 genes to risk nicotine dependence. Mol Psychiatry 20:1467

Zhang Y, Wang D, Johnson AD, Papp AC, Sadée W (2005) Allelic expression imbalance of human mu opioid receptor (OPRM1) caused by variant A118G. J Biol Chem 280(38):32618–32624

Zheng GX, Terry JM, Belgrader P, Ryvkin P, Bent ZW et al (2017) Massively parallel digital transcriptional profiling of single cells. Nat Commun 8:14049

Zhu AZ, Zhou Q, Cox LS, David SP, Ahluwalia JS et al (2014) Association of CHRNA5-A3-B4 SNP rs2036527 with smoking cessation therapy response in African-American smokers. Clin Pharmacol Ther 96:256–265

Small Molecule Neuropeptide S and Melanocortin 4 Receptor Ligands as Potential Treatments for Substance Use Disorders

Bruce Blough and Ojas Namjoshi

Contents

1 SUDs Medications Development 62
2 Neuropeptide S (NPS) 63
2.1 Oxazolo[3,4-a]pyrazin-3-ones 64
2.2 Pyranopyrimidine Derivatives 66
2.3 Furo[3,4-c]pyridine Derivatives 67
2.4 Imidazopyridines 68
2.5 Quinolinone Derivatives 69
2.6 Tricyclic Imidazole Derivatives 70
2.7 Indan-1,3-dione and Indan-1-one Derivatives 71
2.8 Pyrroloimidazole Derivatives 71
3 Melanocortin 4 (MC4) 72
3.1 Spiropiperidines 74
3.2 Piperazinebenzylamine 74
3.3 Arylpiperazinylpiperazines 76
3.4 Imidazoles 77
3.5 Pyridazinones 77
3.6 2,4-Difluorophenylpyrrolidines 78
3.7 2-Oxopiperazines 79
References 80

Abstract

There is a vital need for novel approaches and biological targets for drug discovery and development. Treatment strategies for substance use disorders (SUDs) to date have been mostly ineffective other than substitution-like therapeutics. Two such targets are the peptide G-protein-coupled receptors neuropeptide S (NPS) and melanocortin 4 (MC4). Preclinical evidence suggests that antagonists, inverse agonists, or negative allosteric modulators of these receptors

B. Blough (✉) · O. Namjoshi
Center for Drug Discovery, RTI International, Research Triangle Park, NC, USA
e-mail: beb@rti.org

M. A. Nader, Y. L. Hurd (eds.), *Substance Use Disorders*,
Handbook of Experimental Pharmacology 258, https://doi.org/10.1007/164_2019_313

might be novel therapeutics for SUDs. NPS is a relatively unexplored receptor with high potential for treating SUD. MC4 has a strong link to early-onset obesity, and emerging evidence suggests significant overlap between food-maintained and drug-maintained behaviors making MC4 an intriguing target for SUD. This chapter provides an overview of the literature in relation to the roles of NPS and MC4 in drug-seeking behaviors and then provides a medicinal chemistry-based survey of the small molecule ligands for each receptor.

Keywords
Drug abuse · Medicinal chemistry · Melanocortin 4 · Neuropeptide S · Peptide GPCR

1 SUDs Medications Development

Treatments for substance use disorders (SUDs) remain an unmet clinical need despite several decades of efforts to find suitable solutions. Strategies targeting the receptor systems with drugs have worked in some cases, such as the discovery of varenicline for smoking cessation which targets the nicotinic receptors activated by nicotine (Beard et al. 2016), but in general these strategies have not been very successful. Significant efforts were made to repurpose existing medications as well, but, to date, successful treatments for SUDs remain elusive. There is a significant need for novel targets for SUD therapeutic drug discovery and development. There are many biological targets that have undergone significant medicinal chemistry and show promise in initial efficacy testing, but which need further preclinical study in order to justify additional drug development for SUDs. This chapter describes two such targets: neuropeptide S (NPS) and melanocortin 4 (MC4). While limited, the preclinical data supporting their roles in drug abuse are clear and both appear to be legitimate targets for SUD treatment discovery. A short description of their significance in relation to drug-seeking behavior is provided, followed by an overview of the small molecule ligands developed to date, including agonists and antagonists. In both cases, inhibition of these receptors appears to be the medications development strategy; therefore, antagonists, inverse agonists, and negative allosteric modulators may be effective at reducing drug-seeking behaviors, but additional investigations are needed. Partial agonists may be effective as well, as was the case with varenicline. The potential abuse liability of agonists has not been fully vetted, so agonist scaffolds are also of interest. Both of these receptors are peptide G-protein-coupled receptors (GPCRs) with substantial peptide ligand development, but the focus here is on small molecules since they are more likely to be developed as drugs for treating SUDs and the medicinal chemistry development of peptidomimetic ligands being more difficult.

2 Neuropeptide S (NPS)

NPS is a 20-amino acid peptide which has been identified as the endogenous ligand (subnanomolar K_d) for formerly orphan GPCR, GPR154, which is now referred to as the NPS receptor (NPSR). This NPS/NPSR neuropeptide system was originally identified in 2002 by Sato et al. (2002), but Xu and co-workers delineated the in vivo roles of NPS in 2004 (Xu et al. 2004). The name of the peptide is due to the presence of a serine (S) residue in the N-terminal position of the molecule (primary sequence in *Homo sapiens*: SFRNGVGTGMKKTSFQRAKS). NPS is encoded as a prepropeptide, and its expression is limited to a few discrete brain areas, such as in isolated cells of the amygdala and the dorsomedial hypothalamic nucleus, and particularly confined to specific regions of the brainstem, including the area proximal to the locus coeruleus (LC) region, the principal sensory trigeminal nucleus, and the lateral parabrachial nucleus (Liu et al. 2011; Xu et al. 2004, 2007). The NPSR, on the other hand, is widely distributed in the brain particularly in regions that are associated with regulation of stress response, memory, the olfactory system, and regulation of arousal (Leonard and Ring 2011; Xu et al. 2007). It has been demonstrated that NPS stimulates intracellular calcium levels as well as cAMP accumulation in cells expressing the recombinant NPSR. This indicates that the NPSR can signal via both Gq and Gs to increase cellular excitability (Xu et al. 2004). NPS regulates several biological functions including wakefulness (Xu et al. 2004), stress and anxiety (Leonard et al. 2008; Rizzi et al. 2008; Xu et al. 2004), locomotor activity (Leonard et al. 2008; Xu et al. 2004), food intake (Beck et al. 2005; Smith et al. 2006), and, importantly, drug abuse (Badia-Elder et al. 2008; Cannella et al. 2009; Li et al. 2009; Paneda et al. 2009).

Earlier reports have shown that the most commonly used or abused psychostimulants, such as caffeine and nicotine, modulate NPS and NPSR mRNA expression, which suggests a potential role for NPS in the effects of these drugs as well (Lage et al. 2006, 2007). Patient relapse into drug-seeking and use is a key component of the SUD. Several reports in the literature support the possibility that increased NPS activity may play a role in shaping vulnerability to addiction, especially to relapse. NPSR activation has been shown to modulate reward circuits and is expressed in brain areas associated with reward processing such as the ventral tegmental area (VTA), amygdala, and substantia nigra (Clark et al. 2011). Intracerebroventricular (ICV) administration of NPS stimulates dopamine release in the medial prefrontal cortex (Si et al. 2010). Local intra-VTA microinjections of NPS enhance dopamine release in the nucleus accumbens (Mochizuki et al. 2010), linking NPS to the mesolimbic dopamine system, which is presumed to be a major neuronal pathway modulating reward. When rats were injected ICV with NPS, cocaine self-administration under a fixed-ratio schedule of reinforcement was not affected by the NPS treatment, indicating that it does not play a role in cocaine reward (Kallupi et al. 2010); however, NPS involvement in reinstatement of cocaine-seeking and relapse has been reported (Paneda et al. 2009). Further, ICV injections of NPS appear to have reward-like effects, facilitating seeking and enhance reinforcement (Cao et al. 2011). It has been demonstrated that ICV injection of NPS

(0.45 nmol) reinstated previously extinguished lever pressing for cocaine in mice (Paneda et al. 2009). It has also been demonstrated that rats increased lever presses leading to intraventricular administration of a low dose of NPS (3.4–34 pmol per infusion), in a dose-dependent manner, suggesting that NPS itself may have reinforcing properties (Cao et al. 2011). This increase in cocaine self-administration caused by NPS injection is mediated by activation of the corticotropin-releasing factor (CRF) system (Cao et al. 2011; Paneda et al. 2009). Further, NPS also potently reinstated cocaine-seeking behavior following ICV or intra-lateral hypothalamus (LH) microinfusion (Kallupi et al. 2010). In addition, NPS has also been linked to alcohol intoxication and withdrawal (Ruggeri et al. 2010). Activation of NPS receptors in the LH has been shown to facilitate relapse to ethanol-seeking induced by environmental conditioning factors (Cannella et al. 2009).

Due to these finding, the NPS/NPSR neuropeptide system has been targeted by various research groups as a potential treatment for SUD. Structure activity relationship (SAR) studies on peptide as well as non-peptide ligands have been carried out in order to understand the structural requirements for blockade of the NPSR. In the case of peptide ligands, studies on various analogs of the NPS peptide have been published resulting in partial agonist or antagonist profiles. It has been demonstrated that the 5-position of NPS is a key point for structural modification for NPSR antagonism (Camarda et al. 2008; Cifani et al. 2011; Guerrini et al. 2009, 2010; Nepomuceno et al. 2010; Peng et al. 2010; Tancredi et al. 2007). On the other hand, Clark et al. recently identified a truncated peptide as a potent NPSR agonist exhibiting bias for the calcium mobilization assay over cAMP production (Clark et al. 2017). This compound shows profoundly decreased effect on the locomotor component of the NPS system and provides indication that NPS-mediated anxiolytic-like effects are separable from the effects on locomotion, which may also lead to novel direction in the addiction field. This review, however, is focused on the various classes of non-peptide ligands as NPSR antagonists that have been identified over last 15 years. In humans, multiple single-nucleotide polymorphisms (SNPs), as well as splice variants of the NPSR, have been identified (Reinscheid et al. 2005). One of these polymorphisms produces an Asn-Ile exchange (N107I) in the first extracellular loop of the receptor protein, and the 107I variant displays higher agonist efficacy for both calcium mobilization and cAMP accumulation with no difference in binding affinity. Hence compounds are typically evaluated using both NPSR 107N and NPSR 107I variants. Eight classes of novel antagonists have been reported. Continued development of such novel molecules with potent and selective NPSR antagonist activity and with improved drug-like properties will help further understand the NPS/NPSR system as an emerging target for the treatment of drug abuse.

2.1 Oxazolo[3,4-a]pyrazin-3-ones

The hexahydro-oxazolo[3,4-a]pyrazine scaffold was first described in a patent from Takeda Pharmaceuticals in 2005, but no pharmacological or biological data were

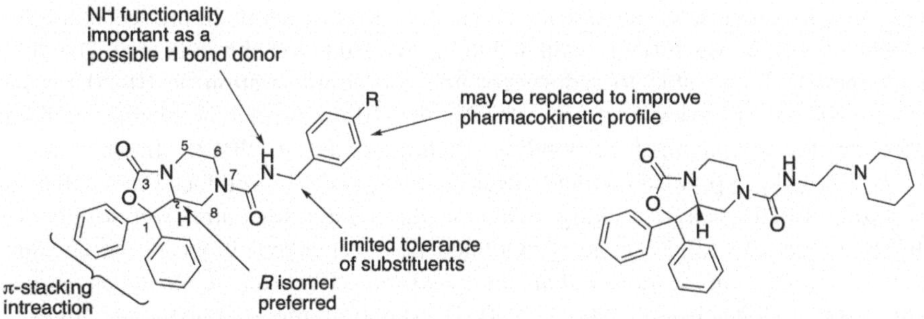

SHA-66 (**1**): R = H; NPSR 107I K_b = 32.6 nM
SHA-68 (**2**): R = F; NPSR 107I K_b = 27.9 nM

(*R*)-RTI-118 (**3**)
NPSR 107I K_e = 36 nM

Fig. 1 Oxazolo[3,4-a]pyrazin-3-one SAR

presented (Fukatsu et al. 2005). Substitution at the 1-position with methyl, cyclopropyl, cyclohexyl, and benzyl moieties or (substituted) phenyl rings has been disclosed in the patent (Fig. 1). Compounds with 1,1-diphenyl substituents were reported to be the most potent NPSR antagonists; hence, most reports thereafter have been focused on the 1,1-diphenyl substituents. The chemical space around the piperazine nitrogen N^7 has been explored to a much larger extent, with the introduction of a wide range of substituents. Two compounds (Fig. 1), SHA-66 (**1**) and SHA-68 (**2**), with N′-(substituted)benzylurea at the 7-position, were synthesized and tested by Okamura et al. and were found to be potent and selective competitive antagonists of both the Asn107 and Ile107 variants of the NPSR with IC_{50} values in the two-digit nanomolar range (Okamura et al. 2008). Pharmacological evaluation of the enantiomers of **2** revealed that the *R* enantiomer of **2** is the active enantiomer in the racemic mixture and is much more potent than the *S* enantiomer (Trapella et al. 2011). Various 7-position substituents in hexahydro-oxazolo[3,4-a]pyrazin-3-one series of compounds were explored by Zhang et al. to understand the structural requirements for NPSR antagonistic activity (Zhang et al. 2008). This study highlighted the importance of NH residue of the urea moiety for antagonistic activity as alkylation of the urea nitrogen or replacement with a carbon or oxygen resulted in reduced potency. This observation has been corroborated by molecular docking studies on **2** in the NPSR binding pocket, in which it was observed that the NH residue of the urea moiety acts as a potential hydrogen bond donor in an interaction with the side chain of Asp297 of the NPSR (Dal Ben et al. 2010). It also appears that 1,1-diphenyl substituent of **2** would engage in π-stacking interactions (non-covalent attractive interactions between two aromatic rings), with a pocket formed by aromatic residues (Phe 177, Tyr 290, Phe 293) (Dal Ben et al. 2010). Zhang et al. observed that the alkyl substituent on the methylene spacer between the urea function and the 4-fluorophenyl group or the elongation of the spacer resulted in reduced potency indicating a limited tolerance for the 7-position substituents (Zhang et al. 2008). RTI-118 (**3**), a racemic mixture (Fig. 1) reported by Zhang et al. (2008), with an ethylpiperidine substituent at the 7-position, and an improved solubility compared with **2**, was further evaluated in in vivo studies (Schmoutz et al. 2012). In a rat model, **3** was able to reduce cocaine self-administration at 10–20 mg/kg, i.p. (much lower doses compared to **2**), in a dose-dependent manner without affecting food-maintained responding (Schmoutz et al. 2012). In this study, **3** (10–20 mg/kg, i.p.) also blocked cocaine-, cue-, and stress-induced reinstatement of extinguished cocaine-seeking behavior. In a rat intracranial self-stimulation (ICSS) model, **3** (3.2–32 mg/kg) exhibited dose-dependent blockade of cocaine-induced facilitation at doses that produced no effect on ICSS when **3** was administered alone (Bonano et al. 2014). Hassler et al. reported a study to improve pharmacokinetic properties of **2**, as well as potency of **3** (Hassler et al. 2014). Replacement of the benzyl moiety of **2** with ionizable 2-anilino moiety afforded a compound with similar potency as **2**, while other substituents such as various pyridyl analogs resulted in reduced potency. On the other hand, any attempt to further modify **3** resulted in a substantial loss of activity. As was observed in the case of **2**, the *R* enantiomer of **3** was the active compound and was about four-fold more potent than the racemic mixture in CHOK1 cells expressing human NPSR 107I, while the (*S*)-**3** was inactive up to high micromolar concentrations (Hassler et al. 2014). In addition, (*R*)-**3** exhibited superior pharmacokinetic properties with rapid systemic absorption with an apparent half-life of 34 min and satisfactory brain penetration.

2.2 Pyranopyrimidine Derivatives

Using a novel homogeneous time-resolved fluorescence (HTRF) assay that measures cAMP responses, McCoy et al. identified a novel substituted napthopyranopyrimidine lead **4** (Fig. 2) with antagonistic activity against NPS in the low micromolar range for both the cAMP and calcium pathways (McCoy et al. 2010). Several analogs were synthesized to understand the SAR and were evaluated in both cAMP and calcium assays. The ability of a particular substituent to increase the antagonistic activity with respect to cAMP did not always correspond with an equivalent effect on calcium signaling. It was found that the replacement of the morpholinoethyl moiety at the 10-position with an aromatic ring increased the potency of the molecule. Disubstitution on the aromatic ring at 12-position leads to improved potency in calcium assay, with compound **5** having a 2,3-dihydrobenzo[b][1,4]dioxin-6-yl substituent being the most potent while compound **6**, with a phenyl group at 12-position, exhibiting superior activity in cAMP assay (Fig. 2). Substitution at the 8 or 9 position of the lead compound resulted in loss of potency in both assays. Similarly, replacement of the naphthyl moiety with substituted aromatic rings or variation in the orientation of the naphthyl group is detrimental for activity. Insertion of an alkyl spacer between the phenyl and the pyrimidine rings leads to retention of the potency in the cAMP assay while loss of potency in the calcium assay. Introduction of small substituents on the 10-phenyl ring leads to reduction in potency in cAMP assay while retaining the potency in calcium assay. Further development of these

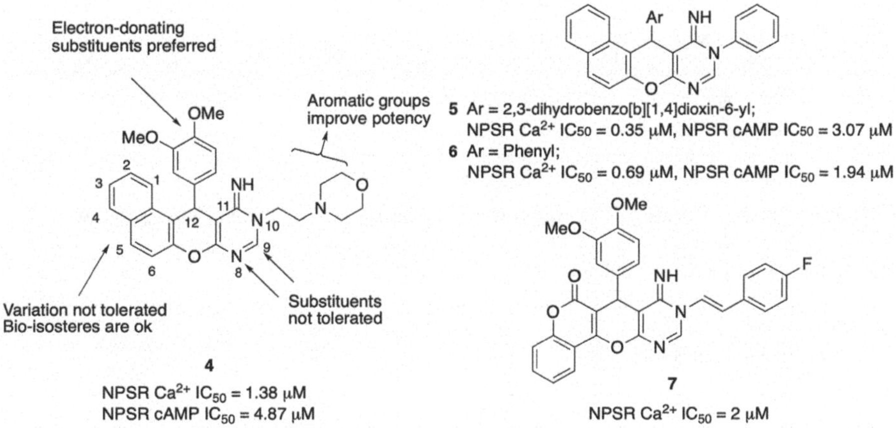

Fig. 2 Pyranopyrimidine SAR

selective analogs may lead to interesting probes to study the involvement of different G coupling pathways in the neurobiology of the NPSR. Recently Batran et al. developed another series of compounds designed by replacing the naphthalene moiety of the lead naphthopyranopyrimidine scaffold by the bioisosteric coumarin moiety (Batran et al. 2017). The rationale was to increase the H-bonding interactions with the NPSR active site. A limited number of analogs with hybridized substitutions such as Schiff's bases and isosteric heterocyclic rings as triazole and tetrazole moieties at the 10- and 11-positions were synthesized. The compounds exhibited antagonistic activity at single-digit micromolar concentration in the calcium assay with **7** being the most potent analog (Fig. 2). The authors further rationalized the activity of these ligands using molecular docking studies, which may be utilized for designing other ligands active at NPSR (Batran et al. 2017).

2.3 Furo[3,4-c]pyridine Derivatives

Runyon et al. disclosed a series of 4,5,6,7-tetrahydrofuro[3,4-c]pyridine-1(3H)-one derivatives as NPSR antagonists (Runyon et al. 2013). Substituents at the C^3 and N^5 positions have been explored. Efficacy curves of three representative compounds **8–10** (Fig. 3) have been disclosed. Compound **10** exhibits K_e of 30 nM against NPSR 107I. This novel scaffold appears to mimic the oxazolo[3,4-a]pyrazine-3-one core described earlier, and one of the phenyl rings in the oxazolo[3,4-a]pyrazine-3-ones can be replaced with an isobutyl group.

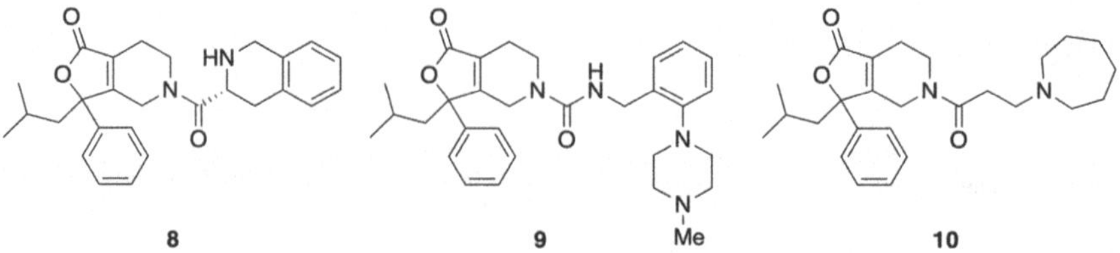

Fig. 3 Furo[3,4-c]pyridine analogs

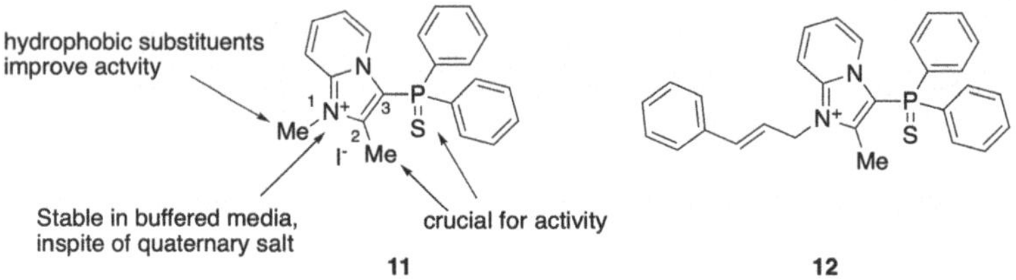

Fig. 4 Imidazopyridines SAR

2.4 Imidazopyridines

Using a HTRF assay that measures the formation of cAMP upon binding of NPS to NPSR using CHO cells stably expressing NPSR, Marugan et al. disclosed a structurally novel lead 3-(diphenylphosphorothioyl)-1,2-dimethylimidazo[1,2-a]pyridin-1-ium iodide **11** (Fig. 4), as an antagonist to the NPS/NPSR neurocircuitry (Marugan et al. 2011). Although this lead is a quaternary ammonium salt and with a diphenyl phosphorothionyl moiety, it was found to be quite stable in buffered media (Patnaik et al. 2013). In the SAR study published by Patnaik et al., it was observed that the 2-methyl and the diphenyl phosphorothionyl moiety were important for their activity (Patnaik et al. 2013). From the molecular modeling studies, it was determined that a hydrophobic substituent at the N^1 position may improve the activity. In line with this prediction, the best compound was **12** with a cinnamyl group at the N^1 position (Fig. 4). This compound exhibited an IC_{50} values of 45 nM and 0.96 nM in the cAMP assay and calcium assay, respectively. It also inhibited activation of ERK at 1.3 nM concentration. Further substitution at the pendant phenyl moiety did not afford any improvement in potency, probably underlining the capacity of the hydrophobic pocket at the binding site. In spite of this, it appears that compound **12** may not be selective as it exhibited >90% inhibition of control in seven targets (out of 55 tested), including the μ-opioid receptor. In in vivo studies, when administered via ICV route, in rats, a single 10 μg dose of **12** was able to reverse the suppression of food intake induced by NPS. It has also been reported that in mice (10 mg/kg; i.p.), **12** crosses the blood-brain barrier (Patnaik et al. 2013).

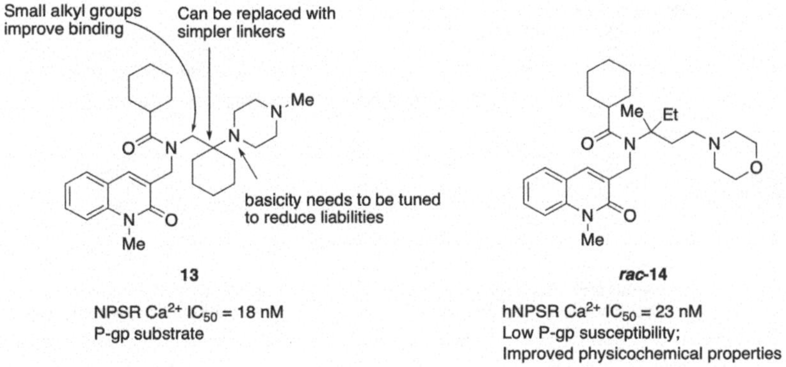

Fig. 5 Quinolinone SAR

2.5 Quinolinone Derivatives

A novel quinolinone-based lead, **13** (Fig. 5), was identified as a potent ($IC_{50} = 18$ nM) NPSR antagonist by Melamed et al. using a dual sequence fluorometric imaging plate reader (FLIPR) calcium mobilization assay (Melamed et al. 2010). Unfortunately, this compound is a substrate for P-glycoprotein (P-gp), thus with a lower chance for crossing the blood-brain barrier. Hence the aim of this study was to reduce the P-gp susceptibility while retaining the NPSR antagonistic potency. The authors claim that the SAR at the cycloheximide moiety is very narrow and wouldn't afford any improvement in the desired properties. Several analogs at the piperazinylcyclohexyl moiety were incorporated based on computational algorithm. The first iteration of SAR identified the 1,3-propanediamine substructure as a viable replacement for the piperazinecyclohexyl moiety, which was probably responsible for the undesired P-gp activity. Cyclic amine such as piperidine at the end of the propyl linker resulted in improved potency. Reducing the basicity of the piperidine nitrogen by the addition of fluorine substituents resulted in reduced P-gp substrate activity, but increased plasma protein binding. Similarly, a gem-dimethyl group as well as an ethyl-methyl substituent at 1-position of the propyl linker provided a significant boost in potency compared with monomethyl-substituted compounds; however, it resulted in a significant increase in plasma protein binding. In this study, compound *rac*-**14** (Fig. 5), with a morpholine substituent at the end of the propyl linker with an ethyl, methyl substituent at the 1-position afforded a better combination of potency and P-gp susceptibility. Resolution of the *rac*-**14** resulted in the potent antipode NPSR-QA1 (undisclosed enantiomer), which exhibited desired physicochemical properties with improved potency at NPSR compared with the other enantiomer as well as the *rac*-**14**. Further evaluation of NPSR-QA1 has been done by Melamed et al. to demonstrate its ability to achieve acceptable CNS concentrations after IP administration in rats. On the other hand, Camarda et al. found that NPSR-QA1 was poorly active in in vivo assays sensitive to NPS effects. In this study, IP administration of NPSR-QA1 (30 mg/kg) resulted only in partial

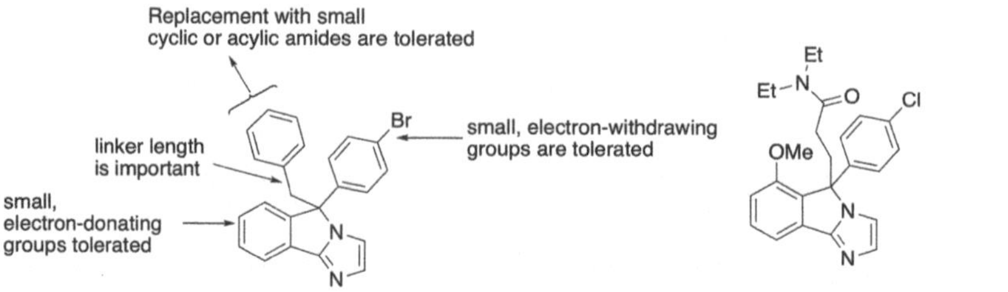

15

hNPSR Ca^{2+} IC_{50} = 380 nM
Poor physicochemical properties

16

hNPSR Ca^{2+} IC_{50} = 43 nM
Improved physicochemical properties

Fig. 6 Tricyclic imidazole SAR

reversal of arousal promoting effect caused by NPS in the righting reflex assay, while it was ineffective in blocking the stimulant effect of NPS in the locomotor activity test (Camarda et al. 2013). This lack of effectiveness in mice may be attributed to the interspecies differences in the pharmacokinetic properties.

2.6 Tricyclic Imidazole Derivatives

A novel high-throughput screening-derived tricyclic imidazole scaffold **15** (Fig. 6) was reported by Trotter et al. (2010). Given to its high lipophilicity, most effort was focused on improving its polarity and potency. Replacement of the benzyl moiety with a tetrahydropyran moiety resulted in improved potency, but with rapid plasma clearance in rat. Various substituents on the 4-bromophenyl group did not afford much improvement in potency, while replacement with a 4-cyanophenyl group resulted in improved pharmacokinetic profile of the compound while retaining its potency. Various combinations of the substituents at the benzyl and 4-bromophenyl moieties afforded compounds with slightly improved potency, but no significant improvements in pharmacokinetic properties. In another series in the tricyclic imidazole scaffold containing a piperidine amide group (instead of benzyl moiety), it was observed that the length of the linker between the amide and the tricyclic scaffold played an important role in improving potency as well as P-gp activity, with a propionamide linker providing the optimum activity. Further SAR on the amide functionality led to the observation that small cyclic and acyclic amides were potent NPSR antagonists. Reducing the basicity of the nitrogen resulted in P-gp non-substrates, but with slight loss in potency. On the other hand, a compound with a diethylamide moiety resulted in optimum activity, with IC_{50} of 90 nM against NPSR and low P-gp susceptibility, but with low CNS exposure in rats. Addition of a methoxy group at the 7-position on the tricyclic scaffold resulted in identification of NPSR-PI1 (**16**), with excellent potency and pharmacokinetic properties (Fig. 6). Intriguingly, Camarda et al. found that **16** was inactive in mouse models of righting reflex and locomotor activity tests at 30 mg/kg in rats (Camarda et al. 2013).

Fig. 7 Indan-1,3-dione SAR

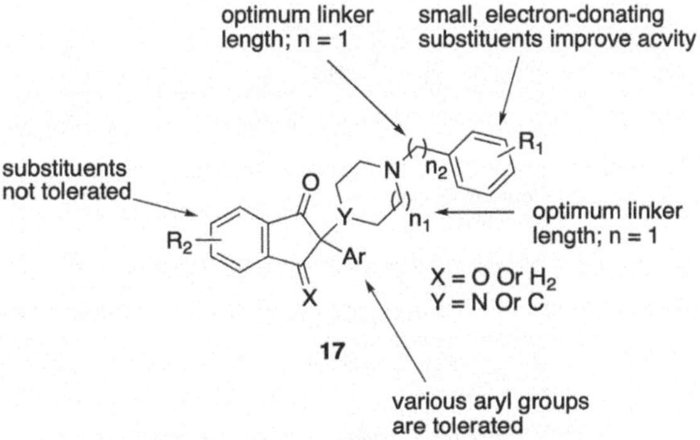

2.7 Indan-1,3-dione and Indan-1-one Derivatives

Recently, Fretz et al. disclosed a series of substituted indan-1,3-diones and indan-1-ones **17** (Fig. 7) as potent NPSR antagonists (Fretz et al. 2013). Several analogs have been synthesized and evaluated in calcium assay for NPSR activity leading to the SAR. Any substitution on the indan-1,3-dione aryl ring leads to lower antagonistic effects. Small, electron-donating substituents on the benzyl ring attached to the piperazine moiety lead to improvement of potency, while bulkier and electron-withdrawing substituents were detrimental for activity. Increasing the length of the linker between the phenyl ring and piperazine moiety leads to reduced potency. On the other hand, various substituents on the 2-phenyl ring are tolerated, with small, electron-donating substituents at the meta-position improving potency against NPSR. Substitution of the 2-phenyl ring with various heteroaryl rings was detrimental to the activity. Finally, while a piperazine ring can be substituted with a piperidine moiety, a six-membered cyclic linker was the ideal linker between the indan-1,3-dione and the benzyl group. Any larger or smaller ring linkers resulted in lower potency. Corresponding indan-1-ones ($X = H_2$) appear to retain potency, probably indicating that this carbonyl may not be involved in any interaction at the receptor site. The compounds reported in this patent appear to be very potent, with IC_{50} values in the nanomolar range against hNPSRAsn107.

2.8 Pyrroloimidazole Derivatives

Micheli et al. described a design strategy based on a screening hit compound **18** (Fig. 8) as a competitive NPSR antagonist (Micheli et al. 2010). The ^{1}HNMR of **18** and molecular modeling studies of this compound indicated a presence of an intramolecular hydrogen bond interaction between the amino group and the furyl oxygen. Based on this information, conformationally locked analogs of **18** were designed by replacing the furyl ring with a pyrrole moiety and then inserting an alkyl bridge between the amine and pyrrole nitrogen atoms. This resulted in a potent novel

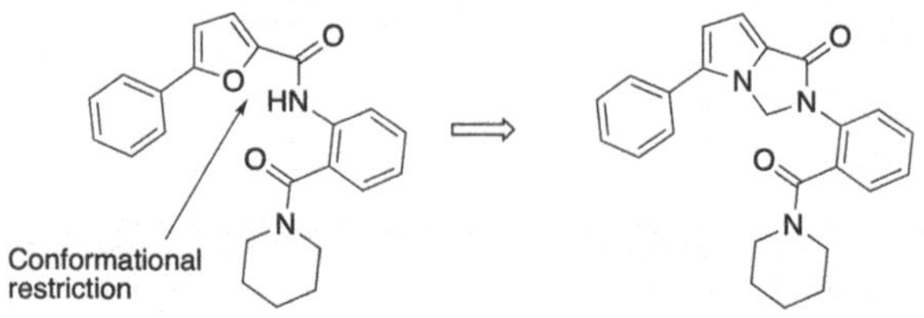

18

hNPSR $pIC_{50} = 7.5$
Low selectivity;
High lipophilicity

19

hNPSR $pIC_{50} = 8.0$
Improved selectivity;
Improved physocichemical properties

Fig. 8 Conformationally locked pyrroloimidazole

derivative **19** (Fig. 8), with pIC_{50} of 8.0 against NPSR in calcium assay with improved selectivity profile (Micheli et al. 2010).

In summary, literature evidence shows that increased NPS activity may play a role in shaping vulnerability to addiction, especially to relapse. Hence selective ligands have been successfully designed that target the NPS/NPSR neuropeptide system as treatments for drug abuse. Several preclinical development studies have also been focused to improve the pharmacokinetic properties and improve bioavailability of these compounds. However, at this stage, none of the NPSR ligands have entered clinical trials. The NPS/NPSR system is still an emerging target in the drug abuse field and further medicinal chemistry campaigns will help identify novel therapeutics for SUDs.

3 Melanocortin 4 (MC4)

The melanocortin system consists of five GPCRs, with the melanocortin 3 receptor (MC3R) and melanocortin 4 receptor (MC4R) being expressed primarily in the brain (Caruso et al. 2014; Tao 2010). MC4R plays a role in a variety of biological functions, including energy homeostasis (Cui and Lutter 2013), food intake (Cabeza de Vaca et al. 2002), pain (Kalange et al. 2007; Starowicz et al. 2005), learning and memory (Caruso et al. 2014; Giuliani et al. 2017), neuroinflammation (Lasaga et al. 2008), and neuroprotection (Giuliani et al. 2014). MC4R gene mutations have been strongly linked to early-onset obesity (Tao 2010), and these findings have made MC4R a target for anti-obesity drug discovery (Emmerson et al. 2007). The development of weight loss medications remains a significant unmet clinical need, so interest in MC4R ligands has been strong.

Increasing evidence suggests that dopaminergic (DAergic) neurons and forebrain circuitry drive both food- and drug-maintained behaviors (Wise 2013); therefore, the role of MC4R in food-seeking behavior makes it a potential target for modifying drug-seeking behavior (Navarro 2017). Indeed, the melanocortin and dopaminergic systems appear to have significant overlap (Lindblom et al. 2002). MC4R mRNA expression is enriched in the nucleus accumbens, an area of the striatum known to be involved with drug reinforcement (Alvaro et al. 1996, 1997). Expression of MC4Rs in D1-like receptor-containing neurons appears to regulate food intake and locomotor sensitization to cocaine (Cui and Lutter 2013). D2-like receptors and MC4Rs are co-expressed in neurons associated with food reward (Yoon and Baik 2015). The melanocortin and dopaminergic systems can also affect each other. MC4R ligands, including the melanocortin peptides and small molecule agonists, can affect the activity of DAergic neurons (Navarro 2017). Chronic cocaine exposure increased MC4R mRNA expression in the striatum and hippocampus (Alvaro et al. 2003; Cabeza de Vaca et al. 2002; Hsu et al. 2005). There appears to be a strong connection between the melanocortin and dopaminergic systems.

Despite these strong connections, MC4R ligands have not been thoroughly vetted as potential treatments for drug abuse. Research has been somewhat sporadic. The selective MC4R antagonist peptides HS014 and HS024 have been shown to prevent nicotine-induced reinstatement (Qi et al. 2015). The MC4R antagonist peptide SHU-9119 blocked the reinforcing, motivational, and locomotor sensitization effects of cocaine (Alserda et al. 2013; Hsu et al. 2005). Melanotan II (MTII), a nonselective melanocortin peptide agonist, enhanced the rewarding effects of amphetamine (Cabeza de Vaca et al. 2002). The MC4R antagonist HS014 enhanced the analgesic effects of opioids while delaying the development of tolerance and preventing withdrawal hyperalgesia (Ercil et al. 2005; Kalange et al. 2007). The MC4R antagonist peptide JKC-363 also delayed the development of opioid tolerance when co-administered with morphine (Starowicz et al. 2005). While a more systematic study of MC4R ligands is lacking, it is clear that the melanocortin system, in particular MC4R, can affect drug-seeking behaviors.

MC4R also plays a role in other related comorbid conditions to chronic drug use, including depression and anxiety, making it even more intriguing as a target for SUD mediations development. Repeated administration of MCL0129, a selective small molecule MC4R antagonist, increased social interactions in an open field test suggesting it has anxiolytic-like effects (Shimazaki and Chaki 2005). The selective MC4R antagonist MCL0042 produced anxiolytic- and antidepressant-like effects in rodent models (Chaki et al. 2005). MC4R antagonists MCL0020 and MCL0129 lowered anxiety in a light/dark test (Chaki and Okuyama 2005); MCL0129 showed antidepressant-like effects in a forced swim test (Chaki and Okuyama 2005). Collectively, the evidence suggests MC4R antagonists, inverse agonists, and/or negative allosteric modulators may be effective therapeutics for treating SUDs.

While the development of MC4R antagonists for drug abuse looks promising based on existing evidence, the wide range of clinical effects observed with MC4R ligands has caused many to remain skeptical. As noted, MC4R ligands affect fundamental processes including weight, energy homeostasis, and sexual function. MC4R deletion in rodents appears to have altered glucose metabolism, lowered energy utilization, and gain weight in certain circumstances (Krashes et al. 2016). These effects would be detrimental for a drug abuse treatment. But these issues remain unresolved and not well understood. The human genetic mutations do not appear to have any deleterious effects, other than the propensity to cause early-onset obesity (Yeo et al. 1998). MC4R knockout animals appear normal as well (Krashes et al. 2016). The effects of a

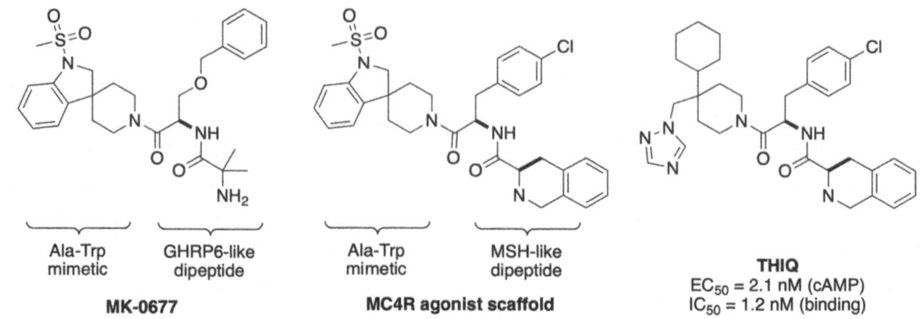

Fig. 9 Spiropiperidine development

pharmacological intervention are difficult to predict. In addition, the signaling cascade is quite complex. MC4R can signal through Gs, Gi/o, and Gq, as well as several G-protein-independent mechanisms including β-arrestins and inwardly rectifying potassium channels (Buch et al. 2009; Gantz and Fong 2003; Newman et al. 2006; Rodrigues et al. 2015). Little is known about how each of these pathways relate to the plethora of effects caused by MC4R ligands. It seems that MC4R could be an ideal system for the development of signaling pathway biased ligands.

3.1 Spiropiperidines

The first small molecule ligands described for MC4R were agonists reported by Merck in 2002 (Sebhat et al. 2002) (Fig. 9). The Merck group had noticed a similarity between the pharmacophores of the growth hormone secretagogue peptide GHRP-6 and melanocortin peptides ACTH and a-MSH (Trp-Ala-DTrp-His vs Trp-Arg-DPhe-His). Modeling on that project had suggested a spiroindanyl piperidine moiety as an Ala-Trp mimetic which was used to develop peptidomimetic small molecule ligands leading to the development of compounds such as MK-0677 (Nargund et al. 1998), so the same approach was applied in the development of MC4R ligands (Fig. 9). An initial core scaffold was developed, which used the same spiroindanyl piperidine moiety linked to a dipeptide comprised of a p-chlorophenylalanine and a Tic group (Fig. 9). The spiro moiety was then explored eventually leading to the discovery of a potent and selective agonist THIQ, with an $EC_{50} = 2.1$ nM.

3.2 Piperazinebenzylamine

Neurocrine Biosciences began to report on the development of the piperazinebenzylamine MC4R ligands in 2003 (Fig. 10). The scaffold was originally identified and developed as an MC4R agonist (Dyck et al. 2003; Pontillo et al. 2004) following the development of THIQ at Merck. Chemists at Neurocrine reasoned that the

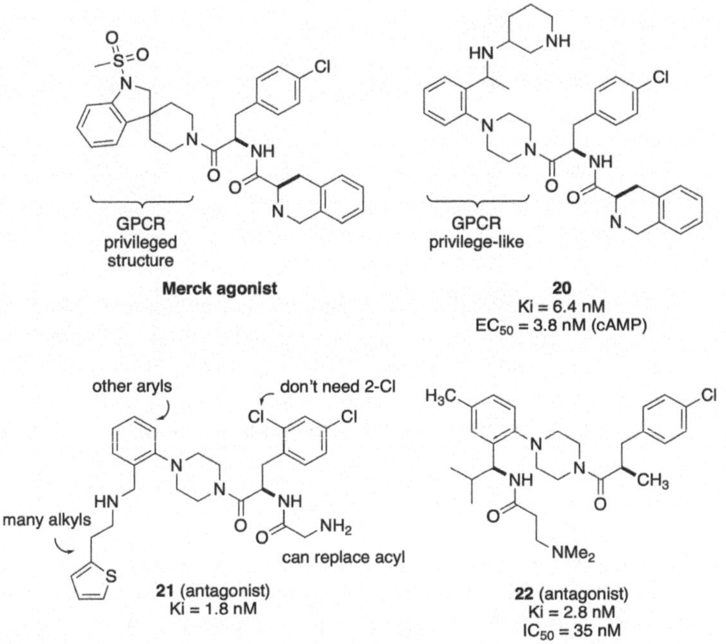

Fig. 10 Piperazinebenzylamine agonists and antagonists

spiropiperidine moiety was a GPCR privileged structure, so they decided to place it with another GPCR privileged structure: a 2-substituted phenylpiperazine group. These changes eventually produced selective and potent MC4R agonists, such as **20** (Fig. 10), which had an EC_{50} of 3.8 nM in a cAMP assay and a binding Ki of 6.4 nM.

To get antagonists, a combination of mutagenesis, peptide SAR, small molecule MC4R SAR, and receptor modeling was employed (Chen et al. 2004). Modeling suggested an interaction between Asp122 of MC4R and polar functionalities off the phenyl group. This prompted the synthesis of a benzylamine analog to enhance this interaction. Modeling suggested that there were lipophilic areas close by, so the benzylamine was alkylated which greatly increased the binding to a $Ki = 10.8$ nM (35-fold) without substantially increasing agonist efficacy to an EC_{50} of 290 nM (three-fold). The group believed the R-Tic residue was important for receptor activation, so it was replaced with a series of other acyl groups. A β-alanine group was found to have good binding properties, but reduced agonist efficacy. Finally, the p-chlorophenyl group was replaced with a more lipophilic 2,4-dichlorophenyl group because it had been known that the agonist activity of the MC4R peptide MT-II could be switched off by replacing the phenyl group with a more lipophilic 2′-naphthyl group. Indeed, this resulted in the first good antagonist lead **21** (Fig. 10) with a $Ki = 1.8$ nM and which had no agonist activity (cAMP) at 10 μM.

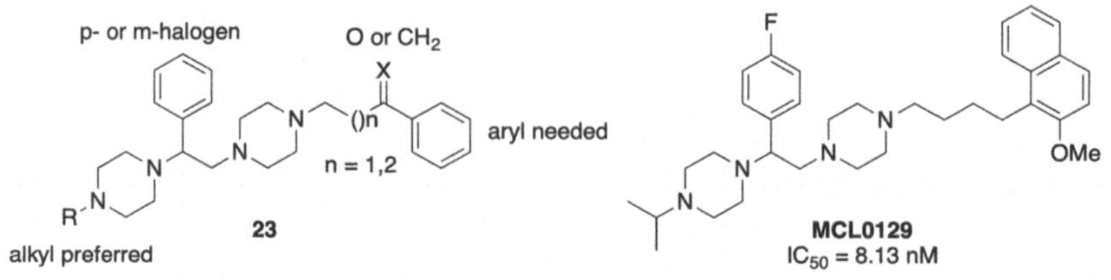

Fig. 11 Arylpiperazinylpiperazines

Neurocrine then spent several years optimizing the antagonist. Many strategies were employed, most centered around the piperazinebenzylamine core. The phenyl group could be replaced with a pyridine (Tran et al. 2006, 2007a) or a cyclohexyl group (Tucci et al. 2005), the thionyl group could be replaced with a 1-methoxy-2-propyl group (Pontillo et al. 2005), and the dipeptide was placed with various acyl functionalities (Jiang et al. 2006). A substantial amount of SAR has been done around the core structure, leading MC4R antagonists such as **22** (Fig. 10), which is highly selective for MC4R with a $Ki = 2.8$ nM, an IC_{50} of 35 nM, good bioavailability (43%), and good pharmacokinetic properties (Chen et al. 2006, 2007a; Tran et al. 2007b). Compound **22** was studied in a tumor model of cachexia (Chen et al. 2007a). Both 5 and 20 mg/kg doses significantly increased food intake compared to vehicle.

3.3 Arylpiperazinylpiperazines

The arylpiperazinylpiperazine class of MC4R antagonists was published in 2003 by Amgen (Arasasingham et al. 2003) (Fig. 11). The scaffold was identified by high-throughput screening starting with a compound active with an IC_{50} of 2.8 μM. Their goal was to find antagonists that blocked the binding of agouti-related protein compared to other melanocortin peptides like α-MSH. While unsuccessful, suggesting that the two binding domains overlap, general MC4R antagonists were developed from the scaffold. A small study of both phenyl substituents showed that halogens were preferred and in the para position. The original compounds also had a ketone adjacent to the phenyl ring which was required for binding. Smaller alkyl groups in the piperazine ring were also preferred. Later, Taisho Pharmaceuticals found that the original phenylketone moiety could be replaced with a naphthyl group or biphenyl group, the linker extended from three carbons to four carbons (n = 2), and the ketone removed (Nozawa et al. 2007a, b, c). Their work identified MCL0129 (Fig. 11), the first antagonist with an IC_{50} value in the low nanomolar range (8.13 nM).

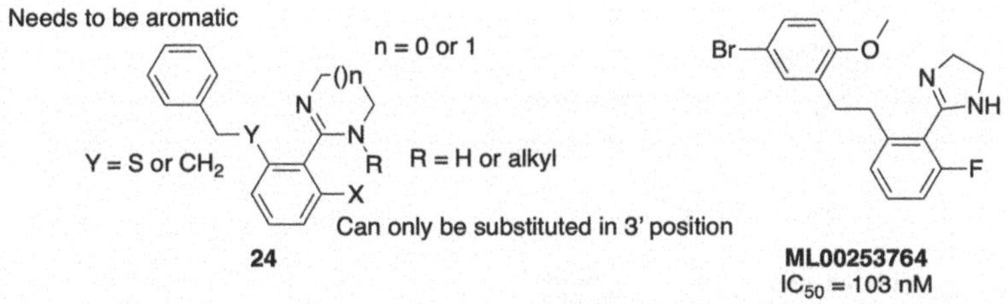

Fig. 12 Imidazole SAR

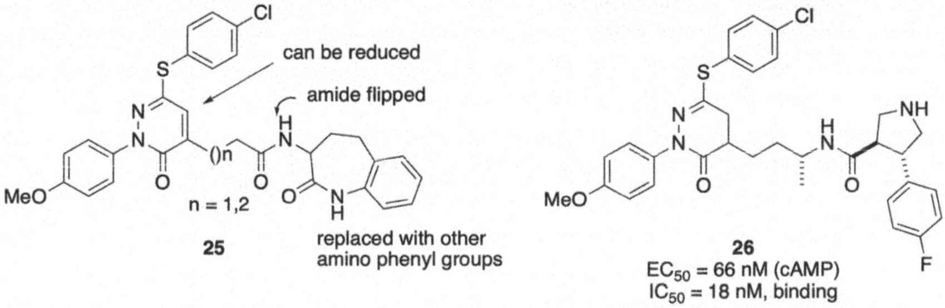

Fig. 13 Pyridazinone SAR

3.4 Imidazoles

The imidazole class of MC4R antagonists was first described in 2004 by Millennium Pharmaceuticals (Marsilje et al. 2004; Vos et al. 2004) (Fig. 12). The scaffold was identified by a high-throughput screening campaign and then optimized which resulted in the identification of ML00253764 (Fig. 12), with an IC_{50} of 103 nM. The initial optimization effort identified the 5-bromo-2-methoxyphenyl group which was two orders of magnitude more potent than the screening hit. The sulfur group was replaced with a methylene without a loss of activity, but the carbon linker was more metabolically stable. Later, the same group replaced the amidine with an acyl guanidine and was able to optimize that scaffold to about the same potency as ML00253764 (Vos et al. 2006). Interestingly, several of those analogs had IC_{50} values in the 100 nM range, but with subnanomolar binding affinities.

3.5 Pyridazinones

The pyridazinone class of MC4R agonist was first reported in 2003 (Ujjainwalla et al. 2003, 2005) (Fig. 13). The origin of the lead structure **25** was not described and may have come from a high-throughput screening effort. Most of the medicinal chemistry effort focused on the 1,3,4,5-tetrahydro-2H-1-benzazepin-2-one moiety. The linker to the pyridazinone could be extended, the entire group could be replaced with other phenyl containing cyclic amines including piperidines and pyrrolidines,

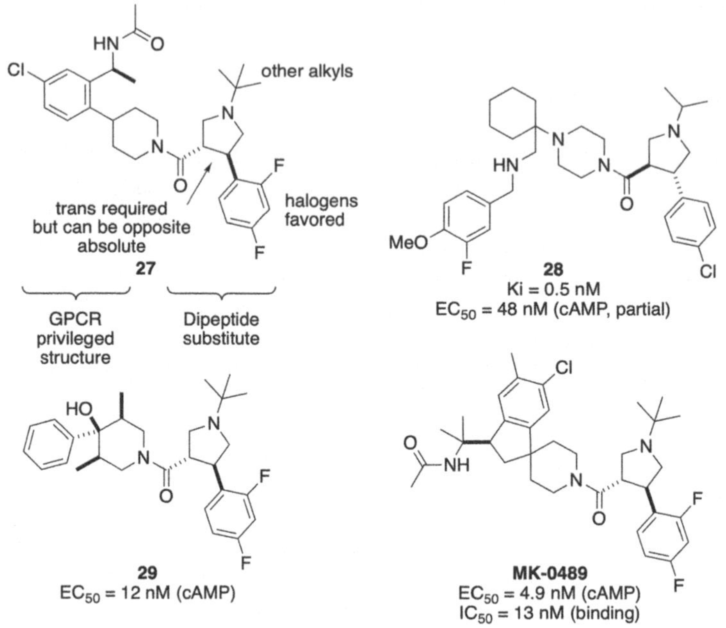

Fig. 14 2,4-Difluorophenylpyrrolidine development

and the pyridazinone could be reduced. A survey of aromatic substituents on the phenylpyrrolidines found that a p-fluoro group provided the best binding and agonist efficacy, resulting in agonist **26** with an EC_{50} of 66 nM (cAMP) and a binding IC_{50} of 18 nM.

3.6 2,4-Difluorophenylpyrrolidines

The 2,4-difluorophenylpyrrolidines class of MC4R agonists evolved from work on the pyridazinones at Merck where the agonist **27** was reported (Guo et al. 2008; Hong et al. 2010) (Fig. 14). The medicinal chemistry strategy here was to use the 2,4-difluorophenylpyrrolidine core as a substitute for the MC4R dipeptide (Fig. 14) and then link it to various phenyl amines, which could be loosely considered to be GPCR "privileged structures" and Ala-Trp mimics. Chemists began to link every phenylamine core structure they could find, resulting in analogs like **28** (Chen et al. 2007b, 2008) and 4-phenylpiperidinols like **29** (Lansdell et al. 2010) (Fig. 14). This class was thoroughly explored by Merck (Guo et al. 2010; He et al. 2010a, c), which eventually developed the highly selective, potent, orally bioavailable MC4R agonist MK-0489 (He et al. 2010b). MK-0489 has an EC_{50} of 4.9 nM (cAMP) and a binding IC_{50} of 13 nM, with a 33% bioavailability in rat (53% in monkey). MK-0489 is erectogenic in rats and shows mechanism-based food intake reduction in diet-induced obesity rats (He et al. 2010b, c).

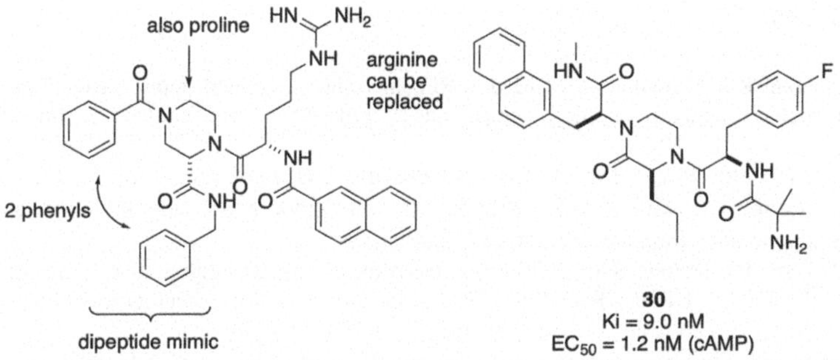

30
Ki = 9.0 nM
EC_{50} = 1.2 nM (cAMP)

Fig. 15 2-Oxopiperazine SAR

3.7 2-Oxopiperazines

In 2005, Procter & Gamble began to report a series of proline- and piperazine-based MC4R ligands based on a piperazine-2-carboxamide scaffold (Fig. 15) designed to capture key recognition elements from the melanocortin peptides. They observed that aromatic side chains at the 2,4-positions of a carboxypiperazine linked to an arginine were common to compounds with binding affinities to MC4Rs. While the binding affinities were weak ($Ki = 376$ nM), they began to probe the scaffold to develop selective MC4R agonists (Tian et al. 2005, 2006a). They found the carboxypiperazine core could be replaced with a proline, but while activity was good in the low nanomolar range at MC4R, the compounds lacked selectivity. Eventually, Procter & Gamble developed the oxopiperazines, culminating in the discovery of compounds such as **30** (Fig. 15), with an EC_{50} of 1.2 nM and a *Ki* of 9.0 nM (Tian et al. 2006b, 2008). Oxopiperazine **30** was orally bioavailable in dog (20.6%) and showed activity in a diet-induced obesity rat model at 30 mg/kg.

In summary, literature evidence shows that MC4R plays a role in modulating drug-maintained behaviors, as well as comorbid conditions including depression and anxiety. MC4R antagonists have shown efficacy in preclinical studies targeting nicotine, cocaine, amphetamine, and opioid use, but this work is limited in scope and needs to be significantly expanded. The role of MC4R in early-onset obesity made it an attractive biological target for the pharmaceutical industry resulting in a significant amount of medicinal chemistry and drug development, including the development of clinical candidates. On-target side effects have limited enthusiasm for the therapeutic development, but it may be possible to remove unwanted side effects through the development of biased ligands or allosteric modulators. The MC4R system is still an emerging target in the drug abuse field, and further assessment of existing compounds in assays targeting drug-seeking behaviors will help drive the validation of MC4R as a biological target for SUD.

References

Alserda E, Adan RA, Ramakers GM (2013) Repeated agouti related peptide (83-132) injections inhibit cocaine-induced locomotor sensitisation, but not via the nucleus accumbens. Eur J Pharmacol 719:187–191

Alvaro JD, Tatro JB, Quillan JM, Fogliano M, Eisenhard M, Lerner MR, Nestler EJ, Duman RS (1996) Morphine down-regulates melanocortin-4 receptor expression in brain regions that mediate opiate addiction. Mol Pharmacol 50:583–591

Alvaro JD, Tatro JB, Duman RS (1997) Melanocortins and opiate addiction. Life Sci 61:1–9

Alvaro JD, Taylor JR, Duman RS (2003) Molecular and behavioral interactions between central melanocortins and cocaine. J Pharmacol Exp Ther 304:391–399

Arasasingham PN, Fotsch C, Ouyang X, Norman MH, Kelly MG, Stark KL, Karbon B, Hale C, Baumgartner JW, Zambrano M, Cheetham J, Tamayo NA (2003) Structure-activity relationship of (1-aryl-2-piperazinylethyl)piperazines: antagonists for the AGRP/melanocortin receptor binding. J Med Chem 46:9–11

Badia-Elder NE, Henderson AN, Bertholomey ML, Dodge NC, Stewart RB (2008) The effects of neuropeptide S on ethanol drinking and other related behaviors in alcohol-preferring and -nonpreferring rats. Alcohol Clin Exp Res 32:1380–1387

Batran RZ, Dawood DH, El-Seginy SA, Maher TJ, Gugnani KS, Rondon-Ortiz AN (2017) Coumarinyl pyranopyrimidines as new neuropeptide S receptor antagonists; design, synthesis, homology and molecular docking. Bioorg Chem 75:274–290

Beard E, Shahab L, Cummings DM, Michie S, West R (2016) New pharmacological agents to aid smoking cessation and tobacco harm reduction: what has been investigated, and what is in the pipeline? CNS Drugs 30:951–983

Beck B, Fernette B, Stricker-Krongrad A (2005) Peptide S is a novel potent inhibitor of voluntary and fast-induced food intake in rats. Biochem Biophys Res Commun 332:859–865

Bonano JS, Runyon SP, Hassler C, Glennon RA, Stevens Negus S (2014) Effects of the neuropeptide S receptor antagonist RTI-118 on abuse-related facilitation of intracranial self-stimulation produced by cocaine and methylenedioxypyrovalerone (MDPV) in rats. Eur J Pharmacol 743:98–105

Buch TR, Heling D, Damm E, Gudermann T, Breit A (2009) Pertussis toxin-sensitive signaling of melanocortin-4 receptors in hypothalamic GT1-7 cells defines agouti-related protein as a biased agonist. J Biol Chem 284:26411–26420

Cabeza de Vaca S, Kim GY, Carr KD (2002) The melanocortin receptor agonist MTII augments the rewarding effect of amphetamine in ad-libitum-fed and food-restricted rats. Psychopharmacology 161:77–85

Camarda V, Trapella C, Calo G, Guerrini R, Rizzi A, Ruzza C, Fiorini S, Marzola E, Reinscheid RK, Regoli D, Salvadori S (2008) Synthesis and biological activity of human neuropeptide S analogues modified in position 2. J Med Chem 51:655–658

Camarda V, Ruzza C, Rizzi A, Trapella C, Guerrini R, Reinscheid RK, Calo G (2013) In vitro and in vivo pharmacological characterization of the novel neuropeptide S receptor ligands QA1 and PI1. Peptides 48:27–35

Cannella N, Economidou D, Kallupi M, Stopponi S, Heilig M, Massi M, Ciccocioppo R (2009) Persistent increase of alcohol-seeking evoked by neuropeptide S: an effect mediated by the hypothalamic hypocretin system. Neuropsychopharmacology 34:2125–2134

Cao J, de Lecea L, Ikemoto S (2011) Intraventricular administration of neuropeptide S has reward-like effects. Eur J Pharmacol 658:16–21

Caruso V, Lagerstrom MC, Olszewski PK, Fredriksson R, Schioth HB (2014) Synaptic changes induced by melanocortin signalling. Nat Rev Neurosci 15:98–110

Chaki S, Okuyama S (2005) Involvement of melanocortin-4 receptor in anxiety and depression. Peptides 26:1952–1964

Chaki S, Oshida Y, Ogawa S, Funakoshi T, Shimazaki T, Okubo T, Nakazato A, Okuyama S (2005) MCL0042: a nonpeptidic MC4 receptor antagonist and serotonin reuptake inhibitor with anxiolytic- and antidepressant-like activity. Pharmacol Biochem Behav 82:621–626

Chen C, Pontillo J, Fleck BA, Gao Y, Wen J, Tran JA, Tucci FC, Marinkovic D, Foster AC, Saunders J (2004) 4-{(2R)-[3-Aminopropionylamido]-3-(2,4-dichlorophenyl)propionyl}-1-{2-[(2-thienyl)ethylaminomethyl]phenyl}piperazine as a potent and selective melanocortin-4 receptor antagonist--design, synthesis, and characterization. J Med Chem 47:6821–6830

Chen CW, Tran JA, Jiang W, Tucci FC, Arellano M, Wen J, Fleck BA, Marinkovic D, White NS, Pontillo J, Saunders J, Madan A, Foster AC, Chen C (2006) Propionylpiperazines as human melanocortin-4 receptor ligands. Bioorg Med Chem Lett 16:4800–4803

Chen C, Jiang W, Tucci F, Tran JA, Fleck BA, Hoare SR, Joppa M, Markison S, Wen J, Sai Y, Johns M, Madan A, Chen T, Chen CW, Marinkovic D, Arellano M, Saunders J, Foster AC (2007a) Discovery of 1-[2-[(1S)-(3-dimethylaminopropionyl)amino-2-methylpropyl]-4-methylphenyl]-4-[(2R)-methyl-3-(4-chlorophenyl)-propionyl]piperazine as an orally active antagonist of the melanocortin-4 receptor for the potential treatment of cachexia. J Med Chem 50:5249–5252

Chen CW, Tran JA, Fleck BA, Tucci FC, Jiang W, Chen C (2007b) Synthesis and characterization of trans-4-(4-chlorophenyl)pyrrolidine-3-carboxamides of piperazinecyclohexanes as ligands for the melanocortin-4 receptor. Bioorg Med Chem Lett 17:6825–6831

Chen C, Jiang W, Tran JA, Tucci FC, Fleck BA, Markison S, Wen J, Madan A, Hoare SR, Foster AC, Marinkovic D, Chen CW, Arellano M, Saunders J (2008) Identification and characterization of pyrrolidine diastereoisomers as potent functional agonists and antagonists of the human melanocortin-4 receptor. Bioorg Med Chem Lett 18:129–136

Cifani C, Micioni Di Bonaventura MV, Cannella N, Fedeli A, Guerrini R, Calo G, Ciccocioppo R, Ubaldi M (2011) Effect of neuropeptide S receptor antagonists and partial agonists on palatable food consumption in the rat. Peptides 32:44–50

Clark SD, Duangdao DM, Schulz S, Zhang L, Liu X, Xu YL, Reinscheid RK (2011) Anatomical characterization of the neuropeptide S system in the mouse brain by in situ hybridization and immunohistochemistry. J Comp Neurol 519:1867–1893

Clark SD, Kenakin TP, Gertz S, Hassler C, Gay EA, Langston TL, Reinscheid RK, Runyon SP (2017) Identification of the first biased NPS receptor agonist that retains anxiolytic and memory promoting effects with reduced levels of locomotor stimulation. Neuropharmacology 118:69–78

Cui H, Lutter M (2013) The expression of MC4Rs in D1R neurons regulates food intake and locomotor sensitization to cocaine. Genes Brain Behav 12:658–665

Dal Ben D, Antonini I, Buccioni M, Lambertucci C, Marucci G, Vittori S, Volpini R, Cristalli G (2010) Molecular modeling studies on the human neuropeptide S receptor and its antagonists. ChemMedChem 5:371–383

Dyck B, Parker J, Phillips T, Carter L, Murphy B, Summers R, Hermann J, Baker T, Cismowski M, Saunders J, Goodfellow V (2003) Aryl piperazine melanocortin MC4 receptor agonists. Bioorg Med Chem Lett 13:3793–3796

Emmerson PJ, Fisher MJ, Yan LZ, Mayer JP (2007) Melanocortin-4 receptor agonists for the treatment of obesity. Curr Top Med Chem 7:1121–1130

Ercil NE, Galici R, Kesterson RA (2005) HS014, a selective melanocortin-4 (MC4) receptor antagonist, modulates the behavioral effects of morphine in mice. Psychopharmacology 180:279–285

Fretz H, Gatfield J, Isler M, Kimmerlin T, Koberstein R, Lyothier I, Monnier L, Pothier J, Valdenaire A (2013) In: Organization WIP (ed) Indanone and indandione derivatives and heterocyclic analogs. Actelion Pharmaceuticals, Allschwil

Fukatsu K, Nakayama Y, Tarui N, Mori M, Matsumoto H, Kurasawa O, Banno H (2005) In: Application WP (ed) Bicyclic piperazine compound and use thereof. Takeda Pharmaceutical Company, Tokyo

Gantz I, Fong TM (2003) The melanocortin system. Am J Physiol Endocrinol Metab 284:E468–E474

Giuliani D, Galantucci M, Neri L, Canalini F, Calevro A, Bitto A, Ottani A, Vandini E, Sena P, Sandrini M, Squadrito F, Zaffe D, Guarini S (2014) Melanocortins protect against brain damage and counteract cognitive decline in a transgenic mouse model of moderate Alzheimers disease. Eur J Pharmacol 740:144–150

Giuliani D, Ottani A, Neri L, Zaffe D, Grieco P, Jochem J, Cavallini GM, Catania A, Guarini S (2017) Multiple beneficial effects of melanocortin MC4 receptor agonists in experimental neurodegenerative disorders: therapeutic perspectives. Prog Neurobiol 148:40–56

Guerrini R, Camarda V, Trapella C, Calo G, Rizzi A, Ruzza C, Fiorini S, Marzola E, Reinscheid RK, Regoli D, Salvadori S (2009) Synthesis and biological activity of human neuropeptide S analogues modified in position 5: identification of potent and pure neuropeptide S receptor antagonists. J Med Chem 52:524–529

Guerrini R, Salvadori S, Rizzi A, Regoli D, Calo G (2010) Neurobiology, pharmacology, and medicinal chemistry of neuropeptide S and its receptor. Med Res Rev 30:751–777

Guo L, Ye Z, Ujjainwalla F, Sings HL, Sebhat IK, Huber J, Weinberg DH, Tang R, MacNeil T, Tamvakopoulos C, Peng Q, MacIntyre E, van der Ploeg LH, Goulet MT, Wyvratt MJ, Nargund RP (2008) Synthesis and SAR of potent and orally bioavailable tert-butylpyrrolidine archetype derived melanocortin subtype-4 receptor modulators. Bioorg Med Chem Lett 18:3242–3247

Guo L, Ye Z, Liu J, He S, Bakshi RK, Sebhat IK, Dobbelaar PH, Hong Q, Jian T, Dellureficio JP, Tsou NN, Ball RG, Weinberg DH, MacNeil T, Tang R, Tamvakopoulos C, Peng Q, Chen HY, Chen AS, Martin WJ, MacIntyre DE, Strack AM, Fong TM, Wyvratt MJ, Nargund RP (2010) Discovery of potent, selective, and orally bioavailable 3H-spiro[isobenzofuran-1,4′-piperidine] based melanocortin subtype-4 receptor agonists. Bioorg Med Chem Lett 20:4895–4900

Hassler C, Zhang Y, Gilmour B, Graf T, Fennell T, Snyder R, Deschamps JR, Reinscheid RK, Garau C, Runyon SP (2014) Identification of neuropeptide S antagonists: structure-activity relationship studies, X-ray crystallography, and in vivo evaluation. ACS Chem Neurosci 5:731–744

He S, Ye Z, Dobbelaar PH, Bakshi RK, Hong Q, Dellureficio JP, Sebhat IK, Guo L, Liu J, Jian T, Lai Y, Franklin CL, Reibarkh M, Holmes MA, Weinberg DH, MacNeil T, Tang R, Tamvakopoulos C, Peng Q, Miller RR, Stearns RA, Chen HY, Chen AS, Strack AM, Fong TM, Wyvratt MJ Jr, Nargund RP (2010a) Discovery of highly potent and efficacious MC4R agonists with spiroindane N-Me-1,2,4-triazole privileged structures for the treatment of obesity. Bioorg Med Chem Lett 20:6524–6532

He S, Ye Z, Dobbelaar PH, Sebhat IK, Guo L, Liu J, Jian T, Lai Y, Franklin CL, Bakshi RK, Dellureficio JP, Hong Q, Tsou NN, Ball RG, Cashen DE, Martin WJ, Weinberg DH, Macneil T, Tang R, Tamvakopoulos C, Peng Q, Miller RR, Stearns RA, Chen HY, Chen AS, Strack AM, Fong TM, Macintyre DE, Wyvratt MJ Jr, Nargund RP (2010b) Discovery of a spiroindane based compound as a potent, selective, orally bioavailable melanocortin subtype-4 receptor agonist. Bioorg Med Chem Lett 20:2106–2110

He S, Ye Z, Dobbelaar PH, Sebhat IK, Guo L, Liu J, Jian T, Lai Y, Franklin CL, Bakshi RK, Dellureficio JP, Hong Q, Weinberg DH, Macneil T, Tang R, Strack AM, Tamvakopoulos C, Peng Q, Miller RR, Stearns RA, Chen HY, Chen AS, Fong TM, Wyvratt MJ Jr, Nargund RP (2010c) Spiroindane based amides as potent and selective MC4R agonists for the treatment of obesity. Bioorg Med Chem Lett 20:4399–4405

Hong Q, Bakshi RK, Dellureficio J, He S, Ye Z, Dobbelaar PH, Sebhat IK, Guo L, Liu J, Jian T, Tang R, Kalyani RN, Macneil T, Vongs A, Rosenblum CI, Weinberg DH, Peng Q, Tamvakopoulos C, Miller RR, Stearns RA, Cashen D, Martin WJ, Chen AS, Metzger JM, Chen HY, Strack AM, Fong TM, MacIntyre E, van der Ploeg LH, Wyvratt MJ, Nargund RP (2010) Optimization of privileged structures for selective and potent melanocortin subtype-4 receptor ligands. Bioorg Med Chem Lett 20:4483–4486

Hsu R, Taylor JR, Newton SS, Alvaro JD, Haile C, Han G, Hruby VJ, Nestler EJ, Duman RS (2005) Blockade of melanocortin transmission inhibits cocaine reward. Eur J Neurosci 21:2233–2242

Jiang W, Tucci FC, Chen CW, Arellano M, Tran JA, White NS, Marinkovic D, Pontillo J, Fleck BA, Wen J, Saunders J, Madan A, Foster AC, Chen C (2006) Arylpropionylpiperazines as antagonists of the human melanocortin-4 receptor. Bioorg Med Chem Lett 16:4674–4678

Kalange AS, Kokare DM, Singru PS, Upadhya MA, Chopde CT, Subhedar NK (2007) Central administration of selective melanocortin 4 receptor antagonist HS014 prevents morphine tolerance and withdrawal hyperalgesia. Brain Res 1181:10–20

Kallupi M, Cannella N, Economidou D, Ubaldi M, Ruggeri B, Weiss F, Massi M, Marugan J, Heilig M, Bonnavion P, de Lecea L, Ciccocioppo R (2010) Neuropeptide S facilitates cue-induced relapse to cocaine seeking through activation of the hypothalamic hypocretin system. Proc Natl Acad Sci U S A 107:19567–19572

Krashes MJ, Lowell BB, Garfield AS (2016) Melanocortin-4 receptor-regulated energy homeostasis. Nat Neurosci 19:206–219

Lage R, Dieguez C, Lopez M (2006) Caffeine treatment regulates neuropeptide S system expression in the rat brain. Neurosci Lett 410:47–51

Lage R, Gonzalez CR, Dieguez C, Lopez M (2007) Nicotine treatment regulates neuropeptide S system expression in the rat brain. Neurotoxicology 28:1129–1135

Lansdell MI, Hepworth D, Calabrese A, Brown AD, Blagg J, Burring DJ, Wilson P, Fradet D, Brown TB, Quinton F, Mistry N, Tang K, Mount N, Stacey P, Edmunds N, Adams C, Gaboardi S, Neal-Morgan S, Wayman C, Cole S, Phipps J, Lewis M, Verrier H, Gillon V, Feeder N, Heatherington A, Sultana S, Haughie S, Martin SW, Sudworth M, Tweedy S (2010) Discovery of a selective small-molecule melanocortin-4 receptor agonist with efficacy in a pilot study of sexual dysfunction in humans. J Med Chem 53:3183–3197

Lasaga M, Debeljuk L, Durand D, Scimonelli TN, Caruso C (2008) Role of alpha-melanocyte stimulating hormone and melanocortin 4 receptor in brain inflammation. Peptides 29:1825–1835

Leonard SK, Ring RH (2011) Immunohistochemical localization of the neuropeptide S receptor in the rat central nervous system. Neuroscience 172:153–163

Leonard SK, Dwyer JM, Sukoff Rizzo SJ, Platt B, Logue SF, Neal SJ, Malberg JE, Beyer CE, Schechter LE, Rosenzweig-Lipson S, Ring RH (2008) Pharmacology of neuropeptide S in mice: therapeutic relevance to anxiety disorders. Psychopharmacology 197:601–611

Li W, Gao YH, Chang M, Peng YL, Yao J, Han RW, Wang R (2009) Neuropeptide S inhibits the acquisition and the expression of conditioned place preference to morphine in mice. Peptides 30:234–240

Lindblom J, Kask A, Hagg E, Harmark L, Bergstrom L, Wikberg J (2002) Chronic infusion of a melanocortin receptor agonist modulates dopamine receptor binding in the rat brain. Pharmacol Res 45:119–124

Liu X, Zeng J, Zhou A, Theodorsson E, Fahrenkrug J, Reinscheid RK (2011) Molecular fingerprint of neuropeptide S-producing neurons in the mouse brain. J Comp Neurol 519:1847–1866

Marsilje TH, Roses JB, Calderwood EF, Stroud SG, Forsyth NE, Blackburn C, Yowe DL, Miao W, Drabic SV, Bohane MD, Daniels JS, Li P, Wu L, Patane MA, Claiborne CF (2004) Synthesis and biological evaluation of imidazole-based small molecule antagonists of the melanocortin 4 receptor (MC4-R). Bioorg Med Chem Lett 14:3721–3725

Marugan JJ, Patnaik S, Heilig MA, Southall NT, Zheng W (2011) In: Organization WIP (ed) United States Department of Health and Human Services. Small molecule neuropeptide S antagonists for the treatment of addictive disorders, mood, anxiety and sleep disorders. National Institutes of Health

McCoy JG, Marugan JJ, Liu K, Zheng W, Southall N, Huang W, Heilig M, Austin CP (2010) Selective modulation of Gq/Gs pathways by Naphtho Pyrano pyrimidines as antagonists of the neuropeptide S receptor. ACS Chem Neurosci 1:559–574

Melamed JY, Zartman AE, Kett NR, Gotter AL, Uebele VN, Reiss DR, Condra CL, Fandozzi C, Lubbers LS, Rowe BA, McGaughey GB, Henault M, Stocco R, Renger JJ, Hartman GD, Bilodeau MT, Trotter BW (2010) Synthesis and evaluation of a new series of neuropeptide S receptor antagonists. Bioorg Med Chem Lett 20:4700–4703

Micheli F, Di Fabio R, Giacometti A, Roth A, Moro E, Merlo G, Paio A, Merlo-Pich E, Tomelleri S, Tonelli F, Zarantonello P, Zonzini L, Capelli AM (2010) Synthesis and pharmacological characterization of 5-phenyl-2-[2-(1-piperidinylcarbonyl)phenyl]-2,3-dihydro-1H-pyrrolo[1,2-c]imidazol-1-ones: a new class of neuropeptide S antagonists. Bioorg Med Chem Lett 20:7308–7311

Mochizuki T, Kim J, Sasaki K (2010) Microinjection of neuropeptide S into the rat ventral tegmental area induces hyperactivity and increases extracellular levels of dopamine metabolites in the nucleus accumbens shell. Peptides 31:926–931

Nargund RP, Patchett AA, Bach MA, Murphy MG, Smith RG (1998) Peptidomimetic growth hormone secretagogues. Design considerations and therapeutic potential. J Med Chem 41:3103–3127

Navarro M (2017) The role of the Melanocortin system in drug and alcohol abuse. Int Rev Neurobiol 136:121–150

Nepomuceno D, Sutton S, Yu J, Zhu J, Liu C, Lovenberg T, Bonaventure P (2010) Mutagenesis studies of neuropeptide S identify a suitable peptide tracer for neuropeptide S receptor binding studies and peptides selectively activating the I(107) variant of human neuropeptide S receptor. Eur J Pharmacol 635:27–33

Newman EA, Chai BX, Zhang W, Li JY, Ammori JB, Mulholland MW (2006) Activation of the melanocortin-4 receptor mobilizes intracellular free calcium in immortalized hypothalamic neurons. J Surg Res 132:201–207

Nozawa D, Okubo T, Ishii T, Chaki S, Okuyama S, Nakazato A (2007a) Synthesis of diphenylmethyl analogues and their affinity for the melanocortin-4 receptor and the serotonin transporter. Chem Pharm Bull (Tokyo) 55:1044–1050

Nozawa D, Okubo T, Ishii T, Kakinuma H, Chaki S, Okuyama S, Nakazato A (2007b) Structure-activity relationships of novel piperazines as antagonists for the melanocortin-4 receptor. Bioorg Med Chem 15:1989–2005

Nozawa D, Okubo T, Ishii T, Takamori K, Chaki S, Okuyama S, Nakazato A (2007c) Novel piperazines: potent melanocortin-4 receptor antagonists with anxiolytic-like activity. Bioorg Med Chem 15:2375–2385

Okamura N, Habay SA, Zeng J, Chamberlin AR, Reinscheid RK (2008) Synthesis and pharmacological in vitro and in vivo profile of 3-oxo-1,1-diphenyl-tetrahydro-oxazolo[3,4-a]pyrazine-7-carboxylic acid 4-fluoro-benzylamide (SHA 68), a selective antagonist of the neuropeptide S receptor. J Pharmacol Exp Ther 325:893–901

Paneda C, Huitron-Resendiz S, Frago LM, Chowen JA, Picetti R, de Lecea L, Roberts AJ (2009) Neuropeptide S reinstates cocaine-seeking behavior and increases locomotor activity through corticotropin-releasing factor receptor 1 in mice. J Neurosci 29:4155–4161

Patnaik S, Marugan JJ, Liu K, Zheng W, Southall N, Dehdashti SJ, Thorsell A, Heilig M, Bell L, Zook M, Eskay B, Brimacombe KR, Austin CP (2013) Structure-activity relationship of imidazopyridinium analogues as antagonists of neuropeptide s receptor. J Med Chem 56:9045–9056

Peng YL, Han RW, Chang M, Zhang L, Zhang RS, Li W, Han YF, Wang R (2010) Central neuropeptide S inhibits food intake in mice through activation of neuropeptide S receptor. Peptides 31:2259–2263

Pontillo J, Tran JA, Arellano M, Fleck BA, Huntley R, Marinkovic D, Lanier M, Nelson J, Parker J, Saunders J, Tucci FC, Jiang W, Chen CW, White NS, Foster AC, Chen C (2004) Structure-activity relationships of piperazinebenzylamines as potent and selective agonists of the human melanocortin-4 receptor. Bioorg Med Chem Lett 14:4417–4423

Pontillo J, Marinkovic D, Tran JA, Arellano M, Fleck BA, Wen J, Tucci FC, Nelson J, Saunders J, Foster AC, Chen C (2005) Optimization of piperazinebenzylamines with a N-(1-methoxy-2-propyl) side chain as potent and selective antagonists of the human melanocortin-4 receptor. Bioorg Med Chem Lett 15:4615–4618

Qi X, Yamada H, Corrie LW, Ji Y, Bauzo RM, Alexander JC, Bruijnzeel AW (2015) A critical role for the melanocortin 4 receptor in stress-induced relapse to nicotine seeking in rats. Addict Biol 20:324–335

Reinscheid RK, Xu YL, Okamura N, Zeng J, Chung S, Pai R, Wang Z, Civelli O (2005) Pharmacological characterization of human and murine neuropeptide s receptor variants. J Pharmacol Exp Ther 315:1338–1345

Rizzi A, Vergura R, Marzola G, Ruzza C, Guerrini R, Salvadori S, Regoli D, Calo G (2008) Neuropeptide S is a stimulatory anxiolytic agent: a behavioural study in mice. Br J Pharmacol 154:471–479

Rodrigues AR, Almeida H, Gouveia AM (2015) Intracellular signaling mechanisms of the melanocortin receptors: current state of the art. Cell Mol Life Sci 72:1331–1345

Ruggeri B, Braconi S, Cannella N, Kallupi M, Soverchia L, Ciccocioppo R, Ubaldi M (2010) Neuropeptide S receptor gene expression in alcohol withdrawal and protracted abstinence in postdependent rats. Alcohol Clin Exp Res 34:90–97

Runyon SP, Zhang Y, Hassler C, Gilmour B (2013) Composition and method for neuropeptide S receptor (NPSR) antagonists. Research Triangle Institute, Research Triangle Park

Sato S, Shintani Y, Miyajima N, Yoshimura K (2002) In: Application WP (ed) Novel G protein-coupled receptor protein and DNA thereof. Takeda Pharmaceutical Company Limited, Osaka

Schmoutz CD, Zhang Y, Runyon SP, Goeders NE (2012) Antagonism of the neuropeptide S receptor with RTI-118 decreases cocaine self-administration and cocaine-seeking behavior in rats. Pharmacol Biochem Behav 103:332–337

Sebhat IK, Martin WJ, Ye Z, Barakat K, Mosley RT, Johnston DB, Bakshi R, Palucki B, Weinberg DH, MacNeil T, Kalyani RN, Tang R, Stearns RA, Miller RR, Tamvakopoulos C, Strack AM, McGowan E, Cashen DE, Drisko JE, Hom GJ, Howard AD, MacIntyre DE, van der Ploeg LH, Patchett AA, Nargund RP (2002) Design and pharmacology of N-[(3R)-1,2,3,4-tetrahydroisoquinolinium-3-ylcarbonyl]-(1R)-1-(4-chlorobenzyl)-2-[4-cyclohexyl-4-(1H-1,2,4-triazol-1-ylmethyl)piperidin-1-yl]-2-oxoethylamine (1), a potent, selective, melanocortin subtype-4 receptor agonist. J Med Chem 45:4589–4593

Shimazaki T, Chaki S (2005) Anxiolytic-like effect of a selective and non-peptidergic melanocortin 4 receptor antagonist, MCL0129, in a social interaction test. Pharmacol Biochem Behav 80:395–400

Si W, Aluisio L, Okamura N, Clark SD, Fraser I, Sutton SW, Bonaventure P, Reinscheid RK (2010) Neuropeptide S stimulates dopaminergic neurotransmission in the medial prefrontal cortex. J Neurochem 115:475–482

Smith KL, Patterson M, Dhillo WS, Patel SR, Semjonous NM, Gardiner JV, Ghatei MA, Bloom SR (2006) Neuropeptide S stimulates the hypothalamo-pituitary-adrenal axis and inhibits food intake. Endocrinology 147:3510–3518

Starowicz K, Obara I, Przewlocki R, Przewlocka B (2005) Inhibition of morphine tolerance by spinal melanocortin receptor blockade. Pain 117:401–411

Tancredi T, Guerrini R, Marzola E, Trapella C, Calo G, Regoli D, Reinscheid RK, Camarda V, Salvadori S, Temussi PA (2007) Conformation-activity relationship of neuropeptide S and some structural mutants: helicity affects their interaction with the receptor. J Med Chem 50:4501–4508

Tao YX (2010) The melanocortin-4 receptor: physiology, pharmacology, and pathophysiology. Endocr Rev 31:506–543

Tian X, Field T, Mazur AW, Ebetino FH, Wos JA, Crossdoersen D, Pinney BB, Sheldon RJ (2005) Design, synthesis, and evaluation of proline based melanocortin receptor ligands. Bioorg Med Chem Lett 15:2819–2823

Tian X, Field TB, Switzer AG, Mazur AW, Ebetino FH, Wos JA, Berberich SM, Jayasinghe LR, Obringer CM, Dowty ME, Pinney BB, Farmer JA, Crossdoersen D, Sheldon RJ (2006a) Design, synthesis, and evaluation of proline and pyrrolidine based melanocortin receptor agonists. A conformationally restricted dipeptide mimic approach. J Med Chem 49:4745–4761

Tian X, Mishra RK, Switzer AG, Hu XE, Kim N, Mazur AW, Ebetino FH, Wos JA, Crossdoersen D, Pinney BB, Farmer JA, Sheldon RJ (2006b) Design and synthesis of potent and selective 1,3,4-trisubstituted-2-oxopiperazine based melanocortin-4 receptor agonists. Bioorg Med Chem Lett 16:4668–4673

Tian X, Switzer AG, Derose SA, Mishra RK, Solinsky MG, Mumin RN, Ebetino FH, Jayasinghe LR, Webster ME, Colson AO, Crossdoersen D, Pinney BB, Farmer JA, Dowty ME, Obringer CM, Cruze CA, Burklow ML, Suchanek PM, Dong L, Dirr MK, Sheldon RJ, Wos JA (2008) Discovery of orally bioavailable 1,3,4-trisubstituted 2-oxopiperazine-based melanocortin-4 receptor agonists as potential antiobesity agents. J Med Chem 51:6055–6066

Tran JA, Pontillo J, Fleck BA, Marinkovic D, Arellano M, Tucci FC, Lanier M, Saunders J, Jiang W, Chen CW, Foster AC, Chen C (2006) Design, synthesis, and SAR studies on a series of 2-pyridinylpiperazines as potent antagonists of the melanocortin-4 receptor. Bioorg Med Chem Lett 16:3693–3696

Tran JA, Jiang W, Tucci FC, Fleck BA, Wen J, Sai Y, Madan A, Chen TK, Markison S, Foster AC, Hoare SR, Marks D, Harman J, Chen CW, Arellano M, Marinkovic D, Bozigian H, Saunders J, Chen C (2007a) Design, synthesis, in vitro, and in vivo characterization of phenylpiperazines and pyridinylpiperazines as potent and selective antagonists of the melanocortin-4 receptor. J Med Chem 50:6356–6366

Tran JA, Tucci FC, Jiang W, Marinkovic D, Chen CW, Arellano M, Markison S, Fleck BA, Wen J, White NS, Pontillo J, Saunders J, Marks D, Hoare SR, Madan A, Foster AC, Chen C (2007b) Pyrrolidinones as orally bioavailable antagonists of the human melanocortin-4 receptor with anti-cachectic activity. Bioorg Med Chem 15:5166–5176

Trapella C, Pela M, Del Zoppo L, Calo G, Camarda V, Ruzza C, Cavazzini A, Costa V, Bertolasi V, Reinscheid RK, Salvadori S, Guerrini R (2011) Synthesis and separation of the enantiomers of the neuropeptide S receptor antagonist (9R/S)-3-oxo-1,1-diphenyl-tetrahydro-oxazolo[3,4-a] pyrazine-7-carboxylic acid 4-fluoro-benzylamide (SHA 68). J Med Chem 54:2738–2744

Trotter BW, Nanda KK, Manley PJ, Uebele VN, Condra CL, Gotter AL, Menzel K, Henault M, Stocco R, Renger JJ, Hartman GD, Bilodeau MT (2010) Tricyclic imidazole antagonists of the neuropeptide S receptor. Bioorg Med Chem Lett 20:4704–4708

Tucci FC, White NS, Markison S, Joppa M, Tran JA, Fleck BA, Madan A, Dyck BP, Parker J, Pontillo J, Arellano LM, Marinkovic D, Jiang W, Chen CW, Gogas KR, Goodfellow VS, Saunders J, Foster AC, Chen C (2005) Potent and orally active non-peptide antagonists of the human melanocortin-4 receptor based on a series of trans-2-disubstituted cyclohexyl-piperazines. Bioorg Med Chem Lett 15:4389–4395

Ujjainwalla F, Warner D, Walsh TF, Wyvratt MJ, Zhou C, Yang L, Kalyani RN, MacNeil T, van der Ploeg LH, Rosenblum CI, Tang R, Vongs A, Weinberg DH, Goulet MT (2003) Design and syntheses of melanocortin subtype-4 receptor agonists: evolution of the pyridazinone archetype. Bioorg Med Chem Lett 13:4431–4435

Ujjainwalla F, Warner D, Snedden C, Grisson RD, Walsh TF, Wyvratt MJ, Kalyani RN, Macneil T, Tang R, Weinberg DH, Van der Ploeg L, Goulet MT (2005) Design and syntheses of melanocortin subtype-4 receptor agonists. Part 2: discovery of the dihydropyridazinone motif. Bioorg Med Chem Lett 15:4023–4028

Vos TJ, Caracoti A, Che JL, Dai M, Farrer CA, Forsyth NE, Drabic SV, Horlick RA, Lamppu D, Yowe DL, Balani S, Li P, Zeng H, Joseph IB, Rodriguez LE, Maguire MP, Patane MA, Claiborne CF (2004) Identification of 2-[2-[2-(5-bromo-2- methoxyphenyl)-ethyl]-3-fluorophenyl]-4,5-dihydro-1H-imidazole (ML00253764), a small molecule melanocortin 4 receptor antagonist that effectively reduces tumor-induced weight loss in a mouse model. J Med Chem 47:1602–1604

Vos TJ, Balani S, Blackburn C, Chau RW, Danca MD, Drabic SV, Farrer CA, Patane MA, Stroud SG, Yowe DL, Claiborne CF (2006) Identification and structure-activity relationships of a new series of Melanocortin-4 receptor antagonists. Bioorg Med Chem Lett 16:2302–2305

Wise RA (2013) Dual roles of dopamine in food and drug seeking: the drive-reward paradox. Biol Psychiatry 73:819–826

Xu YL, Reinscheid RK, Huitron-Resendiz S, Clark SD, Wang Z, Lin SH, Brucher FA, Zeng J, Ly NK, Henriksen SJ, de Lecea L, Civelli O (2004) Neuropeptide S: a neuropeptide promoting arousal and anxiolytic-like effects. Neuron 43:487–497

Xu YL, Gall CM, Jackson VR, Civelli O, Reinscheid RK (2007) Distribution of neuropeptide S receptor mRNA and neurochemical characteristics of neuropeptide S-expressing neurons in the rat brain. J Comp Neurol 500:84–102

Yeo GS, Farooqi IS, Aminian S, Halsall DJ, Stanhope RG, O'Rahilly S (1998) A frameshift mutation in MC4R associated with dominantly inherited human obesity. Nat Genet 20:111–112

Yoon YR, Baik JH (2015) Melanocortin 4 receptor and dopamine D2 receptor expression in brain areas involved in food intake. Endocrinol Metab (Seoul) 30:576–583

Zhang Y, Gilmour BP, Navarro HA, Runyon SP (2008) Identifying structural features on 1,1-diphenyl-hexahydro-oxazolo[3,4-a]pyrazin-3-ones critical for neuropeptide S antagonist activity. Bioorg Med Chem Lett 18:4064–4067

Emerging Insights into Mu Opioid Pharmacology

Gavril W. Pasternak, Steven R. Childers, and Ying-Xian Pan

Contents

1 Introduction: Mu Opioids and the Opioid Epidemic 90
2 MOR Tertiary Structure 92
3 Signaling Pathways: Biased and Unbiased Agonists 94
4 Allosteric Agonists 96
5 MOR Heteromers and Bivalent Ligands 97
6 MOR Regulation by Receptor Phosphorylation 99
7 Alternative Splicing of the Mu Opioid Receptor Gene, *OPRM1* 100
7.1 Full-Length 7TM C-Terminal Variants and 3′ Splicing 102
7.2 Truncated 6TM Variants, Alternative Exon 11 Promoter, and 5′ Splicing 104
7.3 Truncated Single TM Variants and Exon Skipping and Insertion 106

This chapter is dedicated to the memory of our dear colleague and friend Dr. Gavril Pasternak (deceased February 22, 2019), whose pioneering work over four decades contributed immensely to our understanding of opioid pharmacology.

Ying-Xian Pan is a co-scientific founder of Sparian Biosciences that is an early stage pharmaceutical company whose first program is to develop a new class of analgesics, the arylepoxamides, for pain management.

Gavril W. Pasternak was a founder of Sparian Biosciences. He was also a consultant and/or speaker of Endo Pharmaceuticals, Confo Therapeutics, Nektar Therapeutics, Collegium Pharmaceuticals and Novartis.

G. W. Pasternak · Y.-X. Pan (✉)
Department of Neurology and Molecular Pharmacology Program, Memorial Sloan Kettering Cancer Center, New York, NY, USA
e-mail: pany@MSKCC.ORG

S. R. Childers (✉)
Department of Physiology/Pharmacology, Wake Forest School of Medicine, Winston-Salem, NC, USA
e-mail: childers@wakehealth.edu

M. A. Nader, Y. L. Hurd (eds.), *Substance Use Disorders*,
Handbook of Experimental Pharmacology 258, https://doi.org/10.1007/164_2019_270

8 Expression and Function of *OPRM1* Splice Variants 107
8.1 mRNA and Protein Expression 107
8.2 Functions of *OPRM1* Full-Length 7TM C-Terminal Variants 109
8.3 Functions of *OPRM1* Truncated 6TM Variants 111
9 Overall Conclusions 116
References 117

Abstract

Opioid analgesics, most of which act through mu opioid receptors, have long represented valuable therapeutic agents to treat severe pain. Concerted drug development efforts for over a 100 years have resulted in a large variety of opioid analgesics used in the clinic, but all of them continue to exhibit the side effects, especially respiratory depression, that have long plagued the use of morphine. The recent explosion in fatalities resulting from overdose of prescription and synthetic opioids has dramatically increased the need for safer analgesics, but recent developments in mu receptor research have provided new strategies to develop such drugs. This chapter reviews recent advances in developing novel opioid analgesics from an understanding of mu receptor structure and function. This includes a summary of the mechanism of agonist binding deduced from the crystal structure of mu receptors. It will also highlight the development of novel agonist mechanisms, including biased agonists, bivalent ligands, and allosteric modulators of mu receptor function, and describe how receptor phosphorylation modulates these pathways. Finally, it will summarize research on the alternative pre-mRNA splicing mechanisms that produces a multiplicity of mu receptor isoforms. Many of these isoforms exhibit different pharmacological specificities and brain circuitry localization, thus providing an opportunity to develop novel drugs with increased therapeutic windows.

Keywords

Allosteric ligands · Analgesics · Biased agonists · Bivalent ligands · Heterodimers · Splice variants

1 Introduction: Mu Opioids and the Opioid Epidemic

When multiple types of opioid receptors were first suggested (Lord et al. 1977; Martin et al. 1976), it was clear that most of the therapeutic and side effects of clinically relevant opioid analgesics were mediated by mu opioid receptors (MOR). These drugs not only included the classical morphine-like analgesics like morphine but also synthetic derivatives like methadone and fentanyl (Armenian et al. 2018). Since then, numerous genetic studies have confirmed the role of MOR in analgesic actions, with genetic knockouts of the MOR gene eliminating behavioral and analgesic effects of mu agonists (Matthes et al. 1996; Raehal and Bohn 2014). But few researchers at the time could have foreseen the unprecedented onslaught of misuse and overuse of mu opioid analgesics that created the current opioid epidemic (Baumann et al. 2018).

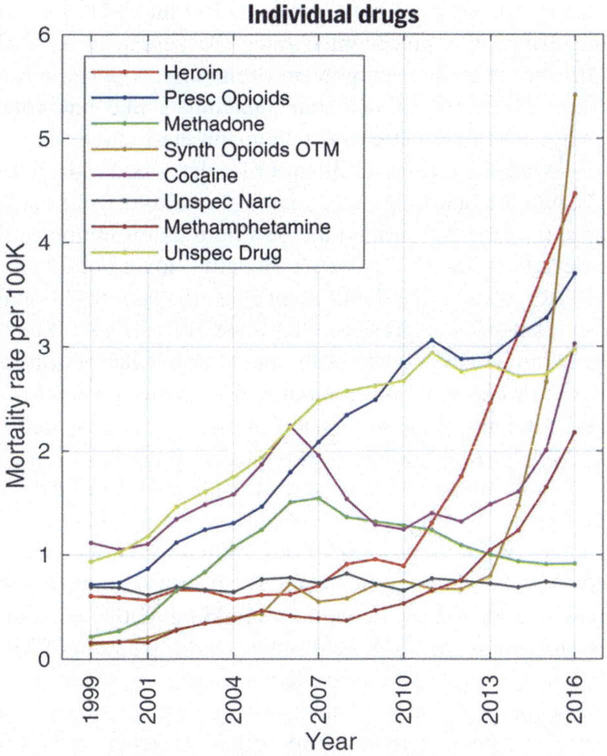

Fig. 1 Mortality rates from drugs of abuse in the USA from 1999 to 2016. Note how the precipitous rise in mortality rates from prescription opioids preceded those from heroin, which then was followed by an alarming increase in mortality rates from synthetic opioids (e.g., fentanyl). From Jalal et al. (2018)

In the USA, the death rate from opioid analgesics nearly quadrupled from 1999 to 2011 (Rudd et al. 2016). In 2016 alone, over 40,000 people in the USA died from opioid overdose (Seth et al. 2018). The course of the opioid epidemic over the past 10 years has occurred in distinct stages, documented in Fig. 1, each stage illustrating various pharmacological properties of mu opioid agonists (Jalal et al. 2018). The first stage was highlighted by overuse of prescription opioids, including codeine, oxycodone, hydrocodone, and oxymorphone. These drugs, widely used clinically for their oral availability as analgesics, as well as their lower DEA schedules compared to morphine, were abused not only by pain patients but also by diversion to the general non-patient population. When prescription opioids became more difficult to obtain, many chronic opioid users turned to heroin, ironically a cheaper option. Because of its rapid uptake into the brain and conversion into morphine, heroin has long been the drug of choice among opioid users, and the availability of cheap heroin on the street made it easy for users to switch from prescription drugs. An even more deadly phase of the epidemic occurred with the widespread availability of illicit fentanyl, whose high potency in vivo (up to 100 times more potent than morphine) makes it easy for clandestine laboratories to synthesize and ship across borders. Now, with the availability on the street of even more potent fentanyl analogs like carfentanil, novel illicit fentanyl analogs like alpha-methyl fentanyl and methyl fentanyl, and potent synthetic opioids like U-47700 and MT-45, opioid overdose fatalities are occurring at unprecedented rates (Armenian et al. 2018). Because of their high affinities at MOR, antagonism of the effects of these highly potent agonists require larger doses of classical mu antagonists like naloxone, as well as longer-acting antagonists like naltrexone (Baumann et al. 2018).

100 years ago, Sir William Osler described morphine as “God’s own medicine.” Despite the alarming progression of fatalities from the current opioid epidemic, mu opioid analgesics remain the best options for treating severe pain. The challenge of researchers has always been to identify novel opioid analgesics that retain analgesic efficacy without the debilitating side effects of traditional opioid agonists, especially the respiratory depression that leads to overdose. For the past 100 years, this has been an elusive goal, with many unfulfilled promises. For example, in 1895, diacetylmorphine (more commonly known as heroin) was introduced as a “non-addicting morphine substitute.” However, new research on the structure and function of MOR has provided novel pathways that not only help understand MOR agonist signaling but also devise new strategies for drug development that could improve treatment of pain while decreasing overdose (Valentino and Volkow 2018). In this chapter, we review some of the MOR mechanisms that have catalyzed these novel strategies, including the detailed structure of agonist binding sites on mu receptors, biased and unbiased agonist signaling pathways, allosteric activators, bivalent ligands acting at MOR heteromers, and regulation of MOR signaling by phosphorylation. The first half of the chapter focuses on the traditional MOR isoform, while in the second half of this chapter, we focus on alternative splicing of mu opioid receptor gene, *OPRM1*, and resulting splice variants or isoforms that mediate different agonist effects of mu opioid analgesics and provide more alternative strategies for drug development.

2 MOR Tertiary Structure

From the early radioligand binding studies (Blume 1978; Childers and Snyder 1980), it was clear that MOR belongs to the superfamily of G-protein-coupled receptors (GPCR) (Satoh and Minami 1995), specifically the γ subfamily of Class A (rhodopsin-like) GPCRs (Manglik et al. 2016). As in any GPCR, MOR has seven transmembrane (TM) α-helices, with an extracellular N-terminal tail and an intracellular C-terminal tail, connected with three intracellular and three extracellular loops. The first crystal structure of MOR (Manglik et al. 2012) was obtained using a lysozyme fusion protein strategy that had been successful in determining structures of other GPCRs (Rosenbaum et al. 2007). In this first report of MOR structure, data were obtained from receptor protein bound to β-FNA, a mu-selective irreversible antagonist. Because these findings were obtained from the antagonist binding conformation of the receptor, these results are often described as the inactive state of the receptor. These data revealed that mu receptors were arranged in dimers tightly associated through TM5 and TM6. The binding pocket for β-FNA was relatively wide and exposed to the extracellular environment. This structure of the

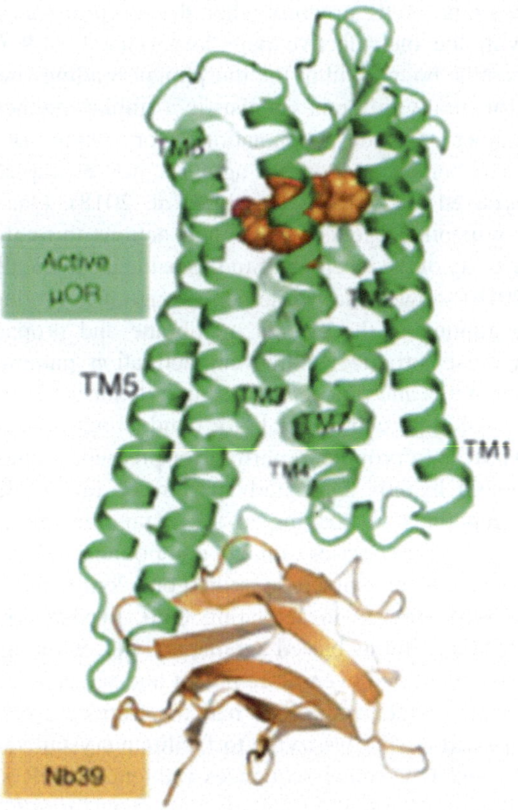

Fig. 2 Structure of the agonist binding site of the active state of MOR, showing the binding of the mu agonist BU72 along with the single-domain antibody fragment (nanobody) Nb39 that mimics Gi/o. From Huang et al. (2015)

antagonist binding site may explain why potent mu antagonists have relatively fast dissociation kinetics, a characteristic highly relevant in the treatment of opioid overdose victims with antagonists like naloxone. The problem with studies of receptor tertiary structure using antagonists like β-FNA is that GPCRs exist in different states when bound to agonists or antagonists (Nygaard et al. 2013). Therefore, data from the antagonist (or inactive) state of MOR (Manglik et al. 2012) may not accurately define MOR structure when the receptor is activated by agonists (Manglik et al. 2016). The agonist/antagonist states of MOR were first recognized by early radioligand binding experiments showing that sodium allosterically inhibited agonist, but not antagonist, binding to MOR (Pert et al. 1973). Using this information, along with single-domain antibody fragments (nanobodies) that mimic the structure of Gα subunits to stabilize the active conformation of MOR, an agonist-activated structure for MOR was reported (Fig. 2) using the potent mu agonist BU72 (Huang et al. 2015; Manglik et al. 2017). These data revealed similarities between the inactive and active forms of MOR, with subtle differences in binding pockets for agonist and antagonist. However, in both studies, the opioids used for binding were closely related to morphinan structures (i.e., closely related to the classical structure of morphine and related opioids). More recent studies (Koehl et al. 2018; Maeda et al. 2018) used high-resolution cryo-electron microscopy to examine MOR structure when the receptor was bound to the Gi heterotrimer along with the mu-selective peptide agonist DAMGO. These results showed that the peptide bound within the morphinan binding site, suggesting that MOR recognizes structurally different agonists in a similar manner. Models derived from all of these studies provide explanations for many of the observed pharmacological characteristics of opioid agonists, for example, the high potency of a series of cyclized enkephalins (Koehl et al. 2018). One novel way in which peptide and non-peptide agonists exert their actions through MOR is via different subcellular activity of the receptors. Studies using a genetically encoded biosensor (Stoeber et al. 2018) showed that while peptide agonists produce an activation pattern in neurons beginning in the plasma membrane and propagating to endosomes, non-peptide agonists produce a different activation pattern beginning in the somatic Golgi apparatus and proceeding through dendrites.

An important rationale for conducting these complex structure identifications of MOR is to provide a scaffold for predicting binding affinities for known and novel opioid ligands. One study performed an in silico analysis of over three million compounds in docking to the antagonist binding site of MOR (Manglik et al. 2016). From a series of novel compounds with significant affinity for MOR binding, specific stereoisomers identified one compound, PZM21, with high affinity and full agonist efficacy in activating Gi/o. Further studies (described below) show that PZM21 exhibits biased agonist activity, while more recent studies (Ma et al. 2019) have identified even more potent and selective analogs of PZM21.

The crystalized MOR had the truncated N- and C-termini of MOR and also inserted the T4 lysozyme to facilitate crystallization, raising the questions how the N- and C-terminal sequences influence MOR structures associated with different signaling. This is particularly important for *OPRM1* splice variants with alternative N- and C-terminal sequences (see below).

3 Signaling Pathways: Biased and Unbiased Agonists

The early discovery that mu receptor agonists inhibit adenylyl cyclase (Sharma et al. 1975), inhibit Ca^{+2} channel activity (Schroeder et al. 1991; Seward et al. 1991), and activate inwardly rectifying K^{+} channels (North and Williams 1985) firmly established that MOR intracellular signaling is mediated by Gi/o-dependent signaling pathways. A feature of GPCRs, in general, is that chronic occupation of receptors by agonists produces receptor internalization in a multistep process that begins with phosphorylation of intracellular amino acid residues by G-protein receptor kinase (GRK) and binding to the intracellular trafficking proteins arrestins, particularly the β-arrestins (Lohse et al. 1990). In some cases, this internalization is followed by degradation of receptors via clathrin-dependent endocytosis (Claing et al. 2002). But in addition to its role in mediating GPCR internalization, β-arrestin also mediates receptor signaling in G-protein independent pathways (Raehal and Bohn 2014). A biased agonist can preferentially activate either the G-protein pathway or a G-protein independent pathway (see Fig. 2 in Williams et al. 2013), and if side effects of mu agonists are preferentially mediated by either of these pathways, development of biased agonists has the potential for production of safer analgesics. Numerous recent reviews of MOR-biased agonists have been published (Kelly 2013; Raehal and Bohn 2014; Siuda et al. 2017; Urits et al. 2019), and the history of biased agonist for GPCRs, in general, is summarized by Madariaga-Mazon et al. (2017). The first description of β-arrestin-mediated signaling mechanisms for mu analgesics came from β-arrestin-2 knockout (KO) studies in mice (Bohn et al. 1999, 2000; Raehal et al. 2005). These studies showed β-arrestin KO mice developed less analgesic tolerance to chronic morphine treatment, as well as less physical dependence and constipation and, most importantly, less respiratory depression. These findings suggest that mu agonists selectively biased toward Gi/o pathways, and not activating β-arrestin mediated pathways, may provide enhanced analgesic efficacy with diminished side effects, including lethality due to respiratory depression (Raehal and Bohn 2014). The development of specific β-arrestin recruitment assays to complement direct assays of Gi/o activation (e.g., Manglik et al. 2016) allows researchers to directly calculate a bias ratio that indicates the preferred selectivity of an agonist for one pathway compared to the other (Kenakin 2014; Schmid et al. 2017). A study that calculated bias ratios for a number of compounds at the human MOR (Schmid et al. 2017) showed a strong correlation between the bias ratio and the therapeutic window between analgesic potency and respiratory depression.

One of the first mu-biased agonists to be reported was herkinorin, a compound derived from the potent selective kappa opioid Salvinorin A (Groer et al. 2007). This compound activated Gi/o signaling in cell culture but did not recruit β-arrestin-1 or β-arrestin-2. Not only was herkinorin active at similar doses as morphine in the formalin rat paw withdrawal test, a model of peripheral antinociception in inflammatory pain, but it did not produce significant tolerance after 5 days of chronic treatment (Lamb et al. 2012). Unfortunately, the ADME properties of herkinorin itself, including low solubility and poor CNS penetration, limit its clinical development as a systemic analgesic (Groer et al. 2007), and efforts are underway to identify analogs with improved bioavailability.

Another promising biased agonist is TRV130, which also activates Gi/o signaling without recruiting β-arrestin (DeWire et al. 2013). While TRV130 was five times more potent than morphine in antinociception tests, it produced less constipation and respiratory depression than morphine at equianalgesic doses (DeWire et al. 2013); the effects of TRV130 on constipation were, however, complicated (Altarifi et al. 2017). Currently, TRV130 (oliceridine) is undergoing clinical trials for treatment of moderate to severe pain. In Phase IIb trials that evaluated preliminary safety and efficacy of IV TRV130 in selected pain patients (Singla et al. 2017), TRV130 exhibited similar analgesic efficacy compared to morphine but fewer adverse effects including nausea, vomiting, and respiratory depression. A follow-up Phase III study in a different set of pain patients (Viscusi et al. 2019) revealed similar results. The status of the safety and efficacy of TRV130 has been recently reviewed (Urits et al. 2019): both respiratory depression and sedation from administration of TRV130 appear to be markedly reduced compared to morphine, and the effects of TRV130 are readily reversed by naloxone, suggesting that potential overdoses from this drug could be reversed with mu antagonists.

Another potentially promising biased mu agonist is PZM21, identified (as described above) from in silico predictions from docking studies of the antagonist binding site of MOR (Manglik et al. 2012). Although PZM21 exhibited 70% of full efficacy in Gi/o activation, it produced little significant recruitment of β-arrestin (Manglik et al. 2016). It produced full analgesic efficacy in several antinociception assays in mice, produced less constipation than morphine, and showed no significant respiratory depression.

What are the structural features of MOR that mediate Gi/o-dependent signaling compared to β-arrestin recruitment? The general features of three GPCRs (adenosine A2A, opsin, and MOR) that contribute to these two separate signaling pathways have been reviewed in detail (Carpenter and Tate 2017). In comparing the binding of TRV130 and morphine to MOR, results showed that binding of TRV130 allowed communication between the binding pocket and the intracellular end of TM3, while morphine allowed communication with both TM3 and TM6 (Altarifi et al. 2017). Single-site mutation studies revealed that residues W320 and Y328, both situated within the MOR binding pocket, were critical in regulating β-arrestin recruitment (Hothersall et al. 2017).

While biased mu agonists may hold potential as analgesics with reduced liability for respiratory depression and constipation, an important question is whether they also exhibit similar abuse potential compared to traditional mu agonists (Negus and Freeman 2018). Opioid conditioned place preference tests performed in β-arrestin KO mice demonstrated that rewarding effects of morphine were not mediated by β-arrestin-2 signaling (Bohn et al. 2003), thus suggesting that reward mechanisms were likely mediated by Gi/o signaling. In support of this concept, several detailed reinforcement studies in rats using TRV130 and PZM21, including opioid self-administration, revealed that these biased agonists produced abuse potential similar to that of traditional mu agonists (Altarifi et al. 2017; Schwienteck et al. 2019; Siuda et al. 2017). At this stage, studies in humans with biased mu agonists are just beginning, but one study comparing subjective effects of TRV130 with morphine in humans suggested that the two drugs exhibited similar abuse potential (Soergel et al. 2014).

While studying the single MOR isoform revealed different biased and unbiased agonists (Williams et al. 2013), the identification of many OPRM1 alternatively spliced C-terminal variants open questions regarding biased signaling of a single agonist at the level of multiple MOR C-terminal variants. Specifically, differences in C-terminal sequences encoded by alternative coding exons may have significant impact on agonist-induced signaling. Increasing evidence from both in vitro and in vivo studies strongly supports this hypothesis (see below).

4 Allosteric Agonists

Classical mu agonists, whether they are biased or unbiased, are regarded as orthosteric agonists; i.e., they bind to the orthosteric ligand-binding pocket of MOR where the endogenous agonist binds, as described in both antagonist and agonist-bound forms of MOR (Huang et al. 2015; Manglik et al. 2012, 2017). In contrast, allosteric ligands bind to sites on MOR that are spatially distinct from orthosteric sites. Allosteric ligands have the capability to modulate the effects of orthosteric agonists. Negative allosteric modulators (NAMs) can inhibit binding of orthosteric agonists or decrease efficacy of their signal transduction. Positive allosteric modulators (PAMs) activate receptors in the presence of an orthosteric agonist. Lastly, silent allosteric activators (SAMs) do not affect binding or efficacy of the orthosteric agonist directly but instead block the allosteric binding site to inhibit activity of NAMs or PAMs. These allosteric sites are often located within the non-conserved regions of a receptor (Remesic et al. 2017); this potentially allows for selectivity among GPCR subtypes that is not feasible for orthosteric agonists. Development of allosteric modulators potentially has advantages over that of orthosteric modulators, allowing for more subtle activation of agonist effects in target tissues by increasing the efficacy of endogenous opioids while at the same time reducing potential negative side effects (Burford et al. 2015; Livingston and Traynor 2018).

Although most interest in this area has focused on PAMs of MOR, at least two NAMs have been identified. The non-intoxicating cannabinoid cannabidiol acts as a NAM at MOR by increasing dissociation of orthosteric agonist binding (Kathmann et al. 2006), but this effect occurs at high concentrations of cannabidiol. The highly selective kappa opioid receptor agonist Salvinorin A also decreases MOR agonist binding and acts as an uncompetitive inhibitor of mu-stimulated [^{35}S]GTPγS binding, albeit at much higher concentrations than its affinity at kappa receptors (Rothman et al. 2007).

Because of their potential as novel analgesics, there has been significant interest in developing mu PAMs. Two ligands, BMS-986121 and BNS-986122, were shown to increase mu orthosteric agonist activation of G-proteins, increasing agonist efficacy at both Gi/o and β-arrestin signaling pathways (Burford et al. 2013). The proposed mechanism of BMS-98612's PAM action is to decrease the ability of sodium to inhibit agonist binding (Livingston and Traynor 2014). Unfortunately, the complexity of the synthesis of these compounds may make them impractical for further drug development (Burford et al. 2013). Another mu PAM, MS1, also increased the efficacy of orthosteric mu agonists, but it had a biased action, showing preferential recruitment of β-arrestin signaling as opposed to Gi/o pathways (Bisignano et al. 2015).

5 MOR Heteromers and Bivalent Ligands

The idea that agonists and/or antagonists of other receptors can modulate the effects of mu agonists is not new. For example, it has long been known that delta opioid receptor (DOR) antagonists can block analgesic tolerance and dependence produced by chronic administration of morphine (Abdelhamid et al. 1991), and DOR KO mice show reduced tolerance to chronic morphine treatment (Nitsche et al. 2002; Zhu et al. 1999). There are several potential explanations for such findings, but a number of laboratories have focused on opioid receptor dimerization as a mechanism for modulating mu receptor function. For example, formation of mu/delta heteromers has been demonstrated in the cell culture and brain (Fujita et al. 2015). Mu/delta heteromers have different pharmacological properties compared to mu receptor monomers, with the former having increased affinity for opioid peptides compared to the latter (George et al. 2000). In addition, a series of studies suggested that disruption of mu/delta heteromers prevented development of antinociceptive tolerance from chronic treatment with morphine (He et al. 2011). Together, these findings are consistent with the idea that interactions between mu and delta receptors as heteromers mediate development of tolerance to mu agonists. For this reason, several laboratories have synthesized bifunctional ligands that act as MOR agonists/DOR antagonists (Cunningham et al. 2019). For example, in one study, an analog of a cyclic tetrapeptide, modified to produce increased bioavailability, produced antinociception with no apparent acute tolerance (Mosberg et al. 2014). However, this study did not explore potential chronic tolerance produced by this analog. A more recent study with another bivalent compound, UFP-505, showed that although UFP-505 was active in antinociception tests, it also produced tolerance like morphine after chronic administration (Dietis et al. 2018). These findings illustrate the point that bivalent ligands are complicated and often produce results that are difficult to interpret (Cunningham et al. 2019).

The dimerization of MORs with other GPCRs suggests that several different signaling pathways with distinct pharmacological properties can be identified using specific bivalent ligands that bind to both receptors. Perhaps the best studied of these systems are the potential heteromers composed of MOR and nociception/orphanin FQ peptide (NOP) receptors (Cunningham et al. 2019; Toll et al. 2016). The NOP receptor is often called the fourth opioid receptor since it exhibits significant homology with mu, delta, and kappa receptors, despite the fact that it doesn't bind most traditional opioid ligands with high affinity (Toll et al. 2016). NOP receptor activation can modulate the function of mu agonists; for example, prolonged treatment with NOP in neuroblastoma cells reduced mu agonist inhibited cAMP (Thakker and Standifer 2002), and MOR/NOP receptor heterodimers have been identified by co-immunoprecipitation and immunofluorescence (Evans et al. 2010; Pan et al. 2002). A number of groups have synthesized novel MOR/NOP receptor bivalent ligands to identify potential analgesics with fewer side effects, with a special focus on using partial mu agonists as part of the ligand design (Cunningham et al. 2019; Toll et al. 2016). One strategy utilized analogs of buprenorphine, a partial agonist activity at both MOR and NOP receptors, to produce BU08028, a compound that exhibits high affinity at all three opioid receptor types as well as NOP receptors (Khroyan et al. 2011). Results in monkeys (Ding et al. 2016) revealed that BU08028 produced potent antinociceptive effects with less reinforcement compared to traditional mu agonists and no signs of physical dependence. Another bifunctional MOR/NOP receptor agonist is AT-121, a partial agonist at both MOR and NOP receptors. This compound produced potent analgesia with low levels of respiratory depression and physical dependence in monkeys (Ding et al. 2018). Finally, cebranopadol (GRT-6005) is a bifunctional ligand with full agonist effects at

MOR, DOR, and NOP receptors (Raffa et al. 2017). It is more potent than morphine in several acute and chronic models of pain in rodents, and it displays little respiratory depression, along with delayed tolerance. It has completed several Phase II clinical trials and is currently in Phase III clinical trials for acute and chronic pain.

6 MOR Regulation by Receptor Phosphorylation

GPCRs undergo desensitization after chronic agonist exposure by uncoupling from G-proteins in a process mediated by phosphorylation of specific residues on the C-terminal tail and third intracellular loop. The phosphorylated receptor can then bind to β-arrestins, thus leading to a complex series of events that include activation of intracellular signaling mechanisms as well as clathrin-induced internalization. A complete review of the large literature of MOR phosphorylation, desensitization, and internalization, as these processes relate to opioid tolerance (Williams et al. 2013), is beyond the scope of this chapter. Instead, we focus on the role of receptor phosphorylation in mediating various aspects of agonist signaling relevant to the ligand development summarized in the previous sections.

Chronic agonist exposure with a variety of drugs uncouples mu receptors from Gi/o proteins both in cell culture and in brain (Breivogel et al. 1997; Sim-Selley et al. 2000); this process of G-protein uncoupling is mediated by agonist-dependent phosphorylation of specific intracellular serine and threonine residues (Williams et al. 2013). The C-terminal tail of MOR contains 11 ser and thr residues capable of being phosphorylated (Kliewer et al. 2019). Morphine (which has low efficacy in stimulating phosphorylation and G-protein uncoupling) stimulates phosphorylation of S375, while higher efficacy agonists like DAMGO stimulate phosphorylation not only of S375 but also residues T370, T376, and T379, all mediated by activation of GRK2 and GRK3 (Gluck et al. 2014; Just et al. 2013; Miess et al. 2018). These phosphorylation events in turn stimulate recruitment of β-arrestin and receptor internalization (Just et al. 2013; Miess et al. 2018), with phosphorylation of S375 crucial for β-arrestin recruitment. The phosphorylation of these different residues by the higher efficacy agonists is a stepwise process, with S375 phosphorylated more rapidly than T370 (Doll et al. 2011).

The role of specific phosphorylated residues in mediating different effects of mu agonists can be studied by genetic mouse models in which specific ser or thr residues on MOR are replaced by ala, thus preventing phosphorylation. Where phosphorylation of S375 is eliminated with the S375A mutation (Grecksch et al. 2011), efficacies of antinociceptive response by morphine were increased, while development of tolerance was unchanged. In contrast, the S375A mutation decreased tolerance to the higher efficacy agonists like DAMGO. These results suggest that tolerance to the antinociceptive effects of mu agonists with different efficacies in stimulating phosphorylation occur through different pathways.

A recent study (Kliewer et al. 2019) used this genetic strategy to examine the roles of different ser and thr residues on MOR to mediate opioid analgesia and side effects. Eliminating phosphorylation of S375 increased fentanyl-induced analgesia and had no effect on morphine-induced analgesia; there was no effect on the potency of morphine or fentanyl to produce respiratory depression or constipation. Since phosphorylation of S375 is critical for β-arrestin recruitment but has little effect on G-protein signaling, these results question the concept that these undesirable opioid effects are mediated by β-arrestin signaling pathways. Therefore, it is possible that the increase in the safety profile of biased mu agonists may be caused by pharmacological factors other than pure agonist bias (Kliewer et al. 2019). At any rate, such findings emphasize the difficulty in interpreting results in a system where multiple signaling pathways exert different effects through complex mechanisms.

7 Alternative Splicing of the Mu Opioid Receptor Gene, *OPRM1*

Molecular cloning of the mu opioid receptor cDNA (MOR-1) led to isolation and characterization of its gene structure, *OPRM1*, from mouse to human (Belknap et al. 1995; Giros et al. 1995; Kozak et al. 1994; Wang et al. 1994). However, only a single copy of the *OPRM1* gene was identified, which was hard to reconcile with mu subtypes suggested by the early pharmacological studies (Cherny et al. 2001; Chou et al. 2009; Inturrisi 2002; Pasternak 2001). Over 90% of human and mouse genes have alternative pre-mRNA splicing, creating great diversity at mRNA and protein levels. One obvious hypothesis is that the *OPRM1* gene alternative splicing generates multiple mu opioid receptors. Driven by this hypothesis, many efforts have been made by several laboratories to successfully identify an array of *OPRM1* alternatively spliced variants or isoforms from mouse and rat to human. Although it is still challenging to correlate these splice variants to the subtypes, such as mu_1 and mu_2, defined by early pharmacological studies, growing evidence suggests that some of these splice variants play important roles in mu opioid pharmacology, particularly providing new insights into biased signaling at multiple mu receptor levels and leading to development of novel opioid analgesics potentially lacking many side effects commonly associated with traditional opiates.

Common patterns of alternative splicing include exon skipping, alternative 5′ and 3′ splicing, intron retention, mutually exclusive exons, and alternative promoter and poly(A) (Black 2003). The *OPRM1* gene adopts all these patterns to create multiple and diverse splice variants. *OPRM1* alternative splicing is conserved from rodent to human in terms of their splicing patterns, location of alternative exons, and types of splice variants, as well as sequences in some variants (see detailed *OPRM1* gene structures and alternative splicing in reviews: Pan 2005; Pasternak and Pan 2013). Based on the predicted structures, the *OPRM1* splice variants can be categorized into three main types: full-length 7TM C-terminal splice variants, truncated 6TM variants, and single TM variants (Table 1 and Fig. 3).

Table 1 List of alternatively spliced variants of mu opioid receptor gene, *OPRM1*

Species	7TM Variant	6TM Variant	1TM Variant
Mouse	mMOR-1	mMOR-1G	mMOR-1Q
	mMOR-1A	mMOR-1K	mMOR-1R
	mMOR-1B1	mMOR-1L	mMOR-1S
	mMOR-1B2	mMOR-1M	mMOR-1T
	mMOR-1B3	mMOR-1N	mMOR-1Z
	mMOR-1B4		
	mMOR-1B5		
	mMOR-1C		
	mMOR-1D		
	mMOR-1E		
	mMOR-1Eii/Eiii/Eiv		
	mMOR-1F		
	mMOR-1H		
	mMOR-1i		
	mMOR-1J		
	mMOR-1*O*		
	mMOR-1P		
	mMOR-1V-Vii		
	mMOR-1U		
	mMOR-1W		
	mMOR-1T		
Rat	rMOR-1	rMOR-1G1	rMOR-1S
	rMOR-1A	rMOR-1G2	rMOR-1Z
	rMOR-1B1		
	rMOR-1B2		
	rMOR-1C1		
	rMOR-1C2		
	rMOR-1D		
	rMOR-1H1/H2		
	rMOR-1i1/i2/i3		
	rMOR-1P		
Human	hMOR-1	hMOR-1G1	hMOR-1S
	hMOR-1A	hMOR-1G2	hMOR-1Z
	hMOR-1B1	hMOR-1K	SV1
	hMOR-1B2		SV2
	hMOR-1B3		
	hMOR-1B4		
	hMOR-1B5		
	hMOR-1*O*		
	hMOR-1X		
	hMOR-1Y		
	hMOR-1i		

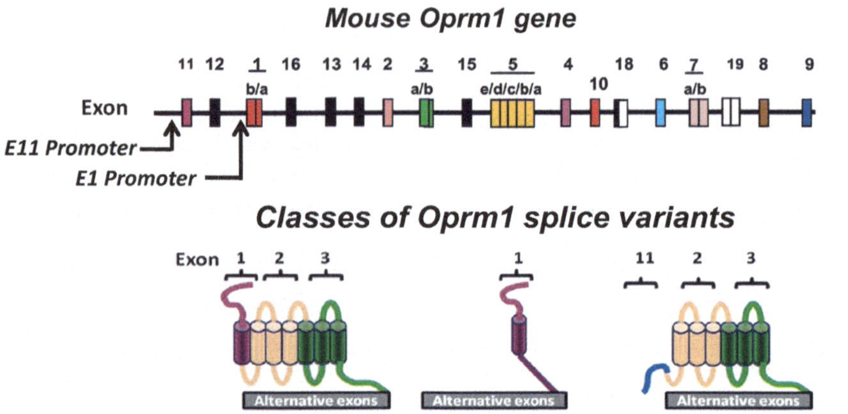

OPRM1 Variants	C-terminal 7TM	Truncated 1TM	Truncated 6TM
Promoter	E1	E1	E11
Mouse variants(n)	22	5	5
Rat variants (n)	13	2	2
Human variants(n)	12	4	4

Knockout model	C-terminal 7TM	Truncated 1TM	Truncated 6TM
E1-KO	Lost	Lost	Retained
E11-KO	Retained	Retained	Lost
E1/E11-KO	Lost	Lost	Lost
Triple KO (E1+DOR-1+KOR-1)	Lost	Lost	Retained

Fig. 3 Schematic of the *Oprm1* gene structure, classes of *Oprm1* splice variants and related knockout mouse models. The mouse *Oprm1* gene structure reported in the literature is shown on the top; adapted from Pasternak and Pan (2013). Exons and introns are indicated by colored boxes and horizontal lines, respectively. Promoters are shown by arrows. Intron sizes are indicated as kilobases (kb). Exons are numbered based on the published data. The exon and intron distances are not drawn to scale. Three classes of the variants based on predicted structure, C-terminal 7TM, truncated 1TM, and 6TM, are shown in the middle; adapted from Lu et al. (2018). The associated promoter and number of the variants from mouse, rat and human in each class are provided in the table under the predicted structures. Knockout mouse models targeting these variants are shown in the lower panel of the table

7.1 Full-Length 7TM C-Terminal Variants and 3′ Splicing

All the *OPRM1* full-length 7TM C-terminal variants contain exons 1/2/3 that encode major parts of the receptor, including the N-terminus, 7-TM domains, three intracellular and three extracellular loops, and part of C-terminus. However, they have a distinct C-terminal tail that is generated through 3′ splicing from exon 3 to an alternative exon downstream of exon 3. Extensive *OPRM1* 3′ splicing generates 22 full-length 7TM C-terminal variants in mouse, 13 in rat, and 12 in human.

The first two C-terminal variants, hMOR-1A (Bare et al. 1994) and rMOR-1B (Zimprich et al. 1995), were identified in the human and rat *Oprm1* genes, respectively. Further 3′ RACE and PCR cloning have isolated many 3′ exons and their associated C-terminal variants in mouse, rat and human (Doyle et al. 2007a, b; Kvam et al. 2004; Pan et al. 1999a, 2000, 2003, 2005a, b; Pasternak et al. 2004). Currently, 22 C-terminal variants in the mouse *Oprm1* gene, 13 in the rat *Oprm1* gene, and 12 in the human OPRM1 gene have been isolated (Fig. 3). The predicted sequences and lengths of the amino acids of the C-terminal tail are unique for each of these C-terminal variants. Several potential phosphorylation sites, such as protein kinase C, GRKs, cAMP- and cGMP-dependent protein kinase, and Casein kinase II, were identified in these C-terminal tails. In vitro studies in cell models suggested the functional relevance of these C-terminal variants in mu agonist-induced receptor phosphorylation, internalization, post-endocytic sorting, and G-protein coupling (see below). Gene targeting mouse models further demonstrated that these alternatively spliced C-termini play important roles in morphine actions (see below).

Among the C-terminal variants, mMOR-1A, rMOR-1A, hMOR-1A, and mMOR-1O were intron retention variants. Loss of splicing from exon 3a to the downstream exons produces MOR-1A. Exon 3b, an intron region in the other variants, is maintained to encode four amino acids, which are identical in mMOR-1A and hMOR-1A. An alternative poly(A) was identified in both mouse and human exon 3b (Lu et al. 2014), which may contribute to the intron retention. Silencing of exon 7a donor site leads to extension from exon 7a to exon 7b, which predicts 30 amino acids from exon 7a and immediately terminates in exon 7b. hMOR-1O has a 3′ exon, exon O that is the homolog of mouse exon 7a, and predicts 30 amino acids, which share 67% identity with those from the mouse exon 7a (Pan et al. 2003). Human exon O has potential donor site which is like that seen in the splice joint of the mouse exons 7a/7b. However, no additional exons downstream of exon O have been identified so far.

Alternative 3′ splicing is a type of splicing that selects different splice acceptor sites along the exon from a common upstream donor site. The MOR-1B series in the mouse, human, and rat *OPRM1* genes are the products from this type of splicing. Splicing from exons 1/2/3 to different splice acceptor sites within exon 5 (exons 5a, 5b, 5c, 5d, and 5e) generates five C-terminal variants (mMOR-1B1–mMOR-1B5 and hMOR-1B1–hMOR-1B5) in mouse and human, and two (rMOR-1B1 and rMOR-1B2) in rat (Pan et al. 2005a, b; Pasternak et al. 2004; Pasternak and Pan 2013). The predicted five amino acids from exon 5a in mMOR-1B1 and rMOR-1B1 are identical. Although the first five amino acids from exon 5a in hMOR-1B1 are the same as those from mMOR-1B1 and rMOR-1B1, hMOR-1B1 had an additional 13 amino acids from the exon 5a (Pan et al. 2005a). Predicted amino acid sequences from the mouse exons 5b, 5c, 5d, and 5e had no homology with those from the corresponding human exons. mMOR-1V and mMOR-1W are another two mouse variants that have alternative 3′ splicing within exon 18 (Doyle et al. 2007a).

Using exon inclusion or skipping, *OPRM1* produces eight variants of the mouse *Oprm1* gene, mMOR-1C, mMOR-1D, mMOR-1E, mMOR-1F, mMOR-1P, mMOR-1U, mMOR-1V, and mMOR-1W; four variants of the rat *Oprm1* gene, rMOR-1C1, rMOR-1C2, rMOR-1D, and rMOR-1P; and three variants of the human *OPRM1* gene, hMOR-1O, hMOR-1X, and mMOR-1Y. Exon inclusion/skipping also generates several variants containing a premature termination codon, which can be targeted by nonsense-mediated mRNA degradation (NMD). NMD degrades a mRNA with a premature termination codon located more than 50 nt upstream of the last exon-exon junction (Chang et al. 2007; Lejeune and Maquat 2005). Thus, mMOR-1E, mMOR-1F, mMOR-1V, mMOR-1W, rMOR-1D, and hMOR-1Y are considered as the NMD target.

Two alternative splicing patterns can be seen in several *OPRM1* C-terminal variants. For example, hMOR-1Y is generated by both exon inclusion of exon Y and alternative 3′ splicing at exon 5c (Pan et al. 2005a). mMOR-1O has both exon skipping and intron retention.

7.2 Truncated 6TM Variants, Alternative Exon 11 Promoter, and 5′ Splicing

Exon 11 was originally identified ~30 kb upstream of exon 1 in the mouse *Oprm1* gene using a modified 5′ RACE approach (Pan et al. 2001). Subsequent cloning isolated eight exon 11-associated splice variants that are generated through 5′ splicing defined by splicing from exon 11 to different downstream exons (Pan et al. 2001). An exon 11 promoter that controls the expression of these exon 11-associated variants was identified and characterized soon after exon 11-associated variants were isolated (Pan 2002). The exon 11 homolog and its associated splice variants were isolated from rat and human *OPRM1* genes (Xu et al. 2009, 2011), indicating the conservation of the 5′ splicing.

The mouse exon 11 promoter contains a functional TATA box and its associated cis-acting elements, favoring a eukaryote class II promoter, which is distinguished from the exon 1 promoter without the TATA box, copying a "housekeeping" gene mode commonly for constitutive genes. Exon 11 promoter activity starts at mouse embryonic day 13.5 (E13.5), 4 days later than the exon 1 promoter activity 9.5 (E9.5) (Xu et al. 2006). Exon 11 promoter and exon 1 promoter were shown to have differential expression in brain regions such as hippocampus and substantia nigra in a transgenic mouse model, suggesting region-specific promoter activity (Xu et al. 2006). More importantly, each promoter controls the expression of a unique set of splice variants. The exon 11 promoter drives the transcription of all truncated 6TM variants, while the exon 1 promoter controls the transcription of all full-length 7TM C-terminal variants and single TM variants. A similar exon 11 promoter activity is found in the rat and human *OPRM1* genes (unpublished observation).

There are five truncated 6TM variants in mouse, all of which are produced by exon inclusion/skipping. Splicing from exon 11 to exon 2 by skipping exon 1 generates mMOR-1G, mMOR-1M and mMOR-1N in mouse (Pan et al. 2001), rMOR-1G1 and rMOR-1G2 in rat (Xu et al. 2011), and hMOR-1G1 and hMOR-1G2 in human (Xu et al. 2009), while splicing from exon 11 to exon 13 or exon 14 in mouse produced mMOR-1K and mMOR-1L (Pan et al. 2001). All these 6TM variants have exons 2 and 3 that encode TM2–TM7 but exclude exon 1 that encodes TM1. Since exons 11, 13, and 14, as well as exons downstream of exon 3, do not predict any TM domains, these variants have a similar receptor core structure with six TM domains, adjoining different C-terminal tails generated through 3′ splicing from exon 3 to downstream exons. These variants are designated as truncated 6TM variants.

The mouse exon 11 predicts 27 amino acids in mMOR-1G, mMOR-1M, and mMOR-1N, whereas the rat and human exon 11a encodes 7 and 16 amino acids in rMOR-1G2 and hMOR-1G2, respectively. These sequences are translated in frame with exons 2, 3, and 4 or 7/8/9 or 8/9 in these variants. Translation using exon 11 AUG in mMOR-1K and mMOR-1L predicts a short peptide with less than 10 kDa due to early translation termination within exon 13 and exon 14, respectively. However, translation from an AUG codon at the beginning of the exon 2 still predicts a truncated 6TM receptor in mMOR-1K and mMOR-1L. Similar scenarios are seen in rMOR-1G1 and hMOR-1G1.

Two human variants, hMOR-1K (Shabalina et al. 2009) and mu_3 (Cadet et al. 2003), were isolated as a truncated 6TM variant that uses the exon 2 AUG as the translational start codon. hMOR-1K was identified by homologous PCR cloning based on identification of human exon 13, a mouse exon 13 homolog in the human *OPRM1* gene. Although it does not have predicted coding sequence, human exon 13 predicts an internal ribosome entry site that can controls translation of hMOR-1K. hMOR-1K is implicated in morphine-induced excitatory cellular effects, such as the increase of intracellular Ca^{2+} and nitric oxide release (Gris et al. 2010). Mu_3 has an exon composition of 2/3 new exon (149 bases)/partial exon 4 (202 bases). The function of the mu $variant_3$ was suggested to involve the nitric oxide regulatory pathway (Cadet et al. 2007; Stefano et al. 1995; Zhu et al. 2004). No upstream exon was identified in hMOR-1K and mu_3, raising the possibility that they have their own promoter, probably located in their upstream regions.

Exon 11-associated variants also contain several full-length 7TM MOR-1 variants, including three in mouse, mMOR-1H, mMOR-1I, and mMOR-1J (Pan et al. 2001); four in rat, rMOR-1H1, rMOR-1I1, rMOR-1I2, and rMOR-1I3 (Xu et al. 2011); and one in human, hMOR-1H (Xu et al. 2009). They all have the same coding exons 1/2/3/4 and predict the same receptor sequences as the original MOR-1 but comprise different 5′ untranslated regions derived from alternative splicing from exon 11 to downstream exons. Therefore, the MOR-1 receptor protein can be generated by multiple transcripts controlled by two distinct promoters, raising the question how these variant mRNAs are distributed and expressed. Although these variants can predict a short peptide due to early termination of translation when the exon 11 AUG is used, it remains unknown if these short peptides are expressed in vivo.

7.3 Truncated Single TM Variants and Exon Skipping and Insertion

Exon skipping or insertion creates another set of splice variants that predict a truncated protein containing a single TM domain. All these variants contain exon 1 that encodes the first TM. However, exon skipping or insertion in these transcripts causes reading-frame shifting and terminates translation early, generating a truncated protein having N-terminus and the first TM identical to MOR-1, but with a different C-terminal tail due to different splicing patterns.

The first two single TM variants, hMOR-1S and hMOR-1Z, were isolated from the human *OPRM1* gene (Du et al. 1997; Pan 2005). Direct splicing from exon 1 to exon 4 by skipping exons 2/3 produces hMOR-1S that encodes a protein containing the first TM by exon 1 with only one serine residue translated from exon 4 due to reading-frame shift. The human hMOR-1S homologs, mMOR-1S and rMOR-1S, were also isolated in mouse and rat *Oprm1* genes, respectively (Xu et al. 2013). hMOR-1Z is generated by skipping exon 2 with exon composition of 1/3/4. Skipping exon 2 shifts the reading frame in exon 3, predicting 90 amino acids in exon 3 that are entirely different from the original 173 amino acids encoded by exon 3 in hMOR-1, and do not contain any transmembrane domains. Thus, hMOR-1Z encodes a single TM protein with a long C-terminal tail. However, hMOR-1Z is considered a target for NMD due to the stop codon located more than 50 nt from exons 3/4 junction. The human hMOR-1Z homologs, mMOR-1Z and rMOR-1Z, were also identified in mouse and rat, respectively (Xu et al. 2013), suggesting conservation of exon 2 skipping. Exon 3 in mMOR-1Z and rMOR-1Z predicts even longer C-terminal tails with128 amino acids containing no transmembrane domain.

There are three additional single TM variants, mMOR-1Q, mMOR-1R, and mMOR-1T, in the mouse *Oprm1* gene. Both mMOR-1Q and mMOR-1R are exon 2 skipping variants and predict the same single TM protein as mMOR-1Z. However, they have different 3′ UTRs due to alternative 3′ splicing that is identical to those seen in mMOR-1O and mMOR-1D. mMOR-1T is an exon 11-associated variant with an exon composition of 11/1a/16/2. Translation from the exon 1 AUG generates a single TM protein with a unique C-terminal tail containing 20 amino acids predicted from exon 16. Two additional human single TM variants, SV1 and SV2, were isolated from human neuroblastoma NMB cells (Choi et al. 2006). Both SV1 and SV2 are exon insertion or alternative 3′ splicing variants. Translation in exon B or A/B from exon 1 predicts a single TM protein with a C-terminal tail of 32 amino acids in SV1 or 5 amino acids in SV2. All these additional single TM variants are potential targets for NMD due to the presence of the premature termination codon.

8 Expression and Function of *OPRM1* Splice Variants

8.1 mRNA and Protein Expression

Initial Northern blot analysis to detect RNA levels using individual exon or combined exon probes and total RNAs from whole brain or human neuroblastoma cell line showed multiple bands with different sizes and intensities, suggesting different lengths of the splice variants associated with the probed exon or exons (Pan et al. 1999b, 2001, 2005a, b; Raynor et al. 1995; Thompson et al. 1993). Further real-time (RT)-PCR showed differential expression of some variant mRNAs among the brain regions, suggesting region-specific alternative splicing (Pan et al. 1999b, 2000, 2001; Xu et al. 2009, 2011, 2013). Leveraging real-time quantitative PCR (qPCR) which provides a more accurate measurement of mRNAs, recent results analyzing *Oprm1* splice variant mRNA expression in ten different brain regions of four different inbred mouse strains suggested that the *Oprm1* alternative splicing is not only region-specific but also strain-specific (Xu et al. 2014) (Fig. 4). This provided insights into the role of genetic background on the regulation of the *Oprm1* gene and mu opioid pharmacology. Furthermore, dramatic alternation of the *Oprm1* variant mRNAs was associated with stabilization of morphine tolerance in a mouse model, raising the possibility that the expression levels of the *Oprm1* splice variants contribute to morphine tolerance stabilization (Xu et al. 2015).

Since most individual exons are shared by more than one variant, it is difficult to develop an antibody against a specific variant. However, several exon-specific antisera were produced to investigate the distribution of the related variants at the protein level in brain. For instance, antisera against an exon 7/8 epitope distinctively labeled several regions, such as the medial eminence and nucleus ambiguous, which were different from those labeled by antisera against the exon 4 epitope (Abbadie et al. 2000a, b). Antisera against an exon 8 epitope specifically hybridized in the dentate gyrus, the mossy fibers of the hippocampal formation, and the nucleus of the solitary tract (Abbadie et al. 2000b). These results suggested region-specific processing of the *Oprm1* variant mRNAs and/or proteins. Yet, the interpretation of these data should consider what types of the variants are involved. For instance, seven variants, including four 7TM variants, mMOR-1, mMOR-1H, mMOR-1I, and mMOR-1J, and three 6TM variants, mMOR-1K, mMOR-1L, and mMOR-1G, have same exon 4 coding sequence and can be labeled by the same antisera against the exon 4 epitope. Similarly, the antisera against the exon 7/8 epitope can label both 7TM variant mMOR-1C and 6TM variant mMOR-1M. Intriguingly, labeling by the antisera against the exon 7/8 epitope was mainly seen at presynaptic membrane, where the antisera against the exon 4 epitope equally labeled both presynaptic and postsynaptic membranes (Abbadie et al. 2001), suggesting differential regulation of variant expression at synapse via mRNA and protein trafficking and local protein synthesis.

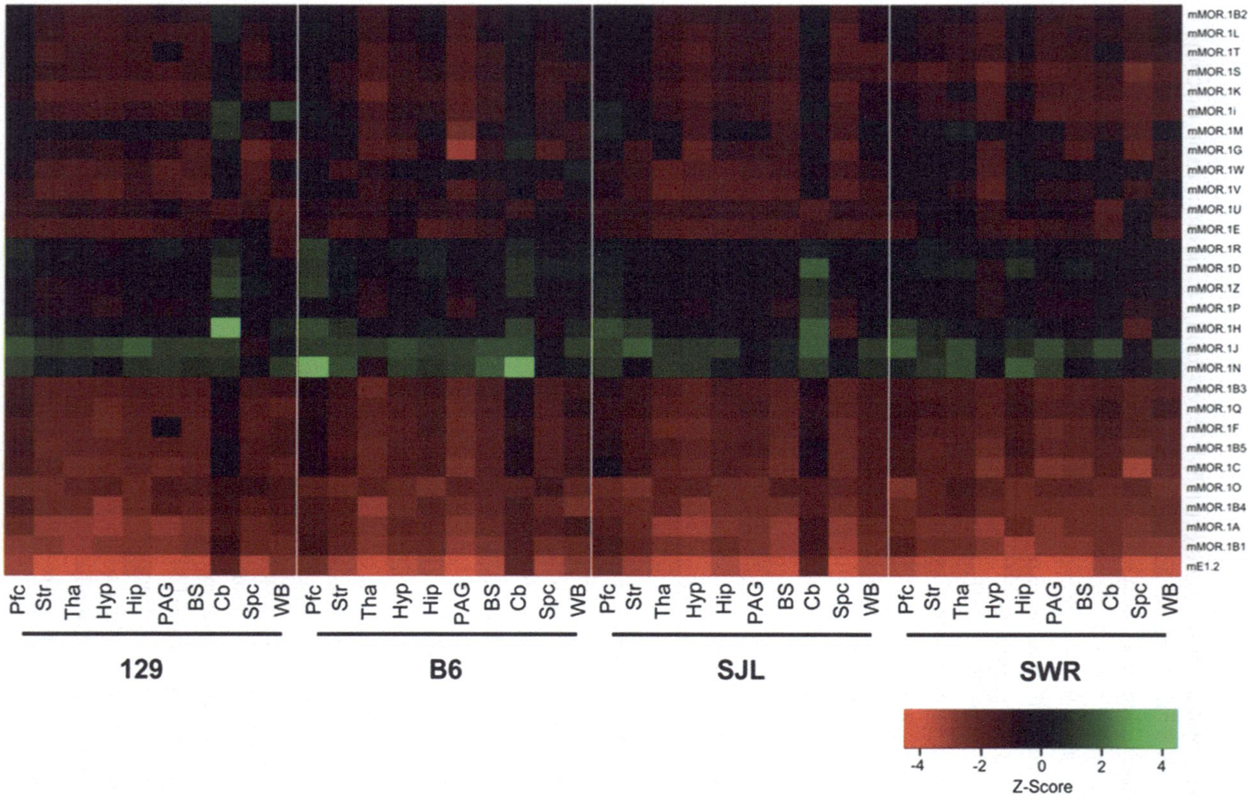

Fig. 4 Regional expression *OPRM1* splice variant mRNAs. The heatmap was generated from RT-qPCR data using total RNAs from ten brain regions (*Pfc* prefrontal cortex, *Str* striatum, *Tha* thalamus, *Hyp* hypothalamus, *Hip* hippocampus, *PAG* periaqueductal gray, *BS* brainstem, *Cb* cerebellum, *Spc* spinal cord, *WB* whole brain) of four inbred mouse strains (129, 129P3/J; B6, C56BL/6J; SJL, SJL/J; SWR, SWR/J) by clustering Z-scores calculated from the values (Log_2 ($E^{-\Delta}C$ (t)) of individual variants across different strains/regions using R statistical language (2.15.0) (www.r-project.org). Expression level was indicated by Z-score. Adapted from Xu et al. (2014)

8.2 Functions of *OPRM1* Full-Length 7TM C-Terminal Variants

8.2.1 In Vitro Studies Using Cell Models: Radioligand Binding, Signaling, Phosphorylation

CHO cell lines stably expressing each individual full-length C-terminal variant were initially established to examine their opioid binding profiles. All the C-terminal variants showed high affinity toward [^{3}H] DAMGO, a full mu agonist, while competition studies further confirmed their mu binding selectivity. These results were not surprising since all the full-length C-terminal variants have the same receptor binding pocket. However, competition studies revealed some subtle but significant differences, particularly in the binding affinities for the endogenous opioid peptides such as β-endorphin and dynorphin A among some variants. For instance, mMOR-1D showed higher affinities for β-endorphin and dynorphin A than mMOR-1 (Pan et al. 1999a). These results raised the possibility that different C-terminal tails may modulate the receptor configuration, contributing to the altered binding affinities.

Intracellular location of alternatively spliced C-terminal tails raises questions regarding their role in influencing signaling molecules such as G-protein activation and adenylyl cyclase inhibition. [^{35}S] GTPγS binding assays are commonly used for assessing overall receptor-G-protein coupling. [^{35}S]GTPγS binding using the same stable CHO cell membranes revealed dramatic differences of mu agonist-induced G-protein activation in both potency and efficacy among the C-terminal variants (Bolan et al. 2004; Pan et al. 2005a, b; Pasternak et al. 2004). Different agonists displayed various efficacies toward different C-terminal variants. For instance, morphine and morphine-6-glucuronide (M6G), a major active metabolite of morphine, are full agonists for hMOR-1A, but partial agonists for other C-terminal variants, such as hMOR-1B1, hMOR-1B3, and hMOR-1B5 (Pan et al. 2005a). On the other hand, β-endorphin is a full agonist for hMOR-1B5 and a partial agonist for hMOR-1A (Pan et al. 2005a). Also, different C-terminal variants showed various intrinsic activities toward the agonists, as indicated by complete lack of correlation between the mu opioid binding affinities and the potency in [^{35}S]GTPγS binding assay (Pan et al. 2005a; Pasternak et al. 2004). Similarly, C-terminal variants showed remarkable differences in both potency and efficacy of mu agonists in inhibiting mu agonist-induced forskolin-stimulated cAMP accumulation among the human C-terminal variants (Pan et al. 2005a). However, there was no correlation between changes in G-protein coupling and adenylyl cyclase inhibition. These results suggested that the C-terminal tails can greatly influence mu agonist-induced G-protein coupling and adenylyl cyclase inhibition.

Mu agonist-induced receptor phosphorylation, desensitization, and internalization have been considered to be involved in mu opioid tolerance and physical dependence (Deng et al. 2000; Koch et al. 1998; Law et al. 2000; Von Zastrow et al. 2003; Waldhoer et al. 2004). A number of consensus phosphorylation sites for GRKs, protein kinase C, casein kinase, tyrosine kinase, and cAMP- and cGMP-dependent protein kinases are predicted from different C-terminal tails, providing potential mechanisms for mu agonist-induced receptor desensitization and internalization. For instance, morphine induced different levels of receptor phosphorylation of mMOR-1, mMOR-1C, mMOR-1D, and mMOR-1E, which correlated with various degrees of morphine-induced receptor internalization among these variants (Koch et al. 1998). The threonine 394 within exon 4-encoded C-terminal tail was crucial for DAMGO-induced receptor phosphorylation in rMOR-1 (Deng et al. 2000). Intracerebroventricular administration of morphine induced robust internalization of mMOR-1C, but not mMOR-1, in the mouse lateral septum (Abbadie and Pasternak 2001). The C-terminal tail encoded by exon 4 contains a MOR1-derived recycling sequence (MRS) that promotes internalized mMOR-1 recycling back to the plasma membrane and plays an important role on mu agonist-induced receptor post-endocytic sorting process (Tanowitz and von Zastrow 2003). Lacking MRS in mMOR-1B, mMOR-1D, and mMOR-1E led to their lysosomal sorting and subsequent degradation (Tanowitz et al. 2008).

8.2.2 In Vivo Studies Using Animal Models

Antisense Oligonucleotides

In vivo administration of antisense oligonucleotides is a commonly used approach to downregulate gene expression. Although these agents produce only a partial knockdown for a short period of time, they provide a means of selectively targeting different exons or exon/exon junctions for studying in vivo function of splice variants. Initially, the function of C-terminal variants in mu opioid analgesia was examined using antisense approaches with short oligonucleotides targeting individual exons in mice (Pasternak and Pan 2000). An antisense oligonucleotide targeting exon 1 eliminated morphine-induced analgesia (Rossi et al. 1994). Antisense oligonucleotides targeting exons 6, 7, 8, 9, and 10 also reduced supraspinal morphine analgesia (Pan et al. 1999a, 2000). These antisense studies suggested that the C-terminal variants are important for morphine analgesia. Antisense mapping studies with oligonucleotides targeting four individual exons in mMOR-1 revealed the divergent role of each exons in morphine and M6G analgesia, implying existence of alternatively spliced variants (Rossi et al. 1995).

C-Terminal Truncation Mouse Models

Several C-terminal truncation mouse models were generated to further explore in vivo functions of alternatively spliced C-termini in opioid pharmacology (Xu et al. 2017). A stop codon strategy was used to create these C-terminal truncation models. Unlike knocking out an exon at the genomic DNA level, this strategy truncates a designated coding exon at the translational level with limited complementary effects on overall *Oprm1* transcription and alternative splicing.

Three C-terminal truncation models were made in two different inbred mouse strains, C57BL/6J (B6) and 129/SvEv (129), because these two strains of mice displayed significant differences in responses to mu opioids (Kest et al. 2002a, b; Klein et al. 2008). The first mouse model truncated all C-termini downstream of exon 3 (mE3M), while the other two selectively truncated the C-terminal tails encoded by either exon 4 (mE4M) or exon 7 (mE7M). These mice revealed divergent roles for the C-termini in various morphine-induced behaviors, highlighting the importance of C-terminal variants in complex morphine actions. For instance, the E7-encoded C-terminal truncation in B6 mice (mE7M-B6) diminished morphine tolerance and reward without altering physical dependence, whereas the E4-encoded C-terminal truncation (mE4M-B6) facilitated morphine tolerance and reduced morphine dependence without affecting morphine reward (Fig. 5). Furthermore, the loss of morphine-induced receptor desensitization in the hypothalamus and brain stem of mE7M-B6 mutant mice implicated the involvement of E7-associated variants in morphine-induced receptor desensitization and tolerance.

Intriguingly, several morphine-induced responses in β-arrestin-2 KO mice were similar to those in mE7M-B6 mutant mice, such as reduced morphine tolerance (Bohn et al. 2000, 2002), no change of physical dependence (Bohn et al. 2000; Raehal and Bohn 2011) and GI transit inhibition (Raehal et al. 2005), and loss of receptor desensitization in the brain stem (Bohn et al. 2000). Although some different responses were also seen between these two models, the similarities that were noted suggest a physical and functional interaction of the E7-encoded C-terminal tails with β-arrestin-2 in producing morphine-induced receptor desensitization in specific regions and morphine tolerance. This hypothesis was further supported by in vitro cell-based studies indicating that several mu agonists displayed greater β-arrestin bias against E7-associated variants than against the E4-associated mMOR-1 (Xu et al. 2017) (Fig. 6). The E7-encoded sequences contain a predicted phosphorylation code, PxPxxE/D or PxxPxxE/D, for high-affinity β-arrestin binding that interacts with positively charged residues at the N-terminus of β-arrestin based on homology modeling with the crystal structure of GPCR-arrestin complex (Zhou et al. 2017) (Fig. 6). It will be interesting to determine if the predicted code is critical for β-arrestin-2 binding to the E7-associated C-terminal variants. Together, the differential effects of C-terminal truncation illustrate the pharmacological significance of *OPRM1* C-terminal splice variants.

8.3 Functions of *OPRM1* Truncated 6TM Variants

8.3.1 Loss of Function Studies: Exon 11 KO Mouse Model

When expressed in CHO or HEK293 cells, the truncated 6TM variants do not bind any available radiolabeled opioids, raising the concerns about their functional relevance in opioid pharmacology despite the differential expression of their mRNAs among brain regions (Pan et al. 2001). The functions of these truncated 6TM variants were detected only when an exon 11 KO (mE11-KO) mouse model was established (Pan et al. 2009). In mE11-KO mice, morphine and methadone analgesia was normal, but the analgesic actions of heroin, M6G, and fentanyl were greatly diminished. Although the mE11-KO model targeted all exon 11-associated variants, including three full-length 7TM variants – five 6TM variants and one single TM variant – the reduced analgesia toward heroin and M6G was most likely mediated by loss of the 6TM variants because heroin and M6G were still active in E1-KO mice. These results strongly suggested that the E11-associated 6TM variants

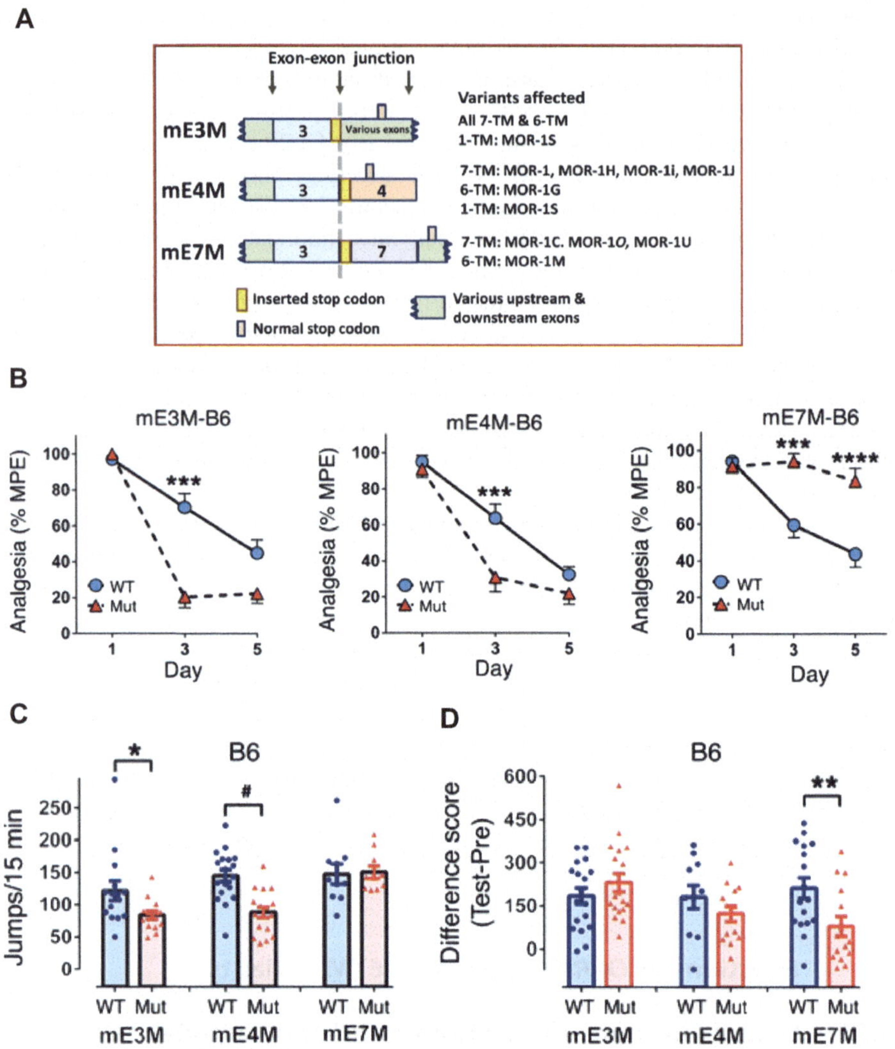

Fig. 5 *Oprm1* C-terminal truncation mouse models; adapted from Xu et al. (2017). (**a**) Schematic of generating C-terminal truncation strategy. Three targeted mouse models, mE3M, mE4M, and mE7M, were generated by inserting a stop codon at an appropriate site within indicated exons shown by colored boxes. Inserted and original stop codons are indicated by yellow and pink bars, respectively. In mE3M, a stop codon was inserted at the end of exon 3 to eliminate every C-terminal tails of all 7TM and 6TM variants, as well as 1TM mMOR-1S. In mE4M and mE7M, a stop codon was created at the beginning of exon 4 or exon 7 to eliminate individual C-terminal tails encoded by exon 4 or exon 7 of indicated variants, respectively. (**b**) Morphine tolerance in the mutant mice on C57BL/6J (B6) background was induced by twice daily injections with morphine (10 mg/kg, s.c.) for 5 days. Morphine analgesia was determined 30 min after s.c. injection using a radiant-heat tail-flick assay. Results are shown as the percentage of maximum possible effect (% MPE). WT, wildtype mice; Mut, homozygous mice. (**c**) Morphine physical dependence was assessed on day 5 of chronic morphine treatment with naloxone (s.c., 1.0 mg/kg) injection 3 h after the last morphine treatment to precipitate withdrawal. The number of jumps within 15 min was used for the measurement of withdrawal. (**d**) Morphine reward was assessed using a 6-day conditioned place preference protocol

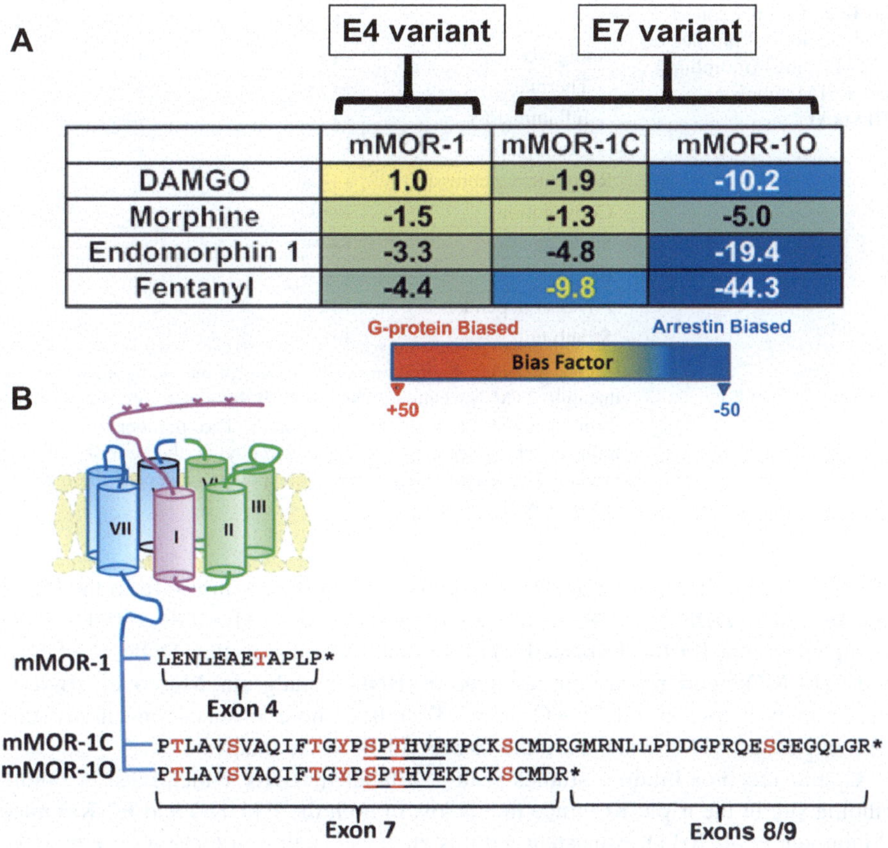

Fig. 6 Biased signaling of *Oprm1* C-terminal splice variants; adapted from Xu et al. (2017). (**a**) Heatmap of biased factors. Biased factors were calculated from β-arrestin-2 recruitment assay (PathHunter enzyme complementation assay) and [^{35}S]GTPγS binding assay using the Black and Leff operational model (Kenakin et al. 2012; van der Westhuizen et al. 2014) and normalized with respect to DAMGO at mMOR-1 for a comparison across variants or drugs. (**b**) Predicted amino acid sequences of different C-terminal tails. Red letter: predicted phosphorylated site. The underlined sequences: phosphorylation code, PxPxxE/D or PxxPxxE/D, predicted from GPCR-arrestin crystal structure for high-affinity β-arrestin binding (Zhou et al. 2017)

are important in mediating the actions of a subset of mu opioids, such as heroin, M6G, and fentanyl.

The functional significance of the truncated 6TM variants has been further defined using a new opioid ligand, 3-iodobenzoylnaltrexamide (IBNtxA) derived from naltrexone (Majumdar et al. 2011, 2012). IBNtxA represents a novel class of opioid analgesics that is potent against thermal, inflammatory, and neuropathic pain but lacks many side effects associated with traditional opiates, including respiratory depression, physical dependence, and reward (Majumdar et al. 2011; Wieskopf et al.

Table 2 Comparison of pharmacological profiles of a 7TM agonist (morphine) and a 6TM agonist (IBNtxA)

	Morphine (7TM)	IBNtxA (6TM)
Analgesia	++++	++++
Thermal	++++	++++
Inflammatory	++	++++
Neuropathic	+	++++
Respiratory depression	++++	–
Constipation	++++	+
Sedation	++++	+
Reward	++++	–
Physical dependence	++++	–
Straub tail	++	–

In vivo pharmacological properties of morphine, an agonist working through 7TM variants (7TM) and IBNtxA, an agonist working through 6TM variants, are compared. The number of + signs indicates the degree of analgesic potency or the severity of side effects. The more + signs, the more potent or severe the effect – not observed

2014) (Table 2). IBNtxA analgesia was active in a triple KO mouse from the Pintar lab, in which DOR-1, KOR-1, and all E1-associated 7TM MOR variants were disrupted except for the truncated 6TM variants, suggesting that DOR-1, KOR-1, and 7TM MOR variants are not involved in IBNtxA analgesia. Moreover, IBNtxA analgesia was lost in mE11-KO mice. Together, these observations imply that E11-associated 6TM variants are the targets for IBNtxA analgesia.

Opioid receptor binding studies with ^{125}I-labeled IBNtxA identifies an opioid binding site in the triple KO mice that is lost in both the E11-KO and E2-KO mice (Majumdar et al. 2011), consistent with its analgesic action in these mouse models. Competition studies revealed that the selectivity of the binding site is unique. Many traditional mu opioid receptor drugs, such as morphine and DAMGO, delta opioid receptor drugs such as DPDPE, and kappa opioid receptor drugs, such as U50,488H, had very poor affinity for the site. However, a large number of established opioid analgesics, such as ketocyclazocine and NalBzoH, showed high affinity toward this site.

8.3.2 Gain of Function Studies: Lentiviral Rescue of IBNtxA Analgesia

To confirm the role of truncated 6TM variants in IBNtxA analgesia, a gain of function study using a lentivirus expressing a 6TM variant mMOR-1G was conducted in a double E1-/E11-KO mouse that did not express any of the *Oprm1* splice variants and had no analgesic responses to all the mu receptor agonists such as morphine and fentanyl, as well as IBNtxA (Lu et al. 2015). Intrathecal administration of the lentivirus expressing mMOR-1G (Lenti-M1G) restored IBNtxA analgesia, which was consistent with lentivirus expression and increased ^{125}I-IBNtxA binding in the spinal cord of E1-/E11-KO mice (Lu et al. 2015). Lenti-M1G also restored ketocyclazocine analgesia. However, Lenti-M1G was unable to restore high doses of the other opioids, such as morphine, fentanyl, and buprenorphine. These results suggest that the 6TM variant mMOR-1G is both necessary and sufficient for IBNtxA analgesia. The mouse *Oprm1* gene has five 6TM variants: mMOR-1G, mMOR-1M, mMOR-1N, mMOR-1K, and mMOR-1L. Further studies using lentivirus expressing individual 6TM variants demonstrated that each of individual 6TM variants rescued IBNtxA analgesia, but not morphine analgesia, confirming the role of 6TM variants in IBNtxA analgesia (Lu et al. 2018). Thus, 6TM variants provide potential therapeutic targets for a distinct type of analgesics that are potent against broad-spectrum pain models without many of the side effects associated with traditional opiates.

8.3.3 Classification of Opioids Based on the *Oprm1* Variant Targets

Studies using gene targeting mouse models and lentiviral rescue provide useful information to classify opioids into three categories based on their receptor targets (Table 3). The first category of opioids is 7TM-dependent or E1-dependent, such as morphine and methadone. Both morphine and methadone analgesia were active in E11-KO mice (Pan et al. 2009) but lost in the E1-KO (Schuller et al. 1999) and E1-/E11-KO mice (Lu et al. 2015). Lentivirus expressing 6TM variants did not restore their analgesia in E1-/E11-KO mice (Lu et al. 2015). These results suggest that these opioid agonists work through 7TM variants, not 6TM variants. The second category is 6TM-dependent or E11-dependent, such as IBNtxA and levorphanol. Although IBNtxA analgesia was eliminated in E11-KO (Majumdar et al. 2011) and E1-/E11-KO mice (Lu et al. 2015), IBNtxA was still active in E1-KO and triple KO mice in which 6TM variants are present (Majumdar et al. 2011). 6TM variants alone were able to restore IBNtxA analgesia in E1-/E11-KO mice (Lu et al. 2015), further confirming that IBNtxA targets 6TM variants. The third category is both 7TM- and 6TM-dependent and E1- and E11-dependent. Buprenorphine and levorphanol belong to this category. Buprenorphine and levorphanol were inactive in both E11-KO (Grinnell et al. 2016) and E1-/E11-KO mice (Lu et al. 2015). Lentivirus expressing 6TM variants rescued buprenorphine and levorphanol analgesia in E11-KO mice that still express 7TM variants (Grinnell et al. 2016) but failed to rescue their analgesia in E1-/E11-KO mice (Lu et al. 2015), suggesting that their analgesia rely on both 7TM and 6TM variants.

Table 3 Classification of mu opioid agonists based on their *Oprm1* variant targets

Group	Variants required for analgesia	Drug
Group 1	7TM-dependent	Morphine Methadone DAMGO
Group 2	6TM-dependent	IBNtxA
Group 3	Both 7TM- and 6TM-dependent	Buprenorphine Levorphanol

8.3.4 The Role of 6TM Variants in Morphine Actions

Truncation of 6TM variants in E11-KO mice did not alter morphine analgesia (Marrone et al. 2017; Pan et al. 2009). However, E11-KO mice failed to develop morphine-induced hyperalgesia (Marrone et al. 2017). In contrast, a triple KO mouse is generated by crossing an E1-KO (Schuller et al. 1999) with delta and kappa receptor KO lost morphine analgesia but retained morphine hyperalgesia (Juni et al. 2007). These results suggest that morphine hyperalgesia requires only 6TM mechanisms, while morphine analgesia is mediated by 7TM receptors. Involvement of a 6TM variant MOR-1K in morphine hyperalgesia was also demonstrated in CXB7/ByJ mice. Downregulating MOR-1K mRNA using chronic intrathecal administration of a siRNA prevented the morphine-induced hyperalgesia (Oladosu et al. 2015). This effect was hypothesized to be mediated through G_s mechanism (Gris et al. 2010).

Truncation of 6TM variants in E11-KO mice also failed to produce morphine-induced hyperlocomotion and developed morphine tolerance more slowly than WT mice, while morphine reward and respiratory depression were not affected (Marrone et al. 2017). These results further illustrate that different morphine actions are mediated through distinct mechanisms.

8.3.5 The Functions of *OPRM1* Truncated Single TM Splice Variants

The abundance of the human single TM variant mRNA was quite high when compared to 7TM MOR-1 in neuroblastoma cells where they were initially isolated (Du et al. 1996), raising questions regarding their function. Using a TET-Off system in CHO cells, the single TM variants have been shown to function as a molecular chaperone for the full-length 7TM MOR-1 through heterodimerization in the ER to facilitate the proper conformation or folding of MOR-1, allowing its escape from the ERAD pathway and thereby increasing its overall expression (Xu et al. 2013). Downregulating a single TM variant mMOR-1S using a specific antisense oligonucleotide reduced both MOR-1 mRNA and receptor protein and also diminished morphine analgesia, suggesting the relevance of this variant in vivo (Xu et al. 2013).

9 Overall Conclusions

The challenge of mu opioid pharmacology today is no different than 100 years ago: develop mu agonists that retain analgesic efficacy but lack the serious side effects of traditional mu agonists. However, the current opioid overdose epidemic makes this goal more imperative than ever. Recent advances in our understanding of mu opioid pharmacology, including the tertiary structure of mu receptors and their ligand binding sites, the identification of biased and unbiased agonists, the heteromeric interaction of mu receptors with other GPCRs, and the discovery that different opioid agonists act through multiple splice variants of the mu receptors that do not mediate some of the side effects of traditional mu opioids, provide for the first time serious opportunities to achieve that goal.

References

Abbadie C, Pasternak GW (2001) Differential in vivo internalization of MOR-1 and MOR-1C by morphine. Neuroreport 12:3069–3072

Abbadie C, Gultekin SH, Pasternak GW (2000a) Immunohistochemical localization of the carboxy terminus of the novel mu opioid receptor splice variant MOR-1C within the human spinal cord. Neuroreport 11:1953–1957

Abbadie C, Pan Y-X, Drake CT, Pasternak GW (2000b) Comparative immunohistochemical distributions of carboxy terminus epitopes from the mu opioid receptor splice variants MOR-1D, MOR-1 and MOR-1C in the mouse and rat central nervous systems. Neuroscience 100:141–153

Abbadie C, Pasternak GW, Aicher SA (2001) Presynaptic localization of the carboxy-terminus epitopes of the mu opioid receptor splice variants MOR-1C and MOR-1D in the superficial laminae of the rat spinal cord. Neuroscience 106:833–842

Abdelhamid EE, Sultana M, Portoghese PS, Takemori AE (1991) Selective blockage of delta opioid receptors prevents the development of morphine tolerance and dependence in mice. J Pharmacol Exp Ther 258:299–303

Altarifi AA, David B, Muchhala KH, Blough BE, Akbarali H, Negus SS (2017) Effects of acute and repeated treatment with the biased mu opioid receptor agonist TRV130 (oliceridine) on measures of antinociception, gastrointestinal function, and abuse liability in rodents. J Psychopharmacol 31:730–739

Armenian P, Vo KT, Barr-Walker J, Lynch KL (2018) Fentanyl, fentanyl analogs and novel synthetic opioids: a comprehensive review. Neuropharmacology 134:121–132

Bare LA, Mansson E, Yang D (1994) Expression of two variants of the human m opioid receptor mRNA in SK-N-SH cells and human brain. FEBS Lett 354:213–216

Baumann MH, Kopajtic TA, Madras BK (2018) Pharmacological research as a key component in mitigating the opioid overdose crisis. Trends Pharmacol Sci 39:995–998

Belknap JK, Mogil JS, Helms ML, Richards SP, O'Toole LA, Bergeson SE, Buck KJ (1995) Localization to chromosome 10 of a locus influencing morphine analgesia in crosses derived from C57BL/6 and DBA/2 strains. Life Sci 57:L117–L124

Bisignano P, Burford NT, Shang Y, Marlow B, Livingston KE, Fenton AM, Rockwell K, Budenholzer L, Traynor JR, Gerritz SW, Alt A, Filizola M (2015) Ligand-based discovery of a new scaffold for allosteric modulation of the mu-opioid receptor. J Chem Inf Model 55:1836–1843

Black DL (2003) Mechanisms of alternative pre-messenger RNA splicing. Annu Rev Biochem 72:291–336

Blume AJ (1978) Interaction of ligands with opiate receptors of brain membranes – regulation by ions and nucleotides. Proc Natl Acad Sci U S A 75:1713–1717

Bohn LM, Lefkowitz RJ, Gainetdinov RR, Peppel K, Caron MG, Lin FT (1999) Enhanced morphine analgesia in mice lacking b-arrestin 2. Science 286:2495–2498

Bohn LM, Gainetdinov RR, Lin FT, Lefkowitz RJ, Caron MG (2000) Mu-opioid receptor desensitization by beta-arrestin-2 determines morphine tolerance but not dependence. Nature 408:720–723

Bohn LM, Lefkowitz RJ, Caron MG (2002) Differential mechanisms of morphine antinociceptive tolerance revealed in (beta)arrestin-2 knock-out mice. J Neurosci 22:10494–10500

Bohn LM, Gainetdinov RR, Sotnikova TD, Medvedev IO, Lefkowitz RJ, Dykstra LA, Caron MG (2003) Enhanced rewarding properties of morphine, but not cocaine, in beta(arrestin)-2 knock-out mice. J Neurosci 23:10265–10273

Bolan EA, Pan YX, Pasternak GW (2004) Functional analysis of MOR-1 splice variants of the mouse mu opioid receptor gene Oprm. Synapse 51:11–18

Breivogel CS, Selley DE, Childers SR (1997) Acute and chronic effects of opioids on delta and mu receptor activation of G proteins in NG108-15 and SK-N-SH cell membranes. J Neurochem 68:1462–1472

Burford NT, Clark MJ, Wehrman TS, Gerritz SW, Banks M, O'Connell J, Traynor JR, Alt A (2013) Discovery of positive allosteric modulators and silent allosteric modulators of the mu-opioid receptor. Proc Natl Acad Sci U S A 110:10830–10835

Burford NT, Traynor JR, Alt A (2015) Positive allosteric modulators of the mu-opioid receptor: a novel approach for future pain medications. Br J Pharmacol 172:277–286

Cadet P, Mantione KJ, Stefano GB (2003) Molecular identification and functional expression of mu 3, a novel alternatively spliced variant of the human mu opiate receptor gene. J Immunol 170:5118–5123

Cadet P, Mantione KJ, Zhu W, Kream RM, Sheehan M, Stefano GB (2007) A functionally coupled mu3-like opiate receptor/nitric oxide regulatory pathway in human multi-lineage progenitor cells. J Immunol 179:5839–5844

Carpenter B, Tate CG (2017) Active state structures of G protein-coupled receptors highlight the similarities and differences in the G protein and arrestin coupling interfaces. Curr Opin Struct Biol 45:124–132

Chang YF, Imam JS, Wilkinson MF (2007) The nonsense-mediated decay RNA surveillance pathway. Annu Rev Biochem 76:51–74

Cherny N, Ripamonti C, Pereira J, Davis C, Fallon M, McQuay H, Mercadante S, Pasternak G, Ventafridda V (2001) Strategies to manage the adverse effects of oral morphine: an evidence-based report. J Clin Oncol 19:2542–2554

Childers SR, Snyder SH (1980) Differential regulation by guanine nucleotides of opiate agonist and antagonist receptor interactions. J Neurochem 34:583–593

Choi HS, Kim CS, Hwang CK, Song KY, Wang W, Qiu Y, Law PY, Wei LN, Loh HH (2006) The opioid ligand binding of human mu-opioid receptor is modulated by novel splice variants of the receptor. Biochem Biophys Res Commun 343:1132–1140

Chou R, Fanciullo GJ, Fine PG, Adler JA, Ballantyne JC, Davies P, Donovan MI, Fishbain DA, Foley KM, Fudin J, Gilson AM, Kelter A, Mauskop A, O'Connor PG, Passik SD, Pasternak GW, Portenoy RK, Rich BA, Roberts RG, Todd KH, Miaskowski C, American Pain Society-American Academy of Pain Medicine Opioids Guidelines Panel (2009) Clinical guidelines for the use of chronic opioid therapy in chronic noncancer pain. J Pain 10:113–130

Claing A, Laporte SA, Caron MG, Lefkowitz RJ (2002) Endocytosis of G protein-coupled receptors: roles of G protein-coupled receptor kinases and beta-arrestin proteins. Prog Neurobiol 66:61–79

Cunningham CW, Elballa WM, Vold SU (2019) Bifunctional opioid receptor ligands as novel analgesics. Neuropharmacology 151:195–207

Deng HB, Yu Y, Pak Y, O'Dowd BF, George SR, Surratt CK, Uhl GR, Wang JB (2000) Role for the C-terminus in agonist-induced mu opioid receptor phosphorylation and desensitization. Biochemistry 39:5492–5499

DeWire SM, Yamashita DS, Rominger DH, Liu G, Cowan CL, Graczyk TM, Chen XT, Pitis PM, Gotchev D, Yuan C, Koblish M, Lark MW, Violin JD (2013) A G protein-biased ligand at the mu-opioid receptor is potently analgesic with reduced gastrointestinal and respiratory dysfunction compared with morphine. J Pharmacol Exp Ther 344:708–717

Dietis N, Niwa H, Tose R, McDonald J, Ruggieri V, Filaferro M, Vitale G, Micheli L, Ghelardini C, Salvadori S, Calo G, Guerrini R, Rowbotham DJ, Lambert DG (2018) In vitro and in vivo characterization of the bifunctional and opioid receptor ligand UFP-505. Br J Pharmacol 175:2881–2896

Ding HP, Czoty PW, Kiguchi N, Cami-Kobeci G, Sukhtankar DD, Nader MA, Husbands SM, Ko MC (2016) A novel orvinol analog, BU08028, as a safe opioid analgesic without abuse liability in primates. Proc Natl Acad Sci U S A 113:E5511–E5518

Ding HP, Kiguchi N, Yasuda D, Daga PR, Polgar WE, Lu JJ, Czoty PW, Kishioka S, Zaveri NT, Ko MC (2018) A bifunctional nociceptin and mu opioid receptor agonist is analgesic without opioid side effects in nonhuman primates. Sci Transl Med 10:eaar3483

Doll C, Konietzko J, Poll F, Koch T, Hollt V, Schulz S (2011) Agonist-selective patterns of mu-opioid receptor phosphorylation revealed by phosphosite-specific antibodies. Br J Pharmacol 164:298–307

Doyle GA, Rebecca SX, Lin SS, Press DM, Grice DE, Buono RJ, Ferraro TN, Berrettini WH (2007a) Identification of three mouse micro-opioid receptor (MOR) gene (Oprm1) splice variants containing a newly identified alternatively spliced exon. Gene 388:135–147

Doyle GA, Sheng XR, Lin SS, Press DM, Grice DE, Buono RJ, Ferraro TN, Berrettini WH (2007b) Identification of five mouse mu-opioid receptor (MOR) gene (Oprm1) splice variants containing a newly identified alternatively spliced exon. Gene 395:98–107

Du Y-L, Pan Y-X, Pasternak GW, Inturrisi CE (1996) Identification of a novel splice variant of the mouse mu opioid receptor. Soc Neurosci 22:1766

Du Y-L, Elliot K, Pan Y-X, Pasternak GW, Inturrisi CE (1997) A splice variant of the mu opioid receptor is present in human SHSY-5Y cells. Soc Neurosci 23:1206

Evans RM, You H, Hameed S, Altier C, Mezghrani A, Bourinet E, Zamponi GW (2010) Heterodimerization of ORL1 and opioid receptors and its consequences for N-type calcium channel regulation. J Biol Chem 285:1032–1040

Fujita W, Gomes I, Devi LA (2015) Heteromers of mu-delta opioid receptors: new pharmacology and novel therapeutic possibilities. Br J Pharmacol 172:375–387

George SR, Fan T, Xie ZD, Tse R, Tam V, Varghese G, O'Dowd BF (2000) Oligomerization of mu- and delta-opioid receptors – generation of novel functional properties. J Biol Chem 275:26128–26135

Giros B, Pohl M, Rochelle JM, Seldin MF (1995) Chromosomal localization of opioid peptide and receptor genes in the mouse. Life Sci 56:PL369–PL375

Gluck L, Loktev A, Mouledous L, Mollereau C, Law PY, Schulz S (2014) Loss of morphine reward and dependence in mice lacking G protein-coupled receptor kinase 5. Biol Psychiatry 76:767–774

Grecksch G, Just S, Pierstorff C, Imhof AK, Gluck L, Doll C, Lupp A, Becker A, Koch T, Stumm R, Hollt V, Schulz S (2011) Analgesic tolerance to high-efficacy agonists but not to morphine is diminished in phosphorylation-deficient S375A mu-opioid receptor knock-in mice. J Neurosci 31:13890–13896

Grinnell SG, Ansonoff M, Marrone GF, Lu Z, Narayan A, Xu J, Rossi G, Majumdar S, Pan YX, Bassoni DL, Pintar J, Pasternak GW (2016) Mediation of buprenorphine analgesia by a combination of traditional and truncated mu opioid receptor splice variants. Synapse 70:395–407

Gris P, Gauthier J, Cheng P, Gibson DG, Gris D, Laur O, Pierson J, Wentworth S, Nackley AG, Maixner W, Diatchenko L (2010) A novel alternatively spliced isoform of the mu-opioid receptor: functional antagonism. Mol Pain 6:33

Groer CE, Tidgewell K, Moyer RA, Harding WW, Rothman RB, Prisinzano TE, Bohn LM (2007) An opioid agonist that does not induce mu-opioid receptor – arrestin interactions or receptor internalization. Mol Pharmacol 71:549–557

He SQ, Zhang ZN, Guan JS, Liu HR, Zhao B, Wang HB, Li Q, Yang H, Luo J, Li ZY, Wang Q, Lu YJ, Bao L, Zhang X (2011) Facilitation of mu-opioid receptor activity by preventing delta-opioid receptor-mediated codegradation. Neuron 69:120–131

Hothersall JD, Torella R, Humphreys S, Hooley M, Brown A, McMurray G, Nickolls SA (2017) Residues W320 and Y328 within the binding site of the mu-opioid receptor influence opiate ligand bias. Neuropharmacology 118:46–58

Huang WJ, Manglik A, Venkatakrishnan AJ, Laeremans T, Feinberg EN, Sanborn AL, Kato HE, Livingston KE, Thorsen TS, Kling RC, Granier S, Gmeiner P, Husbands SM, Traynor JR, Weis WI, Steyaert J, Dror RO, Kobilka BK (2015) Structural insights into mu-opioid receptor activation. Nature 524:315

Inturrisi CE (2002) Clinical pharmacology of opioids for pain. Clin J Pain 18:S3–S13

Jalal H, Buchanich JM, Roberts MS, Balmert LC, Zhang K, Burke DS (2018) Changing dynamics of the drug overdose epidemic in the United States from 1979 through 2016. Science 361: eaau1184

Juni A, Klein G, Pintar JE, Kest B (2007) Nociception increases during opioid infusion in opioid receptor triple knock-out mice. Neuroscience 147:439–444

Just S, Illing S, Trester-Zedlitz M, Lau EK, Kotowski SJ, Miess E, Mann A, Doll C, Trinidad JC, Burlingame AL, von Zastrow M, Schulz S (2013) Differentiation of opioid drug effects by hierarchical multi-site phosphorylation. Mol Pharmacol 83:633–639

Kathmann M, Flau K, Redmer A, Trankle C, Schlicker E (2006) Cannabidiol is an allosteric modulator at mu- and delta-opioid receptors. Naunyn Schmiedebergs Arch Pharmacol 372:354–361

Kelly E (2013) Efficacy and ligand bias at the mu-opioid receptor. Br J Pharmacol 169:1430–1446

Kenakin T (2014) What is pharmacological 'affinity'? Relevance to biased agonism and antagonism. Trends Pharmacol Sci 35:434–441

Kenakin T, Watson C, Muniz-Medina V, Christopoulos A, Novick S (2012) A simple method for quantifying functional selectivity and agonist bias. ACS Chem Neurosci 3:193–203

Kest B, Hopkins E, Palmese CA, Adler M, Mogil JS (2002a) Genetic variation in morphine analgesic tolerance: a survey of 11 inbred mouse strains. Pharmacol Biochem Behav 73:821–828

Kest B, Palmese CA, Hopkins E, Adler M, Juni A, Mogil JS (2002b) Naloxone-precipitated withdrawal jumping in 11 inbred mouse strains: evidence for common genetic mechanisms in acute and chronic morphine physical dependence. Neuroscience 115:463–469

Khroyan TV, Polgar WE, Cami-Kobeci G, Husbands SM, Zaveri NT, Toll L (2011) The first universal opioid ligand, (2S)-2-[(5R,6R,7R,14S)-N-cyclopropylmethyl-4,5-epoxy-6,14-ethano-3-hydroxy-6-methoxymorphinan-7-yl]-3,3-dimethylpentan-2-ol (BU08028): characterization of the in vitro profile and in vivo behavioral effects in mouse models of acute pain and cocaine-induced reward. J Pharmacol Exp Ther 336:952–961

Klein G, Juni A, Waxman AR, Arout CA, Inturrisi CE, Kest B (2008) A survey of acute and chronic heroin dependence in ten inbred mouse strains: evidence of genetic correlation with morphine dependence. Pharmacol Biochem Behav 90:447–452

Kliewer A, Schmiedel F, Sianati S, Bailey A, Bateman JT, Levitt ES, Williams JT, Christie MJ, Schulz S (2019) Phosphorylation-deficient G-protein-biased mu-opioid receptors improve analgesia and diminish tolerance but worsen opioid side effects. Nat Commun 10:367

Koch T, Schulz S, Schroder H, Wolf R, Raulf E, Hollt V (1998) Carboxyl-terminal splicing of the rat mu opioid receptor modulates agonist-mediated internalization and receptor resensitization. J Biol Chem 273:13652–13657

Koehl A, Hu HL, Maeda S, Zhang Y, Qu QH, Paggi JM, Latorraca NR, Hilger D, Dawson R, Matile H, Schertler GFX, Granier S, Weis WI, Dror RO, Manglik A, Skiniotis G, Kobilka BK (2018) Structure of the mu-opioid receptor-G(i) protein complex. Nature 558:547

Kozak CA, Filie J, Adamson MC, Chen Y, Yu L (1994) Murine chromosomal location of the m and kappa opioid receptor genes. Genomics 21:659–661

Kvam TM, Baar C, Rakvag TT, Kaasa S, Krokan HE, Skorpen F (2004) Genetic analysis of the murine mu opioid receptor: increased complexity of Oprm gene splicing. J Mol Med 82:250–255

Lamb K, Tidgewell K, Simpson DS, Bohn LM, Prisinzano TE (2012) Antinociceptive effects of herkinorin, a MOP receptor agonist derived from salvinorin A in the formalin test in rats: new concepts in mu opioid receptor pharmacology: from a symposium on new concepts in mu-opioid pharmacology. Drug Alcohol Depend 121:181–188

Law PY, Wong YH, Loh HH (2000) Molecular mechanisms and regulation of opioid receptor signaling. Annu Rev Pharmacol Toxicol 40:389–430

Lejeune F, Maquat LE (2005) Mechanistic links between nonsense-mediated mRNA decay and pre-mRNA splicing in mammalian cells. Curr Opin Cell Biol 17:309–315

Livingston KE, Traynor JR (2014) Disruption of the Na+ ion binding site as a mechanism for positive allosteric modulation of the mu-opioid receptor. Proc Natl Acad Sci U S A 111:18369–18374

Livingston KE, Traynor JR (2018) Allostery at opioid receptors: modulation with small molecule ligands. Br J Pharmacol 175:2846–2856

Lohse MJ, Benovic JL, Codina J, Caron MG, Lefkowitz RJ (1990) Beta-Arrestin – a protein that regulates beta-adrenergic-receptor function. Science 248:1547–1550

Lord JAH, Waterfield AA, Hughes J, Kosterlitz HW (1977) Endogenous opioid peptides: multiple agonists and receptors. Nature 267:495–499

Lu Z, Xu J, Xu M, Pasternak GW, Pan YX (2014) Morphine regulates expression of mu-opioid receptor MOR-1A, an intron-retention carboxyl terminal splice variant of the mu-opioid receptor (OPRM1) gene via miR-103/miR-107. Mol Pharmacol 85:368–380

Lu Z, Xu J, Rossi GC, Majumdar S, Pasternak GW, Pan YX (2015) Mediation of opioid analgesia by a truncated 6-transmembrane GPCR. J Clin Invest 125:2626–2630

Lu Z, Xu J, Xu M, Rossi GC, Majumdar S, Pasternak GW, Pan YX (2018) Truncated mu-opioid receptors with 6 transmembrane domains are essential for opioid analgesia. Anesth Analg 126:1050–1057

Ma MJ, Sun JL, Li MH, Yu ZX, Cheng JC, Zhong BH, Shi WG (2019) Synthesis and evaluation of novel biased-opioid-receptor (OR) agonists. Molecules 24:259

Madariaga-Mazon A, Marmolejo-Valencia AF, Li YM, Toll L, Houghten RA, Martinez-Mayorga K (2017) Mu-opioid receptor biased ligands: a safer and painless discovery of analgesics? Drug Discov Today 22:1719–1729

Maeda S, Koehl A, Matile H, Hu HL, Hilger D, Schertler GFX, Manglik A, Skiniotis G, Dawson RJP, Kobilka BK (2018) Development of an antibody fragment that stabilizes GPCR/G-protein complexes. Nat Commun 9:3712

Majumdar S, Grinnell S, Le RV, Burgman M, Polikar L, Ansonoff M, Pintar J, Pan YX, Pasternak GW (2011) Truncated G protein-coupled mu opioid receptor MOR-1 splice variants are targets for highly potent opioid analgesics lacking side effects. Proc Natl Acad Sci U S A 108:19778–19783

Majumdar S, Subrath J, Le RV, Polikar L, Burgman M, Nagakura K, Ocampo J, Haselton N, Pasternak AR, Grinnell S, Pan YX, Pasternak GW (2012) Synthesis and evaluation of aryl-naloxamide opiate analgesics targeting truncated exon 11-associated mu opioid receptor (MOR-1) splice variants. J Med Chem 55:6352–6362

Manglik A, Kruse AC, Kobilka TS, Thian FS, Mathiesen JM, Sunahara RK, Pardo L, Weis WI, Kobilka BK, Granier S (2012) Crystal structure of the mu-opioid receptor bound to a morphinan antagonist. Nature 485:321–326

Manglik A, Lin H, Aryal DK, McCorvy JD, Dengler D, Corder G, Levit A, Kling RC, Bernat V, Hubner H, Huang XP, Sassano MF, Giguere PM, Lober S, Duan D, Scherrer G, Kobilka BK, Gmeiner P, Roth BL, Shoichet BK (2016) Structure-based discovery of opioid analgesics with reduced side effects. Nature 537:185

Manglik A, Kobilka BK, Steyaert J (2017) Nanobodies to study G protein-coupled receptor structure and function. Annu Rev Pharmacol 57:19–37

Marrone GF, Le Rouzic V, Varadi A, Xu J, Rajadhyaksha AM, Majumdar S, Pan YX, Pasternak GW (2017) Genetic dissociation of morphine analgesia from hyperalgesia in mice. Psychopharmacology 234:1891–1900

Martin WR, Eades CG, Thompson JA, Huppler RE, Gilbert PE (1976) The effects of morphine and nalorphine-like drugs in the nondependent and morphine-dependent chronic spinal dog. J Pharmacol Exp Ther 197:517–532

Matthes HWD, Maldonado R, Simonin F, Valverde O, Slowe S, Kitchen I, Befort K, Dierich A, Le Meur M, Dollé P, Tzavara E, Hanoune J, Roques BP, Kieffer BL (1996) Loss of morphine-induced analgesia, reward effect and withdrawal symptoms in mice lacking the m-opioid-receptor gene. Nature 383:819–823

Miess E, Gondin AB, Yousuf A, Steinborn R, Mosslein N, Yang YS, Goldner M, Ruland JG, Bunemann M, Krasel C, Christie MJ, Halls ML, Schulz S, Canals M (2018) Multisite phosphorylation is required for sustained interaction with GRKs and arrestins during rapid mu-opioid receptor desensitization. Sci Signal 11:eaas9609

Mosberg HI, Yeomans L, Anand JP, Porter V, Sohczyk-Kojiro K, Traynor JR, Jutkiewicz EM (2014) Development of a bioavailable mu opioid receptor (MOPr) agonist, delta opioid receptor

(DOPr) antagonist peptide that evokes antinociception without development of acute tolerance. J Med Chem 57:3148–3153
Negus SS, Freeman KB (2018) Abuse potential of biased mu opioid receptor agonists. Trends Pharmacol Sci 39:916–919
Nitsche JF, Schuller AGP, King MA, Zengh M, Pasternak GW, Pintar JE (2002) Genetic dissociation of opiate tolerance and physical dependence in delta-opioid receptor-1 and preproenkephalin knock-out mice. J Neurosci 22:10906–10913
North RA, Williams JT (1985) On the potassium conductance increased by opioids in rat locus coeruleus neurons. J Physiol 364:265–280
Nygaard R, Zou YZ, Dror RO, Mildorf TJ, Arlow DH, Manglik A, Pan AC, Liu CW, Fung JJ, Bokoch MP, Thian FS, Kobilka TS, Shaw DE, Mueller L, Prosser RS, Kobilka BK (2013) The dynamic process of beta(2)-adrenergic receptor activation. Cell 152:532–542
Oladosu FA, Conrad MS, O'Buckley SC, Rashid NU, Slade GD, Nackley AG (2015) Mu opioid splice variant MOR-1K contributes to the development of opioid-induced hyperalgesia. PLoS One 10:e0135711
Pan YX (2002) Identification and characterization of a novel promoter of the mouse mu opioid receptor gene (Oprm) that generates eight splice variants. Gene 295:97–108
Pan YX (2005) Diversity and complexity of the mu opioid receptor gene: alternative pre-mRNA splicing and promoters. DNA Cell Biol 24:736–750
Pan YX, Xu J, Bolan E, Abbadie C, Chang A, Zuckerman A, Rossi G, Pasternak GW (1999a) Identification and characterization of three new alternatively spliced mu-opioid receptor isoforms. Mol Pharmacol 56:396–403
Pan YX, Xu J, Bolan E, Abbadie C, Chang A, Zuckerman A, Rossi G, Pasternak GW (1999b) Identification and characterization of three new alternatively spliced mu-opioid receptor isoforms. Mol Pharmacol 56:396–403
Pan YX, Xu J, Bolan E, Chang A, Mahurter L, Rossi G, Pasternak GW (2000) Isolation and expression of a novel alternatively spliced mu opioid receptor isoform, MOR-1F. FEBS Lett 466:337–340
Pan YX, Xu A, Mahurter L, Bolan E, Xu MM, Pasternak GW (2001) Generation of the mu opioid receptor (MOR-1) protein by three new splice variants of the Oprm gene. Proc Natl Acad Sci U S A 98:14084–14089
Pan YX, Bolan E, Pasternak GW (2002) Dimerization of morphine and orphanin FQ/nociceptin receptors: generation of a novel opioid receptor subtype. Biochem Biophys Res Commun 297:659–663
Pan YX, Xu J, Mahurter L, Xu M, Gilbert AK, Pasternak GW (2003) Identification and characterization of two new human mu opioid receptor splice variants, hMOR-1O and hMOR-1X. Biochem Biophys Res Commun 301:1057–1061
Pan L, Xu J, Yu R, Xu MM, Pan YX, Pasternak GW (2005a) Identification and characterization of six new alternatively spliced variants of the human mu opioid receptor gene, Oprm. Neuroscience 133:209–220
Pan YX, Xu J, Bolan E, Moskowitz HS, Xu M, Pasternak GW (2005b) Identification of four novel exon 5 splice variants of the mouse mu-opioid receptor gene: functional consequences of C-terminal splicing. Mol Pharmacol 68:866–875
Pan YX, Xu J, Xu M, Rossi GC, Matulonis JE, Pasternak GW (2009) Involvement of exon 11-associated variants of the mu opioid receptor MOR-1 in heroin, but not morphine, actions. Proc Natl Acad Sci 106:4917–4922
Pasternak GW (2001) The pharmacology of mu analgesics: from patients to genes. Neuroscientist 7:220–231
Pasternak GW, Pan Y-X (2000) Antisense mapping: assessing the functional significance of genes and splice variants. In: Phillips MI (ed) Antisense techniques. Academic Press, Orlando, pp 51–60
Pasternak GW, Pan YX (2013) Mu opioids and their receptors: evolution of a concept. Pharmacol Rev 65:1257–1317

Pasternak DA, Pan L, Xu J, Yu R, Xu MM, Pasternak GW, Pan YX (2004) Identification of three new alternatively spliced variants of the rat mu opioid receptor gene: dissociation of affinity and efficacy. J Neurochem 91:881–890

Pert CB, Pasternak GW, Snyder SH (1973) Opiate agonists and antagonists discriminated by receptor binding in brain. Science 182:1359–1361

Raehal KM, Bohn LM (2011) The role of beta-arrestin2 in the severity of antinociceptive tolerance and physical dependence induced by different opioid pain therapeutics. Neuropharmacology 60:58–65

Raehal KM, Bohn LM (2014) Beta-arrestins: regulatory role and therapeutic potential in opioid and cannabinoid receptor-mediated analgesia. Handb Exp Pharmacol 219:427–443

Raehal KM, Walker JK, Bohn LM (2005) Morphine side effects in beta-arrestin 2 knockout mice. J Pharmacol Exp Ther 314:1195–1201

Raffa RB, Burdge G, Gambrah J, Kinecki HE, Lin F, Lu B, Nguyen JT, Phan V, Ruan A, Sesay MA, Watkins TN (2017) Cebranopadol: novel dual opioid/NOP receptor agonist analgesic. J Clin Pharm Ther 42:8–17

Raynor K, Kong H, Mestek A, Bye LS, Tian M, Liu J, Yu L, Reisine T (1995) Characterization of the cloned human mu opioid receptor. J Pharmacol Exp Ther 272:423–428

Remesic M, Hruby VJ, Porreca F, Lee YS (2017) Recent advances in the realm of allosteric modulators for opioid receptors for future therapeutics. ACS Chem Neurosci 8:1147–1158

Rosenbaum DM, Cherezov V, Hanson MA, Rasmussen SGF, Thian FS, Kobilka TS, Choi HJ, Yao XJ, Weis WI, Stevens RC, Kobilka BK (2007) GPCR engineering yields high-resolution structural insights into beta(2)-adrenergic receptor function. Science 318:1266–1273

Rossi GC, Pan Y-X, Cheng J, Pasternak GW (1994) Blockade of morphine analgesia by an antisense oligodeoxynucleotide against the mu receptor. Life Sci 54:PL375–PL379

Rossi GC, Pan YX, Brown GP, Pasternak GW (1995) Antisense mapping the MOR-1 opioid receptor – evidence for alternative splicing and a novel morphine-6-beta-glucuronide receptor. FEBS Lett 369:192–196

Rothman RB, Murphy DL, Xu H, Godin JA, Dersch CM, Partilla JS, Tidgewell K, Schmidt M, Prisinzano TE (2007) Salvinorin A: allosteric interactions at the mu-opioid receptor. J Pharmacol Exp Ther 320:801–810

Rudd RA, Seth P, David F, Scholl L (2016) Increases in drug and opioid-involved overdose deaths – United States, 2010-2015. MMWR Morb Mortal Wkly Rep 65:1445–1452

Satoh M, Minami M (1995) Molecular pharmacology of the opioid receptors. Pharmacol Ther 68:343–364

Schmid CL, Kennedy NM, Ross NC, Lovell KM, Yue ZZ, Morgenweck J, Cameron MD, Bannister TD, Bohn LM (2017) Bias factor and therapeutic window correlate to predict safer opioid analgesics. Cell 171:1165

Schroeder JE, Fischbach PS, Zheng D, Mccleskey EW (1991) Activation of mu-opioid receptors inhibits transient high-threshold and low-threshold Ca2+ currents, but spares a sustained current. Neuron 6:13–20

Schuller AG, King MA, Zhang J, Bolan E, Pan YX, Morgan DJ, Chang A, Czick ME, Unterwald EM, Pasternak GW, Pintar JE (1999) Retention of heroin and morphine-6 beta-glucuronide analgesia in a new line of mice lacking exon 1 of MOR-1. Nat Neurosci 2:151–156

Schwienteck KL, Faunce KE, Rice KC, Obeng S, Zhang Y, Blough BE, Grim TW, Negus SS, Banks ML (2019) Effectiveness comparisons of G-protein biased and unbiased mu opioid receptor ligands in warm water tail-withdrawal and drug discrimination in male and female rats. Neuropharmacology 150:200–209

Seth P, Scholl L, Rudd RA, Bacon S (2018) Overdose deaths involving opioids, cocaine, and psychostimulants – United States, 2015-2016. MMWR Morb Mortal Wkly Rep 67:349–358

Seward E, Hammond C, Henderson G (1991) Mu-opioid-receptor-mediated inhibition of the N-type calcium-channel current. Proc Biol Sci 244:129–135

Shabalina SA, Zaykin DV, Gris P, Ogurtsov AY, Gauthier J, Shibata K, Tchivileva IE, Belfer I, Mishra B, Kiselycznyk C, Wallace MR, Staud R, Spiridonov NA, Max MB, Goldman D,

Fillingim RB, Maixner W, Diatchenko L (2009) Expansion of the human {micro}-opioid receptor gene architecture: novel functional variants. Hum Mol Genet 18:1037–1051
Sharma SK, Nirenberg M, Klee W (1975) Morphine receptors as regulators of adenylate cyclase activity. Proc Natl Acad Sci U S A 72:590–594
Sim-Selley LJ, Selley DE, Vogt LJ, Childers SR, Martin TJ (2000) Chronic heroin self-administration desensitizes m opioid receptor-activated G-proteins in specific regions of rat brain. J Neurosci 20:4555–4562
Singla N, Minkowitz HS, Soergel DG, Burt DA, Subach RA, Salamea MY, Fossler MJ, Skobieranda F (2017) A randomized, phase IIb study investigating oliceridine (TRV130), a novel mu-receptor G-protein pathway selective (mu-GPS) modulator, for the management of moderate to severe acute pain following abdominoplasty. J Pain Res 10:2413–2424
Siuda ER, Carr R, Rominger DH, Violin JD (2017) Biased mu-opioid receptor ligands: a promising new generation of pain therapeutics. Curr Opin Pharmacol 32:77–84
Soergel DG, Subach RA, Burnham N, Lark MW, James IE, Sadler BM, Skobieranda F, Violin JD, Webster LR (2014) Biased agonism of the mu-opioid receptor by TRV130 increases analgesia and reduces on-target adverse effects versus morphine: a randomized, double-blind, placebo-controlled, crossover study in healthy volunteers. Pain 155:1829–1835
Stefano GB, Hartman A, Bilfinger TV, Magazine HI, Liu Y, Casares F, Goligorsky MS (1995) Presence of the mu3 opiate receptor in endothelial cells. Coupling to nitric oxide production and vasodilation. J Biol Chem 270:30290–30293
Stoeber M, Jullie D, Lobingier BT, Laeremans T, Steyaert J, Schiller PW, Manglik A, von Zastrow M (2018) A genetically encoded biosensor reveals location bias of opioid drug action. Neuron 98:963
Tanowitz M, von Zastrow M (2003) A novel endocytic recycling signal that distinguishes the membrane trafficking of naturally occurring opioid receptors. J Biol Chem 278:45978–45986
Tanowitz M, Hislop JN, von Zastrow M (2008) Alternative splicing determines the post-endocytic sorting fate of G-protein-coupled receptors. J Biol Chem 283:35614–35621
Thakker DR, Standifer KM (2002) Induction of G protein-coupled receptor kinases 2 and 3 contributes to the cross-talk between mu and ORL1 receptors following prolonged agonist exposure. Neuropharmacology 43:979–990
Thompson RC, Mansour A, Akil H, Watson SJ (1993) Cloning and pharmacological characterization of a rat m opioid receptor. Neuron 11:903–913
Toll L, Bruchas MR, Calo G, Cox BM, Zaveri NT (2016) Nociceptin/orphanin FQ receptor structure, signaling, ligands, functions, and interactions with opioid systems. Pharmacol Rev 68:419–457
Urits I, Viswanath O, Orhurhu V, Gress K, Charipova K, Kaye AD, Ngo A (2019) The utilization of mu-opioid receptor biased agonists: oliceridine, an opioid analgesic with reduced adverse effects. Curr Pain Headache Rep 23:31
Valentino RJ, Volkow ND (2018) Untangling the complexity of opioid receptor function. Neuropsychopharmacology 43:2514–2520
van der Westhuizen ET, Breton B, Christopoulos A, Bouvier M (2014) Quantification of ligand bias for clinically relevant beta2-adrenergic receptor ligands: implications for drug taxonomy. Mol Pharmacol 85:492–509
Viscusi ER, Skobieranda F, Soergel DG, Cook E, Burt DA, Singla N (2019) APOLLO-1: a randomized placebo and active-controlled phase III study investigating oliceridine (TRV130), a G protein-biased ligand at the mu-opioid receptor, for management of moderate-to-severe acute pain following bunionectomy. J Pain Res 12:927–943
Von Zastrow M, Svingos A, Haberstock-Debic H, Evans C (2003) Regulated endocytosis of opioid receptors: cellular mechanisms and proposed roles in physiological adaptation to opiate drugs. Curr Opin Neurobiol 13:348–353
Waldhoer M, Bartlett SE, Whistler JL (2004) Opioid receptors. Annu Rev Biochem 73:953–990

Wang JB, Johnson PS, Persico AM, Hawkins AL, Griffin CA, Uhl GR (1994) Human [mu] opiate receptor: cDNA and genomic clones, pharmacologic characterization and chromosomal assignment. FEBS Lett 338:217–222

Wieskopf JS, Pan YX, Marcovitz J, Tuttle AH, Majumdar S, Pidakala J, Pasternak GW, Mogil JS (2014) Broad-spectrum analgesic efficacy of IBNtxA is mediated by exon 11-associated splice variants of the mu-opioid receptor gene. Pain 155:2063–2070

Williams JT, Ingram SL, Henderson G, Chavkin C, von Zastrow M, Schulz S, Koch T, Evans CJ, Christie MJ (2013) Regulation of mu-opioid receptors: desensitization, phosphorylation, internalization, and tolerance. Pharmacol Rev 65:223–254

Xu J, Xu M, Pan YX (2006) Characterizing exons 11 and 1 promoters of the mu opioid receptor (Oprm) gene in transgenic mice. BMC Mol Biol 7:41

Xu J, Xu M, Hurd YL, Pasternak GW, Pan YX (2009) Isolation and characterization of new exon 11-associated N-terminal splice variants of the human mu opioid receptor gene. J Neurochem 108:962–972

Xu J, Xu M, Rossi GC, Pasternak GW, Pan YX (2011) Identification and characterization of seven new exon 11-associated splice variants of the rat mu opioid receptor gene, OPRM1. Mol Pain 7:9

Xu J, Xu M, Brown T, Rossi GC, Hurd YL, Inturrisi CE, Pasternak GW, Pan YX (2013) Stabilization of the mu-opioid receptor by truncated single transmembrane splice variants through a chaperone-like action. J Biol Chem 288:21211–21227

Xu J, Lu Z, Xu M, Rossi GC, Kest B, Waxman AR, Pasternak GW, Pan YX (2014) Differential expressions of the alternatively spliced variant mRNAs of the micro opioid receptor gene, OPRM1, in brain regions of four inbred mouse strains. PLoS One 9:e111267

Xu J, Faskowitz AJ, Rossi GC, Xu M, Lu Z, Pan YX, Pasternak GW (2015) Stabilization of morphine tolerance with long-term dosing: association with selective upregulation of mu-opioid receptor splice variant mRNAs. Proc Natl Acad Sci U S A 112:279–284

Xu J, Lu Z, Narayan A, Le Rouzic VP, Xu M, Hunkele A, Brown TG, Hoefer WF, Rossi GC, Rice RC, Martinez-Rivera A, Rajadhyaksha AM, Cartegni L, Bassoni DL, Pasternak GW, Pan YX (2017) Alternatively spliced mu opioid receptor C termini impact the diverse actions of morphine. J Clin Invest 127:1561–1573

Zhou XE, He Y, de Waal PW, Gao X, Kang Y, Van Eps N, Yin Y, Pal K, Goswami D, White TA, Barty A, Latorraca NR, Chapman HN, Hubbell WL, Dror RO, Stevens RC, Cherezov V, Gurevich VV, Griffin PR, Ernst OP, Melcher K, Xu HE (2017) Identification of phosphorylation codes for arrestin recruitment by G protein-coupled receptors. Cell 170:457–469.e13

Zhu YX, King MA, Schuller AGP, Nitsche JF, Reidl M, Elde RP, Unterwald E, Pasternak GW, Pintar JE (1999) Retention of supraspinal delta-like analgesia and loss of morphine tolerance in d *opioid receptor* knockout mice. Neuron 24:243–252

Zhu W, Ma Y, Bell A, Esch T, Guarna M, Bilfinger TV, Bianchi E, Stefano GB (2004) Presence of morphine in rat amygdala: evidence for the mu3 opiate receptor subtype via nitric oxide release in limbic structures. Med Sci Monit 10:BR433–BR439

Zimprich A, Simon T, Hollt V (1995) Cloning and expression of an isoform of the rat m opioid receptor (rMOR 1 B) which differs in agonist induced desensitization from rMOR1. FEBS Lett 359:142–146

Behavioral Pharmacology of Drugs Acting at Mu Opioid Receptors

Lisa R. Gerak, David R. Maguire, and Charles P. France

Contents

1 Introduction 128
2 Pharmacodynamics and Pharmacokinetics of Drugs Acting at Opioid Receptors 128
3 Pharmacological Efficacy 130
3.1 Preclinical Assessment of Efficacy Differences 130
3.2 Therapeutic Considerations for Drugs that Vary in Efficacy 133
4 Drug-Receptor Interactions 136
4.1 Reversible Interactions and Surmountability 136
4.2 Allosteric Modulation of Mu Opioid Receptors 139
4.3 Biased Agonism 139
5 Selectivity for Opioid Receptor Types 140
6 Conclusions 141
References 141

Abstract

Despite the therapeutic utility of opioids for relieving pain, other behavioral effects, including their potential for abuse and overdose, can be quite detrimental

L. R. Gerak · D. R. Maguire
Department of Pharmacology, University of Texas Health Science Center at San Antonio, San Antonio, TX, USA

Addiction Research, Treatment and Training Center of Excellence, University of Texas Health Science Center at San Antonio, San Antonio, TX, USA

C. P. France (✉)
Department of Pharmacology, University of Texas Health Science Center at San Antonio, San Antonio, TX, USA

Addiction Research, Treatment and Training Center of Excellence, University of Texas Health Science Center at San Antonio, San Antonio, TX, USA

Department of Psychiatry, University of Texas Health Science Center at San Antonio, San Antonio, TX, USA
e-mail: france@uthscsa.edu

M. A. Nader, Y. L. Hurd (eds.), *Substance Use Disorders*,
Handbook of Experimental Pharmacology 258, https://doi.org/10.1007/164_2019_265

to individuals as well as society and have contributed to the ongoing opioid crisis. The dramatic escalation in overdose deaths over the last 15 years was initially driven by abuse of prescription opioids, although abuse of heroin, fentanyl, and fentanyl analogs has been increasing, largely due to increased availability and lower cost compared with prescription opioids. All of these opioids share pharmacological properties, acting as agonists at mu opioid receptors, and produce similar behavioral effects, including abuse-related, pain-relieving, dependence-producing, and respiratory-depressant effects. Despite their similarities, opioids are not pharmacologically identical. In fact, drugs that act at mu opioid receptors, including abused opioids, can vary on a number of dimensions, including pharmacological efficacy, drug-receptor interactions, receptor selectivity, and pharmacokinetics. Overall, these differences impact behavioral effects of drugs acting at mu opioid receptors, and this chapter describes variations in those behavioral effects and how these differences continue to provide new strategies that can be developed to address the ongoing opioid epidemic.

Keywords

Behavioral pharmacology · Drug-receptor interactions · Efficacy · Mu opioid receptors · Opioid abuse · Treatments

1 Introduction

Opioids have been used therapeutically (e.g., to relieve pain) and recreationally for centuries. In fact, widespread overuse of prescription opioids for pain relief has contributed to the current opioid crisis in the USA (Volkow and McLellan 2016). The common feature of opioids that are used therapeutically for pain and abused is that they act as agonists at mu opioid receptors. This shared mechanism of action results in qualitatively similar behavioral effects, although the effects of opioids are not identical. Since morphine was first isolated from opium in 1805, many other opioids have been synthesized and the pharmacology of these drugs can vary on a number of dimensions. These differences among drugs acting at opioid receptors impact their behavioral effects and have been exploited to improve treatment, to reduce adverse effects, and for recreational use. This chapter describes several dimensions on which opioids can vary, such as pharmacological efficacy, selectivity for mu over other opioid receptors, and the nature of the interaction between these drugs and their receptors. In addition to these pharmacodynamic differences, opioids can vary pharmacokinetically, which can alter their behavioral effects and impact their clinical and recreational use.

2 Pharmacodynamics and Pharmacokinetics of Drugs Acting at Opioid Receptors

While drugs acting at opioid receptors have been used for a long time, the opioid receptors themselves were identified and cloned much more recently (Chen et al. 1993; Gioannini et al. 1985; Pert et al. 1973; Simon et al. 1973; Terenius 1973).

Mu opioid receptors belong to the superfamily of G-protein-coupled receptors (GPCR), which is characterized by seven transmembrane-spanning regions and G-protein coupling; mu opioid receptors couple to G_i/G_o proteins. Receptor activation results in inhibition of adenylate cyclase and decreased levels of intracellular cAMP along with inhibition of voltage-gated Ca^{+2} channels, greater phosphorylation of mitogen-activated protein kinase (MAPK), and increased activity of inwardly rectifying K^+ channels and phospholipase C beta (Waldhoer et al. 2004). More recently, it has been shown that opioid receptors can interact with other second messenger systems in addition to G-proteins. For example, opioid receptor agonists can recruit β-arrestin signaling pathways, which can uncouple the receptor from G-proteins; the relative contribution of these and likely other second messenger systems depends on the agonist (e.g., Filizola 2019; Suida et al. 2017). This phenomenon by which agonists can bind to one receptor and differentially activate second messenger systems is called biased agonism and might account for some differences in the behavioral effects of agonists acting at mu opioid receptors, including abuse-related, pain-relieving, dependence-producing, and respiratory-depressant effects.

Although pharmacodynamic properties of mu opioid receptor agonists, including pharmacological efficacy, selectivity, and drug-receptor interactions, are primarily responsible for the behavioral effects of these drugs, pharmacokinetic properties can also play a role. For example, route of administration can affect the potency, effectiveness, and onset of action of drugs. Heroin and buprenorphine are self-administered by and produce positive subjective effects in humans, although the potency of heroin and the effectiveness of buprenorphine are significantly greater when the drugs are used intravenously (i.v.) compared with intranasally (i.n.; Comer et al. 1999; Jones et al. 2014). Moreover, route of administration can alter the time to peak plasma concentration, which can impact onset of action and lead to greater abuse. For example, peak plasma concentrations are achieved quicker when heroin and cocaine are smoked or taken i.v. compared with i.n. administration (Cone 1998). Another pharmacokinetic factor that can impact the behavioral effects of drugs, including abuse liability, is duration of action (Farré and Camí 1991; Vocci 1991); although fentanyl and remifentanil produce similar subjective and physiologic effects in humans, the very short duration of action of remifentanil makes it less appealing to drug abusers, who consistently report that they prefer to take drugs that last longer than remifentanil (Baylon et al. 2000). Duration of action can also affect the development of physical dependence. Other things being equal, drugs with long durations of action tend to produce physical dependence that is more robust than that produced by drugs with shorter durations of action, thereby resulting in the emergence of more severe withdrawal symptoms upon discontinuation of treatment. Paradoxically, however, discontinuation of treatment with drugs that have exceptionally long durations of action can result in a more mild withdrawal syndrome because the slow offset of these drugs prevents the abrupt changes in drug-receptor binding that are responsible for the emergence of severe withdrawal (e.g., Wolf and Griffiths 1991). Thus, pharmacokinetic factors can impact the behavioral effects of drugs, including abuse and physical dependence liability.

3 Pharmacological Efficacy

Efficacy is a property of a drug that indicates the level of effect that the drug can impart on the biological system once it is bound to the receptor. Drugs, including opioids, can vary along a continuum of efficacy, which means that the effects of drugs with affinity for a particular receptor can vary dramatically. For example, commonly used opioids, including heroin, oxycodone, and fentanyl, have high pharmacological efficacy at mu opioid receptors and are abused by humans, relieve moderate to severe pain, and decrease respiration. In contrast, other drugs used in the clinic have affinity at mu opioid receptors but no efficacy; these drugs, including naloxone and naltrexone, antagonize the effects of opioid receptor agonists and are used to block the effects of abused opioids and to reverse respiratory depression, thereby reducing the number of overdose deaths. Finally, some drugs that bind to mu opioid receptors have low efficacy, and these drugs can produce some, but not all, of the effects of the high-efficacy mu opioid receptor agonists. For example, the low-efficacy mu opioid receptor agonist buprenorphine is abused and can relieve pain; however, its effects on respiration are much more limited than those of high-efficacy agonists.

3.1 Preclinical Assessment of Efficacy Differences

Currently, there are three pharmacotherapies for opioid use disorder, methadone, buprenorphine, and naltrexone, and the primary difference among these drug treatments is efficacy. These differences are evident preclinically using behavioral procedures that model drug abuse, pain relief, and respiratory depression. For example, drug self-administration has been used to model aspects of drug abuse, providing face and predictive validity of human drug taking as well as informing on the molecular and neurobiological mechanisms of abuse-related behaviors (Spanagel 2017). Under a variety of conditions, mu opioid receptor agonists, including heroin, methadone, and buprenorphine, are self-administered by a variety of species, including humans and monkeys (Comer et al. 2005; Gerak et al. 2009; Jones et al. 2014; Maguire and France 2016; Mello et al. 1981a, b). In contrast, mu opioid receptor antagonists, like naltrexone, are not self-administered although they attenuate heroin self-administration (Maguire et al. 2019; Mello et al. 1981b). Thus, self-administration procedures can reveal efficacy differences between mu opioid receptor agonists and antagonists when these drugs are given alone or in combination, with the drug interactions predicted accurately by receptor theory (e.g., Kenakin 2008).

While opioid receptor antagonists can be differentiated from agonists using self-administration procedures, the efficacy requirements of many self-administration procedures are relatively low meaning that, under some experimental conditions, opioid receptor agonists with low efficacy are self-administered in a manner that is indistinguishable from high-efficacy agonists. However, variations in efficacy can be detected among mu opioid receptor agonists by changing the experimental conditions. For example, in monkey self-administration procedures, when the number of lever presses needed for delivery of an infusion of drug is relatively small, the low-efficacy mu opioid receptor agonist buprenorphine maintains high response rates, similar to those produced by opioids with higher efficacy; however, when a larger number of lever presses are required, buprenorphine differs from higher-efficacy drugs and maintains much lower responses rates, reflecting the higher-efficacy requirements of the assay and the low efficacy of buprenorphine (Balster and Lukas 1985). In those studies, the number of lever presses required for delivery of an infusion remained constant throughout the session (i.e., a fixed-ratio schedule). Another way to increase the efficacy requirements of self-administration procedures is to use a progressive-ratio schedule of reinforcement such that the number of lever presses required for delivery of an infusion increases across the session; under this schedule, the dependent variable is often reported as the largest ratio completed before subjects stop responding, or breakpoint. In monkeys, the largest ratio completed when buprenorphine is available for self-administration is two- to threefold lower than the largest ratio completed when heroin is available for self-administration (Mello et al. 1988). Efficacy requirements of self-administration procedures can also change as a result of chronic treatment with a mu opioid receptor agonist. In addition to the development of physical dependence, chronic treatment can also result in the development of tolerance (Young et al. 1991). With small treatment doses, self-administration of low-efficacy drugs like buprenorphine would be expected to decrease to a greater extent than self-administration of higher-efficacy drugs. Larger treatment doses would be needed to alter self-administration of drugs with higher efficacy, including heroin and fentanyl. Thus, the parameters of self-administration procedures, as well as the treatment conditions under which self-administration procedures are conducted, can be varied to examine efficacy differences among mu opioid agonists, although other factors, such as pharmacokinetics, can make interpretation more challenging for results of self-administration studies. Methadone was also examined in the progressive-ratio procedure with buprenorphine and heroin, and the largest ratio completed was similar to that of buprenorphine and lower than that of heroin (Mello et al. 1988). While one possibility is that methadone has less pharmacological efficacy than heroin, another possibility is that pharmacokinetics (e.g., delayed onset) might contribute to the reduced reinforcing effects of methadone compared with heroin. In cases where the results of self-administration studies suggest differences, other studies are needed to distinguish among factors that can influence drug self-administration.

Drug discrimination is another procedure that has contributed to the assessment of abuse and physical dependence liability of psychoactive substances, including opioids, and it can be helpful in identifying efficacy differences. In these procedures, subjects are trained to detect the presence of a particular drug with responding on one lever reinforced after administration of the training drug and responding on a second lever reinforced after administration of vehicle; thereafter, other drugs can be tested to determine whether they share discriminative stimulus effects with the training drug (i.e., produce responding on the training drug-associated lever). Discriminative stimulus effects measure a different aspect of abuse liability, compared with the reinforcing effects, and drug discrimination procedures have some important advantages over self-administration procedures. For example, drug discrimination experiments can be designed to distinguish between pharmacodynamic and pharmacokinetic differences. Like self-administration procedures, some drug discrimination procedures have low-efficacy requirements. In rats discriminating 3.2 mg/kg morphine, mu opioid receptor agonists that vary in efficacy, including fentanyl, methadone, and buprenorphine, produce maximal morphine-lever responding (Walker et al. 1994; Young et al. 1992). Increasing the efficacy requirements of the drug discrimination assay, for example by increasing the training dose, changes the ability of some mu opioid receptor agonists to produce drug-lever responding. Under these conditions, there is no change in maximal effect produced by opioids with high efficacy (e.g., morphine, methadone) whereas opioids with low efficacy (e.g., buprenorphine, nalbuphine) no longer produce a maximal effect (Young et al. 1992; Zhang et al. 2000). These studies are consistent with buprenorphine and nalbuphine having lower efficacy than other mu opioid receptor agonists, including morphine, fentanyl, and methadone.

Other behavioral procedures that can detect efficacy differences among mu opioid receptor agonists are antinociception procedures that use thermal stimuli. These effects are related to one of the most important clinical effects of opioids: pain relief. For these procedures, changing the intensity of the stimulus can determine the capacity of drugs acting at opioid receptors to produce antinociceptive effects. One procedure that is used frequently is the warm water tail withdrawal procedure, which measures the latency for an animal to remove its tail from warm water. Efficacy differences across agonists can be detected by examining latencies from water maintained at different temperatures. When the tails of monkeys are placed in water maintained at 50°C, many mu opioid receptor agonists, including nalbuphine, dose-dependently increase tail-withdrawal latency to more than 80% of the maximum possible effect; however, when the water temperature is increased to 54°C, latencies for monkeys to remove their tails are still increased after administration of fentanyl and morphine but are no longer increased by administration of the low-efficacy agonist nalbuphine (Maguire and France 2014). In another study in monkeys, buprenorphine increased tail-withdrawal latencies from water maintained at 48°C and not water at 55°C (Walker et al. 1995). These results are consistent with nalbuphine and buprenorphine having low efficacy at mu opioid receptors. Further evidence that these effects of nalbuphine and buprenorphine are due to low efficacy at mu opioid receptors can be obtained by showing that these low-efficacy drugs attenuate the antinociceptive effects of drugs with higher efficacy. Indeed, under conditions where nalbuphine and buprenorphine do not increase tail-withdrawal latency, they antagonize the antinociceptive effects of mu opioid receptor agonists with higher efficacy such as fentanyl and morphine (Gerak et al. 1994; Walker et al. 1995), thereby demonstrating that nalbuphine and buprenorphine are acting at mu receptors and their inability to produce a maximal effect is due to limited efficacy. In antinociception procedures, the potency and effectiveness of mu opioid receptor agonists are affected by the sex of the subject with the relative efficacy of opioids appearing to be greater in males compared with females (Barrett et al. 2001; Cook et al. 2000).

The ability to vary stimulus intensity (e.g., water temperature) in these antinociception studies has provided evidence of a direct relationship between stimulus intensity and the efficacy needed to produce an antinociceptive effect. Another way to detect efficacy differences among mu opioid receptor agonists is to examine respiratory-depressant effects. The consequences of decreased respiration produced by opioids have been well documented with more than 42,000 Americans dying from an overdose involving opioids in 2016 and the rate of fatalities involving an opioid increasing by 19% per year between 2013 and 2017 (CDC 2018). When given alone, most mu opioid receptor agonists can decrease respiration; however, only those with high efficacy can eliminate respiration. Thus, comparing changes in respiration provides another indication of agonist efficacy. Morphine, fentanyl, and heroin markedly and steadily decrease minute volume (V_E) in rhesus monkeys; in contrast, buprenorphine decreases V_E to only 60% of control, and this effect asymptotes such that a 100-fold larger dose of buprenorphine does not further change V_E (Gerak et al. 1998; Kishioka et al. 2000; Vivian et al. 1998). Under these conditions, buprenorphine antagonizes the respiratory-depressant effects of morphine and heroin, further indicating that buprenorphine is acting at mu opioid receptors and its limited effects on respiration are due to its lower pharmacological efficacy compared with morphine, fentanyl, and heroin. Importantly, the effects of a drug in one assay predict those in other assays, with buprenorphine and nalbuphine consistently shown to have less efficacy than morphine, methadone, and fentanyl. This reliability across drug discrimination, antinociception, and respiratory depression assays strengthens the supposition about the findings with methadone in the progressive-ratio self-administration procedure. Under those conditions, the reinforcing effects of methadone were more similar to those of buprenorphine than to the reinforcing effects of heroin (Mello et al. 1988), and these apparent limited reinforcing effects of methadone are thought to be due to pharmacokinetic, rather than pharmacodynamic, differences between methadone and heroin.

3.2 Therapeutic Considerations for Drugs that Vary in Efficacy

The primary difference among drugs that are currently used to treat opioid use disorder is efficacy at mu opioid receptors. One treatment strategy is to replace abused opioids with a therapeutic drug that mimics some effects of the drug used illicitly. Methadone has high efficacy at mu opioid receptors, shares behavioral effects with abused opioids, including reinforcing, antinociceptive, and respiratory-depressant effects, and has been used for many years as a replacement therapy. The primary advantage of methadone is that it mimics the effects of abused opioids, which includes its ability to prevent the emergence of withdrawal regardless of the level of physical dependence. However, the disadvantages of using methadone to treat opioid use disorder are also related to its ability to mimic the effects of abused opioids. Methadone is abused and diverted; consequently, it is regulated to limit diversion with methadone dispensed only by certified opioid treatment programs. Because of this regulation, patients are required to report to the clinic every day to receive their daily dose, which can be burdensome to many and virtually impossible to those living in rural areas. Another disadvantage is the ability of methadone to decrease markedly respiration. Overdose can occur if large doses are used or if methadone is combined with other drugs that decrease respiration, including other mu opioid receptor agonists as well as drugs like alcohol and benzodiazepines. These limitations impact the clinical usefulness of this treatment.

A second treatment option is the opioid receptor antagonist naltrexone. It works by blocking the effects of mu opioid receptor agonists, including the reinforcing effects of abused opioids, and can be effective in reducing opioid use. The primary advantage of naltrexone is that it does not have the same adverse effects as methadone, making naltrexone a much safer option. Because it has no pharmacological efficacy, naltrexone does not have reinforcing effects, it is not abused or diverted, and it does not decrease respiration when it is given alone or with other drugs. Moreover, naltrexone can be prescribed by any licensed provider, which makes it more accessible than methadone. On the other hand, naltrexone has its own limitations. For example, naltrexone precipitates withdrawal in patients who are physically dependent on opioids; consequently, treatment with naltrexone does not begin for 7–10 days after patients discontinue opioid use. Compliance can be a problem with patients not taking their medication to avoid withdrawal or so that the reinforcing effects of abused opioids are not attenuated. An extended-release injectable formulation of naltrexone (Vivitrol®) can be used to reduce some compliance issues and extend the duration of action of naltrexone, although some patients who intend to initiate treatment with this formulation never begin and many who start discontinue treatment prematurely (Jarvis et al. 2018). Nevertheless, this formulation provides an advantage by extending the duration of action of naltrexone, which is rather short and would require administration multiple times each day to maintain a constant therapeutic effect. While some limitations of naltrexone use can be overcome using a special formulation and beginning treatment only after opioid use is discontinued, one concern that persists is that the antagonist effects of naltrexone are surmountable, which means that the reinforcing and respiratory-depressant effects of opioids can emerge even in the presence of naltrexone after taking additional opioids. Another opioid receptor antagonist, naloxone, is used clinically to reverse opioid overdose; its effects are very similar to those of naltrexone, including its short duration of action and surmountability. While it can be effective in reversing the respiratory-depressant effects of opioids and it is safe, its antagonist effects can wane sooner than those of the opioid that produced the overdose, and respiratory depression can reemerge after rescue with naloxone (Dahan et al. 2010). Because its effects are surmountable, the blockade produced by naloxone can be overcome if patients continue to take opioids. In addition, naloxone will precipitate withdrawal in patients who are dependent on opioids.

Naltrexone and naloxone have similar pharmacological profiles and are effective in treating opioid abuse and overdose, respectively; however, treatment might be improved with opioid receptor antagonists that are not surmountable.

The third treatment option, buprenorphine, acts as a low-efficacy mu opioid receptor agonist and this property makes it an attractive treatment option for drug abuse because it has advantages of both methadone and naltrexone. Like methadone, some effects of buprenorphine mimic those of abused opioids, including reinforcing effects; however, the lower efficacy of buprenorphine limits its effects and buprenorphine is less likely than methadone to produce euphoric effects. Not only does the low efficacy of buprenorphine reduce the likelihood of diversion and abuse; it also increases safety compared with methadone by producing only modest respiratory-depressant effects when taken alone. Thus, buprenorphine has enough efficacy to serve as a replacement therapy by mimicking some effects of abused opioids but is much less likely to result in overdose. In addition to these agonist effects of buprenorphine that are similar to those of methadone, the low efficacy of buprenorphine means that it also shares some effects with naltrexone. For example, buprenorphine can block the severe respiratory-depressant effects of higher-efficacy mu opioid receptor agonists that are abused, thereby providing protection against overdose. While buprenorphine has some clear advantages over methadone and naltrexone, there are some limitations. For example, the modest decreases in respiration produced by buprenorphine can be exacerbated by drugs acting at sites other than opioid receptors. Deaths attributed to buprenorphine overdose remain relatively low, compared with deaths from overdose of abused opioids, although the number of buprenorphine fatalities has been steadily increasing, largely due to the concurrent use of other drugs, including alcohol and benzodiazepines, (Kintz 2001; Martin 2011; Pelissier-Alicot et al. 2010; Pirnay et al. 2004; Reynaud et al. 1998). Because of its mu opioid receptor agonist effects, prescribing of buprenorphine is regulated with special training required, and each medical provider can treat a limited number of patients (Jarvis et al. 2018). Extended-release formulations of buprenorphine are available, which eliminates the need for frequent office visits; however, these formulations must be surgically implanted and explanted, which requires even more training and further limits the number of providers willing to prescribe buprenorphine. Other limitations associated with the therapeutic use of buprenorphine are similar to those of naltrexone. Because buprenorphine has relatively low efficacy at mu opioid receptors, it can precipitate withdrawal in patients who are highly dependent on opioids, and treatment guidelines recommend that buprenorphine therapy be initiated only after withdrawal signs have begun to emerge. Buprenorphine has enough efficacy to prevent the emergence of severe signs of opioid withdrawal; while treatment with naltrexone should begin only after patients are completely detoxified (i.e., 7–10 days after discontinuing opioid use), treatment with buprenorphine can start within 1–3 days of discontinuing opioid use, thereby avoiding severe opioid withdrawal. Thus, buprenorphine shares some advantages with methadone and some with naltrexone, making it more effective than naltrexone and safer than methadone.

Efficacy differences among drugs acting at mu opioid receptors have been exploited to provide several options for treating opioid use disorder with each pharmacotherapy having benefits and limitations; however, these drugs also vary on dimensions other than pharmacological efficacy. For example, one reason that methadone is used as a replacement therapy, as opposed to any other mu opioid receptor agonist with high efficacy, is that it has a duration of action that is long enough to allow for once daily dosing. Similarly, buprenorphine is not the only mu opioid receptor agonist with limited efficacy; it is used to treat opioid use disorder because it dissociates very slowly from mu opioid receptors (Hambrook and Rance 1976) resulting in a long duration of action (Bullingham et al. 1982; Dykstra 1983; France et al. 1984; Walsh et al. 1994). This slow dissociation has been termed pseudoirreversible and suggests that factors involving the kinetics of the drug-receptor interaction also contribute to the pharmacological profile and clinical effects of drugs acting at opioid receptors.

4 Drug-Receptor Interactions

The primary differences among the pharmacotherapies currently approved for opioid use disorder are pharmacological efficacy and duration of action, and while these drugs are effective, each has limitations. In addition to pharmacological efficacy, drugs can vary on other dimensions, and ongoing research is investigating the possibility of improving treatment by exploiting some of the other differences among drugs acting at mu opioid receptors. Evidence of these differences is only beginning to emerge as the complexity of opioid receptor structure, signaling, and interaction with drugs becomes better understood. Thus, several strategies are currently being employed to identify drugs with novel pharmacological profiles that could be developed to improve treatment of opioid use disorder and opioid overdose. One approach is to start with a drug that is effective, such as buprenorphine for opioid use disorder and naloxone for overdose, and find novel compounds that retain their advantages while reducing some of the limitations. For example, a drug that is safer than buprenorphine, especially when combined with other drugs like alcohol, might provide a novel approach for treating opioid abuse whereas an antagonist whose effects cannot be surmounted by taking more opioids might be useful in patients who have overdosed. A second strategy for identifying novel pharmacotherapies is to develop drugs based on the emerging understanding of opioid receptor function, which might take advantage of allosteric sites on opioid receptors or drugs that selectively activate some signaling cascades.

4.1 Reversible Interactions and Surmountability

Most opioids that are used clinically produce their effects by binding reversibly to the orthosteric site on mu opioid receptors. The orthosteric site is the site to which endogenous opioids bind, and reversible interactions at this site occur when the dissociation rate of the drug is similar to its association rate. For reversible drugs, including methadone, naltrexone, and naloxone, their duration of action is governed by their pharmacokinetics (e.g., metabolism and elimination). In contrast, the interaction between some drugs and mu opioid receptors is irreversible; these drugs form a covalent bond with receptors such that the dissociation rate of the drug is zero. Drugs that bind irreversibly to mu opioid receptors, such as β-FNA, have a long duration of antagonist action, insurmountably blocking the behavioral effects of mu opioid receptor agonists until those receptors are replaced with newly synthesized ones (Gmerek and Woods 1985; Hayes et al. 1986). These drugs have not been developed for clinical use, in part due to their effects at other types of opioid receptors (i.e., kappa and delta), including unwanted effects that could impact the clinical usefulness of these drugs.

In addition to differences in efficacy, buprenorphine also differs from the other drugs used to treat opioid use disorder in the way that it binds to mu opioid receptors. The interaction between buprenorphine and mu opioid receptors has been termed pseudoirreversible, meaning that, while buprenorphine does not form a covalent bond with mu opioid receptors, its rate of offset is so slow that it is functionally irreversible. Because of this type of interaction with mu opioid receptors, buprenorphine has a long duration of action that is not governed by pharmacokinetics. Under conditions where buprenorphine produces agonist effects, such as antinociception and modest respiratory depression, its agonist effects are evident for at least 2 days. Similarly, when buprenorphine is combined with more efficacious mu opioid receptor agonists under conditions where it does not produce a maximal agonist effect (e.g., when a higher water temperature is used in antinociception studies), buprenorphine produces a long-lasting and often insurmountable (depending on the mu opioid receptor agonist) antagonism (Kishioka et al. 2000; Walker et al. 1995). These persistent effects of buprenorphine provide a clinical benefit because it does not need to be given daily to maintain its therapeutic effect. In addition, buprenorphine will block insurmountably the respiratory-depressant effects of abused opioids, providing protection against overdose if patients continue to abuse opioids during treatment. However, the pseudoirreversible nature of the interaction between buprenorphine and mu opioid receptors can also be a limitation. Specifically, buprenorphine is insensitive to reversal by naloxone and other mu opioid receptor antagonists. For drugs like buprenorphine with wide safety margins, inability to reverse effects is generally not a concern; however, when combined with other drugs such as alcohol or benzodiazepines, buprenorphine can markedly decrease respiration, and this effect is not reversed by naloxone (Kintz 2001; Sansone and Sansone 2015).

Given the advantages of buprenorphine as a treatment for opioid use disorder, additional compounds related to buprenorphine were synthesized in an attempt to reduce its adverse effects (Broadbear et al. 2000). These efforts resulted in the discovery of the mu opioid receptor antagonist methocinnamox (MCAM). Like buprenorphine, MCAM binds pseudoirreversibly to mu opioid receptors; however, it does not appear to produce agonist effects at mu opioid receptors under any conditions. Instead, MCAM produces long-lasting antagonism at mu opioid receptors, as evidenced by attenuation of the antinociceptive effects of morphine in rodents, with the morphine dose-effect curve shifted up to hundredfold rightward (Peckham et al. 2005) and antagonist effects evident for at least 2 days after administration (Broadbear et al. 2000). Because of its pharmacological profile, MCAM might improve upon currently available treatments. It is expected to be safer than buprenorphine because it does not have agonist effects (i.e., no pharmacological efficacy), and there would be no interaction with nonopioids like alcohol or benzodiazepines. Moreover, MCAM would also have advantages over the currently available opioid receptor antagonists naltrexone and naloxone; its pseudoirreversible interaction with mu opioid receptors would be expected to provide long-lasting and insurmountable protection from both the abuse-related and respiratory-depressant effects of opioid receptor agonists. Like naltrexone, MCAM decreased responding for heroin and choice of remifentanil over food in monkeys; however, in contrast to the antagonist effects of naltrexone, which were gone in less than 1 day, this antagonism of opioid self-administration by an acute injection of MCAM lasted several days (Maguire et al. 2019). Similarly, while both naloxone and MCAM reversed heroin-induced respiratory depression in monkeys, the antagonist effects of naloxone were gone by the next day whereas MCAM continued to provide protection against heroin-induced respiratory depression for at least 4 days after MCAM administration; a single dose of MCAM shifted the heroin dose-effect curve at least tenfold rightward and made normally toxic doses of heroin safe (Gerak et al. 2019). These persistent effects of MCAM would be expected to block the reinforcing effects of abused opioids and to protect patients from respiratory depression produced by use of very large doses of abused opioids, including those taken subsequent to rescue, for a much longer period than naltrexone and naloxone.

These proof-of-principle studies demonstrate the potential clinical utility of MCAM; however, relatively little is known about MCAM, and there are potentially important issues that need to be investigated. For example, although minute volume (V_E) recovers slightly within 15 min, it is not restored to control values until 30 min after MCAM administration (Gerak et al. 2019). Full reversal of the respiratory-depressant effects of abused opioids might not be required to protect patients from lethal overdose, and the much longer duration of action of MCAM would likely provide a distinct clinical advantage over naloxone. In fact, the short duration of action of naloxone is its primary clinical limitation because the opioid causing the overdose often lasts longer than naloxone (e.g., Dahan et al. 2010; Gatewood et al. 2016; Tomassoni et al. 2017), resulting in the reemergence of respiratory depression after rescue. Although rapid reversal of the lethal effects of abused opioids would be needed to save lives, it does not necessarily mean that respiration must be fully restored to control values to provide adequate protection. Partial reversal might be sufficient to protect patients from fatal respiratory depression and the slower onset of action of MCAM would provide an additional benefit. In patients who receive an opioid receptor antagonist as an antidote for overdose, withdrawal symptoms often emerge (Avetian et al. 2018); a slower onset of recovery from overdose appears to reduce withdrawal symptoms (Wermeling 2015). Thus, MCAM might effectively reverse overdose in a manner that minimizes the emergence of withdrawal.

While MCAM can precipitate withdrawal in morphine-dependent rats, withdrawal is no more severe or prolonged than withdrawal precipitated by naloxone (Gerak et al. under review), suggesting that MCAM could be used to treat opioid overdose or opioid use disorder in a manner that is not different from the current clinical use of naloxone or naltrexone, although with a much longer period of protection.

4.2 Allosteric Modulation of Mu Opioid Receptors

Opioids that are used clinically and/or abused act at the orthosteric site on mu opioid receptors; however, increasing evidence suggests that there are other binding sites on G-protein-coupled receptors, including mu opioid receptors. Drugs acting at these distinct sites would modulate the actions of opioids by changing the affinity of agonists acting at the orthosteric site or the responsiveness of the receptor to these agonists. Consequently, allosteric modulators are only effective when an orthosteric agonist is present and effects produced by allosteric modulators reach an asymptote when all allosteric sites are occupied. These features of allosterism are appealing for the treatment of opioid use disorder because, for example, the effects of these drugs would be limited, possibly reducing the likelihood of overdose. Moreover, there is speculation that adverse effects, particularly the development of tolerance and physical dependence, would be less likely to occur for an allosteric, compared with an orthosteric, modulator (Burford et al. 2013). Allosterism at mu opioid receptors has been documented previously. Salvinorin A has been shown to act as a positive allosteric modulator of mu opioid receptors (Rothman et al. 2007); however, its actions at kappa opioid receptors limit its usefulness as a pharmacological tool to elucidate the effects of drugs acting at this unique binding site on mu opioid receptors or as a possible pharmacotherapy for opioid use disorder. In addition, high-throughput screening was used to identify two positive allosteric modulators of mu opioid receptors, providing proof-of-principle that could lead to the development of novel therapeutics targeting this site (Burford et al. 2013). Finally, there has been some speculation that the persistent and insurmountable effects of MCAM might be due to actions at an allosteric site on mu opioid receptors, where it would negatively modulate the receptor (W Clarke, personal communication). Development of additional allosteric modulators that act at mu opioid receptors has been slow; however, additional methods are being utilized to aid in the identification and evaluation of these drugs (Valentino and Volkow 2018).

4.3 Biased Agonism

It is well established that mu opioid receptors can interact with multiple signaling pathways, recruiting G-proteins and/or β-arrestin, depending on the agonist that initiates the signaling cascade (Filizola 2019; Suida et al. 2017). This differential activation of second messenger systems results in different cellular responses and ultimately in different behavioral effects. For example, the antinociceptive effects of mu opioid receptor agonists are believed to be mediated through G-protein-dependent pathways, whereas other effects, such as respiratory depression, constipation, and tolerance, are believed to be mediated through recruitment of β-arrestin (Bohn et al. 1999, 2000; Maguma et al. 2012; Raehal et al. 2005). Not surprisingly, a proposed strategy for improving the treatment of pain has been to identify and develop biased agonists that activate mu opioid receptors and selectively recruit G-protein, and not β-arrestin, signaling pathways. One drug, TRV130, shows a strong bias for G_i coupling and is currently in clinical trials for moderate to severe pain; however, it has also been shown to produce reinforcing effects similar to those of oxycodone in terms of potency and effectiveness along with other abuse-related effects (Negus and Freeman 2018; Zamarripa et al. 2018). An agonist with a bias toward G_i coupling might not reduce its abuse liability, which would likely limit its therapeutic utility for treating pain, although it might be effective in treating opioid use disorder with fewer adverse effects, such as respiratory depression (Negus and Freeman 2018). The usefulness of biased agonists in treating opioid use disorder remains to be determined, although the possibility of having a pharmacotherapy that selectively produces a therapeutic effect warrants further investigation. Regardless of whether these drugs provide a clinical advantage in reducing opioid abuse, biased agonists might impact the opioid epidemic indirectly by relieving pain without the development of tolerance or the possibility of overdose.

5 Selectivity for Opioid Receptor Types

Mu opioid receptors are the primary target for therapeutic and abused opioids, although they are not the only type of opioid receptor. Two other distinct receptors (kappa and delta) have been cloned (Knapp et al. 1994; Meng et al. 1993). Mu, kappa, and delta opioid receptors bind differentially to the three endogenous opioid peptides, which are encoded by different genes. Some behavioral effects mediated by these three receptor types are similar, such as the antinociceptive effects of mu and kappa opioid receptor agonists. In contrast, some effects are completely opposite, like euphoria or dysphoria produced by activation of mu or kappa receptors, respectively. Although selective kappa opioid receptor agonists produce antinociception that, in many cases, is equivalent to antinociception produced by mu opioid receptor agonists, the dysphoria that accompanies the pain-relieving effects of agonists acting at kappa receptors precludes their clinical use. While kappa and delta receptors are not the primary target for drugs that are currently available clinically or abused, some pharmacotherapies act at these receptors. For example, buprenorphine has low-efficacy actions at mu receptors and antagonist actions at kappa receptors (Hambrook and Rance 1976). In addition, the opioid antagonists naltrexone and naloxone are only modestly selective and likely bind to other opioid receptors even at therapeutic doses. In contrast, the long-lasting effects of MCAM, which might be useful for treating opioid use disorder and opioid overdose, are selective for mu opioid receptors (Broadbear et al. 2000), and although the consequences of long-term blockade of kappa and delta receptors is not known, the selectivity of MCAM might provide another advantage for this novel compound.

6 Conclusions

Drugs acting at mu opioid receptors have long been used therapeutically and recreationally, although the increasing use of opioids over the last 20 years has resulted in the current national crisis. This ongoing opioid epidemic is a complicated challenge because of the magnitude of the problem as well as the many dimensions on which opioids can vary. In addition, a wide variety of opioids are currently used and abused, including prescription opioids, heroin, fentanyl, and ultra-potent analogs of fentanyl. These drugs are qualitatively the same, activating mu opioid receptors to produce their behavioral effects. Despite the similarities, drugs that act at opioid receptors can vary on a number of pharmacodynamic and pharmacokinetic dimensions. These differences among drugs can be exploited to improve treatment of opioid use disorder and opioid overdose while simultaneously reducing adverse effects. Pharmacological efficacy, unique drug-receptor interactions, allosterism, biased agonism, and selectivity for mu over other opioid receptors pharmacology are being investigated to identify novel treatment options to decrease opioid abuse and overdose deaths.

Acknowledgments This work was supported by the National Institutes of Health, National Institute on Drug Abuse [Grants R01 DA005018, R01 DA048417, and R21 DA 046805], and the Welch Foundation [Grant AQ-0039]. The authors have no conflict of interest. The content is solely the responsibility of the authors and does not necessarily represent the official views of the National Institutes of Health or the National Institute on Drug Abuse.

References

Avetian GK, Fiuty P, Mazzella S, Koppa D, Heye V, Hebbar P (2018) Use of naloxone nasal spray 4 mg in the community setting: a survey of use by community organizations. Curr Med Res Opin 34:573–576

Balster RL, Lukas SE (1985) Review of self-administration. Drug Alcohol Depend 14:249–261

Barrett AC, Cook CD, Terner JM, Craft RM, Picker MJ (2001) Importance of sex and relative efficacy at the mu opioid receptor in the development of tolerance and cross-tolerance to the antinociceptive effects of opioids. Psychopharmacology (Berl) 158:154–164

Baylon GJ, Kaplan HL, Somer G, Busto UE, Sellers EM (2000) Comparative abuse liability of intravenously administered remifentanil and fentanyl. J Clin Psychopharmacol 20:597–606

Bohn LM, Lefkowitz RJ, Gainetdinov RR, Peppel K, Caron MG, Lin FT (1999) Enhanced morphine analgesia in mice lacking beta-arrestin 2. Science 286:2495–2498

Bohn LM, Gainetdinov RR, Lin FT, Lefkowitz RJ, Caron MG (2000) Mu-opioid receptor desensitization by beta-arrestin-2 determines morphine tolerance but not dependence. Nature 408:720–723

Broadbear JH, Sumpter TL, Burke TF, Husbands SM, Lewis JW, Woods JH, Traynor JR (2000) Methocinnamox is a potent, long-lasting, and selective antagonist of morphine-mediated antinociception in the mouse: comparison with clocinnamox, β-funaltrexamine, and β-chlornaltrexamine. J Pharmacol Exp Ther 294:933–940

Bullingham R, McQuay H, Porter E, Allen H, Moore R (1982) Sublingual buprenorphine used postoperatively: ten hour plasma drug concentration analysis. Br J Clin Pharmacol 13:665–673

Burford NT, Clark MJ, Wehrman TS, Gerritz SW, Banks M, O'Connell J, Traynor JR, Alt A (2013) Discovery of positive allosteric modulators and silent allosteric modulators of the μ-opioid receptor. Proc Natl Acad Sci U S A 110:10830–10835

Centers for Disease Control and Prevention (CDC) (2018) Annual surveillance report of drug-related risks and outcomes – United States. Surveillance special report. Centers for Disease Control and Prevention, U.S. Department of Health and Human Services. Published August 31, 2018. https://www.cdc.gov/drugoverdose/pdf/pubs/2018-cdc-drug-surveillance-report.pdf. Accessed 28 Sept 2018

Chen Y, Mestek A, Liu J, Hurley JA, Yu L (1993) Molecular cloning and functional expression of a mu-opioid receptor from rat brain. Mol Pharmacol 44:8–12

Comer SD, Collins ED, MacArthur RB, Fischman MW (1999) Comparison of intravenous and intranasal heroin self-administration by morphine-maintained humans. Psychopharmacology (Berl) 143:327–338

Comer SD, Sullivan MA, Walker EA (2005) Comparison of intravenous buprenorphine and methadone self-administration by recently detoxified heroin-dependent individuals. J Pharmacol Exp Ther 315:1320–1330

Cone EJ (1998) Recent discoveries in pharmacokinetics of drugs of abuse. Toxicol Lett 102–103:97–101

Cook CD, Barrett AC, Roach EL, Bowman JR, Picker MJ (2000) Sex-related differences in the antinociceptive effects of opioids: importance of rat genotype, nociceptive stimulus intensity, and efficacy at the mu opioid receptor. Psychopharmacology (Berl) 130:430–442

Dahan A, Aarts L, Smith TW (2010) Incidence, reversal, and prevention of opioid-induced respiratory depression. Anesthesiology 112:226–238

Dykstra LA (1983) Behavioral effects of buprenorphine and diprenorphine under a multiple schedule of food presentation in squirrel monkeys. J Pharmacol Exp Ther 226:317–323

Farré M, Camí J (1991) Pharmacokinetic considerations in abuse liability evaluation. Br J Addict 86:1601–1606

Filizola M (2019) Insights from molecular dynamics simulations to exploit new trends for the development of improved opioid drugs. Neurosci Lett 700:50–55

France CP, Jacobson AE, Woods JH (1984) Discriminative stimulus effects of reversible and irreversible opiate agonists: morphine, oxymorphazone and buprenorphine. J Pharmacol Exp Ther 230:652–657

Gatewood AK, Van Wert MJ, Andrada AP, Surkan PJ (2016) Academic physicians' and medical students' perceived barriers toward bystander administered naloxone as an overdose prevention strategy. Addict Behav 61:40–46

Gerak LR, Butelman ER, Woods JH, France CP (1994) Antinociceptive and respiratory effects of nalbuphine in rhesus monkeys. J Pharmacol Exp Ther 271:993–999

Gerak LR, Brandt MR, France CP (1998) Studies on benzodiazepines and opioids administered alone and in combination in rhesus monkeys: ventilation and drug discrimination. Psychopharmacology (Berl) 137:164–174

Gerak LR, Galici R, France CP (2009) Self administration of heroin and cocaine in morphine-dependent and morphine-withdrawn rhesus monkeys. Psychopharmacology (Berl) 204:403–411

Gerak LR, Maguire DR, Woods JH, Husbands SM, Disney A, France CP (2019) Reversal and prevention of the respiratory-depressant effects of heroin by the novel μ opioid receptor antagonist methocinnamox in rhesus monkeys. J Pharmacol Exp Ther 368:229–236

Gerak LR, Minervini V, Latham E, Ghodrati S, Lillis KV, Wooden J, Disney A, Husbands SM, France CP (under review) Methocinnamox (MCAM) produces long-lasting antagonism of the behavioral effects of μ opioid receptor agonists but not prolonged precipitated withdrawal in rats. J Pharmacol Exp Ther

Gioannini TL, Howard AD, Hiller JM, Simon EJ (1985) Purification of an active opioid-binding protein from bovine striatum. J Biol Chem 260:15117–15121

Gmerek DE, Woods JH (1985) Effects of beta-funaltrexamine in normal and morphine-dependent rhesus monkeys: observational studies. J Pharmacol Exp Ther 235:296–301

Hambrook J, Rance M (1976) The interaction of buprenorphine with the opiate receptor: lipophilicity as a determining factor in drug-receptor kinetics. In: Kosterlitz H (ed) Opiates and endogenous peptides. North Holland, Amsterdam, pp 295–301

Hayes AG, Skingle M, Tyers MB (1986) Reversal by beta-funaltrexamine of the antinociceptive effect of opioid agonists in the rat. Br J Pharmacol 88:867–872

Jarvis BP, Holtyn AF, Subramaniam S, Tompkins DA, Oga EA, Bigelow GE, Silverman K (2018) Extended-release injectable naltrexone for opioid use disorder: a systematic review. Addiction 113:1188–1209

Jones JD, Madera G, Comer SD (2014) The reinforcing and subjective effect of intravenous and intranasal buprenorphine in heroin users. Pharmacol Biochem Behav 122:299–306

Kenakin T (2008) Receptor theory. Curr Protoc Pharmacol 41:1.2.1–1.2.28

Kintz P (2001) Deaths involving buprenorphine: a compendium of French cases. Foren Sci Int 121:65–69

Kishioka S, Paronis CA, Lewis JW, Woods JH (2000) Buprenorphine and methoclocinnamox: agonist and antagonist effects on respiratory function in rhesus monkeys. Eur J Pharmacol 391:289–297

Knapp RJ, Malatynska E, Fang L, Li X, Babin E, Nguyen M, Santoro G, Varga EV, Hruby VJ, Roeske WR (1994) Identification of a human delta opioid receptor: cloning and expression. Life Sci 54:L463–L469

Maguire DR, France CP (2014) Impact of efficacy at the mu-opioid receptor on antinociceptive effects of combinations of mu-opioid receptor agonists and cannabinoid receptor agonists. J Pharmacol Ther Exp 351:383–389

Maguire DR, France CP (2016) Effects of daily delta-9-tetrahydrocannabinol treatment on heroin self-administration in rhesus monkeys. Behav Pharmacol 27:249–257

Maguire DR, Gerak LR, Woods JH, Husbands SM, Disney A, France CP (2019) Long-lasting effects of methocinnamox on heroin self-administration in rhesus monkeys. J Pharmacol Exp Ther 368:88–99

Maguma HT, Dewey WL, Akbarali HI (2012) Differences in the characteristics of tolerance to μ-opioid receptor agonists in the colon from wild type and β-arrestin2 knockout mice. Eur J Pharmacol 685:133–140

Martin HA (2011) The possible consequences of combining lorazepam and buprenorphine/naloxone: a case review. J Emerg Nurs 37:200–202

Mello NK, Bree MP, Mendelson JH (1981a) Buprenorphine self-administration by rhesus monkey. Pharmacol Biochem Behav 15:215–225

Mello NK, Mendelson JH, Kuehnle JC, Sellers MS (1981b) Operant analysis of human heroin self-administration and the effects of naltrexone. J Pharmacol Exp Ther 216:45–54

Mello NK, Lukas SE, Bree MP, Mendelson JH (1988) Progressive ratio performance maintained by buprenorphine, heroin and methadone in Macaque monkeys. Drug Alcohol Depend 21:81–97

Meng F, Xie GX, Thompson RC, Mansour A, Goldstein A, Watson SJ, Akil H (1993) Cloning and pharmacological characterization of a rat kappa opioid receptor. Proc Natl Acad Sci U S A 90:9954–9958

Negus SS, Freeman KB (2018) Abuse potential of biased mu opioid receptor agonists. Trends Pharmacol Sci 39:916–919

Peckham EM, Barkley LM, Divin MF, Cicero TJ, Traynor JR (2005) Comparison of the antinociceptive effect of acute morphine in female and male Sprague-Dawley rats using the long-lasting mu-antagonist methocinnamox. Brain Res 1058:137–147

Pelissier-Alicot A-L, Sastre C, Baillif-Couniou V, Gaulier J-M, Kintz P, Kuhlmann E, Perich P, Bartoli C, Piercecchi-Marti M-D, Leonetti G (2010) Buprenorphine-related deaths: unusual forensic situations. Int J Leg Med 124:647–651

Pert CB, Pasternak GW, Snyder SH (1973) Opiate agonists and antagonists discriminated by receptor binding in brain. Science 182:1359–1361

Pirnay S, Borron SW, Giudicelli CP, Tourneau J, Baud FJ, Ricordel I (2004) A critical review of the causes of death among post-mortem toxicological investigations: analysis of 34 buprenorphine-associated and 35 methadone-associated deaths. Addiction 99:978–988

Raehal KM, Walker JM, Bohn LM (2005) Morphine side effects in beta-arrestin 2 knockout mice. J Pharmacol Exp Ther 314:1195–1201

Reynaud M, Tracqui A, Petit G, Potard D, Courty P (1998) Six deaths linked to misuse of buprenorphine-benzodiazepine combinations. Am J Psychiatry 155:448–449

Rothman RB, Murphy DL, Xu H, Godin JA, Dersch CM, Partilla JS, Tidgewell K, Schimidt M, Prisinzano TE (2007) Salvinorin A: allosteric interactions at the μ-opioid receptor. J Pharmacol Exp Ther 320:801–810

Sansone RA, Sansone LA (2015) Buprenorphine treatment for narcotic addiction: not without risks. Innov Clin Neurosci 12:32–36

Simon EJ, Hiller JM, Edelman I (1973) Stereospecific binding of the potent narcotic analgesic [^{3}H] etorphine to rat-brain homogenate. Proc Natl Acad Sci 70:1947–1949

Spanagel R (2017) Animal models of addiction. Dialogues Clin Neurosci 19:247–258

Suida ER, Carr R, Rominger DH, Violin JD (2017) Biased mu-opioid receptor ligands: a promising new generation of pain therapeutics. Curr Opin Pharmacol 32:77–84

Terenius L (1973) Stereospecific interaction between narcotic analgesics and a synaptic plasma membrane fraction of rat cerebral cortex. Acta Pharmacol Toxicol 32:317–320

Tomassoni AJ, Hawk KF, Jubanyik K, Nogee DP, Durant T, Lynch KL, Patel R, Dinh D, Ulrich A, D'Onofrio GD (2017) Multiple fentanyl overdoses – New Haven, Connecticut, June 23, 2016. MMWR Morb Mortal Wkly Rep 66:107–111

Valentino RJ, Volkow ND (2018) Untangling the complexity of opioid receptor function. Neuropsychopharmacology 43:2514–2520

Vivian JA, Kishioka S, Butelman ER, Broadbear J, Lee KO, Woods JH (1998) Analgesic, respiratory and heart rate effects of cannabinoid and opioid agonists in rhesus monkeys: antagonist effects of SR 141716A. J Pharmacol Exp Ther 286:697–703

Vocci F (1991) The necessity and utility of abuse liability testing in human subjects. Br J Addict 12:1537–1542

Volkow ND, McLellan AT (2016) Opioid abuse in chronic pain – misconceptions and mitigation strategies. N Engl J Med 374:1253–1256

Waldhoer M, Bartlett SE, Whistler JL (2004) Opioid receptors. Annu Rev Biochem 73:953–990

Walker EA, Makhay MM, House JD, Young AM (1994) In vivo apparent pA_2 analysis for naltrexone antagonism of discriminative stimulus and analgesic effects of opiate agonists in rats. J Pharmacol Exp Ther 271:959–968

Walker EA, Zernig G, Woods JH (1995) Buprenorphine antagonism of *mu* opioids in the rhesus monkey tail-withdrawal procedure. J Pharmacol Exp Ther 273:1345–1352

Walsh SL, Preston KL, Stitzer ML, Cosa EJ, Bigelow GE (1994) Clinical pharmacology of buprenorphine: ceiling effects at high doses. Clin Pharmacol Ther 55:569–580

Wermeling DP (2015) Review of naloxone safety for opioid overdose: practical considerations for new technology and expanded public access. Ther Adv Drug Saf 6:20–31

Wolf B, Griffiths RR (1991) Physical dependence on benzodiazepines: differences within the class. Drug Alcohol Depend 29:153–156

Young AM, Kapitsopoulos G, Makhay MM (1991) Tolerance to morphine-like stimulus effects of *mu* opioid agonists. J Pharmacol Exp Ther 257:795–805

Young AM, Masaki MA, Geula C (1992) Discriminative stimulus effects of morphine: effects of training dose on agonist and antagonist effects of *mu* opioids. J Pharmacol Exp Ther 261:246–257

Zamarripa CA, Edwards SR, Qureshi HN, Yi JN, Blough BE, Freeman KB (2018) The G-protein biased mu-opioid agonist, TRV130, produces reinforcing and antinociceptive effects that are comparable to oxycodone in rats. Drug Alcohol Depend 192:158–162

Zhang L, Walker EA, Sutherland J 2nd, Young AM (2000) Discriminative stimulus effects of two doses of fentanyl in rats: pharmacological selectivity and effect of training dose on agonist and antagonist effects of mu opioids. Psychopharmacology (Berl) 148:136–145

The Rise and Fall of Kappa-Opioid Receptors in Drug Abuse Research

Matthew L. Banks

Contents

1 Preclinical Evaluation of Candidate Substance Use Disorder Treatments 148
2 Rationale for Kappa-Opioid Receptors as Candidate SUD Treatments 149
3 KOR Agonist Effects on Preclinical Drug SA 151
   3.1 Preclinical SA of KOR Agonists and Drug of Abuse Combinations 151
   3.2 KOR Agonists as Pretreatments to Preclinical Drug of Abuse SA 156
4 KOR Antagonist Effects on Preclinical Drug Self-Administration 157
   4.1 KOR Antagonist Effects on Preclinical Drug Choice SA 159
   4.2 KOR Antagonist Effects on Human Drug SA Metrics 159
5 Conclusions and Future Directions 160
References 161

Abstract

Substance use disorders represent a global public health issue. This mental health disorder is hypothesized to result from neurobiological changes as a result of chronic drug exposure and clinically manifests as inappropriate behavioral allocation toward the procurement and use of the abused substance and away from other behaviors maintained by more adaptive nondrug reinforcers (e.g., social relationships, work). The dynorphin/kappa-opioid receptor (KOR) is one receptor system that has been altered following chronic exposure to drugs of abuse (e.g., cocaine, opioids, alcohol) in both laboratory animals and humans, implicating the dynorphin/KOR system in the expression, mechanisms, and treatment of substance use disorders. KOR antagonists have reduced drug self-administration in laboratory animals under certain experimental conditions, but not others. Recently, several human laboratory and clinical trials have evaluated the effectiveness of KOR antagonists as candidate pharmacotherapies for cocaine or

M. L. Banks (✉)
Department of Pharmacology and Toxicology, Virginia Commonwealth University, Richmond, VA, USA
e-mail: matthew.banks@vcuhealth.org

M. A. Nader, Y. L. Hurd (eds.), *Substance Use Disorders*,
Handbook of Experimental Pharmacology 258, https://doi.org/10.1007/164_2019_268

tobacco use disorder to test hypotheses generated from preclinical studies. KOR antagonists failed to significantly alter drug use metrics in humans suggesting translational discordance between some preclinical drug self-administration studies and consistent with other preclinical drug self-administration studies that provide concurrent access to an alternative nondrug reinforcer (e.g., food). The implications of this translational discordance and future directions for examining the therapeutic potential of KOR agonists or antagonists as candidate substance use disorder pharmacotherapies are discussed.

Keywords
Cocaine · Ethanol · Kappa opioid receptor · Medication development · Nicotine · Opioid

1 Preclinical Evaluation of Candidate Substance Use Disorder Treatments

Substance use disorders (SUDs; i.e., drug addiction) are an insidious and global public health issue. This complex and multifaceted mental health disorder is most commonly modeled in the laboratory using a drug self-administration (SA) procedure to provide an opportunity to measure volitional drug intake. Both preclinical and human laboratory drug SA procedures have made significant contributions to improving our understanding of psychoactive compounds for more than 50 years. In general, preclinical drug SA procedures are used to address two main categories of scientific questions. One category is for abuse liability assessment of psychoactive compounds for potential scheduling as controlled substances by the Drug Enforcement Agency, and there are already excellent reviews on the utility of drug SA procedures for this purpose (Ator and Griffiths 2003; Carter and Griffiths 2009). The other category is for understanding the expression, mechanisms, and treatment of drug-taking behavior as a model of SUDs. This chapter will focus on the use of drug SA procedures to address this latter scientific category.

Although there are infinite iterations of drug SA procedures, all use the classic 3-term contingency of operant conditioning to investigate the stimulus properties of drugs (Skinner 1938). This 3-term contingency can be diagrammed as follows in Eq. (1):

$$S^D \rightarrow R \rightarrow S^C \tag{1}$$

where S^D designates a *discriminative stimulus*, R designates a *response* on the part of the organism, and S^C designates a *consequent stimulus*. The arrows specify the contingency that, in the presence of the discriminative stimulus S^D, performance of response R will deliver the consequent stimulus S^C. As a simple example, a rat implanted with a chronic indwelling venous catheter might be connected to an infusion pump containing a dose of a psychoactive drug and placed into an experimental chamber that contains a stimulus light and a response lever. Contingencies can be programmed such that if the stimulus light is illuminated (the discriminative stimulus), then depression of the response lever (the response) will result in delivery of a drug injection (the consequent stimulus). Conversely, if the stimulus light is not illuminated, then responding does not result in the delivery of the drug injection. Under these conditions, subjects typically learn to respond when the discriminative stimulus is present. Consequent stimuli that increase responding leading to their delivery are operationally defined as *reinforcers*, whereas stimuli that decrease responding leading to their delivery are defined as *punishers*. The contingencies that relate discriminative stimuli, responses, and consequent stimuli are defined by the schedule of reinforcement (Ferster and Skinner 1957).

Although there are Food and Drug Administration (FDA)-approved pharmacotherapies for some SUDs (e.g., opioid, nicotine, and ethanol), FDA-approved pharmacotherapies are absent for many other classes of abused drugs (e.g., cocaine, methamphetamine, and cannabis). Moreover, the development of safer and more efficacious medications to treat SUDs remains a priority for both preclinical and human laboratory/clinical drug abuse research. Preclinical evaluation of candidate medication treatment effects on drug SA has demonstrated good, but not perfect, concordance with both medication effects in human laboratory drug SA studies and metrics of drug abuse in clinical trials (Comer et al. 2008; Haney and Spealman 2008a; Mello and Negus 1996).

2 Rationale for Kappa-Opioid Receptors as Candidate SUD Treatments

This chapter will focus on kappa-opioid receptor (KOR) agonist and antagonist effects on preclinical drug SA endpoints. The KOR is a seven transmembrane $G_{i/o}$-protein coupled receptor that is ubiquitously expressed in the central and peripheral nervous system and is hypothesized to be involved in mental health disorders including stress, anxiety, depression, and SUD (for review, see Chavkin and Koob 2015; Crowley and Kash 2015; Tejeda and Bonci 2019; Wee and Koob 2010b). In general, KOR activation results in inhibition of neuronal function and can occur following either endogenous release of the dynorphin peptide (Chavkin et al. 1982; Oka et al. 1982) or synthetic KOR agonist administration. For example, administration of synthetic KOR agonists (e.g., U69,593, U50,488, or salvinorin A) decreases extracellular dopamine levels in the nucleus accumbens (Carlezon et al. 2006; Di Chiara and Imperato 1988; Leitl et al. 2014).

Table 1 lists the most prominent KOR agonists and antagonists used in preclinical and clinical research along with the relative selectivity for the KOR over other similar homology receptors such as the mu-opioid (MOR) and delta-opioid (DOR) receptors. In general, the greater the selectivity for KOR over MOR and DOR, the more confidence the result is due to KOR activation or inhibition and not due to an off-target receptor. In addition, the availability of both selective KOR agonists and antagonists allows for sufficient and necessary experimentation in the role of KOR for a specific pharmacological effect. For example, if you were interested in whether activation of KOR receptors by dynorphin was sufficient to decrease mesolimbic dopamine levels, then you could administer a KOR agonist (e.g., salvinorin A) and

Table 1 Kappa-opioid receptor (KOR) agonists and antagonists that have been most commonly used in preclinical studies examining the potential of KOR ligands as candidate substance use disorder medications

Ligand	KOR (K_i nM)	MOR (K_i nM)	DOR (K_i nM)	NOPR (K_i nM)	Reference
KOR agonists					
Dynorphin A	0.5	32	>1,000	Not determined	(Raynor et al. 1994)
U-50,488	0.12	>1,000	>1,000	Not determined	(Raynor et al. 1994)
U-69,593	0.59	>1,000	>1,000	Not determined	(Raynor et al. 1994)
Salvinorin A	16	>10,000	>10,000	Not determined	(Roth et al. 2002)
Nalfurafine (TRK-820)	0.2	0.6	96.5	Not determined	(Nagase et al. 2012)
Enadoline (CI-977)	0.11	99	1	Not determined	(Hunter et al. 1990)
Spiradoline	0.036	21	>1,000	Not determined	(Raynor et al. 1994)
Bremazocine	0.09	0.75	2.3	Not determined	(Raynor et al. 1994)
KOR antagonists					
Nor-binaltorphimine	4	41	20	4,400	(Munro et al. 2013)
JDTic	1	3	44	12	(Munro et al. 2013)
6′-guanidonaltrindole	3	54	58	2,500	(Munro et al. 2013)
CERC-501 (LY2456302)	0.8	24	155	Not determined	(Rorick-Kehn et al. 2014)

Columns show the affinity (K_i nM) for the ligand at the KOR and three potential off-target receptor affinities mu-opioid receptor (MOR), delta-opioid receptor (DOR), and nociceptin opioid peptide receptor (NOPR). Together, these results provide one index of KOR selectivity

measure mesolimbic dopamine levels. As mentioned above, this is a reported effect of KOR agonists. However, if you were interested in whether KOR were necessary for salvinorin A to decrease mesolimbic dopamine levels, then you would administer a KOR antagonist before salvinorin A to determine whether salvinorin A decreases mesolimbic dopamine levels. The availability of selective agonists and antagonists allows for rigorous experimentation into the mechanisms associated with or involved in SUDs.

Repeated exposure to several drugs of abuse (e.g., cocaine, methamphetamine, mu-opioid receptor agonists) has been shown to activate or sensitize the endogenous dynorphin/KOR system. This engagement of the dynorphin/KOR system by drugs of abuse has been theorized to contribute to the development of compulsive drug use and SUD (Chavkin and Koob 2015; Shippenberg et al. 2007). For example, polymorphisms of prodynorphin have been correlated with increased diagnosis of opioid use disorder (Clarke et al. 2012). In addition, both increased dynorphin expression and KOR density have been observed in cocaine overdose patients (Hurd and Herkenham 1993; Staley et al. 1997). Furthermore, cocaine SA leads to a reduction in KOR availability in humans as measured using positron-emission tomography (Martinez et al. 2019). Consistent with these clinical data, a history of either heroin or cocaine SA under extended access conditions increases prodynorphin expression in the nucleus accumbens shell of rats or monkeys (Daunais et al. 1993; Fagergren et al. 2003; Schlosburg et al. 2013; Solecki et al. 2009). These results have been interpreted to suggest that chronic KOR activation is one key neurobiological system mediating the progression from drug abuse to severe SUD (Koob and Moal 2008; Wee and Koob 2010a). Table 2 summarizes the 34 publications that have examined either acute or chronic (i.e., repeated administration for at least 3 days) treatment effects of KOR agonists or antagonists in preclinical drug SA procedures. The predominant drugs of abuse examined have been cocaine (44%), ethanol (35%), and opioids (24%). The predominant research subjects have been rats (74%) and rhesus monkeys (26%); most studies only involved male subjects (~76%). The results and implication of this literature will be reviewed in more detail below.

3 KOR Agonist Effects on Preclinical Drug SA

KOR agonists and drugs of abuse appear to produce opposing effects on both abuse-related neurochemical and behavioral endpoints. For example, KOR agonists decrease mesolimbic dopamine levels in rats (Devine et al. 1993; Donzanti et al. 1992; Leitl et al. 2014; Spanagel et al. 1990), produce dysphoric subjective effects in humans (Pfeiffer et al. 1986; Walsh et al. 2001), and fail to function as positive reinforcers in rodent and nonhuman primate drug SA procedures (Marinelli et al. 1998; Negus et al. 2008; Tang and Collins 1985; Townsend et al. 2017; Woods and Gmerek 1985). This line of research led to the hypothesis that KOR agonists may have clinical utility as candidate SUD pharmacotherapies by either punishing drug-taking behavior if the KOR agonist and the drug of abuse were combined or antagonizing the abuse-related effects of central nervous system-active drugs if the KOR agonist was administered as an acute or repeated pretreatment to subsequent drug-taking behavior. Two general types of experiments have been conducted examining the effects of KOR agonists on drug SA.

3.1 Preclinical SA of KOR Agonists and Drug of Abuse Combinations

One type of experiment involves combining a KOR agonist and the drug of abuse in the same syringe for SA to determine whether the KOR agonist would function as a punisher (i.e., presentation of the stimulus (KOR agonist) decreases the probability of the preceding behavior). Thus, the research animal would self-administer a

Table 2 Summary of published preclinical manuscripts reporting effects of kappa-opioid receptor (KOR) agonists or antagonists on IV drug self-administration (SA)

#	Self-administered drug (dose)	KOR ligand (dose)	Sex and species	Main effect	Reference
KOR agonists studied					
1	Fentanyl (0.01–1 μg/kg/inj)	U69,593 (fixed proportion based on fentanyl dose)	Male rhesus monkey	Increasing proportions of U69,593 in the U69,593/fentanyl mixture decreased rates of fentanyl self-administration (SA)	(Negus et al. 2008)
2	Oxycodone (0.032–0.18 mg/kg/inj)	Nalfurafine (fixed proportion based on oxycodone dose)	Male Sprague-Dawley (S-D) rat	Increasing proportions of nalfurafine in the nalfurafine/oxycodone mixture decreased rates of oxycodone SA	(Townsend et al. 2017)
3	Cocaine (0.1 mg/kg/inj) Remifentanil (0.1 μg /kg/inj)	Salvinorin A (0.0003–0.01 mg/kg/inj)	Male rhesus monkey	Increasing doses of Salvinorin A decreased both cocaine and remifentanil SA in a drug vs. drug choice procedure	(Freeman et al. 2014)
4	Cocaine (0.4 mg/kg, inj) Morphine (0.04 mg/kg/inj)	U50,488 (2.5–10 mg/kg, IP) Spiradoline (1.25–5 mg/kg, IP) Nor-BNI (10 mg/kg, SC)	Female S-D rat	Acute U50,488 and spiradoline decreased rates of cocaine and morphine SA. Nor-BNI had no effect alone but blocked KOR agonist effects	(Glick et al. 1995)
5	Cocaine (0.007–0.06 mg/kg/inj) Morphine (0.2–2.4 μg/kg/inj)	U50,488 (2.5–10 mg/kg, IP)	Male Wistar rat (cocaine) male mice (morphine)	Repeated U50,488 shifted cocaine and morphine SA dose-effect functions to the left	(Kuzmin et al. 1997)
6	Cocaine (0.0032–0.1 mg/kg/inj)	U50,488 (0.0032–0.1 mg/kg/h, IV) Nor-BNI (3.2 mg/kg, IV)	Male rhesus monkey	Chronic U50,488 increased cocaine choice. Acute nor-BNI did not alter cocaine choice but blocked U50,488 effects	(Negus 2004)
7	Cocaine (0.001–0.3 mg/kg/inj)	Enadoline (0.001–0.01 mg/kg/h, IV)	Male rhesus monkey	Acute enadoline decreased cocaine and food-maintained responding	(Bowen et al. 2003)
8	Cocaine (0.01–0.032 mg/kg/inj)	Enadoline (0.00032–0.0032 mg/kg/h, IV) Spiradoline (0.0032–0.018 mg/kg/h, IV)	Male and female rhesus monkey	Repeated KOR agonist decreased rates of cocaine SA at doses that decreased food SA with one exception. Mr2033 selectively attenuate cocaine SA compared to food SA	(Mello and Negus 1998)

		PD117302 (0.032–0.32 mg/kg/h, IV) Bremazocine (0.0032–0.032 mg/kg/h, IV) Mr2033 (0.0032–0.032 mg/kg/h, IV) Cyclazocine (0.001–0.1 mg/kg/h, IV)			
9	Cocaine (0.01–0.032 mg/kg/inj)	Ethylketocyclazocine (EKC; 0.0032–0.032 mg/kg/h, IV) U50,488 (0.032–0.1 mg/kg/h, IV) Nor-BNI (3.2 mg/kg, IV)	Male and female rhesus monkey	Repeated EKC and U50,488 treatment decreased rates of cocaine SA at doses that also tended to decrease food SA. Nor-BNI did not alter cocaine or food SA	(Negus et al. 1997)
10	Smoke cocaine (1 mg/kg/delivery) PCP (0.25 mg/mL) EtOH (not reported)	Bremazocine (0.00032, 0.001, 0.0025 mg/kg, IM)	Male rhesus monkey	Repeated bremazocine decreased rates of cocaine, EtOH, saccharin, PCP, and food SA	(Cosgrove and Carroll 2002)
11	Cocaine (0.4 mg/kg/inj)	Cyclazocine (0–1 8 mg/kg, PO)	Female Long-Evans rat	Acute racemic, but not enantiomers, cyclazocine decreased rates of cocaine SA but not water-maintained behavior	(Glick et al. 1998)
12	Cocaine (0.015–1 mg/kg/inj)	U69,593 (0, 0.32 mg/kg, SC)	Male S-D rat	Acute U69,593 decreased rates of low dose, but not high-dose cocaine SA	(Schenk et al. 1999)
13	Cocaine (0.5 mg/kg/inj)	U69,593 (0, 0.32 mg/kg, SC)	Male S-D rat	Acute U69,593 decreased rates of cocaine SA when cocaine delivery was paired with a visual stimulus	(Schenk et al. 2001)
14	Nicotine (0.03 mg/kg/inj)	U50,488 (0.3–3 mg/kg, IP)	Male Wistar rat	Repeated U50,488 treatment decreased rates of nicotine self-administration at doses that did not alter food-maintained responding	(Ismayilova and Shoaib 2010)
15	EtOH (10% v/v)	Bremazocine (0.1 mg/kg, SC) U50,488 (10 mg/kg, SC)	Male Wistar rat	Repeated bremazocine produced sustained decrease in EtOH SA. Repeated U50,488 decreased EtOH SA on day 1 only	(Nestby et al. 1999)
16	EtOH (20% v/v)	Enadoline (0.01 mg/kg/h, SC) Nor-BNI (5 mg/kg,IP x 2)	Male Wistar rat	Repeated enadoline increased EtOH SA. Acute enadoline decreased EtOH SA. Acute nor-BNI had no effect	(Hölter et al. 2000)

(continued)

Table 2 (continued)

#	Self-administered drug (dose)	KOR ligand (dose)	Sex and species	Main effect	Reference
KOR antagonists studied					
17	Heroin (0–0.1 mg/kg/inj)	5′-guanidinaltrindole (GNTI; 1.0 mg/kg, IM)	Male rhesus monkey	Acute GNTI did not attenuate withdrawal-associated increases in heroin choice	(Negus and Rice 2009)
18	Heroin (0.06 mg/kg/inj)	Nor-BNI (5 or 10 mg/kg, SC)	Male Wistar rat	Acute nor-BNI did not alter heroin SA	(Negus et al. 1993)
19	Heroin (60 μg/kg/inj)	Nor-BNI (30 mg/kg, SC or 4 μg/side)	Male Wistar rat	Acute nor-BNI blocked increased rates "escalation" of heroin SA	(Schlosburg et al. 2013)
20	Cocaine (0–0.1 mg/kg/inj)	Nor-BNI (3.2–10 mg/kg, IM)	Male rhesus monkey	Nor-BNI did not block or reverse cocaine choice or rates of cocaine SA	(Hutsell et al. 2016)
21	Cocaine (0.03, 0.06 mg/kg/inj)	Nor-BNI (30 mg/kg, SC)	Male Wistar rat	Acute nor-BNI decreased rates of cocaine SA at 0.03, but not 0.06 mg/kg/inj cocaine	(Kuzmin et al. 1998)
22	Cocaine (0.5 mg/kg/inj)	Nor-BNI (15, 30 mg/kg, SC)	Male Wistar rat	Nor-BNI blocked increased "escalated" rates of cocaine SA	(Wee et al. 2009)
23	Cocaine (0.5 mg/kg/inj)	Buprenorphine (3 mg/kg alone or in combination with 0.3–10 mg/kg, naltrexone)	Male Wistar rat	Repeated 2-day Buprenorphine/naltrexone blocked increased rates "escalation" of heroin SA and reduced cocaine PR responding	(Wee et al. 2012)
24	Methamphetamine (0.05 mg/kg/inj)	Nor-BNI (30 mg/kg, SC)	Male Wistar rat	Acute nor-BNI blocked increased rates "escalation" of methamphetamine SA	(Whitfield et al. 2015)
25	Nicotine (0.03 mg/kg/inj)	GNTI (0–1 mg/kg, IP)	Male S-D rat	GNTI pretreatment failed to alter rates of nicotine self-administration	(Liu and Jernigan 2011)
26	EtOH (10% v/v)	Nor-BNI (10 mg/kg, SC)	Male Lewis rat	Acute nor-BNI increased EtOH consumption	(Mitchell et al. 2005)
27	EtOH (10% v/v) w/ sucrose	Nor-BNI (0 or 20 mg/kg, SC)	Male Long-evans rat	Acute nor-BNI did not alter EtOH SA	(Doyon et al. 2006)
28	EtOH (10% v/v)	Nor-BNI (5 mg/kg, SC)	Male Wistar rat	Nor-BNI blocked increased "escalated" rates of EtOH SA	(Walker et al. 2011)

29	EtOH (10% v/v)	JDTic (0–10 mg/kg, IP) Nor-BNI (0, 30 mg/kg, SC)	Male Wistar rat	JDTic and nor-BNI decreased rates of EtOH SA	(Schank et al. 2012)
30	EtOH (15% v/v)	JDTic (0–10 mg/kg, SC)	Female alcohol-preferring (P) rat	JDTic did not alter EtOH SA	(Deehan et al. 2012)
31	EtOH (15% v/v)	LY2456302 (3–10 mg/kg, PO)	Female P rat	Acute LY2456302 decreased the amount of EtOH consumed	(Rorick-Kehn et al. 2014)
32	EtOH/saccharin/sucrose (10%/0.125%/3%)	Nor-BNI (0–10 mg/kg, SC)	Male and female S-D rat	Nor-BNI increased ethanol/saccharin consumption in male rats, decreased in female rats. Nor-BNI had no effect on adolescent EtOH/saccharin consumption	(Morales et al. 2014)
33	EtOH (10% v/v)	Compound 5 (0.0031–0.0125 mg/kg, SC)	Male P rat	Acute compound 5 (KOR antagonist) decreased rates of EtOH SA	(Cashman and Azar 2014)
34	EtOH (20% v/v)	CERC-501 (0–10 mg/kg, PO)	Male Wistar rat	Acute CERC-501 decreases rates of EtOH SA	(Domi et al. 2018)

Columns show the self-administered drug, the specific KOR ligand, the sex and species in which the studies were conducted, the primary effect reported in the study, and the reference. Numbers in parentheses indicate unit drug doses in μg or mg/kg/injection for the self-administered drug and drug doses for the KOR ligand mixture of KOR agonist and drug of abuse. Based on the literature cited above, the hypothesis for these studies would be that the KOR agonist mixed with the drug of abuse would lead to a decrease in rates of drug SA. Three studies (#1–3 in Table 2) have examined combining a KOR agonist and cocaine (Freeman et al. 2014) or a MOR agonist (Negus et al. 2008; Townsend et al. 2017). All three studies reported that mixtures of the abused drug and KOR agonist were less reinforcing (i.e., maintained lower rates of operant responding) than the abused drug alone. These results have been interpreted to suggest that clinical combinations of MOR agonists and KOR agonists might retain the therapeutic desirable effects (e.g., analgesia) of MOR agonists with reduced undesirable effects (e.g., abuse liability). However, illicit drug manufacturers or dealers are unlikely to adulterate their product with something that would deter abuse liability.

3.2 KOR Agonists as Pretreatments to Preclinical Drug of Abuse SA

A second type of experiment has examined either acute KOR agonist pretreatment to a single drug SA or repeated KOR agonist treatment effects across multiple days of drug SA. The studies that employed a repeated dosing procedure were modeling aspects of repeated candidate medication administration utilized in human laboratory studies, clinical trials, and clinical prescribing patterns for current FDA-approved treatments for SUDs (e.g., buprenorphine, methadone, varenicline, and naltrexone). Thirteen studies (#4–16 in Table 2) have examined the effects of either acute or repeated KOR agonist treatment on drug SA in mice, rats, and rhesus monkeys. Acute administration of U50,488 (Glick et al. 1995), U69,593 (Schenk et al. 1999; Schenk et al. 2001), cyclazocine (Glick et al. 1998), spiradoline (Glick et al. 1995), and enadoline (Bowen et al. 2003; Hölter et al. 2000) has been reported to decrease rates of cocaine, morphine, and ethanol SA in both rats and rhesus monkeys. These results were interpreted as evidence that KOR agonists may have clinical utility as candidate medications for SUD treatment.

However, when KOR agonist effects on drug SA were examined under repeated dosing conditions, a more complicated profile of effects emerged compared to the acute KOR agonist pretreatment studies described above. For example, repeated ethylketocyclazine, U50,488, enadoline, spiradoline, PD117302, bremazocine, and cyclazocine treatments all produced sustained decreases in rates of cocaine and ethanol SA in rhesus monkeys (Cosgrove and Carroll 2002; Mello and Negus 1998; Negus et al. 1997). Repeated bremazocine, but not U50,488, produced sustained decreases in rates of ethanol SA in rats (Nestby et al. 1999). Repeated U50,488 treatment significantly decreased rates of nicotine SA in rats on the third day of treatment and without altering food-maintained responding (Ismayilova and Shoaib 2010). However, the KOR agonist doses that decreased drug SA also decreased rates of food-maintained responding when food-maintained responding was assessed (Cosgrove and Carroll 2002; Mello and Negus 1998; Negus et al. 1997). Thus, repeated KOR agonist treatment effects were not behaviorally selective for drug vs. nondrug reinforcers and suggestive of overall depression of behavior. In contrast to these results, repeated enadoline treatment increased rates of ethanol SA in rats (Hölter et al. 2000) and repeated U50,488 treatment shifted both cocaine and morphine SA dose-effect functions to the left in rats (Kuzmin et al. 1997). Furthermore, when repeated U50,488 treatment effects were examined on cocaine SA in rhesus monkeys under conditions where there was an alternative nondrug food reinforcer available concurrently to intravenous cocaine injections, repeated U50,488 increased cocaine "choice" and decreased food "choice" (Negus 2004). Consistent with these later results, repeated enadoline treatment failed to attenuate cocaine vs. money choice in humans, and there was a trend for increased cocaine choice at the largest enadoline dose examined (Walsh et al. 2001). No double-blind, placebo-controlled clinical trials examining KOR agonists as candidate pharmacotherapies for SUD treatment have been published.

In summary, the effects of KOR agonists on preclinical drug SA studies and the single human laboratory drug SA study have thus far generated three main findings. First, when KOR agonists are mixed with the abuse drug and co-administered, KOR agonists can function as punishers and decrease SA of the abused drug. Second, acute pretreatment with a KOR agonist decreased rates of drug SA across a broad range of abused drug classes (e.g. cocaine, ethanol, morphine). Lastly, repeated KOR agonist treatment either decreased rates of abused drug SA typically at doses that also decreased rates of food-maintained responding or increases rates of drug SA including under a drug vs. food choice procedure. Overall, this body of preclinical literature does not support the clinical utility of KOR agonists as candidate SUD treatments.

4 KOR Antagonist Effects on Preclinical Drug Self-Administration

One prominent and emerging SUD theory is that chronic exposure to drugs of abuse and withdrawal produces a "motivational withdrawal syndrome" that increases the magnitude and alters the mechanisms of drug reinforcement and serves as "one of the driving factors of compulsivity in addiction" (Koob and Mason 2016). Chronic exposure to drugs of abuse is hypothesized to alter the state of the patient or research subject and thereby alter the mechanisms of and increase the magnitude of drug reinforcement. For example, opioid abuse often leads to physical dependence, and opioid withdrawal in dependent subjects increases the reinforcing effects of opioids, decreases the reinforcing efficacy of nondrug reinforcers like food, and promotes a maladaptive allocation of behavior toward further drug use at the expense of behaviors maintained by more adaptive behaviors. Specifically, chronic drug exposure has been shown to (1) decrease basal activity of dopamine and/or opioid reward systems and (2) recruit activation of other neural systems, sometimes described as "stress" or "anti-reward" systems, that involve neurotransmitters including corticotropic releasing factor (CRF) and dynorphin (Koob and Mason 2016; Koob and Moal 2008; Koob and Volkow 2009). Overall, consumption of any abused drug dose is hypothesized to produce an initial increase in dopamine/opioid signaling as drug levels rise and peak, followed by a longer period of depressed dopamine/opioid signaling and enhanced stress hormone signaling that together mediate negative affective states of drug withdrawal. Increasingly intensive regimens of abused drug exposure are hypothesized to produce a cumulative increase in the later effects and increasingly intense aversive subjective states. Under these circumstances, drug-induced reinforcing effects are often described as "negative," because the drug is now hypothesized to produce its reinforcing effects not by increasing dopamine/opioid signaling from a normal basal level but rather by alleviating the aversive state produced by a depressed reward system and activated stress system; however, this interpretation is not consistent with the operational definition of negative reinforcement (i.e., response requirement completion results in removal of S^C proposed by Skinner (1938)). The subject in a drug SA procedure is responding to receive the drug injection (S^C) which is positive reinforcement and not the removal of some hypothesized internal state (Negus and Banks 2018).

Evidence to support this hypothesized transition comes in part from preclinical rat drug SA studies that have used single-operant drug SA procedures in which the primary dependent measure is the rate of drug SA. Two observations have been seminal in support of this hypothesized transition. *First*, the recruitment of negative reinforcement processes that occurs with extended drug SA is hypothesized to not only modify the mechanisms of drug reinforcement but also to increase its magnitude (i.e., by summing positive and negative reinforcement mechanisms). In support of this hypothesis, regiments of "extended access" (produced by increasing the number of hours per day that subjects can self-administer drug) have been shown to increase rates of SA, a phenomenon referred to as "escalation" (Koob and Kreek 2007). *Second*, the recruitment of these negative reinforcement processes is also hypothesized to render drug SA sensitive to experimental manipulations that attenuate the KOR/stress system signaling. For example, dynorphin acting at KOR is one stress-related neurotransmitter implicated in "negative reinforcement" processes, and KOR antagonists such as nor-binaltorphimine (nor-BNI) and CERC-501 have been reported to block escalated rates of cocaine, methamphetamine, heroin, and ethanol SA in rats (Domi et al. 2018; Schlosburg et al. 2013; Walker et al. 2011; Wee et al. 2009; Wee et al. 2012; Whitfield et al. 2015). Furthermore, KOR antagonists do not attenuate cocaine, methamphetamine, or heroin SA under more limited (~1–2 h) drug access conditions in both rats (Deehan et al. 2012; Doyon et al. 2006; Glick et al. 1995; Hölter et al. 2000; Liu and Jernigan 2011; Negus et al. 1993) and rhesus monkeys (Negus 2004; Negus et al. 1997) suggesting that the recruitment of the dynorphin/KOR system only occurs during extended drug access conditions. Although the effectiveness of KOR antagonists to alter drug SA appears to be dependent on the length of the drug SA session for MOR agonists and monoamine transporter ligands (cocaine and methamphetamine; Table 2), the literature suggests the same principle does not necessarily hold true for ethanol. For example, under limited ethanol access conditions, KOR antagonists have been shown to increase

(Mitchell et al. 2005), have no effect (Deehan et al. 2012; Doyon et al. 2006), or decrease (Cashman and Azar 2014; Rorick-Kehn et al. 2014; Schank et al. 2012) ethanol SA in rats. Overall, one implication of this literature is that different classes of abused drugs might recruit the dynorphin/KOR system in different manners.

4.1 KOR Antagonist Effects on Preclinical Drug Choice SA

However, these KOR antagonist treatment effects on preclinical drug SA endpoints have not translated when evaluated in nonhuman primates or humans. For example, in opioid-dependent rhesus monkeys, the KOR antagonist 5′-guanidinaltrindole (GNTI) failed to attenuate opioid withdrawal-associated increases in opioid vs. food choice (Negus and Rice 2009). In addition, nor-BNI failed to attenuate both rates of cocaine SA during extended cocaine access sessions and cocaine vs. food choice in rhesus monkeys self-administering cocaine 22-h per day (Hutsell et al. 2016). Whether these differences in KOR antagonist effects are due to species differences between rats and rhesus monkeys or procedural differences in the drug SA schedule or reinforcement remain unexplored scientific space.

4.2 KOR Antagonist Effects on Human Drug SA Metrics

In humans, buprenorphine plus naloxone and naltrexone maintenance, combined to produce a KOR antagonist effect, failed to attenuate cocaine use in a double-blind, placebo-controlled, multi-centered clinical trial (Ling et al. 2016). Repeated LY2456302 treatment also failed to attenuate cocaine craving in humans (Reed et al. 2017). Furthermore, CERC-501 (i.e., LY2456301) failed to attenuate cigarette smoking, craving, or nicotine withdrawal in humans (Jones et al. 2019). Moreover, a recent positron-emission tomography study examining KOR binding in healthy controls and cocaine abusers reported no significant differences in KOR binding in any brain region examined (Martinez et al. 2019). These results suggest that a history of repeated cocaine exposure and a diagnosis of cocaine use disorder were not sufficient to alter KOR binding in humans and are in contrast to previous results in cocaine overdose patients using autoradiography methods (Hurd and Herkenham 1993; Staley et al. 1997). Reasons for differences between the in vivo positron-emission tomography study and the postmortem mRNA and autoradiography study are not presently clear but could be related to the affinity of the ligands for different KOR subtypes or states (i.e., high vs. low affinity). In summary, the promising results of KOR antagonists in preclinical rodent models of cocaine use disorder have so far failed to translate when evaluated in higher-order species such as nonhuman primates or humans and on endpoints that focus on behavioral allocation between drug and nondrug reinforcers instead of rates of drug-taking behavior.

5 Conclusions and Future Directions

Over the past two decades, preclinical research has improved our understanding of the role of KOR in the expression, mechanisms, and treatment of SUD. Converging lines of evidence from both preclinical and human studies support the conclusion that chronic abused drug exposure changes the dynorphin/KOR system. Furthermore, mixtures of MOR and KOR agonists (Freeman et al. 2014; Negus et al. 2008; Townsend et al. 2017) or mixed-action MOR/KOR agonists such as pentazocine (Hoffmeister 1979) appear to have reduced abuse-related effects compared to MOR agonists. However, both KOR agonist and KOR antagonist treatments have thus far failed to significantly alter metrics of cocaine use in humans. Unfortunately, there are no published human laboratory drug SA studies or clinical trials evaluating KOR agonist or antagonist effects on other SUDs, such as methamphetamine, opioids, ethanol, or tobacco. CERC-501 is currently being evaluated in clinical trials as a candidate medication for tobacco smoking and smoking relapse (Helal et al. 2017). The evaluation of candidate medication effects in SUD patients provides critical reverse translational feedback to improve the predictive validity of preclinical SUD models. However, the results of KOR agonists and antagonists in cocaine use disorder and tobacco use disorder patients thus far fail to support the continued development and evaluation of novel chemical entities targeting the dynorphin/KOR system as candidate SUD pharmacotherapies. There are presently no published clinical data on the effectiveness of KOR antagonists for alcohol or opioid use disorder.

In the broader preclinical drug abuse literature, there are two experimental features that appear to promote accurate translation of preclinical-to-clinical results. First, repeated treatment with the candidate medication to match the subchronic-to-chronic treatment regimens commonly employed in clinical SUD treatment (Czoty et al. 2016; Haney and Spealman 2008b; Mello and Negus 1996). The effects of acute vs. repeated KOR agonists on preclinical drug SA endpoints reviewed above are consistent with this conclusion. However, the examination of repeated KOR antagonist effects on drug SA endpoints has been problematic because most currently available KOR antagonists are irreversible or receptor-inactivating antagonists (Butelman et al. 1993, 1998; Schmid et al. 2013). The long duration of action of irreversible KOR antagonists complicates dose titration and potentially increases the risk of off-target undesirable effects. The development of short-acting KOR antagonists CERC-501 (i.e., LY2456302) (Helal et al. 2017; Reed et al. 2017) has facilitated clinical SUD research to provide necessary feedback regarding hypotheses developed using preclinical drug SA procedures. Second, assessment of candidate medication effects in preclinical drug SA procedures that use behavioral allocation between the target drug of abuse and an alternative nondrug reinforcer (e.g., food or social) rather than rates of drug SA behavior has shown strong translational concordance with clinical results (for review, see Banks et al. 2015; Banks and Negus 2012, 2017). A critical step in efficiently evaluating candidate SUD medications is the utilization of preclinical testing procedures that are both sensitive to FDA-approved medications (if available) and selective for those positive controls in comparison to active negative controls known to be clinically ineffective (Banks et al. 2019). Given the human laboratory and clinical literature cited above in Sects. 3 and 4, both KOR agonists and KOR antagonists could function as active negative controls, but should not continued to be evaluated as candidate OUD medications (Rasmussen et al. 2019).

References

Ator NA, Griffiths RR (2003) Principles of drug abuse liability assessment in laboratory animals. Drug Alcohol Depend 70:S55–S72

Banks ML, Negus SS (2012) Preclinical determinants of drug choice under concurrent schedules of drug self-administration. Adv Pharmacol Sci 2012:281768

Banks ML, Negus SS (2017) Insights from preclinical choice models on treating drug addiction. Trends Pharmacol Sci 38:181–194

Banks ML, Hutsell BA, Schwienteck KL, Negus SS (2015) Use of preclinical drug vs. food choice procedures to evaluate candidate medications for cocaine addiction. Curr Treat Options Psychiatry 2:136–150

Banks ML, Townsend EA, Negus SS (2019) Testing the 10 most wanted: a preclinical algorithm to screen candidate opioid use disorder medications. Neuropsychopharmacology

Bowen CA, Negus SS, Zong R, Neumeyer JL, Bidlack JM, Mello NK (2003) Effects of mixed-action κ/μ opioids on cocaine self-administration and cocaine discrimination by rhesus monkeys. Neuropsychopharmacology 28:1125–1139

Butelman ER, Negus SS, Ai Y, de Costa BR, Woods JH (1993) Kappa opioid antagonist effects of systemically administered nor-binaltorphimine in a thermal antinociception assay in rhesus monkeys. J Pharmacol Exp Ther 267:1269–1276

Butelman ER, Ko M-C, Sobczyk-Kojiro K, Mosberg HI, Van Bemmel B, Zernig G, Woods JH (1998) Kappa-opioid receptor binding populations in rhesus monkey brain: relationship to an assay of thermal antinociception. J Pharmacol Exp Ther 285:595–601

Carlezon WA, Béguin C, DiNieri JA, Baumann MH, Richards MR, Todtenkopf MS, Rothman RB, Ma Z, Lee DY-W, Cohen BM (2006) Depressive-like effects of the κ-opioid receptor agonist salvinorin A on behavior and neurochemistry in rats. J Pharmacol Exp Ther 316:440–447

Carter LP, Griffiths RR (2009) Principles of laboratory assessment of drug abuse liability and implications for clinical development. Drug Alcohol Depend 105(Suppl 1):S14–S25

Cashman JR, Azar MR (2014) Potent inhibition of alcohol self-administration in alcohol-preferring rats by a κ-opioid receptor antagonist. J Pharmacol Exp Ther 350:171–180

Chavkin C, Koob GF (2015) Dynorphin, dysphoria, and dependence: the stress of addiction. Neuropsychopharmacology 41:373

Chavkin C, James I, Goldstein A (1982) Dynorphin is a specific endogenous ligand of the kappa opioid receptor. Science 215:413–415

Clarke T-K, Ambrose-Lanci L, Ferraro TN, Berrettini WH, Kampman KM, Dackis CA, Pettinati HM, O'Brien CP, Oslin DW, Lohoff FW (2012) Genetic association analyses of PDYN polymorphisms with heroin and cocaine addiction. Genes Brain Behav 11:415–423

Comer SD, Ashworth JB, Foltin RW, Johanson CE, Zacny JP, Walsh SL (2008) The role of human drug self-administration procedures in the development of medications. Drug Alcohol Depend 96:1–15

Cosgrove KP, Carroll ME (2002) Effects of bremazocine on self-administration of smoked cocaine base and orally delivered ethanol, phencyclidine, saccharin, and food in rhesus monkeys: a behavioral economic analysis. J Pharmacol Exp Ther 301:993–1002

Crowley NA, Kash TL (2015) Kappa opioid receptor signaling in the brain: circuitry and implications for treatment. Prog Neuro-Psychopharmacol Biol Psychiatry 62:51–60

Czoty PW, Stoops WW, Rush CR (2016) Evaluation of the "Pipeline" for development of medications for cocaine use disorder: a review of translational preclinical, human laboratory, and clinical trial research. Pharmacol Rev 68:533–562

Daunais JB, Roberts DC, McGinty JF (1993) Cocaine self-administration increases preprodynorphin, but not c-fos, mRNA in rat striatum. Neuroreport 4:543–546

Deehan GA, McKinzie DL, Carroll FI, McBride WJ, Rodd ZA (2012) The long-lasting effects of JDTic, a kappa opioid receptor antagonist, on the expression of ethanol-seeking behavior and the relapse drinking of female alcohol-preferring (P) rats. Pharmacol Biochem Behav 101:581–587

Devine DP, Leone P, Pocock D, Wise RA (1993) Differential involvement of ventral tegmental mu, delta and kappa opioid receptors in modulation of basal mesolimbic dopamine release: in vivo microdialysis studies. J Pharmacol Exp Ther 266:1236–1246

Di Chiara G, Imperato A (1988) Drugs abused by humans preferentially increase synaptic dopamine concentrations in the mesolimbic system of freely moving rats. Proc Natl Acad Sci U S A 85:5274–5278

Domi E, Barbier E, Augier E, Augier G, Gehlert D, Barchiesi R, Thorsell A, Holm L, Heilig M (2018) Preclinical evaluation of the kappa-opioid receptor antagonist CERC-501 as a candidate therapeutic for alcohol use disorders. Neuropsychopharmacology 43:1805–1812

Donzanti BA, Althaus JS, Payson MM, Von Voigtlander PF (1992) Kappa agonist-induced reduction in dopamine release: site of action and tolerance. Res Commun Chem Pathol Pharmacol 78:193–210

Doyon WM, Howard EC, Shippenberg TS, Gonzales RA (2006) κ-Opioid receptor modulation of accumbal dopamine concentration during operant ethanol self-administration. Neuropharmacology 51:487–496

Fagergren P, Smith HR, Daunais JB, Nader MA, Porrino LJ, Hurd YL (2003) Temporal upregulation of prodynorphin mRNA in the primate striatum after cocaine self-administration. Eur J Neurosci 17:2212–2218

Ferster C, Skinner B (1957) Schedules of reinforcement. Appleton-Century-Croft, New York

Freeman KB, Naylor JE, Prisinzano TE, Woolverton WL (2014) Assessment of the kappa opioid agonist, salvinorin A, as a punisher of drug self-administration in monkeys. Psychopharmacology 231:2751–2758

Glick SD, Maisonneuve IM, Raucci J, Sydney A (1995) Kappa opioid inhibition of morphine and cocaine self-administration in rats. Brain Res 681:147–152

Glick SD, Visker KE, Maisonneuve IM (1998) Effects of cyclazocine on cocaine self-administration in rats. Eur J Pharmacol 357:9–14

Haney M, Spealman R (2008a) Controversies in translational research: drug self-administration. Psychopharmacology 199:403–419

Haney M, Spealman R (2008b) Controversies in translational research: drug self-administration. Psychopharmacology 199:403–419

Helal MA, Habib ES, Chittiboyina AG (2017) Selective kappa opioid antagonists for treatment of addiction, are we there yet? Eur J Med Chem 141:632–647

Hoffmeister F (1979) Progressive-ratio performance in the rhesus monkey maintained by opiate infusions. Psychopharmacology 62:181–186

Hölter SM, Henniger MSH, Lipkowski AW, Spanagel R (2000) Kappa-opioid receptors and relapse-like drinking in long-term ethanol-experienced rats. Psychopharmacology 153:93–102

Hunter JC, Leighton GE, Meecham KG, Boyle SJ, Horwell DC, Rees DC, Hughes J (1990) CI-977, a novel and selective agonist for the κ-opioid receptor. Br J Pharmacol 101:183–189

Hurd YL, Herkenham M (1993) Molecular alterations in the neostriatum of human cocaine addicts. Synapse 13:357–369

Hutsell BA, Cheng K, Rice KC, Negus SS, Banks ML (2016) Effects of the kappa opioid receptor antagonist nor-binaltorphimine (nor-BNI) on cocaine versus food choice and extended-access cocaine intake in rhesus monkeys. Addict Biol 00:360–373

Ismayilova N, Shoaib M (2010) Alteration of intravenous nicotine self-administration by opioid receptor agonist and antagonists in rats. Psychopharmacology 210:211–220

Jones JD, Babalonis S, Marcus R, Vince B, Kelsh D, Lofwall MR, Fraser H, Paterson B, Martinez S, Martinez DM, Nunes EV, Walsh SL, Comer SD (2019) A randomized, double-blind, placebo-controlled study of the kappa opioid receptor antagonist, CERC-501, in a human laboratory model of smoking behavior. Addict Biol 0: e12799

Koob GF, Kreek MJ (2007) Stress, dysregulation of drug reward pathways, and the transition to drug dependence. Am J Psychiatr 164:1149–1159

Koob GF, Mason BJ (2016) Existing and future drugs for the treatment of the dark side of addiction. Ann Rev Pharmacol Toxicol 56:299–322

Koob GF, Moal ML (2008) Addiction and the brain antireward system. Annu Rev Psychol 59:29–53

Koob GF, Volkow ND (2009) Neurocircuitry of addiction. Neuropsychopharmacology 35:217

Kuzmin AV, Semenova S, Gerrits MAFM, Zvartau EE, Van Ree JM (1997) κ-Opioid receptor agonist U50,488H modulates cocaine and morphine self-administration in drug-naive rats and mice. Eur J Pharmacol 321:265–271

Kuzmin AV, Gerrits MA, Van Ree JM (1998) Kappa-opioid receptor blockade with nor-binaltorphimine modulates cocaine self-administration in drug-naive rats. Eur J Pharmacol 358:197–202

Leitl MD, Onvani S, Bowers MS, Cheng K, Rice KC, Carlezon WA Jr, Banks ML, Negus SS (2014) Pain-related depression of the mesolimbic dopamine system in rats: expression, blockade by analgesics, and role of endogenous kappa-opioids. Neuropsychopharmacology 39:614–624

Ling W, Hillhouse MP, Saxon AJ, Mooney LJ, Thomas CM, Ang A, Matthews AG, Hasson A, Annon J, Sparenborg S, Liu DS, McCormack J, Church S, Swafford W, Drexler K, Schuman C, Ross S, Wiest K, Korthuis PT, Lawson W, Brigham GS, Knox PC, Dawes M, Rotrosen J (2016) Buprenorphine + naloxone plus naltrexone for the treatment of cocaine dependence: the cocaine use reduction with buprenorphine (CURB) study. Addiction 111:1416–1427

Liu X, Jernigan C (2011) Activation of the opioid μ1, but not δ or κ, receptors is required for nicotine reinforcement in a rat model of drug self-administration. Prog Neuro-Psychopharmacol Biol Psychiatry 35:146–153

Marinelli M, Barrot M, Simon H, Oberlander C, Dekeyne A, Moal ML, Piazza PV (1998) Pharmacological stimuli decreasing nucleus accumbens dopamine can act as positive reinforcers but have a low addictive potential. Eur J Neurosci 10:3269–3275

Martinez D, Slifstein M, Matuskey D, Nabulsi N, Zheng M-Q, Lin S-f, Ropchan J, Urban N, Grassetti A, Chang D, Salling M, Foltin R, Carson RE, Huang Y (2019) Kappa-opioid receptors, dynorphin, and cocaine addiction: a positron emission tomography study. Neuropsychopharmacology

Mello NK, Negus SS (1996) Preclinical evaluation of pharmacotherapies for treatment of cocaine and opioid abuse using drug self-administration procedures. Neuropsychopharmacology 14:375–424

Mello NK, Negus SS (1998) Effects of kappa opioid agonists on cocaine- and food-maintained responding by rhesus monkeys. J Pharmacol Exp Ther 286:812–824

Mitchell JM, Liang MT, Fields HL (2005) A single injection of the kappa opioid antagonist norbinaltorphimine increases ethanol consumption in rats. Psychopharmacology 182:384–392

Morales M, Anderson RI, Spear LP, El V (2014) Effects of the kappa opioid receptor antagonist, norbinaltorphimine, on ethanol intake: impact of age and sex. Dev Psychobiol 56:700–712

Munro TA, Huang X-P, Inglese C, Perrone MG, Van't Veer A, Carroll FI, Béguin C, Carlezon WA Jr, Colabufo NA, Cohen BM, Roth BL (2013) Selective κ opioid antagonists nor-BNI, GNTI and JDTic have low affinities for non-opioid receptors and transporters. PLoS One 8:e70701

Nagase H, Imaide S, Hirayama S, Nemoto T, Fujii H (2012) Essential structure of opioid κ receptor agonist nalfurafine for binding to the κ receptor 2: synthesis of decahydro(iminoethano)phen-anthrene derivatives and their pharmacologies. Bioorg Med Chem Letts 22:5071–5074

Negus SS (2004) Effects of the kappa opioid agonist U50,488 and the kappa opioid antagonist nor-binaltorphimine on choice between cocaine and food in rhesus monkeys. Psychopharmacology 176:204–213

Negus SS, Banks ML (2018) Modulation of drug choice by extended drug access and withdrawal in rhesus monkeys: implications for negative reinforcement as a driver of addiction and target for medications development. Pharmacol Biochem Behav 164:32–39

Negus SS, Rice KC (2009) Mechanisms of withdrawal-associated increases in heroin self-administration: pharmacologic modulation of heroin vs food choice in heroin-dependent rhesus monkeys. Neuropsychopharmacology 34:899–911

Negus SS, Henriksen SJ, Mattox A, Pasternak GW, Portoghese PS, Takemori AE, Weinger MB, Koob GF (1993) Effect of antagonists selective for mu, delta and kappa opioid receptors on the reinforcing effects of heroin in rats. J Pharmacol Exp Ther 265:1245–1252

Negus SS, Mello NK, Portoghese PS, Lin C-E (1997) Effects of kappa opioids on cocaine self-administration by rhesus monkeys. J Pharmacol Exp Ther 282:44–55

Negus SS, Schrode K, Stevenson GW (2008) Mu/kappa opioid interactions in rhesus monkeys: implications for analgesia and abuse liability. Exp Clin Psychopharmacol 16:386–399

Nestby P, Schoffelmeer ANM, Homberg JR, Wardeh G, De Vries TJ, Mulder AH, Vanderschuren LJMJ (1999) Bremazocine reduces unrestricted free-choice ethanol self-administration in rats without affecting sucrose preference. Psychopharmacology 142:309–317

Oka T, Negishi K, Suda M, Sawa A, Fujino M, Wakimasu M (1982) Evidence that dynorphin-(1–13) acts as an agonist on opioid κ-receptors. Eur J Pharmacol 77:137–141

Pfeiffer A, Brantl V, Herz A, Emrich H (1986) Psychotomimesis mediated by kappa opiate receptors. Science 233:774–776

Rasmussen K, White DA, Acri JB (2019) NIDA's medication development priorities in response to the opioid crisis: ten most wanted. Neuropsychopharmacology 44:657–659

Raynor K, Kong H, Chen Y, Yasuda K, Yu L, Bell GI, Reisine T (1994) Pharmacological characterization of the cloned kappa-, delta-, and mu-opioid receptors. Mol Pharmacol 45:330–334

Reed B, Butelman ER, Fry RS, Kimani R, Kreek MJ (2017) Repeated administration of opra kappa (LY2456302), a novel, short-acting, selective KOP-r antagonist, in persons with and without cocaine dependence. Neuropsychopharmacology 43:739

Rorick-Kehn LM, Witkin JM, Statnick MA, Eberle EL, McKinzie JH, Kahl SD, Forster BM, Wong CJ, Li X, Crile RS, Shaw DB, Sahr AE, Adams BL, Quimby SJ, Diaz N, Jimenez A, Pedregal C, Mitch CH, Knopp KL, Anderson WH, Cramer JW, McKinzie DL (2014) LY2456302 is a novel, potent, orally-bioavailable small molecule kappa-selective antagonist with activity in animal models predictive of efficacy in mood and addictive disorders. Neuropharmacology 77:131–144

Roth BL, Baner K, Westkaemper R, Siebert D, Rice KC, Steinberg S, Ernsberger P, Rothman RB (2002) Salvinorin A: a potent naturally occurring nonnitrogenous κ opioid selective agonist. Proc Natl Acad Sci U S A 99:11934–11939

Schank JR, Goldstein AL, Rowe KE, King CE, Marusich JA, Wiley JL, Carroll FI, Thorsell A, Heilig M (2012) The kappa opioid receptor antagonist JDTic attenuates alcohol seeking and withdrawal anxiety. Addict Biol 17:634–647

Schenk S, Partridge B, Shippenberg TS (1999) U69593, a kappa-opioid agonist, decreases cocaine self-administration and decreases cocaine-produced drug-seeking. Psychopharmacology 144:339–346

Schenk S, Partridge B, Shippenberg TS (2001) Effects of the kappa-opioid receptor agonist, U69593, on the development of sensitization and on the maintenance of cocaine self-administration. Neuropsychopharmacology 24:441

Schlosburg JE, Whitfield TW, Park PE, Crawford EF, George O, Vendruscolo LF, Koob GF (2013) Long-term antagonism of κ opioid receptors prevents escalation of and increased motivation for heroin intake. J Neurosci 33:19384–19392

Schmid CL, Streicher JM, Groer CE, Munro TA, Zhou L, Bohn LM (2013) Functional selectivity of 6′-guanidinonaltrindole (6′-GNTI) at κ opioid receptors in striatal neurons. J Biol Chem 288:22387–22398

Shippenberg TS, Zapata A, Chefer VI (2007) Dynorphin and the pathophysiology of drug addiction. Pharmacol Ther 116:306–321

Skinner B (1938) The behavior of organisms. Appleton-Century-Crofts, New York

Solecki W, Ziolkowska B, Krowka T, Gieryk A, Filip M, Przewlocki R (2009) Alterations of prodynorphin gene expression in the rat mesocorticolimbic system during heroin self-administration. Brain Res 1255:113–121

Spanagel R, Herz A, Shippenberg TS (1990) The effects of opioid peptides on dopamine release in the nucleus accumbens: an in vivo microdialysis study. J Neurochem 55:1734–1740

Staley JK, Rothman RB, Rice KC, Partilla J, Mash DC (1997) κ2 opioid receptors in limbic areas of the human brain are upregulated by cocaine in fatal overdose victims. J Neurosci 17:8225–8233

Tang AH, Collins RJ (1985) Behavioral effects of a novel kappa opioid analgesic, U-50488, in rats and rhesus monkeys. Psychopharmacology 85:309–314

Tejeda HA, Bonci A (2019) Dynorphin/kappa-opioid receptor control of dopamine dynamics: Implications for negative affective states and psychiatric disorders. Brain Res 1713:91–101

Townsend EA, Naylor JE, Negus SS, Edwards SR, Qureshi HN, McLendon HW, McCurdy CR, Kapanda CN, do Carmo JM, da Silva FS, Hall JE, Sufka KJ, Freeman KB (2017) Effects of nalfurafine on the reinforcing, thermal antinociceptive, and respiratory-depressant effects of oxycodone: modeling an abuse-deterrent opioid analgesic in rats. Psychopharmacology 234:2597–2605

Walker BM, Zorrilla EP, Koob GF (2011) Systemic κ-opioid receptor antagonism by nor-binaltorphimine reduces dependence-induced excessive alcohol self-administration in rats. Addict Biol 16:116–119

Walsh SL, Geter-Douglas B, Strain EC, Bigelow GE (2001) Enadoline and butorphanol: evaluation of κ-agonists on cocaine pharmacodynamics and cocaine self-administration in humans. J Pharmacol Exp Ther 299:147–158

Wee S, Koob G (2010a) The role of the dynorphin–κ opioid system in the reinforcing effects of drugs of abuse. Psychopharmacology 210:121–135

Wee S, Koob GF (2010b) The role of the dynorphin–κ opioid system in the reinforcing effects of drugs of abuse. Psychopharmacology 210:121–135

Wee S, Orio L, Ghirmai S, Cashman J, Koob G (2009) Inhibition of kappa opioid receptors attenuated increased cocaine intake in rats with extended access to cocaine. Psychopharmacology 205:565–575

Wee S, Vendruscolo LF, Misra KK, Schlosburg JE, Koob GF (2012) A combination of buprenorphine and naltrexone blocks compulsive cocaine intake in rodents without producing dependence. Science Transl Med 4:146ra110

Whitfield TW, Schlosburg JE, Wee S, Gould A, George O, Grant Y, Zamora-Martinez ER, Edwards S, Crawford E, Vendruscolo LF, Koob GF (2015) κ opioid receptors in the nucleus accumbens shell mediate escalation of methamphetamine intake. J Neurosci 35:4296–4305

Woods JH, Gmerek DE (1985) Substitution and primary dependence studies in animals. Drug Alcohol Depend 14:233–247

Clinical Trials for Opioid Use Disorder

Esther Blessing, Sanya Virani, and John Rotrosen

Contents

1 Background 168
2 Current OUD Pharmacotherapies 169
3 Novel Pharmacotherapies Under Study 174
3.1 Opioid Receptor Modulators 174
3.2 Cannabidiol, THC, and Cannabis 174
3.3 Psychedelics 177
3.4 Neuropeptides and Neuropeptide Receptor Modulators 178
3.5 Serotonin Receptor Modulators 180
3.6 Anti-inflammatory and Immunomodulatory Agents 180
3.7 Other: Analgesics, Calcium Channel Blockers, and Acetyl-Cholinesterase Inhibitors 182
4 Vaccines 184
5 New Formulations of Existing Drugs 185
6 Trials to Expand Use of Existing Marketed Agents, New Models of Care 186
7 Helping to End Addiction Long-Term (HEAL) 189
8 Initiatives for Special Populations 192
9 Devices, Apps, and Behavioral Interventions 193
10 Summary, Conclusions, and New Directions 194
References 195

Abstract

This chapter describes recent clinical trials for opioid use disorder (OUD), an area that has rapidly accelerated in response to the opioid overdose crisis in the USA and newly appropriated funding. Trials involve a wide range of compounds including cannabinoids and psychedelics, new and existing compounds targeting

E. Blessing (✉) · J. Rotrosen
Department of Psychiatry, NYU School of Medicine, New York, NY, USA
e-mail: esther.blessing@nyumc.org

S. Virani
Department of Psychiatry, Maimonides Medical Center, Brooklyn, NY, USA

M. A. Nader, Y. L. Hurd (eds.), *Substance Use Disorders*,
Handbook of Experimental Pharmacology 258, https://doi.org/10.1007/164_2019_304

domains emerging from addiction neuroscience, agents repurposed from other indications, and novel strategies including vaccines, enzymes, and other biologicals. In parallel, new formulations of existing compounds offer immediate promise, as do a variety of web-based interventions and smartphone-delivered apps. Trials focused on implementing existing effective interventions in mainstream healthcare settings, and others focused on special populations, e.g., adolescents, criminal justice, pregnant women, native Americans, etc., have the potential to vastly expand treatment in the near term. Given the range of ongoing and recent trials, this chapter is not intended to be an exhaustive review but rather to present an overview of approaches within the framework of the opioid treatment cascade and the context of current OUD pharmacotherapies.

Keywords
Addiction · Clinical trial · Opioid · Opioid use disorder

1 Background

Well before modern pharmacology, and even pharmacology itself, opioids were widely used, and it is likely that the ancients had an intuitive grasp of concepts now described as tolerance, dependence, withdrawal, and craving, which now form the underpinnings of our understanding of addiction and its treatment. More deliberate, empirical behavioral and pharmacological approaches to understanding and treating opioid addiction began with work in the early part of the past century led largely by the Addiction Research Center in Lexington, KY, and work done in the middle of the past century at The Rockefeller University in NY (Kreek et al. 2002; Kreek and Vocci 2002; Stimmel and Kreek 2000; Kreek 2000). Much of the current impetus and funding for treatment development stems from the present opioid crisis, which is not the first in the USA and, while devastating, of lesser magnitude than that in China in the early to mid-nineteenth century which led to the opium wars.

The present opioid crisis in the USA is really a combination of an urban minority heroin epidemic dating back to the mid-1900s and a more recent epidemic affecting all sociodemographic groups and rural and suburban communities, largely attributable to opioid painkiller overprescribing. Recent widespread availability of exceptionally potent fentanyl(s), which currently contributes to more than 80% of deaths in some regions of the country, has greatly increased overdose fatalities. This is also a global problem: the World Health Organization reported that roughly 450,000 people died worldwide as a result of drug use in 2015, and of those deaths, about 160,000 were directly associated with drug use disorders and about 118,000 with opioid use disorders (WHO 2019).

Currently, drug overdoses (most of them opioid-related) are killing more Americans each year than died at the peak of the HIV epidemic or during the entire 20-year duration of the Vietnam conflict. Geographic hotspots include northern New England, Appalachia and the Ohio Valley, Florida and the Gulf Coast, the Southwest, Northern California and the Pacific Northwest, and the Canadian border, but virtually every state has pockets of high use and high morbidity. Over the past decade, painkiller prescribing and related overdose fatalities have declined as its causative role has become more widely recognized; however prescription opioids continue to play a role in initiation. Many of those starting on pills now switch to heroin and fentanyl(s), largely because of the scarcity and high "street" cost of the former and the increased availability and lower cost of the latter (heroin prices are nearly an order of magnitude lower than a decade ago).

This led to the launch of a broad effort supported by federal, state, and local agencies and by industry, philanthropy, and public-private partnerships to develop new molecular entities working via opioid and non-opioid mechanisms; to develop new formulations of existing effective pharmacotherapies; to develop behavioral interventions, devices, and mHealth applications; and to vastly expand access to effective interventions by expanding their implementation from addiction specialty settings to mainstream healthcare settings such as primary care, HIV clinics, and emergency departments and also to criminal justice and other community settings. While this chapter will focus primarily on pharmaceutical clinical trials, we will touch on all of these areas insofar as other approaches may have equal or greater public health impact.

This chapter will first review currently used OUD treatments to contextualize recent and current clinical trials. The latter encompass a diverse suite of interventions, reviewed in the following order: novel pharmacotherapies, including new compounds and repurposing of drugs approved for other indications; vaccines and other biologicals; new formulations of existing compounds aimed to improve drug delivery; trials to expand use of existing marketed agents and new models of care; the National Institutes of Health (NIH) Helping to End Addiction Long-term (HEAL) initiative; trials aimed at special risk populations; and devices, apps, and behavioral interventions intended to expand and improve treatment. This is not an exhaustive review of all OUD clinical trials but rather is intended to include the major and, in our opinion, most promising drugs and interventions. Throughout, current and developing OUD treatments are contextualized in terms of molecular targets (e.g., opioid receptors, dopamine receptors, transporters, etc.), clinical targets (e.g., craving, withdrawal, relapse, etc.), and targets defined by the "opioid treatment cascade" (Williams et al. 2018) (e.g., treatment engagement, initiation, retention, re-engagement, etc.). For novel drugs, findings are included that are relevant to how these agents impact neurobiological addiction domains such as negative affect or cognitive and emotional regulation (Koob and Volkow 2016; Volkow et al. 2018). A summary then discusses the scope of current treatments and clinical trials and highlights limitations and areas for further development.

2 Current OUD Pharmacotherapies

Current OUD pharmacotherapies are nearly all opioid based, i.e., their efficacy depends on actions at the mu opioid receptor. These include methadone, a full mu receptor agonist; buprenorphine (BUP), a partial mu receptor agonist; and naltrexone (NTX) and naloxone (NX), full mu receptor antagonists. Methadone and BUP are the cornerstones of opioid *maintenance therapy*. In contrast, NTX, particularly in its extended-release formulation, is approved for *relapse prevention*. NX, a short-acting mu antagonist, is used primarily for acute *overdose reversal*. Beyond these, there are a handful of non-opioid medications that are often used to mitigate the aversive symptoms of opioid withdrawal and to facilitate detoxification. These include clonidine and lofexidine, both alpha-2 agonists, muscle relaxants, and sleep medications. Methadone, BUP, and NTX are sometimes referred to as "MAT" for "medication-assisted therapy". This terminology is rejected by some who believe that medication *is* therapy in and of itself, instead preferring to rebrand MAT as "medication addiction therapy"; this term then evolved to "MOUD" for "medication for opioid use disorder". We will also use the term "addiction pharmacotherapy."

Although all three of the opioid addiction pharmacotherapies owe their efficacy to actions at the mu receptor, there are striking pharmacological, philosophical, logistical, economic, and societal differences between them. Agonists (methadone and BUP) replace opioids at the receptor, thereby preventing craving, withdrawal, and other effects of addiction while at the same time maintaining tolerance and dependence and leading to withdrawal on discontinuation. At high doses, methadone, due to its full agonist properties, blocks the effects of all but extremely high doses of heroin or other opioids and blunts the "rush" even from high doses (Kreek et al. 2002; Kreek and Vocci 2002; Stimmel and Kreek 2000; Kreek 2000). BUP accomplishes the same due to its high mu receptor affinity and its partial mu agonist and kappa antagonist properties (Gowing et al. 2017; Nielsen et al. 2016; Mattick et al. 2014). In contrast, naltrexone, a full mu receptor antagonist with no agonist properties, is devoid of opioid-like effects and does not maintain tolerance or dependence, i.e., in contrast to agonists, there are no subjective consequences upon discontinuation (Krupitsky et al. 2011).

There are striking and important differences in transitioning from opioid misuse to treatment with each of these medications ("induction"). Because it is a full receptor agonist, patients misusing opioids can simply begin taking methadone at a low dose and begin to increase toward a "blocking" dose, usually considered to be in the 80–100 mg/day range. BUP, a partial agonist, has a very high affinity for the mu receptor and will displace most full agonists, precipitating withdrawal symptoms; hence BUP shouldn't be started until a patient has abstained from opioid use for hours to a day or so (depending on the half-life of the opioid being used) and is experiencing at least mild to moderate withdrawal symptoms, at which point BUP can be administered and escalated to an effective dose, usually considered to be in the 8–24 mg/day range. At the other extreme is NTX which should not be administered until all or nearly all opioid is washed out, usually requiring several days to several weeks of detoxification. The need for full or nearly full detoxification adds costs (frequently including inpatient care), and because many patients don't tolerate detoxification and walk away, a substantial proportion of patients intending to start naltrexone are lost before they get a first dose. Fortunately, there are recent and ongoing clinical trials aimed at facilitating and hastening NTX induction.

Because agonists can be abused, there are diversion risks and controlled substance restrictions (in some cases quite burdensome); neither is the case for antagonists. From a societal and a family perspective, it is sometimes perceived to be important to be "drug-free" meaning "opioid agonist-free" which precludes methadone and BUP and which can only be achieved via "abstinence-based" or "drug-free" programs or with a full antagonist (i.e., naltrexone). Some countries (e.g., Russia) and some systems (e.g., criminal justice systems (CJS) in some jurisdictions) discourage or absolutely prohibit agonist therapy.

These pharmacological and societal differences have led to regulatory restrictions that limit widespread treatment. Methadone is typically administered only in tightly controlled settings that don't and likely won't exist in many parts of the USA and the Russian Federation and, even where they do, are often off-putting to patients. In the USA, BUP can only be prescribed by providers who complete intensive training and obtain a special waiver, a significant barrier, particularly for busy primary care providers. Extended-release NTX (XR-NTX) can be prescribed by any provider and therefore provides a way around this barrier. However, because of the induction hurdle, the absence (until recently) of comparative effectiveness data and high cost, XR-NTX has only infrequently been prescribed. It should come as no surprise that there are long-standing controversies in the field – fueled in part by the absence of data – as to whether pharmacologically and conceptually quite opposite agonist or antagonist approaches are preferable or even acceptable. This is one of many lenses through which clinical trials, development, marketing, and regulation of these three pharmacotherapies should be viewed and the foundation upon which new opioid and non-opioid medications, behavioral therapies, and devices and applications will be built.

Methadone was initially developed in Germany in 1937 by Hoechst chemists seeking synthetic opioids to address Germany's opium shortage. It was marketed shortly thereafter and used widely during the World War II. Following the war, the patent was confiscated by the US Department of Commerce Intelligence and brought to the USA. In 1947 Eli Lilly (and subsequently Roxane Laboratories and Mallinckrodt Pharmaceuticals) began manufacturing methadone as an analgesic under the trade name Dolophine. Yet it was not until the heroin crisis of the 1960s that it was developed as a treatment for opioid addiction, largely by Drs. Vincent Dole, Marie Nyswander, and Mary Jeanne Kreek at The Rockefeller University, often in collaboration with Robert Newman and others at Beth Israel Hospital in NY City (Kreek et al. 2002; Kreek and Vocci 2002; Stimmel and Kreek 2000; Kreek 2000). Methadone is by far the best-studied OUD pharmacotherapy and is the gold standard for treatment. It is used both for short-term detoxification, usually 3–5 days in inpatient or outpatient settings, and for long-term, sometimes lifetime, opioid maintenance therapy in methadone maintenance treatment programs (MMTPs). Methadone maintenance is associated with reduced illicit opioid use, reduced criminality, reduced HIV transmission, reduced morbidity and mortality, and improved physiological and health outcomes, societal functioning, and employment. In the USA and in many other parts of the world, methadone can only be dispensed through highly regulated MMTPs which limits access geographically and which is perceived by some as being overly controlling and stigmatizing.

Buprenorphine (BUP) was synthesized by Reckitt and Colman (now Reckitt Benckiser) in 1969. It was initially developed as an analgesic lacking some of the undesirable properties of full mu agonists. Clinical trials began in 1971 leading to approval in the UK in 1978 of an injectable formulation and in 1982 for sublingual use. BUP is a partial mu receptor agonist and an antagonist at kappa and delta receptors. Development to treat OUD was begun in the 1990s, initially as a monotherapy (Subutex) and later in combination with naloxone (Suboxone) to prevent diversion. Many of the clinical trials were supported by NIDA in partnership with Reckitt Benckiser and the Department of Veterans Affairs Cooperative Studies Program, through VA CSP trials CS-999, CS-1008, and CS-1018, leading to approval for the present OUD indication in 2002. A specific goal was to develop BUP for "office-based" treatment (in contrast to MMTP clinic-type treatment with all its associated constraints) made possible by its partial agonist properties and the formulation including naloxone, both of which were expected to reduce overdose risk and diversion risk. Current labeling in the USA reflects involvement from the FDA, Drug Enforcement Administration (DEA), Substance Abuse and Mental Health Services Administration (SAMHSA), and other federal and local agencies and, while permitting office-based use, imposes regulatory burdens that are hurdles to more widespread use. In contrast, France (and other countries) allows widespread essentially unrestricted prescribing which had a rapid and dramatic impact on OUD-associated overdose fatalities (Auriacombe et al. 1994; Dupouy et al. 2017). Like methadone, BUP is used both for detoxification (several days) and for long-term maintenance. A focus of much ongoing and planned work is to expand BUP treatment in the community.

Methadone and BUP are classified as Schedule II and III drugs, respectively. While methadone is available by prescription as a pain medication, and commonly used for brief inpatient medical supervised withdrawal in hospital settings, it can be dispensed only at an outpatient opioid treatment program certified by SAMHSA and registered with the DEA or to a hospitalized patient in an emergency. BUP on the other hand is relatively less restricted and is available for outpatient use, and refills can also be provided.

Naltrexone (NTX) was first synthesized in 1963, and although it received FDA approval for opioid dependence in 1984 and for alcohol dependence in 1994, its use and effectiveness in the form of once-a-day tablets for oral administration have been sharply limited by poor adherence. To address this, a longer-acting formulation consisting of NTX embedded in polylactide-co-glycolide microspheres for once-monthly injection (extended-release NTX, XR-NTX) was developed in the 1990s and tested in clinical trials in the USA leading to approval for alcoholism in 2006 (Garbutt et al. 2005). A single trial in Russia led to US approval for opioid addiction in 2010 (Krupitsky et al. 2011). XR-NTX (Vivitrol) is administered by deep intramuscular injection following which naltrexone plasma concentrations rise to a transient initial peak in a few hours, followed 2–3 days later with a second peak. Plasma concentrations then gradually decrease but usually maintain therapeutic levels for about 4 weeks. It is important to recognize that XR-NTX's FDA labeling is for "relapse prevention," a contrast to BUP's labeling for "maintenance treatment of opioid dependence." There is good efficacy and effectiveness data from across a number of trials conducted in the CJS (Lee et al. 2016; McDonald et al. 2016; Murphy et al. 2017; Lee et al. 2015) which largely rejects agonist interventions, from a large NIDA Clinical Trials Network (NIDA CTN) trial comparing XR-NTX to buprenorphine/naloxone (Lee et al. 2018) and from a smaller parallel Norwegian trial (Tanum et al. 2017) with a similar design. Current clinical trials focus on improving and accelerating induction so as not to lose patients before a first injection and improving retention rates following initial treatment. Additional challenges remain around detoxification costs, XR-NTX costs, and providers' interest and perceived competence in treating OUD.

Naloxone (NX) is a rapidly acting and short-acting opioid receptor antagonist developed in 1961 and approved for use in treating opioid overdose in 1971 (Chou et al. 2017; Robinson and Wermeling 2014; Kim and Nelson 2015; Strang et al. 2016). Until recently it was available primarily in injectable form and used primarily in emergency department settings. Naloxone administration rapidly reverses the effects of opioid agonists and precipitates an acute withdrawal syndrome. As its effects wear off, signs and symptoms of overdose – most importantly respiratory depression, which can be fatal – re-emerge, sometimes requiring repeated administration or constant slow infusion, particularly in the case of overdose from long-acting opioids. More recently, NX has been reformulated for administration via intranasal spray and widely distributed to opioid users (including both addicts and those prescribed potent opioids), families, first responders (fire, police, EMS), and others in affected communities. Ongoing studies including clinical trials are focused on how best to distribute and educate the community to optimize outcomes, i.e., overdose reversals and overall reduction in overdose fatalities. Naloxone in usual doses may not be sufficient in reversing overdose from fentanyl and even higher-potency fentanyl derivatives, and the effects of NX also wear off rapidly. In highly affected regions of the USA, this has strained the budgets of first responder agencies. Wristwatch-like devices in development use biosensors to detect changes in heart rate and respiration and use algorithms to ascertain overdose and activate naloxone auto-injection. These have the potential to save lives in cases of unobserved overdose, yet fear of accidental auto-injection and precipitated withdrawal may sharply limit use.

Clonidine and Lofexidine are alpha-2 adrenergic receptor agonists used to modulate symptoms of opioid withdrawal. Clonidine has been marketed as an antihypertensive agent in the USA since 1966. Clonidine is not approved for opioid withdrawal but has been widely used off-label for this indication since the early 1980s (Gold et al. 1979, 1980a, b; Gold 1993), particularly in settings where opioid detoxification (methadone or BUP) is not available. Lofexidine (Gorodetzky et al. 2017; Cox and Alcorn 1995; Gowing et al. 2009) was also developed and initially used as an antihypertensive but received FDA approval in 2018 for "mitigation of withdrawal symptoms to facilitate abrupt discontinuation of opioids." Lofexidine was developed for this indication by US WorldMeds and is the first non-opioid approved for use in treating withdrawal symptoms of OUD. Both agents are used for periods of a few days to two weeks. Lofexidine may be less sedating and produce less orthostasis than clonidine, but otherwise there is little difference except in cost.

3 Novel Pharmacotherapies Under Study

3.1 Opioid Receptor Modulators

Nalmefene is a mu opioid receptor antagonist which contrasts with naloxone in also being a delta opioid receptor antagonist and partial kappa opioid receptor agonist. Intravenous (IV) nalmefene was FDA approved in 1995 to treat opioid overdose and then withdrawn from the market in 2008 due to low sales, with no significant safety issues. Nalmefene is also currently approved to treat alcohol use disorder (AUD) in France and the UK. Given nalmefene's longer half-life (6–8 h) and ~5× higher affinity at mu opioid receptors compared with NX (Krieter et al. 2019), it has the potential to address the important goal of developing stronger and longer-acting opioid antagonists (Volkow and Collins 2017) – this need stems from NX's relatively short half-life, necessitating repeated doses in overdose rescue situations. Evidence for the potential of nalmefene in treating opioid overdose in humans is currently limited to IV formulations. A double-blind study in patients reporting to the emergency department with suspected narcotic overdose compared IV nalmefene (1 or 2 mg) with naloxone (2 mg), given every 5 min as needed for up to 4 doses. Nalmefene and NX treatment led to a similar reduction in opioid withdrawal scale scores and improvement in respiratory depression and more nonfatal adverse events in the nalmefene 2 mg group (Kaplan et al. 1999). Toward intranasal (IN) nalmefene formulations, a recent Phase I study (NCT03129347) compared the pharmacokinetic properties of IN nalmefene (3 mg) in the presence of an absorption enhancer dodecyl maltoside to intramuscular nalmefene (1.5 mg) (Krieter et al. 2019). Results showed IN nalmefene with the enhancer had a relatively long half-life compared to NX and a comparable time to peak plasma level, making it suitable for reversing overdose. Studies are also underway to develop a much longer-acting (>28 days) nalmefene prodrug (NRS-033) for OUD treatment as (opposed to overdose reversal) (Grant number UG3DA048234).

3.2 Cannabidiol, THC, and Cannabis

Cannabidiol (CBD) is a phytocannabinoid present in *Cannabis sativa* that is non-psychotomimetic and nonintoxicating and pharmacologically distinct from tetrahydrocannabinol (THC), the major psychoactive constituent in cannabis. CBD has broad-spectrum pharmacological actions that are not yet fully understood (Zuardi 2008). Those linked to anti-addictive or anxiolytic actions relevant to its potential for treating OUD are detailed below. Several pharma companies have developed purified formulations of CBD with negligible THC content for oral or transdermal delivery; synthetic forms also exist. Epidiolex (pure oral CBD manufactured by GW Pharmaceuticals) was recently FDA approved for the treatment of childhood seizures.

CBD has been evaluated in Phase II and III trials for diverse medical and neuropsychiatric disorders, including nicotine (Morgan et al. 2013) and alcohol addiction (NCT03252756), and showed anxiolytic effects in human laboratory studies (Blessing et al. 2015). Completed clinical trials confirmed CBD's lack of psychotomimetic, intoxicating, and other adverse effects (apart from possible mild sedation and diarrhea) up to high (1,200 mg) repeated doses (Iffland and Grotenhermen 2017). Animal model, human laboratory and clinical trial evidence suggests potential for multiple therapeutic effects, including anti-addictive, anticonvulsive, anxiolytic, antipsychotic, anti-inflammatory, and neuroprotective (Fasinu et al. 2016; Crippa et al. 2018). CBD did not exhibit abuse liability in cannabis users (Babalonis et al. 2017).

CBD has not yet been evaluated for reducing substance use in OUD clinical trials, but has shown promising effects for reducing heroin craving and anxiety in abstinent heroin users. Hurd et al. recently assessed the acute (1, 2, and 24 h), short-term (3 consecutive days), and protracted (7 days after the last of three consecutive daily administrations) effects of oral CBD (400 or 800 mg, once daily for 3 consecutive days) on drug cue-induced craving and anxiety in drug-abstinent individuals with heroin use disorder in a double-blind randomized placebo-controlled trial (Hurd et al. 2019): CBD (vs placebo) substantially and significantly reduced both craving and anxiety induced by the presentation of drug cues, with protracted effects. This study replicated results from a smaller pilot study with a similar design (Hurd et al. 2015).

The human laboratory studies add to highly promising rodent model evidence showing CBD's potential to reduce behavioral vulnerabilities that drive relapse. Ren et al. demonstrated that CBD inhibited cue-induced heroin drug-seeking and reinstatement of this behavior in rats, with long-lasting effects (2 weeks) (Ren et al. 2009). In another study, CBD reduced cocaine and ethanol reinstatement with long-lasting effects (months) beyond drug action and also reduced context- and stress-induced ethanol seeking, anxiety, and impulsivity (Gonzalez-Cuevas et al. 2018). Receptor mechanisms linked to CBD's anxiolytic and pro-fear extinction effects include 5-HT_{1a} receptor agonist and indirect cannabinoid 1 receptor (CB1R) agonist actions in the extended amygdala, hippocampus, and medial prefrontal cortex (Blessing et al. 2015). Mechanisms underlying anti-addictive actions are less well studied; however one study showed correction of dependence-related neuroplasticity involved in normalization of α-amino-3-hydroxy-5-methyl-4-isoxazolepropionic acid (AMPA) GluR1 and CB1Rs in the nucleus accumbens (Ren et al. 2009). More broadly, CBD has multiple actions within the endocannabinoid system, which plays a central role in activity-dependent neuroplasticity and closely interacts with the opioid system (Scavone et al. 2013); CBD is also an allosteric modulator of the mu and delta opioid receptors (Kathmann et al. 2006).

Overall, CBD seems to offer promise for reducing relapse and anxiety in OUD, as will likely be explored in further clinical trials. Potential challenges include CBD's capacity, demonstrated in vitro, to inhibit cytochrome P450 enzymes that metabolize several prescribed and recreational opioids including fentanyl (CYP2D6 and CYP34A and others) (Yamaori et al. 2011a, b). Given the genetic variation in these enzymes, rigorous Phase I trials would be necessary to investigate the potential for CBD to increase opioid levels. Clinical trials to address these issues are in planning.

THC (Dronabinol) has also been investigated in humans for treating withdrawal in OUD, based upon findings in animal models showing that CB1 receptor agonists reduce opioid withdrawal symptoms. THC is a partial agonist at the CB1 receptor and, like CBD, is also an allosteric modulator of the mu and delta opioid receptors. Synthetic forms of THC or its analogues (dronabinol) are approved for neuropathic pain and treating nausea and vomiting associated with chemotherapy. In a study of opioid-dependent participants, dronabinol (30 mg/day for 5 weeks) was found to be superior to placebo in reducing withdrawal symptoms during detoxification but did not increase rates of induction onto XR-NTX or treatment retention relative to placebo (Bisaga et al. 2015). In another study of physically dependent opioid users, moderate-to-high doses of dronabinol were associated with elevated heart rate, anxiety, and panic raising safety concerns (Jicha et al. 2015; Lofwall et al. 2016).

Whole Cannabis Pharmacologically, cannabis includes the actions of CBD, THC, and other cannabinoids present in lower amounts. Most recreational cannabis (marijuana) contains minimal CBD and high levels of THC, whereas other cannabis varieties such as hemp (classified as cannabis containing less than 0.3% of THC according to the Agriculture Improvement Act of 2018) can contain upward of 50% CBD. Medical use of cannabis from a designated dispensary for a specified range of conditions is legal in 33 states. Very few or no clinical trials have been conducted with medical cannabis, and limited data are available on the potential therapeutic effects of recreational marijuana use. One clinical trial in 63 opioid-dependent users reported that intermittent marijuana use was associated with greater adherence with naltrexone treatment compared to no use or consistent use (Raby et al. 2009). Several epidemiological studies have suggested that overdose rates and opioid use may be lower in states where cannabis is legalized (Bachhuber et al. 2014; Liang et al. 2018); however, a recent prospective study in the USA showed that cannabis use (according to National Epidemiological Survey on Alcohol and Related Conditions data) was associated with a substantial increase in opioid use 3 years later (Olfson et al. 2018). Ongoing clinical trials are exploring subjective and safety interactions between cannabis and opioid use (NCT03705559); medical marijuana for reducing opioid analgesic use in HIV patients (NCT03268551), and the effects of naltrexone on cannabis use (NCT00403117).

3.3 Psychedelics

Ketamine and Other NMDA Antagonists Ketamine is a nonselective noncompetitive NMDA receptor antagonist (Zorumski et al. 2016) that is approved for use in general anesthesia. Long-lasting (post-drug) therapeutic effects that are observed in treating depression and other disorders suggest disease-modifying effects that are not currently understood (Strong and Kabbaj 2018). Three published studies have evaluated the efficacy of ketamine for OUD-related measures. Krupitsky et al. (Krupitsky et al. 2002) conducted a randomized controlled trial of ketamine-assisted psychotherapy in heroin-dependent participants. They compared the efficacy of high (2 mg/kg IM)- vs low (0.2 mg/kg IM)-dose ketamine with psychotherapy for maintaining abstinence from heroin, delivered at intervals over 24 months. The higher dose was associated with higher rates of abstinence (85%) compared to the lower dose (55%) and a greater reduction in craving. The same authors conducted a follow-up study in which they evaluated single vs repeated sessions of ketamine-assisted psychotherapy for maintaining heroin abstinence (Krupitsky et al. 2007). Repeated treatments were associated with 50% abstinence at 1-year follow-up, compared to 22% of single treatments, and a greater reduction in craving. In 58 opiate-dependent patients, Jovaisa et al. (2006) studied the effects of ketamine (0.5 mg/kg/h infusion) vs placebo on withdrawal symptoms following rapid opiate antagonist induction under general anesthesia, assessed immediately, at 48 h, and at 4 months. Ketamine was associated with reduced immediate and 48 h withdrawal symptoms. At 4 months, there was no difference from placebo. A trial is near completion for CI-581, an NMDA receptor antagonist, to facilitate induction into naltrexone (NCT02437344).

Ibogaine is a psychedelic alkaloid extracted from the root bark of *Tabernanthe iboga* or bark of *Voacanga africana* that has been in tribal ritual use for many centuries. Interest in ibogaine as a treatment for addiction including OUD is long-standing (>50 years), and it was marketed in France (Lambrene) until ~1970, but has never been approved in Europe or the USA for clinical trials, in part because of neuro- and cardiotoxic effects, especially QTc prolongation (Litjens and Brunt 2016; C Mash 2018). It has multiple pharmacological actions that are not fully characterized, including serotonergic, dopaminergic, and glutamatergic, and CYP2D6-mediated drug-drug interactions (Litjens and Brunt 2016). A considerable number of small, uncontrolled, open-label retrospective clinical studies as well as observational studies conducted in countries outside the USA have evaluated the efficacy of ibogaine for reducing withdrawal symptoms and drug use in OUD patients following detoxification. These studies reported promising results: administration of a single ibogaine dose between 10 and 30 mg/kg was associated with substantially reduced withdrawal symptoms including physiological measures – Clinical Opioid Withdrawal Scale (COWS) and Subjective Opioid Withdrawal Scale (SOWS) – craving, and drug use, with long-lasting effects (Malcolm et al. 2018; Brown and Alper 2018; Noller et al. 2018). Ibogaine's complex pharmacokinetics and high inter-individual variability in metabolism (Litjens and Brunt 2016;

C Mash 2018) as well as its neuro- and cardiotoxicity remain challenges to further development. Based on preclinical evidence, there is now new focus on 18-methoxycoronaridine (18-MC), an ibogaine analogue specifically developed to be devoid of neuro- and cardiotoxicity. It is an orally active and relatively specific $\alpha3\beta4$ nicotinic cholinergic receptor antagonist which indirectly modulates the dopaminergic mesolimbic pathway via actions in the habenulo-interpeduncular pathway and the basolateral amygdala. There are no clinical trials as yet for 18-MC in OUD.

Lysergic Acid Diethylamide (LSD) is a recreationally used classic hallucinogen, the psychoactive effects of which have been linked to serotonergic 2A agonist actions (Preller et al. 2017). One controlled clinical trial of LSD assisted psychotherapy was conducted in OUD patients in the early 1970s (Savage and McCabe 1973). The study was conducted in an outpatient clinic for paroled heroin addicts. Volunteer inmates with heroin addiction were discharged following release from prison and randomized to either an outpatient abstinence-based treatment program of 4–6 weeks of residential treatment in conjunction with high-dose LSD and psychedelic therapy (37 completers), or a control outpatient abstinence-based treatment-as-usual program with group therapy (37 completers). In both groups urine was monitored daily for opioid use. Results were promising: 25% of the treatment group were continuously abstinent during the 12-month follow-up, compared with 5% of the control group.

3.4 Neuropeptides and Neuropeptide Receptor Modulators

Dynorphin is an endogenous ligand for the kappa opioid receptor (KOR), which is widely distributed in the central nervous system. The dynorphin-KOR system plays a central role in modulation of nociception and the stress response, among other diverse physiological roles (Bruchas et al. 2010). Activation of this system is proposed to drive the addiction cycle by increasing stress and negative valence (Koob and Volkow 2016; Koob 2013; Koob et al. 2014). This hypothesis is consistent with findings that KOR activation consequent to dynorphin release increases corticotropin release in the extended amygdala and increases behaviors consistent with averse, dysphoric states; in addition, KOR activation reduces dopamine release in the VTA and glutamate release in the nucleus accumbens (Bruchas et al. 2010). Accordingly, KOR antagonists have been proposed to potentially combat addiction by reducing hyperactivation of the KOR system associated with stress surfeit in withdrawal states or stress-related psychiatric disorders (Butelman et al. 2012). A study evaluating the efficacy of a single dose of IV dynorphin (porcine fragment A 1-13) for reducing craving and other measures during acute withdrawal is near completion (NCT00000244). The rationale for using a partial agonist of the KOR (porcine dynorphin fragment) may be to block activation by endogenous dynorphin and thereby maintain a more constant tone in the dynorphin-KOR system; this hypothesis is based on the understanding that this system is upregulated and sensitized in addiction states (Bruchas et al. 2010; Butelman et al. 2012; Wee and Koob 2010).

Oxytocin is a neuropeptide that is synthesized in the magnocellular neurons of the paraventricular, supraoptic, and accessory magnocellular nuclei of the hypothalamus and released into the bloodstream from the posterior pituitary. Oxytocin regulates a variety of physiological functions and behaviors related to social bonding via dopaminergic interactions, which may contribute to its anti-addictive effects (Kovacs et al. 1998). Results from several clinical trials of oxytocin in AUD and cocaine use disorder have been published but thus far only one study in OUD. In a randomized, double-blind, placebo-controlled crossover study, the efficacy of intranasal oxytocin (40 international units) was evaluated for reducing cue-induced craving and improving measures of social cognition in 36 abstinent heroin-addicted patients who were stable on buprenorphine BUP or methadone (Woolley et al. 2016). Oxytocin did not reduce craving relative to placebo and had mixed effects on social cognition (Woolley et al. 2016). In rodent models of OUD, oxytocin reduced opioid tolerance and stress- and cue-induced drug seeking in dependent animals (Kovacs et al. 1998; Leong et al. 2018). Clinical trials evaluating oxytocin for several OUD indications including craving and withdrawal with concurrent assessment of social cognition are underway (NCT02548728, NCT02028533, NCT03016598, NCT02052258).

Aprepitant is a neurokinin 1 receptor (NK1R) antagonist that is clinically approved as an antiemetic. The NK1R is expressed throughout the reward system and autonomic midbrain and brainstem nuclei (Hargreaves 2002). Aprepitant blocks NK1R activation by the endogenous agonist substance P, which, in addition to reducing the vomiting reflex, modulates nociception (De Felipe et al. 1998), stress responsivity (Commons 2010), and reward behavior (Mannangatti et al. 2017), in part via interactions with opioid, dopaminergic, and serotonergic systems (Sandweiss and Vanderah 2015). Two preliminary human laboratory studies did not support the efficacy of aprepitant for OUD: Walsh et al. assessed subjective and physiologic responses to the mu agonist oxycodone in eight healthy adults who reported prescription opioid misuse, but were not physically dependent, and found that aprepitant (0, 40, and 200 mg, p.o. given as a 2-h pretreatment) substantially *increased* euphoria and liking and physiological effects (Walsh et al. 2013). Jones et al. reported that aprepitant 80 mg p.o. daily over 4 weeks was associated with a trend toward reduction in withdrawal symptoms, but increased methadone liking in 15 OUD subjects maintained on methadone (Jones et al. 2013).

These findings add to mixed results in rodent studies regarding the potential of NK1 antagonists for OUD treatment: these agents reduced naloxone-induced morphine withdrawal syndrome (Maldonado et al. 1993) and attenuated morphine-induced locomotor activity (Placenza et al. 2006), but also increased heroin self-administration (Placenza et al. 2006). Genetic modifications were more promising: NK1R knockout mice had reduced opioid-induced addictive behaviors (Murtra et al. 2000), and ablation of NK1Rs in the amygdala reduced morphine conditioned place preference (CPP) (Gadd et al. 2003). Clinical trials in alcohol use disorder (AUD) have shown some promising results: 4 weeks treatment with 50 mg daily NK1 antagonist LY686017 reduced cue-induced craving and stress-induced cortisol release in detoxified AUD patients with high trait anxiety (George et al. 2008), and aprepitant 125 mg/day daily over 4 weeks increased ventromedial prefrontal activation to aversive stimuli in subjects with comorbid post-traumatic stress disorder (PTSD) and AUD, but did not affect PTSD symptoms or alcohol craving (Kwako et al. 2015). Further trials in OUD, AUD, and cocaine use disorder are in progress, and mixed opioid receptor agonist/NK1R antagonist compounds targeted for nociception without addictive features are in development (Olson et al. 2017).

3.5 Serotonin Receptor Modulators

Buspirone is a 5-HT_{1a} receptor agonist approved for the treatment of anxiety and depression that has shown initial efficacy in treating opioid withdrawal symptoms. In a small double-blind, placebo-controlled trial (Buydens-Branchey et al. 2005), heroin-dependent subjects undergoing a 5-day methadone taper from their opioid pain medications were randomized to either buspirone 30 mg daily, buspirone 45 mg daily, continuing methadone, or placebo over 12 days. Both 30 mg and 40 mg buspirone doses showed similar efficacy to methadone and greater efficacy than placebo in reducing SOWS and COWS scores. A further clinical trial (NCT03521960) evaluating the efficacy of buspirone for reducing withdrawal symptoms during a supervised taper from opioid pain medications is currently underway.

Ondansetron is a 5-HT_3 receptor antagonist that is marketed as an antiemetic. A double-blind randomized crossover study in chronic back pain patients evaluated the efficacy of ondansetron vs placebo pretreatment in reducing withdrawal symptoms induced by naloxone following treatment with sustained-release oral morphine (Chu et al. 2018). No significant treatment vs placebo differences were observed in objective or subjective opioid withdrawal symptoms. A further trial is underway for withdrawal (NCT01549652).

Lorcaserin is an agonist at the 5HT_{2C} receptor that is approved for weight loss. Preclinical studies in nonhuman primate and rodent models show promising effects of lorcaserin: it reduced the reinforcing effects of heroin (Kohut and Bergman 2018) and heroin-induced reinstatement in opioid-dependent rhesus monkeys (Gerak et al. 2019) and reduced naloxone-precipitated withdrawal (Zhao et al. 2016) and oxycodone seeking and reinstatement in mice (Neelakantan et al. 2017). Three studies of lorcaserin are underway in OUD patients: one examining effects on brain activity (NCT03143543), another efficacy when administered in combination with XR-NTX for reducing relapse (NCT03169816), and, a third, subjective responses to oxycodone (NCT03143855).

3.6 Anti-inflammatory and Immunomodulatory Agents

Ibudilast (MN-166), previously AV411, is a proinflammatory cytokine macrophage migration inhibitory factor and phosphodiesterase inhibitor which has been in use for over 20 years in Japan and some other Asian countries for the treatment of asthma, among other conditions, but is not yet approved outside Asia. A series of studies from the Comer lab at Columbia and NYSPI have evaluated ibudilast for OUD. A small human laboratory inpatient study in nontreatment-seeking opioid-dependent subjects with 10 participants per group evaluated the analgesic, subjective, and physiological effects of oxycodone in patients treated with ibudilast (20 or 40 mg, p.o., BID for 7 days) vs placebo-treated groups following 14 days treatment with morphine (Cooper et al. 2017). Compared to placebo, ibudilast increased oxycodone analgesia following the cold pressor test, but did not increase subjective drug ratings. In a follow-up study with a similar design, population, and sample size, ibudilast (50 mg BID for 7 days) was found to significantly reduce subjective liking of oxycodone and heroin craving and to improve analgesic effects of oxycodone (Metz et al. 2017). A third study with a similar population and design evaluated ibudilast (20 or 40 mg, p.o., BID for 7 days) for reducing SOWS and COWS scores, finding a trend in SOWS improvement for the combined treatment arms (Cooper et al. 2016).

These preliminary findings are a promising translation of in vitro and rodent studies that showed, first, that opioids activated microglia (Watkins et al. 2007) and, second, that inhibition of microglial activation decreased opioid tolerance, reward responsivity, and withdrawal symptoms and increased analgesic effects (Watkins et al. 2007; Johnston et al. 2004; Watkins et al. 2005; Hutchinson et al. 2008; Ledeboer et al. 2007) and stress responsivity (Zhao et al. 2016). Therefore drugs with the potential to inhibit microglial activation may be a promising approach to reducing opioid dependence related to pain treatment and to treating OUD in general (Cooper et al. 2012).

Pioglitazone is an agonist at the peroxisome proliferator-activated receptor gamma (PPARγ), which is a nuclear hormone receptor that regulates gene expression as a ligand-activated transcription factor and, in the central nervous system, is expressed on oligodendrocytes and astrocytes as well as neurons in multiple brain areas including the VTA, nucleus accumbens, and hippocampus (de Guglielmo et al. 2015; Sarruf et al. 2009). Pioglitazone is marketed for treatment of diabetes via its peripheral role in adipogenesis and glucose metabolism. In the brain, PPARγ agonists modulate dopaminergic transmission (de Guglielmo et al. 2015) and also inhibit microglial activation (Bernardo and Minghetti 2006). As discussed for ibudilast (see above), this latter process is induced by opioids and may reduce opioid withdrawal and improve opioid analgesia. Three small human laboratory clinical studies have evaluated pioglitazone for opioid addiction indications with mostly negative findings. A nonrandomized crossover study in nondependent users found pioglitazone (up to 45 mg daily p.o. over 3 weeks) did not affect subjective ratings of opioids (Jones et al. 2016). A similar negative result was reported from a placebo-controlled RCT of pioglitazone (45 mg daily p.o. over 3 weeks) in OUD subjects stabilized on BUP (Jones et al. 2018); however pioglitazone did reduce heroin craving and general anxiety. Another recent placebo-controlled RCT in OUD patients found that pioglitazone (45 mg/day for 11 weeks) did not reduce withdrawal symptoms (COWS or SOWS), opioid use, or inflammatory cytokines following discharge from inpatient treatment (Schroeder et al. 2018). No ongoing clinical studies were identified in ClinicalTrials.gov.

These findings contrast with mostly positive findings in rodent studies, in which PPARγ agonists were associated with the following effects: reduced heroin self-administration, reduced heroin-induced VTA neuron activation and extracellular dopamine increase in the nucleus accumbens shell (de Guglielmo et al. 2015), reduced heroin (de Guglielmo et al. 2017) and morphine (Ghavimi et al. 2014, 2015) withdrawal behaviors (although see (Javadi et al. 2013)), reduced heroin seeking (de Guglielmo et al. 2017) and heroin-induced reinstatement (de Guglielmo et al. 2017), as well as reduced stress responsivity in non-opioid-related addiction models (Ryan et al. 2012). This discrepancy with clinical studies may possibly reflect insufficient doses or species differences.

3.7 Other: Analgesics, Calcium Channel Blockers, and Acetyl-Cholinesterase Inhibitors

Pregabalin and Gabapentin Pregabalin (Lyrica) is similar in structure to γ-amino butyric acid (GABA), but is a ligand for the α2δ voltage-gated calcium channel subunit, at which it acts to suppress Ca2+-dependent presynaptic neurotransmitter release (Taylor et al. 2007). Pregabalin is currently approved for the treatment of neuropathic pain and fibromyalgia and as an adjunctive treatment for seizures. To date, results (intermediate analysis) from only one clinical trial in OUD (Krupitsky et al. 2016) have been published. A single-blind randomized symptom-regulated protocol with an active control evaluated withdrawal symptoms (OWS), craving, fatigue, and need for analgesia in inpatients undergoing opioid detoxification. Patients were randomized to either pregabalin (up to 600 mg per day, 19 patients) or clonidine (600 micrograms per day, 15 patients) for 6 days, in addition to as needed medications. While OWS outcomes did not differ, pregabalin showed greater efficacy compared to clonidine in reducing craving, fatigue, and need for analgesia and was associated with a higher detoxification completion rate. This preliminary evidence adds to case reports of pregabalin reducing withdrawal in OUD patients (Kammerer et al. 2012) and to preclinical studies in which it suppressed naloxone-precipitated withdrawal in morphine-dependent mice (Hasanein and Shakeri 2014; Vashchinkina et al. 2018); further, pregabalin was effective in reducing craving, withdrawal symptoms, and relapse in AUD clinical trials (Freynhagen et al. 2016). Finally, a randomized clinical trial in postsurgical patients found that compared to placebo, pregabalin reduced postoperative opioid use (Myhre et al. 2017). While these studies suggest pregabalin has significant promise in treating OUD, this is complicated by evidence of abuse potential (Schjerning et al. 2016; Bonnet and Scherbaum 2017). Further studies for withdrawal in OUD (NCT03017430) are ongoing.

Gabapentin is structurally and pharmacologically similar to pregabalin, and is approved for the treatment of neuropathic pain. In a two-stage double-blind, randomized study, two doses of gabapentin (900 mg/day or 1,600 mg/day) plus methadone were compared with placebo plus methadone for efficacy in reducing opioid withdrawal in heroin-dependent patients (Kheirabadi et al. 2008; Salehi et al. 2011). The higher, but not the lower dose, reduced subjective and physiological manifestations of withdrawal. In another RCT, gabapentin (increased from 200 to 1,600 mg and tapered back down over 5 weeks) was found to be effective in reducing recreational opioid use in OUD patients during a 10-day BUP detoxification protocol (Sanders et al. 2013). In a recent large placebo-controlled RCT, gabapentin (1,200 mg/day for 72 h peri- and postoperatively) was also effective at reducing prescription opiate use following surgery (Hah et al. 2018). Multiple clinical trials are underway evaluating gabapentin for postoperative opioid use. Similar concerns exist regarding gabapentin misuse (Bastiaens et al. 2016).

Tramadol is a centrally acting serotonin-norepinephrine reuptake inhibitor and a mild to moderate agonist at the μ, κ, and δ opioid receptors that is approved as an analgesic. It has relatively less abuse liability than other opioid agonists. Published studies in OUD, all evaluating tramadol for reducing withdrawal symptoms, include controlled RCTs, human laboratory studies, and retrospective reviews. Initial smaller placebo-controlled RCTs evaluating tramadol hydrochloride extended release in heroin- or prescription opioid-dependent patients showed that tramadol was superior to clonidine and placebo and comparable to buprenorphine and methadone for suppressing opioid withdrawal symptoms (Lofwall et al. 2007, 2013; Chattopadhyay et al. 2010; Sobey et al. 2003). Mild withdrawal symptoms following cessation of tramadol were reported in some studies. A recent large RCT (Dunn et al. 2017) involving OUD patients in a residential setting compared the efficacy of tramadol hydrochloride extended release (tapered up to 600 mg/day during a 7-day taper), clonidine, or BUP for withdrawal, after which patients were crossed over to double blind placebo. Results confirmed previous findings, showing tramadol was more effective than clonidine and similar to BUP in reducing SOWS and COWS. Multiple clinical trials with similar designs are in progress (NCT00142896, NCT00301210, NCT00980044, NCT03678792).

Isradipine is a dihydropyridine L-type calcium channel (LTCC) blocker that is approved for treatment of hypertension and is being evaluated as a treatment for several psychiatric conditions including bipolar disorder and schizophrenia. Consistent with the role of LTCCs in modulating the activity of VTA neurons responsible for phasic dopamine signaling in the nucleus accumbens, israpidine was recently shown to attenuate cocaine seeking in rats when injected into the VTA (Addy et al. 2018). A trial is currently nearing completion for evaluating the efficacy of isradipine (10 mg/day) as an adjunct to BUP for reducing opioid withdrawal symptoms, craving, and use (NCT01895270).

Galantamine is a naturally occurring acetylcholinesterase inhibitor used in treating Alzheimer's disease and vascular dementias. An ongoing clinical trial (NCT03547622) is testing galantamine versus placebo, both in combination with web-based cognitive behavioral therapy (CBT4CBT), for preventing relapse to opioid use in patients tapering from opioid receptor agonist maintenance (methadone or BUP). The premise for the trial is that galantamine may enhance the efficacy of cognitive behavioral therapy (CBT), particularly in patients with mild cognitive impairment. Primary outcomes include successful taper, opioid withdrawal symptoms, and opioid use for the 3 months following the completion of taper. A double-blind placebo-controlled trial of galantamine for methadone-maintained individuals with cocaine use disorder conducted by Carroll et al. demonstrated in their secondary analysis of opioid use that a significant main effect for galantamine was seen over placebo on percent of urine specimens that were negative for opioids, both within treatment (77% for galantamine vs 62% for placebo), and through a 6-month follow-up (81% vs 59%, respectively). This effect was seen regardless of whether participants used nonprescribed opioids during the baseline period. Galantamine effects were seen early in treatment, leading to the conclusion that it may hold promise across multiple drugs of abuse, including opioids (Bonnet and Scherbaum 2017).

4 Vaccines

Vaccines for addictive disorders including OUD induce antibodies that bind the drug of abuse in the periphery, preventing it from crossing the blood-brain barrier and activating relevant targets including opioid receptors in the brain. Vaccines generally consist of small molecule haptens that mimic the opioid drug structure conjugated to a larger carrier protein and an adjuvant. This complex stimulates the immune system to generate drug-specific antibodies. The idea of using vaccines to treat addiction was tested in animal models over 40 years ago (Bonese et al. 1974), with incremental progress toward clinical use (Pravetoni 2016; Pravetoni and Comer 2019). For opioid-targeted vaccines in particular, data from only one clinical trial have been published; however several clinical trials are now underway (see next paragraph). In the one published trial (Akbarzadeh et al. 2009), conducted in Iran, safety and tolerability of a morphine-bovine serum albumin conjugate were evaluated in 347 morphine-addicted volunteers, showing that it was well-tolerated with no serious adverse events; efficacy data was not included and has not yet been published from any trial in OUD (Pravetoni and Comer 2019). By contrast, clinical trials of vaccines for nicotine and cocaine use disorders are at a more advanced stage, with Phase II or III clinical trials either underway or completed in both disorders – though none of these have yet produced sufficient titers of high-affinity antibody to be commercialized (Pravetoni 2016). This latter outcome has been a key challenge in vaccine research, owing in large part to substantial inter-individual heterogeneity in immune responses (Pravetoni 2016; Pravetoni and Comer 2019).

Recent preclinical work is promising. Vaccines against heroin were shown to reduce drug-induced reinstatement of drug seeking in rats (Schlosburg et al. 2013) and overdose lethality in mice (Bremer et al. 2016); in rhesus monkeys, a vaccine against fentanyl substantially reduced fentanyl's potency in assays of operant responding and antinociception (Tenney et al. 2019). Several initiatives, still in early stages, have been funded to develop similar vaccines for clinical treatment of OUD; they are current in the early stages of developing and evaluating the safety, immunogenicity, and preliminary efficacy of multivalent vaccines targeting oxycodone, heroin, and morphine (1UGD3DA047711-01), fentanyl and fentanyl derivatives (1UGD3DA047711-01), and prescription opioids oxycodone, hydrocodone and hydromorphone (1UGD3DA047711-01). Given the potential benefits of vaccines, including among other things their capacity to be used without the need for detoxification and to be co-administered with other OUD pharmacotherapies, these approaches remain promising.

5 New Formulations of Existing Drugs

In light of nearly universal problems with treatment adherence, a number of extended-release formulations of BUP and NTX have been and are being developed. Probuphine is a long duration of action implantable rod preparation containing BUP embedded in flexible ethylene vinyl acetate rods from which the BUP elutes over a 6-month period (Brown and Alper 2018; White et al. 2009; Ling et al. 2011; Smith et al. 2017). Probuphine was approved by the FDA in 2016. Each rod contains 80 mg BUP, and up to six rods are usually implanted subcutaneously on the inner aspect of the bicep. Spent rods need to be surgically removed at the end of 6 months, and new rods are then implanted on the other arm. Plasma levels achieved are relatively low, and clinical trials in support of approval were limited to patients on low doses of sublingual BUP, 8 mg/day or less.

There are three new long-acting formulations of BUP for subcutaneous injection. An Indivior formulation (Sublocade) (https://www.sublocade.com) (No Authors Listed 2018) was FDA approved in 2017 and provides a month of coverage. Sublocade is marketed in prefilled syringes containing BUP in a biodegradable 50:50 poly (DL-lactide-co-glycolide) polymer and a biocompatible solvent, *N*-methyl-2-pyrrolidone. Two Braeburn Camurus formulations (CAM2038) (Walsh et al. 2017; Haasen et al. 2017), including a 1-week and a 1-month duration-of-action product, were determined to be approvable by the FDA in 2018, but marketing has been delayed on the basis of and exclusivity determination for Sublocade. CAM2038 is planned to be marketed in prefilled syringes containing BUP in a proprietary FluidCrystal® technology (based on soy phosphatidylcholine and diglyceride lipid) which on injection converts to a crystalline gel which slowly releases the BUP. Sublocade labeling requires that patients be maintained or stabilized on sublingual BUP for at least 7 days prior to an initial injection. In contrast, CAM2038 is expected to be approved without that restriction, perhaps requiring only a single sublingual test dose, making the latter a more ideal preparation for use in emergency department settings. Use in such settings has the potential to provide as long as a month's coverage, protecting patients from relapse and overdose fatalities, while longer-term continuing care is being arranged. Clinical trials in planning for these XR-BUP products include head-to-head comparisons with XR-NTX in clinical justice system (CJS) populations; comparisons with sublingual-buprenorphine

(SL-BUP) in OUD patients on discharge from hospital settings; similar comparisons in pregnant OUD patients with a focus on fetal, neonatal, and maternal outcomes; and studies in rural settings where XR interventions may afford advantages as a consequence of travel burdens. All of the extended-release preparations (BUP and NTX) are substantially more expensive, which is likely to preclude their use as a first-line treatment unless clinical trials can establish favorable cost-effectiveness.

Implantable NTX pellets with durations of action up to about 6 months have been used outside of the USA for several years. A very long-acting subcutaneous implantable pellet formulation of NTX, the O'Neil Long-Acting Naltrexone Implant (OLANI), has been under development for close to two decades, and work is currently underway (NCT03810495) to move it toward FDA approval for OUD relapse prevention. Several formulations have been tested in RCTs and have been used clinically in Australia. The formulation being tested in the US trials has higher drug loading; it is manufactured under GMP conditions and has been used in over 800 patients.

6 Trials to Expand Use of Existing Marketed Agents, New Models of Care

As efficacious as currently approved agents are, there's a vast gap between research and community practice. Only between 5 and 10% of people who would benefit from treatment are ever seen in addiction specialty programs, and many of these are "drug-free," meaning that these programs do not use medication. Bringing effective treatment to a larger proportion of the population by introducing existing established medications into specialty programs and into mainstream healthcare settings, e.g., primary care, emergency departments, and the CJS, can have a greater and certainly more immediate impact than developing new drugs. NIDA has supported numerous clinical trials and implementation studies in these settings, many of them through its Clinical Trials Network (NIDA CTN). Studies deemed most relevant to advances or innovations in clinical trial design will be briefly reviewed here, though there are many others of equal importance.

Buprenorphine for Acute Detoxification NIDA CTN-0001 and CTN-0002 (Ling et al. 2005) compared buprenorphine/naloxone (BUP/NX) to clonidine for inpatient and outpatient detoxification, respectively. Prior to these studies, opioid-based detoxification was largely unavailable outside of the restrictive confines of narcotic treatment programs, and clonidine-based detoxification was of limited value for a large number of patients. In the inpatient setting, 77% of patients assigned to BUP/NX met predefined success criteria compared to 22% of the clonidine cohort. In the outpatient setting, the parallel contrast was 29% vs 5%. These studies supported the benefits of BUP/NX as well as the relative benefits of inpatient settings for detox. The benefits were so striking that a previously "drug-free" program withdrew from the trial and established BUP/NX as "treatment-as-usual" because it was so much more effective in retaining patients, reducing the chaos associated with revolving admissions and discharges, and improving bottom-line revenues. Note the striking success rate differences between inpatient and outpatient settings, which emphasize the need for improved outpatient detoxification strategies.

Buprenorphine Tapering CTN-0003 (Ling et al. 2009) compared a rapid (7 day) versus a gradual (28 day) BUP-NX tapering schedule following 4 weeks of BUP/NX stabilization. Counterintuitively the rapid taper beats the gradual taper insofar as at the end of the taper, 44% of the rapid taper group provided opioid-negative urine samples compared to 30% of the gradual taper group. By the time of 1-month and 3-month follow-up visits, only 12–18% of participants from the rapid taper group provided negative urines highlighting the importance of longer-term treatment.

Buprenorphine for Adolescents and Young Adults Adolescents with heroin use disorder are typically treated with detoxification and counseling. CTN-0010 (Woody et al. 2008) compared a relatively short BUP/NX treatment (9 weeks +3 weeks taper) to a 2-week BUP/NX detox, both conditions with 12 weeks of counseling. The longer BUP/NX treatment was associated with less opioid use, better treatment retention, less injection, and less cocaine and marijuana use.

Buprenorphine Hepatotoxicity and Long-Term Treatment CTN-0027 (Saxon et al. 2013) was a head-to-head comparison of BUP/NX to methadone with a primary focus on hepatotoxicity, a study mandated by the FDA as a condition of initial labeling. A long-term follow-up study of the same patients was completed in CTN-0050 (Hser et al. 2016). The key finding from CTN-0027 was that there was no evidence of hepatotoxicity with 6 months of either treatment, encouraging use of BUP/NX in primary care and other settings. Retention in treatment was better for the methadone cohort. Long-term follow-up occurring between 3 and 10 years after randomization revealed no differences in mortality, but higher opioid use in the BUP/NX group largely owing to lower retention. For those retained in treatment, there were no differences in opioid use across the two medications, highlighting the importance of treatment retention.

Treatment of Prescription Opioid Dependence Until recently, most opioid pharmacotherapy research has focused on heroin addiction. With increasing use of – and addiction to – prescription opioids, CTN-0030 (Weiss et al. 2011) (POATS, Prescription Opioid Addiction Treatment Study) examined whether adding traditional individual drug counseling to BUP/NX in the context of standard lean medical management improved outcomes. The primary findings were that patients reduced opioid use during BUP/NX treatment, individual counseling didn't make any difference, and most importantly within a few weeks of completing BUP/NX treatment, close to 90% of patients were again using, highlighting the importance of long-term treatment.

Comparative Effectiveness: XR-NTX Versus BUP/NX CTN-0051 (Lee et al. 2018) was a head-to-head comparison of 6 months of treatment with two office-based medications, BUP/NX and XR-NTX. Key findings were that it was more difficult to initiate treatment with XR-NTX because of the detoxification hurdle (28% of participants randomized to XR-NTX were not successfully inducted compared to 6% of those assigned to BUP/NX) but that once treatment was initiated, the outcomes did not differ. Over the course of 6 months, more than 50% of participants in each group discontinued treatment. These findings highlight the importance of developing more effective induction procedures for XR-NTX and of developing and testing strategies to improve treatment retention. A smaller and shorter but otherwise almost identical study conducted at the same time in Norway yielded similar findings (Tanum et al. 2017).

Moving Addiction Screening, Assessment, and Treatment into Primary Care Settings: Use of the EHR Without appropriate screening, assessment, training, and resources, it is unlikely that opioid treatment will ever find its way into mainstream healthcare settings. CTN-0059 (McNeely et al. 2016) was a validation study of the TAPS Tool (Tobacco, Alcohol, Prescription Medications, and Substance Use/Misuse Brief Screen/Assessment Tool) in primary care settings, the key findings of which were that the tool has good sensitivity and specificity and that interviewer- and self-administered versions performed similarly in these settings. CTN-0062 builds on this and other screening tools by programming these and other NIDA addiction common data elements (CDEs) into electronic health records (EHRs), implementing these in primary care settings after conducting focus groups and providing training and establishing linkages with addiction specialty settings with the goal of reducing stigma and increasing screening, treatment, and referral. CTN-0074 (PROUD, Primary Care Opioid Use Disorders Treatment Trial) further builds on this by implementing and testing a collaborative care model (Massachusetts Model) (Saitz et al. 2008).

Initiating Buprenorphine in Emergency Department Settings Two NIDA CTN trials build on a recently published single-site study (D'Onofrio et al. 2015) showing that initiating BUP/NX treatment in an academic emergency medicine setting and providing a linkage to continuing care in a primary care setting improve 30-day treatment engagement rates. CTN-0069 (Project ED-Health) (Volkow et al. 2018) is a hybrid implementation-effectiveness study using a stepped wedge design currently being conducted in four large urban academic emergency settings. CTN-0079 (ED-CONNECT) (Koob and Volkow 2016) is a study of the feasibility, acceptability, and impact of introducing a clinical protocol for OUD including BUP/NX in rural and urban settings with high need, limited resources, and different staffing structures.

New Models of Care New models of care have been developed both to enhance initial engagement and to make it feasible for busy primary care practitioners to manage the complexities of an OUD population. Examples include establishing bridge clinics to temporarily treat patients identified (and sometimes initially treated) in emergency settings, the CJS, or elsewhere while they are waiting to be accepted into more structured programs: "interim buprenorphine" (Sigmon et al. 2016) and the Massachusetts model (LaBelle et al. 2016) involving embedding a nurse care manager in primary care practices using a collaborative care approach.

Naloxone Kit Distribution and Training Several studies aim at improving the use and outcomes associated with distribution of naloxone kits. These focus on the need to modify existing training programs, improving accurate identification of opioid overdose, long-term follow-up, and inclusion of friends and family in training. It is expected that enhanced psychosocial interventions will improve outcome, that adverse events will be minimal, and that drug use patterns will not be affected (addressing concerns that the availability of naloxone would increase opioid use) (Grant number 5R01DA035207-05). A second study focuses on pharmacy-based naloxone distribution and training, working in the context of two large retail pharmacy chains (Grant number 1R01DA045745-01). A third study is evaluating the impact of emergency response communities (ERCs) which are "specialized smartphone-based social networks in which members are approved carriers" or users of naloxone and can support intervention in overdose emergencies (Grant number 5R34DA044758-02). The model combines GPS and IP location tracking.

Strategies to Transition Off Buprenorphine Either to Medication-Free Abstinence or to XR-NTX While some OUD patients continue to take BUP indefinitely, there are others who prefer not to remain dependent and are looking for safe, effective strategies to discontinue. These include rapid or slow taper to no medication which is often associated with relapse to opioid use and transition to XR-NTX for short-term or long-term relapse prevention. Recent and ongoing trials are comparing rapid transition strategies (rapid daily escalation from very low dose (0.25 or 0.5 mg) oral naltrexone to 25 mg followed by an initial XR-NTX injection) to more traditional gradual BUP taper. Primary outcomes are the percent of participants successfully transitioned off BUP and abstinent at 6 months; secondary outcomes include measures of withdrawal, sleep, mood, anxiety, opioid, and other drug use (Grant number R21DA042243-02). Transition to XR-NTX is expected to be associated with better outcomes than simple taper. A large about-to-be-initiated NIDA CTN study is CTN-0100 focused on optimizing retention, duration, and discontinuation strategies for medications for OUD.

7 Helping to End Addiction Long-Term (HEAL)

The US Congress's Fiscal Year 2018 Consolidated Appropriations Act designated $500 million for NIH to fund research to combat the opioid crisis, funding which is anticipated to continue as an addition to the NIH base (HEAL initiative). Half of the appropriation is designated for NIDA to address opioid addiction and half for NINDS to address management of chronic pain. The act also authorized the NIH Director to transfer some of these funds "specifically appropriated for opioid addiction, opioid alternatives, pain management, and addiction treatment to other Institutes and Centers of the NIH." Responding to this appropriation, the NIH implemented the HEAL (Helping to End Addiction Long-term) initiative, an overarching and ambitious partnership with other agencies building on a track record of research across the translational spectrum – from basic science to behavioral and pharmacotherapy development and testing and to implementation research. NIDA's focus will be on prevention and treatment of OUD with the goal of achieving sustained recovery. For NIDA which has had a budget of approximately $1 billion annually for nearly the last decade, this represents a greater than 20% increase that will be used to build infrastructure and fund exciting new initiatives many of which involve clinical trials. Amongst these are:

NIH HEAL Vaccine Initiative Recognizing that expertise in vaccine development spans many NIH Institutes and Centers as well as academia and industry, NIAID, NIDA, and ORIP issued NOT-AI-18-0155 calling for administrative supplement requests to fund vaccine work, specifically optimization of immunogens, structural analysis of antibody-immunogen binding, opioid B cell epitopes, carrier platforms to improve immunogenicity, novel haptenation, and development of adjuvants for opioid vaccines. Additional areas of interest include IND-enabling studies, mechanisms of vaccine efficacy and safety, mucosal immunity, immune responsivity in OUD, and development of relevant animal models. In October 2018, these ICs sponsored an NIH symposium that brought together NIDA medications development staff, NIDA-funded addiction vaccine researchers, and staff from NIAID and others with expertise in adjuvants, linkers, and other aspects of vaccine development.

Laboratories for Early Clinical Evaluation of Pharmacotherapies This initiative focuses on building infrastructure and expertise to conduct Phase I and Phase II studies to look at safety, drug interactions, PK and PD studies, and human laboratory studies including proof of concept trials.

Medications Development to Prevent and Treat OUD and Overdose This initiative will expand NIDA's existing medications development program, now housed in NIDA's Division of Therapeutics and Medical Consequences.

Respiratory Stimulants Opioid overdose fatalities are nearly always a consequence of opioid-induced respiratory depression. By blocking opioid receptors, antagonists like naloxone rapidly reverse respiratory depression and save lives. But this is not always the case, and additional approaches are needed, particularly in the context of high-potency fentanyl(s). This initiative seeks to develop non-opioid molecules that can stimulate respiration even in the presence of significant opioid agonists. In addition to potential use in opioid overdose, such respiratory stimulants might be used in alcohol poisoning and for overdoses in combination with alcohol and benzodiazepines. Respiratory stimulants have the added advantage that they may be able to restore breathing without precipitating withdrawal.

Virtual Reality (VR) Tools This initiative focuses on moving beyond traditional technology-driven approaches such as text messaging, smartphone apps, and ecological momentary assessment, to include virtual reality approaches to mimic real social situations in which patients may be more prone to responding to drug cues and are at risk of relapse. VR approaches have the potential to enhance treatment effects by allowing patients to be exposed in realistic settings to extend treatment beyond clinical settings and to support digital phenotyping.

NIDA CTN HEAL Projects NIDA Clinical Trials Network is developing a number of large, high-impact trials including a trial to improve retention in MOUD (medication for opioid use disorder) treatment and to better understand how long treatment needs to continue, and for whom and how best to discontinue treatment when that is warranted; a trial to identify and intervene to prevent subthreshold OUD from progressing; a trial examining best approaches to providing MOUD in rural settings; a trial on interventions following hospitalization for medical/surgical indications; a trial focused on strategies to optimize MOUD in tribal communities; and additional trials focused on introducing addictions treatment, particularly buprenorphine BUP, in emergency department settings. In July 2019, five new nodes were added to the network to enhance clinical trial capacity.

Justice and Community Opioid Innovation Network (JCOIN) See below.

HEALing Communities Study By far the most ambitious, expensive, and far-reaching project is the HEALing Communities Study (http://ctndisseminationlibrary.org/protocols/ctn0080.htm) the goals of which are to "determine if an integrated set of evidence-based interventions within healthcare, behavioral health, justice systems, and community organizations can work to decrease opioid overdoses and to prevent and treat OUD." NIDA is leading this effort in partnership with the Substance Abuse and Mental Health Services Administration (SAMHSA) and coordinating with close to a dozen other federal agencies. NIDA recently funded four research sites in highly impacted states (Kentucky, Ohio, New York, Massachusetts) as well as a Data Coordinating Center. Each research site includes at least 15 communities of which 30% are in rural areas. Goals are to reduce overdose fatalities by 40% over 3 years, as well as to reduce overdose events and incidence of OUD and to increase the number of individuals on medication for OUD and those retained in treatment for over 6 months. Extensive linkages with local agencies and organizations are planned. NIDA expects to commit approximately $100 million in each of FY19, FY20, and FY21, and $50 million in FY22 for the research sites (in aggregate), and $6.5 million in each of the 4 years for the Data Coordinating Center.

8 Initiatives for Special Populations

CJS Involved Populations In the USA, the criminal justice system – which has become a de facto residential setting for those with mental illness and substance use disorders – is an important setting in which to screen for, assess, and initiate treatment. Most arrestees test positive for drugs, and of these, opioids are highly prevalent. Methadone maintenance at reentry to the community is well-established (Tomasino et al. 2001; Kinlock et al. 2007). More recently, BUP initiated in jails and prisons and linked to primary care settings for ongoing care has also been extensively studied and shown to be effective. Jail-released patients do as well in primary care as do community comparison groups in terms of retention, opioid use, and opioid abstinence (Lee et al. 2012). Opioid antagonists are often preferred by the CJS, and in a large multi-site trial in parolees, XR-NTX was found to be superior to treatment-as-usual in time-to-relapse, overall relapse, and opioid-negative urines (Lee et al. 2018). A small pilot study found that initiating XR-NTX just prior to release and linking continuing treatment to a primary care setting was acceptable and was associated with lower relapse rates and more negative urine samples (Lee et al. 2015); a large follow-up study focused on relapse and overdose prevention is just being completed.

The Justice and Community Opioid Innovation Network (JCOIN) JCOIN (https://www.nih.gov/research-training/medical-research-initiatives/heal-initiative/justice-community-opioid-innovation-network) will build infrastructure in the form of a network of collaborating researchers and fund specific trials around improving access to treatment for CJS involved populations. It will also initiate a national survey on addiction services in CJS settings. Current work in this area includes bridging gaps in BUP treatment, improving access to OUD pharmacotherapies for veterans, drug injection surveillance in rural areas, optimizing OUD pharmacotherapies in CJS settings, and mining social media big data to monitor HIV. A head-to-head multi-site trial comparing extended-release BUP to extended-release naltrexone is currently pending review.

Optimizing MOUD in Tribal Communities (AI/AN) See above under HEAL CTN.

Maternal Opioid Management Support (MOMS) NIDA CTN-0080: The MOMS study (http://ctndisseminationlibrary.org/protocols/ctn0080.htm) grows out of the increasing prevalence of neonatal abstinence syndrome (NAS, also referred to as neonatal opioid withdrawal syndrome, NOWS) in the context of the opioid crisis. NAS is associated with compromised health outcomes for infants and with exorbitant costs for neonatal intensive care. The present standard of care for pregnant opioid-dependent women is SL-BUP, although problems like poor adherence and treatment dropout are well known. In addition, once-a-day BUP yields daily peaks and troughs which expose the fetus to cycles of sedation and withdrawal. It is hypothesized that replacing SL-BUP with XR-BUP will eliminate the daily cycling and result in improved fetal and neonatal outcomes, e.g., heart rate variability, birth weight, head circumference, etc., as well as improved maternal outcomes, e.g., retention-in-treatment, opioid misuse, etc., and infant outcomes, e.g., early development.

The ABCD and bBCD Studies While not clinical trials per se, two very large and forward-thinking NIDA initiatives warrant mention because they will accrue populations and data-sets that have the potential to both identify need for future clinical trials and potential candidates for same. The ABCD study (Adolescent Brain and Cognitive Development study) https://abcdstudy.org (Lisdahl et al. 2018) was to some extent spurred by the rapid evolution of state medical and recreational marijuana laws, mostly by referendum. Given that THC has profound effects on the developing brain and that with wider availability and legalization of marijuana, teenagers may be using it more frequently, it is imperative to understand the impact on brain and cognitive development. The ABCD study is a 10-year prospective study enrolling 9–10-year-olds, following them through adolescence and into early adulthood and using a common protocol across 21 sites to collect repeated biological, social, behavioral, cognitive, and neuroimaging measures. Enrollment of 11,875 participants was completed in October 2018, and an initial data-set of de-identified baseline measures from ~4,500 participants, including structural MR, diffusion MR, resting-state MR, and task MR imaging as well as clinical and social data, was released through the NIMH Data Archive. Similar curated data will be released annually. ABCD represents a partnership between NIDA, NIAAA, NCI, NIMH, NICHD, CDC, and others. The bBCD study (babies, Brain and Cognitive Development (https://www.nimh.nih.gov/funding/grant-writing-and-application-process/concept-clearances/2018/the-trans-nih-baby-brain-cognitive-development-bbcd-study.html) is also a trans-NIH initiative stimulated in part by the opioid crisis and the increase in prenatal exposure to opioids and NOWS. The bBCD study is still in planning, but intends to recruit 7,500 pregnant women from highly impacted regions of the USA. Goals are to establish normative developmental trajectories against which to assess affected children.

9 Devices, Apps, and Behavioral Interventions

A large number of apps, web-based interventions, and devices have been and are being developed: widespread use of smart phones, text messaging, and geo-positioning, the relatively very low cost of app development and data analytical approaches including big data analytics, and the potential to use these as research tools and to commercialize them have led to an explosion of new approaches. We mention just a few examples to provide a taste of what's in development. The extent to which these are supported by clinical trials is highly variable. Building on the findings of CTN-0044 (NCT01104805), Pear Therapeutics has developed reSET, and reSET-O, apps that include educational and contingency management approaches. As far as we're aware, this is the only app presently available that has received FDA clearance. Pear is working with Sandoz to commercialize this:

CBT4CBT (www.CBT4CBT.com) is based on years of work showing that cognitive behavioral therapy approaches are effective, particularly in relapse prevention, and that web-based CBT is effective, cost-effective, and of higher fidelity than counselor-administered approaches. It can be used 24/7, requires no scheduling, and is often preferred by patients. Many text messaging approaches have been used to collect EMA (ecological momentary assessment) data which can be used both for research purposes and to drive temporally targeted interventions, including multiple sequential randomizations based on EMA outcome measures. Many apps use geo-mapping to gather information about "safe" and "dangerous" places (i.e., the street corner where your dealer deals, your favorite bar, etc.) and use those data to steer users away from dangerous locales, to safer, more supportive ones. Other apps, e.g., "emocha" (www.emocha.com), use real-time smartphone video apps and facial recognition software to monitor and reward for medication taking and adherence. DynamiCare combines many of these features in a single app. Datacubed (D3) (www.datacubed.com) combines many of the same features with "gamefied" decision science measures derived from neuroeconomics including measures of temporal discounting, risk-taking, and decision-making under ambiguous conditions which may predict vulnerability to relapse and provide opportunities for targeted intervention.

10 Summary, Conclusions, and New Directions

Recent clinical trials and interventions for OUD include diverse new pharmacotherapies, many of which are non-opioid based, enhancement of existing opioid-based medications, modernization of big data collection, and large-scale systemic interventions at the healthcare provider and societal levels to increase access to, and retention in MAT, and to prevent overdose. Novel non-opioid pharmacotherapies that have the potential to mitigate neurobiological alterations underlying addiction have been or are being evaluated for OUD indications, representing a change from current therapeutics, which are almost all opioid based. The outcomes of most of these trials were, or are, craving or withdrawal during or following detoxification, with a few also evaluating retention in MAT. In the context of addiction domains highlighted by Koob and Volkow (Koob and Volkow 2016), many relevant new pharmacotherapies, including CBD, THC, aprepitant, PPARγ agonists, dynorphin/KOPR agents, and buspirone, have the potential to reduce stress and negative affect. Relatively fewer agents – galantamine and potentially CBD – are known to improve prefrontal or executive function. Also prevalent among new OUD pharmacotherapies are medications that are approved for treating pain (ketamine, tramadol, pregabalin, and gabapentin) or are potential analgesics via direct actions, or via interactions with opioid-based nociception. These include ibudilast and pioglitazone via inhibition of glial activation; CBD and low-dose THC via endocannabinoid actions and cannabinoid-opioid interaction; aprepitant via neurokinin-related nociception; or the developing opioid agonist/NK1R antagonist compounds. Anti-inflammatory agents (ibudilast, pioglitazone,

CBD) are also represented. Most of these studies reported positive findings for at least one outcome.

Future directions and potential areas of need include improved strategies to combat the unique challenges raised by the potency and availability of fentanyl and related epidemic of overdose fatalities. Fentanyl is about 50–100 times more potent than morphine, and carfentanil and other fentanyl derivatives an order of magnitude greater or more. As a consequence, naloxone kits are less efficacious, and first responders frequently report needing to use five or ten or more kits for a single overdose. More potent, rapidly acting antagonists with user-friendly packaging need to be developed, possibly with longer durations of action (as noted, naloxone is short-lived and frequently needs to be readministered). In addition to this, fentanyl's potency may produce greater tolerance and greater dependence than do less potent opioids, rendering current agonist and antagonist interventions inadequate or requiring higher methadone or BUP dosing or that XR-NTX be administered every 2 weeks rather than every 4. All of this requires focused clinical trials.

While there are multiple pharmacotherapies that have the potential to reduce prescription opioid use in chronic pain (described above), relatively few trials were identified that included pain, opioid analgesic use, or tolerance as outcomes. Chronic pain is frequently comorbid with OUD and greatly increases the risk for overdose (Volkow et al. 2018). Developing non-opioid-based analgesics to replace opioid use was recently identified as a high priority for combating OUD (Volkow et al. 2018).

Finally, despite recent emphasis on the importance of precision medicine approaches, i.e., strategies for identifying individual patient characteristics that predict response for a given medication (Terry 2015; Litten et al. 2015), few OUD clinical trials to date have reported demographic, psychiatric, or biological measures that were or were not associated with treatment response. To achieve this, future clinical trials would need not only to include these measures, but also to employ statistical analyses that permit these measures to be causally linked to treatment outcome in sufficiently large clinical samples (as opposed to the current practice of testing for group mean differences in studies with relatively small sample sizes). A particularly important patient characteristic that is likely to influence treatment response, but which has been omitted from study in most clinical trials, is psychiatric comorbidity: psychiatric disorders, particularly mood disorders, are highly prevalent in OUD and interact with the addictive cycle in a mutually exacerbating manner that requires integrated treatment of both disorders (Volkow et al. 2018). Precision medicine approaches will also be necessary to incorporate recent findings that genetic and epigenetic variations between individuals both contribute to developing OUD, and may also be treatment targets (Hurd and O'Brien 2018).

References

Addy NA et al (2018) The L-type calcium channel blocker, isradipine, attenuates cue-induced cocaine-seeking by enhancing dopaminergic activity in the ventral tegmental area to nucleus accumbens pathway. Neuropsychopharmacology 43(12):2361–2372

Akbarzadeh A et al (2009) J Pharmacol Toxicol 4(1):30–35
Auriacombe M, O'Brien CP, Tignol J (1994) Buprenorphine in the treatment of opiate dependence. Ann Med Interne (Paris) 145(Suppl 3):27
Babalonis S et al (2017) Oral cannabidiol does not produce a signal for abuse liability in frequent marijuana smokers. Drug Alcohol Depend 172:9–13
Bachhuber MA et al (2014) Medical cannabis laws and opioid analgesic overdose mortality in the United States, 1999-2010. JAMA Intern Med 174(10):1668–1673
Bastiaens L, Galus J, Mazur C (2016) Abuse of gabapentin is associated with opioid addiction. Psychiatry Q 87(4):763–767
Bernardo A, Minghetti L (2006) PPAR-gamma agonists as regulators of microglial activation and brain inflammation. Curr Pharm Des 12(1):93–109
Bisaga A et al (2015) The effects of dronabinol during detoxification and the initiation of treatment with extended release naltrexone. Drug Alcohol Depend 154:38–45
Blessing EM et al (2015) Cannabidiol as a potential treatment for anxiety disorders. Neurotherapeutics 12(4):825–836
Bonese KF et al (1974) Changes in heroin self-administration by a rhesus monkey after morphine immunisation. Nature 252(5485):708–710
Bonnet U, Scherbaum N (2017) How addictive are gabapentin and pregabalin? A systematic review. Eur Neuropsychopharmacol 27(12):1185–1215
Bremer PT et al (2016) Combatting synthetic designer opioids: a conjugate vaccine ablates lethal doses of fentanyl class drugs. Angew Chem Int Ed Engl 55(11):3772–3775
Brown TK, Alper K (2018) Treatment of opioid use disorder with ibogaine: detoxification and drug use outcomes. Am J Drug Alcohol Abuse 44(1):24–36
Bruchas MR, Land BB, Chavkin C (2010) The dynorphin/kappa opioid system as a modulator of stress-induced and pro-addictive behaviors. Brain Res 1314:44–55
Butelman ER, Yuferov V, Kreek MJ (2012) kappa-opioid receptor/dynorphin system: genetic and pharmacotherapeutic implications for addiction. Trends Neurosci 35(10):587–596
Buydens-Branchey L, Branchey M, Reel-Brander C (2005) Efficacy of buspirone in the treatment of opioid withdrawal. J Clin Psychopharmacol 25(3):230–236
C Mash D (2018) Breaking the cycle of opioid use disorder with ibogaine. Am J Drug Alcohol Abuse 44(1):1–3
Chattopadhyay S et al (2010) Tramadol versus clonidine in management of heroin withdrawal. Asian J Psychiatr 3(4):237–239
Chou R et al (2017) Management of suspected opioid overdose with naloxone in out-of-hospital settings: a systematic review. Ann Intern Med 167(12):867–875
Chu LF et al (2018) Ondansetron does not prevent physical dependence in patients taking opioid medications chronically for pain control. Drug Alcohol Depend 183:176–183
Commons KG (2010) Neuronal pathways linking substance P to drug addiction and stress. Brain Res 1314:175–182
Cooper ZD, Jones JD, Comer SD (2012) Glial modulators: a novel pharmacological approach to altering the behavioral effects of abused substances. Expert Opin Investig Drugs 21(2):169–178
Cooper ZD et al (2016) The effects of ibudilast, a glial activation inhibitor, on opioid withdrawal symptoms in opioid-dependent volunteers. Addict Biol 21(4):895–903
Cooper ZD et al (2017) Effects of ibudilast on oxycodone-induced analgesia and subjective effects in opioid-dependent volunteers. Drug Alcohol Depend 178:340–347
Cox S, Alcorn R (1995) Lofexidine and opioid withdrawal. Lancet 345(8962):1385–1386
Crippa JA et al (2018) Translational investigation of the therapeutic potential of cannabidiol (CBD): toward a new age. Front Immunol 9:2009
D'Onofrio G et al (2015) Emergency department-initiated buprenorphine/naloxone treatment for opioid dependence: a randomized clinical trial. JAMA 313(16):1636–1644
De Felipe C et al (1998) Altered nociception, analgesia and aggression in mice lacking the receptor for substance P. Nature 392(6674):394–397

de Guglielmo G et al (2015) PPARgamma activation attenuates opioid consumption and modulates mesolimbic dopamine transmission. Neuropsychopharmacology 40(4):927–937
de Guglielmo G et al (2017) Pioglitazone attenuates the opioid withdrawal and vulnerability to relapse to heroin seeking in rodents. Psychopharmacology (Berl) 234(2):223–234
Dunn KE et al (2017) Efficacy of tramadol extended-release for opioid withdrawal: a randomized clinical trial. JAMA Psychiatry 74(9):885–893
Dupouy J et al (2017) Mortality associated with time in and out of buprenorphine treatment in french office-based general practice: a 7-year cohort study. Ann Fam Med 15(4):355–358
Fasinu PS et al (2016) Current status and prospects for cannabidiol preparations as new therapeutic agents. Pharmacotherapy 36(7):781–796
Freynhagen R et al (2016) Pregabalin for the treatment of drug and alcohol withdrawal symptoms: a comprehensive review. CNS Drugs 30(12):1191–1200
Gadd CA et al (2003) Neurokinin-1 receptor-expressing neurons in the amygdala modulate morphine reward and anxiety behaviors in the mouse. J Neurosci 23(23):8271–8280
Garbutt JC et al (2005) Efficacy and tolerability of long-acting injectable naltrexone for alcohol dependence: a randomized controlled trial. JAMA 293(13):1617–1625
George DT et al (2008) Neurokinin 1 receptor antagonism as a possible therapy for alcoholism. Science 319(5869):1536–1539
Gerak LR et al (2019) Effects of lorcaserin on reinstatement of responding previously maintained by cocaine or remifentanil in rhesus monkeys. Exp Clin Psychopharmacol 27(1):78–86
Ghavimi H et al (2014) Pioglitazone prevents morphine antinociception tolerance and withdrawal symptoms in rats. Naunyn Schmiedebergs Arch Pharmacol 387(9):811–821
Ghavimi H et al (2015) Acute administration of pioglitazone attenuates morphine withdrawal syndrome in rat: a novel role of pioglitazone. Drug Res (Stuttg) 65(3):113–118
Gold MS (1993) Opiate addiction and the locus coeruleus. The clinical utility of clonidine, naltrexone, methadone, and buprenorphine. Psychiatr Clin North Am 16(1):61–73
Gold MS et al (1979) Clonidine detoxification: a fourteen-day protocol for rapid opiate withdrawal. NIDA Res Monogr 27:226–232
Gold MS et al (1980a) Opiate withdrawal using clonidine. A safe, effective, and rapid nonopiate treatment. JAMA 243(4):343–346
Gold MS et al (1980b) Clonidine and opiate withdrawal. Lancet 2(8203):1078–1079
Gonzalez-Cuevas G et al (2018) Unique treatment potential of cannabidiol for the prevention of relapse to drug use: preclinical proof of principle. Neuropsychopharmacology 43 (10):2036–2045
Gorodetzky CW et al (2017) A phase III, randomized, multi-center, double blind, placebo controlled study of safety and efficacy of lofexidine for relief of symptoms in individuals undergoing inpatient opioid withdrawal. Drug Alcohol Depend 176:79–88
Gowing L, Ali R, White JM (2009) Opioid antagonists with minimal sedation for opioid withdrawal. Cochrane Database Syst Rev 4:CD002021
Gowing L et al (2017) Buprenorphine for managing opioid withdrawal. Cochrane Database Syst Rev 2:CD002025
Haasen C, Linden M, Tiberg F (2017) Pharmacokinetics and pharmacodynamics of a buprenorphine subcutaneous depot formulation (CAM2038) for once-weekly dosing in patients with opioid use disorder. J Subst Abuse Treat 78:22–29
Hah J et al (2018) Effect of perioperative gabapentin on postoperative pain resolution and opioid cessation in a mixed surgical cohort: a randomized clinical trial. JAMA Surg 153(4):303–311
Hargreaves R (2002) Imaging substance P receptors (NK1) in the living human brain using positron emission tomography. J Clin Psychiatry 63(Suppl 11):18–24
Hasanein P, Shakeri S (2014) Pregabalin role in inhibition of morphine analgesic tolerance and physical dependency in rats. Eur J Pharmacol 742:113–117
Hser YI et al (2016) Long-term outcomes after randomization to buprenorphine/naloxone versus methadone in a multi-site trial. Addiction 111(4):695–705

Addiction Reserach Center. https://archives.drugabuse.gov/news-events/nida-notes/1995/12/history-addiction-research-center
Present opioid crisis. https://www.drugabuse.gov/drugs-abuse/opioids/opioid-overdose-crisis; https://www.hhs.gov/opioids/about-the-epidemic/index.html
HEAL initiative. https://www.nih.gov/research-training/medical-research-initiatives/heal-initiative/heal-initiative-research-plan
Hurd YL, O'Brien CP (2018) Molecular genetics and new medication strategies for opioid addiction. Am J Psychiatry 175(10):935–942
Hurd YL et al (2015) Early phase in the development of cannabidiol as a treatment for addiction: opioid relapse takes initial center stage. Neurotherapeutics 12(4):807–815
Hurd YL et al (2019) Cannabidiol for the reduction of cue-induced craving and anxiety in drug-abstinent individuals with heroin use disorder: a double-blind randomized placebo-controlled trial. Am J Psychiatry:appiajp201918101191
Hutchinson MR et al (2008) Proinflammatory cytokines oppose opioid-induced acute and chronic analgesia. Brain Behav Immun 22(8):1178–1189
Iffland K, Grotenhermen F (2017) An update on safety and side effects of cannabidiol: a review of clinical data and relevant animal studies. Cannabis Cannabinoid Res 2(1):139–154
Javadi S et al (2013) Pioglitazone potentiates development of morphine-dependence in mice: possible role of NO/cGMP pathway. Brain Res 1510:22–37
Jicha CJ et al (2015) Safety of oral dronabinol during opioid withdrawal in humans. Drug Alcohol Depend 157:179–183
Johnston IN et al (2004) A role for proinflammatory cytokines and fractalkine in analgesia, tolerance, and subsequent pain facilitation induced by chronic intrathecal morphine. J Neurosci 24(33):7353–7365
Jones JD et al (2013) Opioid-like effects of the neurokinin 1 antagonist aprepitant in patients maintained on and briefly withdrawn from methadone. Am J Drug Alcohol Abuse 39(2):86–91
Jones JD et al (2016) The effects of pioglitazone, a PPARgamma receptor agonist, on the abuse liability of oxycodone among nondependent opioid users. Physiol Behav 159:33–39
Jones JD et al (2018) The PPARgamma agonist pioglitazone fails to alter the abuse potential of heroin, but does reduce heroin craving and anxiety. J Psychoactive Drugs 50(5):390–401
Jovaisa T et al (2006) Effects of ketamine on precipitated opiate withdrawal. Medicina (Kaunas) 42 (8):625–634
Kammerer N et al (2012) Pregabalin for the reduction of opiate withdrawal symptoms. Psychiatr Prax 39(7):351–352
Kaplan JL et al (1999) Double-blind, randomized study of nalmefene and naloxone in emergency department patients with suspected narcotic overdose. Ann Emerg Med 34(1):42–50
Kathmann M et al (2006) Cannabidiol is an allosteric modulator at mu- and delta-opioid receptors. Naunyn Schmiedebergs Arch Pharmacol 372(5):354–361
Kheirabadi GR et al (2008) Effect of add-on gabapentin on opioid withdrawal symptoms in opium-dependent patients. Addiction 103(9):1495–1499
Kim HK, Nelson LS (2015) Reducing the harm of opioid overdose with the safe use of naloxone: a pharmacologic review. Expert Opin Drug Saf 14(7):1137–1146
Kinlock TW et al (2007) A randomized clinical trial of methadone maintenance for prisoners: results at 1-month post-release. Drug Alcohol Depend 91(2–3):220–227
Kohut SJ, Bergman J (2018) Lorcaserin decreases the reinforcing effects of heroin, but not food, in rhesus monkeys. Eur J Pharmacol 840:28–32
Koob GF (2013) Addiction is a reward deficit and stress surfeit disorder. Front Psychiatry 4:72
Koob GF, Volkow ND (2016) Neurobiology of addiction: a neurocircuitry analysis. Lancet Psychiatry 3(8):760–773
Koob GF et al (2014) Addiction as a stress surfeit disorder. Neuropharmacology 76(Pt B):370–382
Kovacs GL, Sarnyai Z, Szabo G (1998) Oxytocin and addiction: a review. Psychoneuroendocrinology 23(8):945–962

Kreek MJ (2000) Methadone-related opioid agonist pharmacotherapy for heroin addiction. History, recent molecular and neurochemical research and future in mainstream medicine. Ann N Y Acad Sci 909:186–216

Kreek MJ, Vocci FJ (2002) History and current status of opioid maintenance treatments: blending conference session. J Subst Abuse Treat 23(2):93–105

Kreek MJ, LaForge KS, Butelman E (2002) Pharmacotherapy of addictions. Nat Rev Drug Discov 1(9):710–726

Krieter P et al (2019) Fighting fire with fire: development of intranasal nalmefene to treat synthetic opioid overdose. J Pharmacol Exp Ther 371(2):409–415

Krupitsky E et al (2002) Ketamine psychotherapy for heroin addiction: immediate effects and two-year follow-up. J Subst Abuse Treat 23(4):273–283

Krupitsky EM et al (2007) Single versus repeated sessions of ketamine-assisted psychotherapy for people with heroin dependence. J Psychoactive Drugs 39(1):13–19

Krupitsky E et al (2011) Injectable extended-release naltrexone for opioid dependence: a double-blind, placebo-controlled, multicentre randomised trial. Lancet 377(9776):1506–1513

Krupitsky EM et al (2016) A randomized single blind study of the efficacy of pregabalin in the treatment of opioid withdrawal syndrome. Zh Nevrol Psikhiatr Im S S Korsakova 116(7):29–36

Kwako LE et al (2015) The neurokinin-1 receptor antagonist aprepitant in co-morbid alcohol dependence and posttraumatic stress disorder: a human experimental study. Psychopharmacology (Berl) 232(1):295–304

LaBelle CT et al (2016) Office-based opioid treatment with buprenorphine (OBOT-B): statewide implementation of the Massachusetts Collaborative Care Model in community health centers. J Subst Abuse Treat 60:6–13

Ledeboer A et al (2007) Ibudilast (AV-411). A new class therapeutic candidate for neuropathic pain and opioid withdrawal syndromes. Expert Opin Investig Drugs 16(7):935–950

Lee JD et al (2012) Buprenorphine-naloxone maintenance following release from jail. Subst Abus 33(1):40–47

Lee JD et al (2015) Opioid treatment at release from jail using extended-release naltrexone: a pilot proof-of-concept randomized effectiveness trial. Addiction 110(6):1008–1014

Lee JD et al (2016) Extended-release naltrexone to prevent opioid relapse in criminal justice offenders. N Engl J Med 374(13):1232–1242

Lee JD et al (2018) Comparative effectiveness of extended-release naltrexone versus buprenorphine-naloxone for opioid relapse prevention (X:BOT): a multicentre, open-label, randomised controlled trial. Lancet 391(10118):309–318

Leong KC et al (2018) Oxytocin and rodent models of addiction. Int Rev Neurobiol 140:201–247

Liang D et al (2018) Medical cannabis legalization and opioid prescriptions: evidence on US Medicaid enrollees during 1993-2014. Addiction 113(11):2060–2070

Ling W et al (2005) A multi-center randomized trial of buprenorphine-naloxone versus clonidine for opioid detoxification: findings from the National Institute on Drug Abuse Clinical Trials Network. Addiction 100(8):1090–1100

Ling W et al (2009) Buprenorphine tapering schedule and illicit opioid use. Addiction 104 (2):256–265

Ling W et al (2011) Selective review and commentary on emerging pharmacotherapies for opioid addiction. Subst Abuse Rehabil 2:181–188

Lisdahl KM et al (2018) Adolescent brain cognitive development (ABCD) study: overview of substance use assessment methods. Dev Cogn Neurosci 32:80–96

Litjens RP, Brunt TM (2016) How toxic is ibogaine? Clin Toxicol (Phila) 54(4):297–302

Litten RZ et al (2015) Heterogeneity of alcohol use disorder: understanding mechanisms to advance personalized treatment. Alcohol Clin Exp Res 39(4):579–584

Lofwall MR et al (2007) Modest opioid withdrawal suppression efficacy of oral tramadol in humans. Psychopharmacology (Berl) 194(3):381–393

Lofwall MR et al (2013) Efficacy of extended-release tramadol for treatment of prescription opioid withdrawal: a two-phase randomized controlled trial. Drug Alcohol Depend 133(1):188–197

Lofwall MR et al (2016) Opioid withdrawal suppression efficacy of oral dronabinol in opioid dependent humans. Drug Alcohol Depend 164:143–150

Malcolm BJ, Polanco M, Barsuglia JP (2018) Changes in withdrawal and craving scores in participants undergoing opioid detoxification utilizing ibogaine. J Psychoactive Drugs 50 (3):256–265

Maldonado R, Girdlestone D, Roques BP (1993) RP 67580, a selective antagonist of neurokinin-1 receptors, modifies some of the naloxone-precipitated morphine withdrawal signs in rats. Neurosci Lett 156(1–2):135–140

Mannangatti P et al (2017) Differential effects of aprepitant, a clinically used neurokinin-1 receptor antagonist on the expression of conditioned psychostimulant versus opioid reward. Psychopharmacology (Berl) 234(4):695–705

Mattick RP et al (2014) Buprenorphine maintenance versus placebo or methadone maintenance for opioid dependence. Cochrane Database Syst Rev 2:CD002207

McDonald RD et al (2016) Extended-release naltrexone opioid treatment at jail reentry (XOR). Contemp Clin Trials 49:57–64

McNeely J et al (2016) Performance of the tobacco, alcohol, prescription medication, and other substance use (TAPS) tool for substance use screening in primary care patients. Ann Intern Med 165(10):690–699

Metz VE et al (2017) Effects of ibudilast on the subjective, reinforcing, and analgesic effects of oxycodone in recently detoxified adults with opioid dependence. Neuropsychopharmacology 42 (9):1825–1832

Morgan CJ et al (2013) Cannabidiol reduces cigarette consumption in tobacco smokers: preliminary findings. Addict Behav 38(9):2433–2436

Murphy SM et al (2017) Cost-effectiveness of extended release naltrexone to prevent relapse among criminal justice-involved individuals with a history of opioid use disorder. Addiction 112 (8):1440–1450

Murtra P et al (2000) Rewarding effects of opiates are absent in mice lacking the receptor for substance P. Nature 405(6783):180–183

Myhre M, Romundstad L, Stubhaug A (2017) Pregabalin reduces opioid consumption and hyperalgesia but not pain intensity after laparoscopic donor nephrectomy. Acta Anaesthesiol Scand 61(10):1314–1324

Neelakantan H et al (2017) Lorcaserin suppresses oxycodone self-administration and relapse vulnerability in rats. ACS Chem Nerosci 8(5):1065–1073

Nielsen S et al (2016) Opioid agonist treatment for pharmaceutical opioid dependent people. Cochrane Database Syst Rev 5:CD011117

No Authors Listed (2018) Once-monthly subcutaneous buprenorphine (Sublocade) for opioid use disorder. Med Lett Drugs Ther 60(1541):35–37

Noller GE, Frampton CM, Yazar-Klosinski B (2018) Ibogaine treatment outcomes for opioid dependence from a twelve-month follow-up observational study. Am J Drug Alcohol Abuse 44(1):37–46

Olfson M et al (2018) Cannabis use and risk of prescription opioid use disorder in the United States. Am J Psychiatry 175(1):47–53

Olson KM et al (2017) Novel molecular strategies and targets for opioid drug discovery for the treatment of chronic pain. Yale J Biol Med 90(1):97–110

Placenza FM et al (2006) Effects of central neurokinin-1 receptor antagonism on cocaine- and opiate-induced locomotor activity and self-administration behaviour in rats. Pharmacol Biochem Behav 84(1):94–101

Pravetoni M (2016) Biologics to treat substance use disorders: current status and new directions. Hum Vaccin Immunother 12(12):3005–3019

Pravetoni M, Comer SD (2019) Development of vaccines to treat opioid use disorders and reduce incidence of overdose. Neuropharmacology:107662

Preller KH et al (2017) The fabric of meaning and subjective effects in LSD-induced states depend on serotonin 2A receptor activation. Curr Biol 27(3):451–457

Raby WN et al (2009) Intermittent marijuana use is associated with improved retention in naltrexone treatment for opiate-dependence. Am J Addict 18(4):301–308

Ren Y et al (2009) Cannabidiol, a nonpsychotropic component of cannabis, inhibits cue-induced heroin seeking and normalizes discrete mesolimbic neuronal disturbances. J Neurosci 29 (47):14764–14769

Robinson A, Wermeling DP (2014) Intranasal naloxone administration for treatment of opioid overdose. Am J Health Syst Pharm 71(24):2129–2135

Ryan KK et al (2012) Physiological responses to acute psychological stress are reduced by the PPARgamma agonist rosiglitazone. Endocrinology 153(3):1279–1287

Saitz R et al (2008) The case for chronic disease management for addiction. J Addict Med 2 (2):55–65

Salehi M et al (2011) Importance of gabapentin dose in treatment of opioid withdrawal. J Clin Psychopharmacol 31(5):593–596

Sanders NC et al (2013) Randomized, placebo-controlled pilot trial of gabapentin during an outpatient, buprenorphine-assisted detoxification procedure. Exp Clin Psychopharmacol 21 (4):294–302

Sandweiss AJ, Vanderah TW (2015) The pharmacology of neurokinin receptors in addiction: prospects for therapy. Subst Abuse Rehabil 6:93–102

Sarruf DA et al (2009) Expression of peroxisome proliferator-activated receptor-gamma in key neuronal subsets regulating glucose metabolism and energy homeostasis. Endocrinology 150 (2):707–712

Savage C, McCabe OL (1973) Residential psychedelic (LSD) therapy for the narcotic addict. A controlled study. Arch Gen Psychiatry 28(6):808–814

Saxon AJ et al (2013) Buprenorphine/naloxone and methadone effects on laboratory indices of liver health: a randomized trial. Drug Alcohol Depend 128(1–2):71–76

Scavone JL, Sterling RC, Van Bockstaele EJ (2013) Cannabinoid and opioid interactions: implications for opiate dependence and withdrawal. Neuroscience 248:637–654

Schjerning O et al (2016) Abuse potential of pregabalin: a systematic review. CNS Drugs 30 (1):9–25

Schlosburg JE et al (2013) Dynamic vaccine blocks relapse to compulsive intake of heroin. Proc Natl Acad Sci U S A 110(22):9036–9041

Schroeder JR et al (2018) Assessment of pioglitazone and proinflammatory cytokines during buprenorphine taper in patients with opioid use disorder. Psychopharmacology (Berl) 235 (10):2957–2966

Sigmon SC et al (2016) Interim buprenorphine vs. waiting list for opioid dependence. N Engl J Med 375(25):2504–2505

Smith L et al (2017) Probuphine (buprenorphine) subdermal implants for the treatment of opioid-dependent patients. P T 42(8):505–508

Sobey PW et al (2003) The use of tramadol for acute heroin withdrawal: a comparison to clonidine. J Addict Dis 22(4):13–25

Stimmel B, Kreek MJ (2000) Neurobiology of addictive behaviors and its relationship to methadone maintenance. Mt Sinai J Med 67(5–6):375–380

Strang J et al (2016) Naloxone without the needle – systematic review of candidate routes for non-injectable naloxone for opioid overdose reversal. Drug Alcohol Depend 163:16–23

Strong CE, Kabbaj M (2018) On the safety of repeated ketamine infusions for the treatment of depression: effects of sex and developmental periods. Neurobiol Stress 9:166–175

Tanum L et al (2017) Effectiveness of injectable extended-release naltrexone vs daily buprenorphine-naloxone for opioid dependence: a randomized clinical noninferiority trial. JAMA Psychiatry 74(12):1197–1205

Taylor CP, Angelotti T, Fauman E (2007) Pharmacology and mechanism of action of pregabalin: the calcium channel alpha2-delta (alpha2-delta) subunit as a target for antiepileptic drug discovery. Epilepsy Res 73(2):137–150

Tenney RD et al (2019) Vaccine blunts fentanyl potency in male rhesus monkeys. Neuropharmacology 158:107730
Terry SF (2015) Obama's precision medicine initiative. Genet Test Mol Biomarkers 19(3):113–114
Tomasino V et al (2001) The Key Extended Entry Program (KEEP): a methadone treatment program for opiate-dependent inmates. Mt Sinai J Med 68(1):14–20
Vashchinkina E et al (2018) Addiction-related interactions of pregabalin with morphine in mice and humans: reinforcing and inhibiting effects. Addict Biol 23(3):945–958
Volkow ND, Collins FS (2017) The role of science in addressing the opioid crisis. N Engl J Med 377(4):391–394
Volkow ND et al (2018) Prevention and treatment of opioid misuse and addiction: a review. JAMA Psychiatry 76(2):208–216
Walsh SL et al (2013) Effects of the NK1 antagonist, aprepitant, on response to oral and intranasal oxycodone in prescription opioid abusers. Addict Biol 18(2):332–343
Walsh SL et al (2017) Effect of buprenorphine weekly depot (CAM2038) and hydromorphone blockade in individuals with opioid use disorder: a randomized clinical trial. JAMA Psychiatry 74(9):894–902
Watkins LR et al (2005) Glia: novel counter-regulators of opioid analgesia. Trends Neurosci 28 (12):661–669
Watkins LR et al (2007) "Listening" and "talking" to neurons: implications of immune activation for pain control and increasing the efficacy of opioids. Brain Res Rev 56(1):148–169
Wee S, Koob GF (2010) The role of the dynorphin-kappa opioid system in the reinforcing effects of drugs of abuse. Psychopharmacology (Berl) 210(2):121–135
Weiss RD et al (2011) Adjunctive counseling during brief and extended buprenorphine-naloxone treatment for prescription opioid dependence: a 2-phase randomized controlled trial. Arch Gen Psychiatry 68(12):1238–1246
White J et al (2009) Open-label dose-finding trial of buprenorphine implants (Probuphine) for treatment of heroin dependence. Drug Alcohol Depend 103(1–2):37–43
WHO (2019) https://www.who.int/substance_abuse/information-sheet/en/
Williams AR et al (2018) Developing an opioid use disorder treatment cascade: a review of quality measures. J Subst Abuse Treat 91:57–68
Woody GE et al (2008) Extended vs short-term buprenorphine-naloxone for treatment of opioid-addicted youth: a randomized trial. JAMA 300(17):2003–2011
Woolley JD et al (2016) The effects of intranasal oxytocin in opioid-dependent individuals and healthy control subjects: a pilot study. Psychopharmacology (Berl) 233(13):2571–2580
Yamaori S et al (2011a) Cannabidiol, a major phytocannabinoid, as a potent atypical inhibitor for CYP2D6. Drug Metab Dispos 39(11):2049–2056
Yamaori S et al (2011b) Potent inhibition of human cytochrome P450 3A isoforms by cannabidiol: role of phenolic hydroxyl groups in the resorcinol moiety. Life Sci 88(15–16):730–736
Zhao Q et al (2016) The antidepressant-like effects of pioglitazone in a chronic mild stress mouse model are associated with PPARgamma-mediated alteration of microglial activation phenotypes. J Neuroinflammation 13(1):259
Zorumski CF, Izumi Y, Mennerick S (2016) Ketamine: NMDA receptors and beyond. J Neurosci 36(44):11158–11164
Zuardi AW (2008) Cannabidiol: from an inactive cannabinoid to a drug with wide spectrum of action. Braz J Psychiatry 30(3):271–280

Modelling Differential Vulnerability to Substance Use Disorder in Rodents: Neurobiological Mechanisms

Bianca Jupp, Jolyon A. Jones, and Jeffrey W. Dalley

Contents

1 Introduction 204
2 Behavioural Endophenotypes of SUD 205
  2.1 Relationship Between Impulsivity and SUD-Like Behaviour 205
  2.2 Relationship Between Sensation-Seeking and SUD-Like Behaviour in Rodents ... 207
  2.3 Relationship Between Anxiety and SUD-Like Behaviour in Rodents 208
  2.4 Relationship Between Incentive Salience Attribution and SUD-Like Behaviour ... 209
3 Neural Substrates of SUD-Relevant Behavioural Endophenotypes 210
  3.1 Impulsivity 210
  3.2 Sensation-Seeking 212
  3.3 Anxiety 213
  3.4 Incentive Salience Attribution 214
4 Implications for Neural Mechanisms of SUD Vulnerability 215
5 Conclusions 218
References 219

Abstract

Despite the prevalence of drug use within society, only a subset of individuals actively taking addictive drugs lose control over their intake and develop compulsive drug-seeking and intake that typifies substance use disorder (SUD). Although research in this field continues to be an important and dynamic discipline, the specific neuroadaptations that drive compulsive behaviour in humans addicted to drugs and the neurobiological mechanisms that underlie an individual's innate susceptibility to SUD remain surprisingly poorly understood.

B. Jupp · J. A. Jones
Department of Psychology, University of Cambridge, Cambridge, UK

J. W. Dalley (✉)
Department of Psychology, University of Cambridge, Cambridge, UK

Department of Psychiatry, Addenbrooke's Hospital, Cambridge, UK
e-mail: jwd20@cam.ac.uk

M. A. Nader, Y. L. Hurd (eds.), *Substance Use Disorders*,
Handbook of Experimental Pharmacology 258, https://doi.org/10.1007/164_2019_300

Nonetheless, it is clear from research within the clinical domain that some behavioural traits are recurrently co-expressed in individuals with SUD, thereby inviting the hypothesis that certain behavioural endophenotypes may be predictive, or at least act in some way, to modify an individual's probability for developing this disorder. The analysis of such endophenotypes and their *catalytic* relationship to the expression of addiction-related behaviours has been greatly augmented by experimental approaches in rodents that attempt to capture diagnostically relevant aspects of this progressive brain disorder. This work has evolved from an early focus on aberrant drug reinforcement mechanisms to a now much richer account of the putatively impaired cognitive control processes that ultimately determine individual trajectories to compulsive drug-related behaviours. In this chapter we discuss the utility of experimental approaches in rodents designed to elucidate the neurobiological and genetic underpinnings of so-called risk traits and how these innate vulnerabilities collectively contribute to the pathogenesis of SUD.

Keywords
Anxiety · Cocaine · Impulsivity · Nucleus accumbens · Prefrontal cortex · Reward

1 Introduction

Substance use disorder (SUD) is characterised as a chronically relapsing disorder involving compulsive drug-seeking and intake that endures in the face of mounting adverse consequences for the individual (Koob and Le Moal 2001; Kalivas and Volkow 2005; Everitt and Robbins 2005). Of particular importance, it is widely acknowledged that despite the high prevalence of licit and illicit drug use within society, only a subset of individuals 'switch' from social and recreational use to compulsive forms of drug consumption involving repeated bouts of drug bingeing, withdrawal and relapse (Anthony et al. 1989). The reasons for this are unclear but are thought to result from an interaction between antecedent vulnerability traits and drug-induced neural plasticity mechanisms that subvert the normal control over volitional behaviour, ultimately to drive compulsive drug behaviours and an enduring propensity for relapse (Nestler 2001; Nader et al. 2008; Luscher and Malenka 2011; Everitt et al. 2008). The intricate interplay of interacting genetic, behavioural and psychosocial factors that determine an individual's susceptibility to SUD presents a formidable challenge to understanding the aetiological mechanisms of SUDs (Uhl 2006; Wong and Schumann 2008; Kreek et al. 2012).

Clinically, SUD associates with a number of co-expressed behavioural traits that collectively determine an individual's vulnerability to this disorder. These include the traits of impulsivity (Ersche et al. 2012a; Hamilton et al. 2015; Bickel et al. 2012; Winstanley et al. 2010; de Wit 2009), sensation-seeking (Ersche et al. 2012a), anxiety (Brown and Wolfe 1994) and aberrant attribution of reward cue salience (Robinson and Berridge 2001; Robinson and Flagel 2009). However, in the clinical setting, it is often difficult to separate the causal impacts of co-existing behavioural endophenotypes from the enduring and multivariate effects of chronic drug exposure. As a way to disambiguate causal mechanisms, rats have been widely used to investigate individual propensity for the development of SUD-like behaviours, specifically in the context of clinically translatable behavioural endophenotypes (Jupp and Dalley 2014). Increasingly, these studies have attempted to incorporate sophisticated measures of addiction-like behaviours, integrating aspects of the DSM criteria, including enhanced escalation and motivation for drug and maintained drug use in the face of adverse consequences (compulsive use), in addition to classical measures of drug reinforcement. Consequentially, elucidating the relationship of these traits in rodents to SUD-like behaviours has enabled the identification of novel neural substrates and mechanisms for translatable intervention. In this chapter, we review the various rodent models of behavioural endophenotypes of vulnerability to SUD of several classes of drugs, including stimulants, alcohol and opioids, their underlying neurobiology and the translational relevance of this work for human addiction.

2 Behavioural Endophenotypes of SUD

The notion of an 'addictive personality' is a widespread but rather imprecise description used to explain why some but not all people lose control over their drug intake. The idea of an addictive personality, however, is largely a misnomer as no single personality trait can ever deterministically be responsible for this disorder. Rather, the co-expression of certain risk traits probably reflects shared biological and/or genetic aetiologies that interact with several variables, including the psychosocial and environmental context, and the precise class of drug abused (Badiani et al. 2011). Evidence from clinical studies suggests that behavioural traits can predispose an individual to SUD (Verdejo-Garcia et al. 2008; Blanchard et al. 2009; Belin and Deroche-Gamonet 2012) by modifying disease progression, the frequency and intensity of drug relapse (Muller et al. 2008), as well as treatment outcome (Moeller et al. 2001; Patkar et al. 2004). Significantly, the expression of these traits (e.g. impulsivity, novelty/sensation-seeking, anxiety) varies across the lifespan (e.g. adolescence (Spear 2000)) and during different stages of the addiction cycle (e.g. initiation versus chronic use, Kreek et al. 2005), making it almost impossible to establish how in neural terms these behavioural traits interact with drug exposure and other environmental factors to promote the development of compulsive drug-taking behaviours in humans. This constraint can be overcome by the longitudinal analysis of rodents and other experimental animal species that naturally express recognised vulnerability traits.

2.1 Relationship Between Impulsivity and SUD-Like Behaviour

Impulsivity describes the predisposition of an individual to premature, poorly planned and unduly risky actions and decisions (Dalley and Robbins 2017; Daruna and Barnes 1993). While generally considered an adaptive trait promoting sociability and appropriate risk-taking, the maladaptive expression of impulsivity is often associated with negative consequences for the individual and is co-expressed with a number of neuropsychiatric disorders including SUD (Chamberlain and Sahakian 2007). While impulsivity is suggested to comprise multiple domains of behaviour, this trait can broadly be defined as impaired delayed gratification, rash anticipatory behaviour and impaired action cancellation. The diverse taxonomies of impulsivity are reflected in the variety of scales measured in self-report questionnaires and in various psychometric laboratory-based measures, which capture distinct aspects of the impulsivity phenotype. Many of these psychometric tasks have been translated into operant-based paradigms and enable assessment of behavioural traits in rodents (Winstanley 2011). Such tasks include the Go/No-Go and stop-signal reaction time tasks (SSRTT), which assess action cancellation (Logan et al. 1984; Eagle et al. 2008), delay discounting which examines delayed gratification (Richards et al. 1999) and the five choice serial reaction time task (5CSRTT, Robbins 2002), which assays impulsivity on the basis of anticipatory responding for a food-predictive, visual target cue. Importantly, impulsive performance on these tasks is enhanced in some strains of rodents (e.g. Roman high avoidance rats – RHA (Moreno et al. 2010); spontaneously hypertensive rats – SHR (Adriani et al. 2003)), and further, various outbred rat strains demonstrate 'trait-like' variability in the expression of impulsive responding in the 5CSRTT (Dalley et al. 2007) and delay discounting task (Perry et al. 2005; Broos et al. 2012).

Rodent studies have convincingly demonstrated that enhanced impulsivity predicts several SUD-like behaviours. However, the precise relationship depends on the class of drug administered and the particular impulsivity subtype assessed. Thus elevated levels of impulsive responding in the 5CSRTT are associated with enhanced self-administration (SA) of a range of drugs, including stimulants (Dalley et al. 2007; Marusich and Bardo 2009; Belin et al. 2008; Molander et al. 2011), alcohol (Radwanska and Kaczmarek 2012) and nicotine (Diergaarde et al. 2008) while also predicting increased rates of relapse to cocaine-seeking (Economidou et al. 2009). Similarly, rats displaying impulsive-like behaviours on the delay discounting task show increased alcohol (Oberlin and Grahame 2009; Poulos et al. 1995, but see Stein et al. 2015), cocaine (Perry et al. 2005) and nicotine (Diergaarde et al. 2008; Kayir et al. 2014) SA, as well as an increased resistance to extinction and enhanced propensity for reinstatement to responding for nicotine (Diergaarde et al. 2008) and cocaine (Broos et al. 2012). By contrast, different measures of impulsivity are less clearly related to opiate SA (McNamara et al. 2010; Schippers et al. 2012) with the exception of impulsivity innate to SHRs, which predicts increased opiate SA and relapse (Miller et al. 2018).

While escalation of drug intake defines one aspect of SUD-like behaviour, more relevant for the clinical picture is the persistence of drug taking in the face of punishment. Such behaviour is more closely aligned to the DSM criteria for SUD and has allowed greater opportunities for vertical and back translation between rodents and humans (Belin-Rauscent et al. 2016a). For example, trait-like impulsivity on the 5CSRTT predicts the development of compulsive cocaine SA in rodents (Belin et al. 2008), defined operationally by the persistence of drug SA despite negative consequences associated with this behaviour (Everitt et al. 2008). In keeping with the vulnerability to the development of compulsive behaviours, impulsive SHR and RHA rats develop compulsive water drinking on the schedule-induced polydipsia (SIP) task (Moreno et al. 2010; Ibias and Pellon 2011). Further, enhanced expression of compulsive SIP in rats predicts increased impulsive responding on both delay discounting (Cardona et al. 2011) and the 5CSRTT (Moreno et al. 2012). However, it has yet to be established whether trait impulsivity also predicts compulsive alcohol SA, as measured by recently developed models of this behaviour (e.g. Seif et al. 2013; Giuliano et al. 2018). Taken together, these findings demonstrate that impulsivity in its various forms is a vulnerability marker for both drug escalation and the development of compulsive drug-seeking and taking in rodents.

2.2 Relationship Between Sensation-Seeking and SUD-Like Behaviour in Rodents

Novelty/sensation-seeking is defined as a tendency to pursue novel and intense emotional experiences (Zukerman 1979) and can be divided into a number of dimensions related to novelty-seeking, novelty preference and other behavioural facets including harm avoidance and risk-taking. In humans, the various dimensions of sensation-seeking are usually assessed by questionnaire-based inventories (Whohlwill 1984; Arnett 1994) and are of interest because sensation-seeking often co-exists in individuals with SUD (Noel et al. 2011; Hittner and Swickert 2006; Gerra et al. 2004) and may predict the initiation of drug use (Stephenson and Helme 2006; Sargent et al. 2010; Spillane et al. 2012; Nees et al. 2012). However, it is unclear whether novelty/sensation-seeking truly represents an endophenotype of addiction. Thus although sensation-seeking is present in individuals who regularly abuse drugs, such individuals are nevertheless able to maintain control over drug use (Ersche et al. 2012b). By contrast, individuals with SUD expressed both sensation-seeking and impulsive traits (Ersche et al. 2012b), suggesting the expression of sensation-seeking may affect the onset or initiation of drug use or arise as a consequence of chronic drug exposure.

In rodents, the trait of novelty-/sensation-seeking is typically assessed by increased locomotor activity in a novel, inescapable environment (Blanchard et al. 2009) or by novelty preference, which assays the time spent in novel environment over a familiar one (Hughes 1968). Like impulsivity, particular strains of rodents express high levels of these behaviours (e.g. bred high responders, 'bHR' (Flagel et al. 2014), RHA (Giorgi et al. 2007)) or show individual variability in their expression (high responders, 'HR', Hughes 1968; Piazza et al. 1990). Novelty-reactive rats show an enhanced propensity to self-administer stimulants (Belin et al. 2008; Flagel et al. 2014; Marinelli and White 2000; Piazza et al. 1989), alcohol (Nadal et al. 2002), nicotine (Suto et al. 2001) and morphine (Ambrosio et al. 1995; Swain et al. 2018), but the trait of novelty-seeking is not associated with the development of compulsive cocaine behaviours as defined by resistance to punishment (Belin et al. 2008; Deroche-Gamonet et al. 2004). Conversely, rats showing high novelty preference show enhanced ethanol SA (Pelloux et al. 2015a) and are predisposed to develop compulsive cocaine SA (Belin et al. 2011). Interestingly, no apparent relationship appears to exist between the expression of novelty reactivity and novelty preference (Hughson et al. 2019), suggesting that these traits are independent and model different aspects of addiction-like behaviour.

2.3 Relationship Between Anxiety and SUD-Like Behaviour in Rodents

Anxiety is a naturally expressed response to threatening situations or stressors that is designed to protect the individual from harm. Pathological anxiety involves aberrant emotional processing such that typically nonthreatening or innocuous stimuli provoke a maladaptive prolonged anxiety response and is often co-morbidly expressed in individuals with SUD (Merikangas et al. 1998; Grant et al. 2004). Anxiety has been suggested to underlie the initiation of drug use (Goodwin et al. 2004), subjective drug craving (Sherman et al. 1989) and relapse to drug use (Schellekens et al. 2015). Further, there is evidence that drug exposure causes anxiety disorders (e.g. Johnson et al. 2000), especially associated with withdrawal states (McLaughlin et al. 2017). Clinically, anxiety can be assessed on the basis of maladaptive hyperarousal, often incorporating somatic measures (e.g. palpitations, dyspnea, sweating) in combination with self-report measures (Beck et al. 1988). Although there are inherent anthropomorphic issues in attempting to model emotionality in rodents, a number of tasks are used to assess anxiety in rodents (reviewed Steimer 2011; Harro 2018; Perusini and Fanselow 2015). Such tasks broadly assess anxiety as either a response to a generalised context or fear derived from a distinct threat (Perusini and Fanselow 2015). Ethological models of anxiety generally exploit the innate fear of animals to brightly lit spaces and their natural desire and curiosity to explore novel environments. These include the elevated plus maze (EPM) (Pellow et al. 1985), open field (OF) test (Britton and Britton 1981) and light-dark box (Vogel et al. 1971) and assess anxiety in terms of the time spent exploring or grooming in the safe versus aversive areas of the apparatus. In general, however, anxiety tests in rodents fail to reflect the maladaptive expression of anxiety and generally assay behaviour that falls within a 'normal' range. Thus, the extent to which we can really extrapolate anxiety measures in rodents to pathological anxiety in humans is unclear.

Notwithstanding the above considerations, there is persuasive evidence that anxiety in rodents predicts drug reinforcement. Thus, rats exhibiting anxiety-like behaviour on the EPM more readily escalate cocaine SA than low-anxious rats (Homberg et al. 2002; Dilleen et al. 2012). Critically, however, no relationship was observed between anxiety-like behaviour and the development of compulsive responding for cocaine (Deroche-Gamonet et al. 2004). In a similar vein, OF and EPM anxiety correlates with nicotine SA and relapse (Wang et al. 2018), which more controversially also extends to various alcohol-motivated behaviours. Thus, whereas trait anxiety in rats has been linked with increased alcohol SA (Spanagel et al. 1995; Hayton et al. 2012; Acevedo et al. 2016; Chappell et al. 2013), other studies report a reduction in alcohol drinking (Henniger et al. 2002; Langen and Fink 2004). Further controversies extend to the expression of anxiety-like behaviour in alcohol-preferring rats. In such animals, anxiety-like behaviour is either reduced (Acewicz et al. 2014), no different (Viglinskaya et al. 1995; Tuominen et al. 1990) or increased (Acevedo et al. 2016; Fernandez et al. 2017; Colombo et al. 1995; Ciccocioppo et al. 2006) compared with alcohol non-preferring rats. Finally, and reinforcing the view that risk endophenotypes depend selectively on particular classes of abused drug, there is no convincing evidence that 'trait' anxiety predicts opiate SA in rodents (Swain et al. 2018; Dilleen et al. 2012).

2.4 Relationship Between Incentive Salience Attribution and SUD-Like Behaviour

The attribution of motivational significance to 'cues' in the environment is an important form of learning, guiding behaviour towards rewarding outcomes and away from harmful or unfavourable stimuli. For some individuals, environmental cues may gain aberrant incentive salience, promoting the expression of maladaptive behaviours to drug-associated cues (Robinson and Berridge 2001). These include attentional (reviewed in Field and Cox 2008) and conditioned approach (reviewed in Watson et al. 2012) biases to cues associated with drug availability. However, in general, there have been relatively few studies that have looked at individual variability in the attribution of incentive salience in humans (Martin-Soelch et al. 2007; Mahler and de Wit 2010; Garofalo and di Pellegrino 2015; Styn et al. 2013). In rodents, this behaviour is typically assessed using the Pavlovian conditioned approach paradigm, which measures the development of approach behaviour during repeated presentations of a non-contingent, reward-predictive stimulus (conditioned stimulus, CS). Rats are subsequently divided into either 'goal-tracking' or 'sign-tracking' groups on the basis of their preference for the food reward or the CS. For goal-trackers, presentation of the CS elicits a response towards the location of the reward delivery, while sign-trackers preferentially approach and interact with the CS (Robinson and Flagel 2009). The expression of goal- vs sign-tracking behaviours varies within (Meyer et al. 2012) and between (Dickson et al. 2015; Flagel et al. 2010) different rat strains.

Sign-tracking is considered a maladaptive behaviour, persisting even when associated with delayed or cancelled rewards (e.g. Holland 1979; Chang and Smith 2016). Compared with goal-trackers, sign-trackers show enhanced instrumental responding (Robinson and Berridge 2001) and reinstatement of food-seeking (Yager and Robinson 2010). They also (1) show a greater preference for cocaine over natural reward (Tunstall and Kearns 2015), (2) an increased propensity to acquire cocaine SA (Beckmann et al. 2011), (3) increased motivation to self-administer stimulants and alcohol (Saunders and Robinson 2012; Versaggi et al. 2016; Anderson and Spear 2011) and (4) an increased propensity to reinstate nicotine and cocaine-seeking (Saunders and Robinson 2012). Nevertheless, a recent study reported no significant differences in punishment resistance between sign- and goal-trackers following an intermittent access paradigm of exposure (Kawa et al. 2016), thus calling into question the dichotomy of sign versus goal-tracking as a predictor of individual predisposition to compulsive drug SA.

3 Neural Substrates of SUD-Relevant Behavioural Endophenotypes

Collectively, the studies discussed above indicate that some behavioural endophenotypes in rodents can predict aspects of SUD-like behaviour. However, it is often the case that these traits are co-expressed in animals predisposed to SUD-like behaviour (see Table 1). Thus, novelty-reactive rats are also sign-trackers (Flagel et al. 2010) and show increased impulsivity on the 5CSRTT. Further, novelty-reactive rats are less impulsive on delay discounting tasks (Flagel et al. 2010) and are less anxious (Stead et al. 2006) and interestingly show no relationship with novelty preference (Hughson et al. 2019; Lukkes et al. 2016; Marusich et al. 2011). On the other hand, sign-trackers discount reward more readily than their goal-tracking counterparts (Tomie et al. 1998) and are also more impulsive on the 5CSRTT (Lovic et al. 2011). High-impulsive (HI) rats on the 5CSRTT, however, show no obvious relationship with novelty reactivity (Dalley et al. 2007; Molander et al. 2011), nor do they differentially acquire appetitive conditioned approach compared with low-impulsive rats (Robinson et al. 2009). Nevertheless, HI rats show a preference for novel objects and contexts (Molander et al. 2011; Giorgi et al. 2007), which may reflect a reduction in novelty-induced anxiety in these animals (Duclot et al. 2011). Indeed, anxiety-like behaviours appear to be inversely related to impulsivity on the 5CSRTT (Schneider et al. 2012), a curious relationship given that both traits predict SUD-related outcomes. However, there is no evidence that animals deemed highly impulsive on the 5CSRTT display enhanced measures of anxiety-like behaviour (Loos et al. 2009), suggesting their apparent preference for novelty may reflect an underlying deficit in behavioural inhibition.

3.1 Impulsivity

A number of studies have investigated the neurobiology of ‘trait’ impulsivity in rodents, predominantly in animals displaying enhanced impulsive responding in the 5CSRTT (i.e. the highly impulsive or HI phenotype). Convergent evidence points to abnormalities within the ventral striatum of HI rats, including diminished dopamine (DA) D2/D3 receptor availability in the nucleus accumbens (NAc) (Dalley et al. 2007), consistent with findings in non-human primates (Nader et al. 2006) and humans (Buckholtz et al. 2010). The locus of this deficit was later isolated to the NAc shell subregion of the ventral striatum (Jupp et al. 2013) and was accompanied by reduced transcript expression for this receptor (Besson et al. 2013). While it is not clear whether this reduction in binding capacity represents an effect on autoreceptors and/or on postsynaptic D2/D3 receptors, HI rats additionally exhibited reduced

Table 1 Predictive relationships between distinct behavioural traits in rodents and addiction-relevant behavioural endpoints

	Behaviour														
						Drug SA				Relapse				
Trait	5CSRTT	DD	NR	NP	ST	Anxiety	C	N	A	O	C	N	A	O	Compulsive drug SA
High 5CSRTT	↑	↑	–	↑	–	–	↑	↑	↑	–	↑	–	†	†	Cocaine
High DD	↓	↑	†	–	†	↑	↑	↑	↑	–	↑	↑	†	†	†
HR	↑	↓	↑	–	↑	↓	↑	↑	↑	↑	↑	†	†	†	–
HNP	†	†	↓	↑	†	†	–	†	↑	†	†	†	↑	†	Cocaine
ST	↑	↑	↑	†	↑	–	↑	↑	↑	†	↑	↑	†	†	–
Anxiety	↓	†	↓	–	–	↑	↑	↑	↑/↓	–	†	↑	↑	†	–

↓ Decreased expression of behaviour; ↑ increased expression of behaviour; – no observed relationship; † not assessed. Individual contrasts were made between the extremes of each trait (i.e. low versus high impulsivity on either the 5CSRTT or DD, high versus low novelty reactivity/preference, sign-tracking versus goal-tracking, high versus low anxiety)

5CSRTT 5-choice serial reaction time task, *DD* delay discounting, *HR* high responder or high novelty reactivity, *HNP* high novelty preference, *ST* sign tacking, *C* cocaine, *N* nicotine, *A* alcohol, *O* opiate [See text for citations related to each phenotype]

binding for the DA transporter in the NAc shell (Jupp et al. 2013), reduced D2 receptor transcript expression in the ventral tegmental area (VTA) (Besson et al. 2013) and enhanced electrically stimulated DA release (Diergaarde et al. 2008). Deficits in DA-ergic function were also present in the NAc core of HI rats, specifically diminished DA D1 receptor binding (Jupp et al. 2013) and reduced electrically evoked DA release compared with low-impulsive (LI) rats (Diergaarde et al. 2008).

Using magnetic resonance imaging and voxel-wise morphometry, we reported reduced grey matter density in the NAc core, accompanying reductions in protein levels of dendritic spines and microtubules (Caprioli et al. 2014), and reduced levels of GABA (Sawiak et al. 2016) and glutamate decarboxylase (Caprioli et al. 2014). Based on these findings, we hypothesised that 5CSRTT impulsivity may be mediated by a failure of the NAc core to appropriately gate behavioural responses driven by dysregulated DA function in the NAc shell. Intriguingly, we also found that D2/D3 binding was *higher* in the NAc shell and *lower* in the NAc core of rats exhibiting delay discounting impulsivity (Barlow et al. 2018). Distinct from HI rats, DA release was also diminished in the NAc core of rats showing delay discounting impulsivity (Diergaarde et al. 2008; Moschak and Carelli 2017). Thus, the mesolimbic DA system appears to make regionally selective contributions to different forms of impulsivity, namely, premature responding in the 5CSRTT and the rapid subjective devaluation of delayed rewards (i.e. delay aversion).

One of the original findings with the HI phenotype was reduced serotonin (5-HT) efflux in the prefrontal cortex (PFC) during task performance (Dalley et al. 2002), binding of 5-HT2A (Fink et al. 2015), and expression of 5-HT2C (Besson et al. 2013; Anastasio et al. 2014) receptors. There is also evidence for alterations in GABAergic function of the PFC, with reductions in binding for the GABAA receptor associated with enhanced levels of premature responding on the 5CSRTT (Jupp et al. 2013). Together these studies support the large body of evidence implicating the importance of frontal areas of the cortex in mediating impulse control (reviewed in Kim and Lee 2011). Impulsive responding on the 5CSRTT has also been found to relate to the cortical thickness of the anterior insula (Belin-Rauscent et al. 2016b). Moreover, lesions of the insular cortex selectively reduced impulsivity in HI rats but had no effect in mid- or low-impulsive rats (Belin-Rauscent et al. 2016b), suggesting that the insula may act as a node in the network contributing to these behaviours while not necessarily independently promoting impulse control. Importantly, for the link between impulsivity and vulnerability to compulsive behaviours, lesions of the insula in high-impulsive rats prevented the development of compulsive drinking behaviour in the SIP task (Belin-Rauscent et al. 2016b).

3.2 Sensation-Seeking

Studies examining the neurobiological correlates associated with high trait-like levels of novelty reactivity and novelty preference largely implicate alterations in monoaminergic function within corticostriatal circuitries in the expression of these behaviours (reviewed in Flagel et al. 2014; Arenas et al. 2016). Early studies of HR rats revealed significant effects on DA signalling within the striatum. These findings implicate enhanced baseline and psychostimulant-induced DA release in the ventral striatum (Piazza et al. 1989; Hooks et al. 1991) and reduced D2/D3 receptor density in both the dorsal and ventral striatum (Hooks et al. 1994) of these rats. More recent studies have confirmed the apparent hyperdopaminergic functioning of the striatum and associated circuitries in HR rats. Following up on the initial findings concerning the role of D2 receptors in novelty reactivity, studies by Flagel and colleagues found reduced transcript expression for D2 receptors (Flagel et al. 2010, 2014; Hughson et al. 2019), reflecting an effect of epigenetic regulation of the expression of this receptor within the NAc core (Hughson et al. 2019). Interestingly, a study of the trait of social dominance in rats found these animals to also be novelty-reactive, but found opposite effects on D2 receptor binding, with increased levels observed in the NAc shell, accompanied by increased binding for the DA transporter (Jupp et al. 2016). Further implicating effects on striatal DA function in novelty-reactive rats, there is evidence for enhanced basal firing rates of the VTA (Marinelli and White 2000), increased frequency of spontaneous (Flagel et al. 2010) and cocaine-induced (Mabrouk et al. 2018) DA release and reduced binding for the DA transporter (Chefer et al. 2003) within the NAc. Rats with high trait levels of novelty preference also demonstrate alterations in DA-ergic function, with reduced D2 receptor binding in the NAc and dorsal striatum, and greater behavioural responses after DA administration into the NAc (Hooks et al. 1994).

RHA rats additionally exhibited enhanced novelty preference behaviour and increased basal and amphetamine-induced DA release in the striatum, accompanied by reduced binding for D2 receptors in the substantia nigra/VTA (Tournier et al. 2013). Thus, similar to impulsivity and novelty reactivity, novelty preference implicates a reduction in DA release-regulating autoreceptors and increased DA release in the NAc.

Novelty preference and novelty reactivity further involve deficits in DA (Piazza et al. 1991) in the PFC. These changes were accompanied by increased transcript expression of the 5-HT genes, tyrosine hydroxylase-2 and the 5-HT transporter in brainstem projection nuclei (Kerman et al. 2011), findings that suggest that novelty reactivity is expressed not only by reduced serotonergic tone in the PFC but also by a dysregulation of PFC control over DA release in the NAc and dorsal striatum (Jackson et al. 2001; Katsidoni et al. 2011).

3.3 Anxiety

Despite numerous pharmacological and lesion-based studies seeking to understand the neural basis of anxiety (reviewed in Perusini and Fanselow 2015; Luthi and Luscher 2014), the neural substrates of individual variation in anxiety-like behaviours have been relatively neglected. In broad terms, anxiety encompasses primarily limbic cortico-hippocampal-amygdala circuitries and output from the periaqueductal grey and bed nucleus of the stria terminalis (Perusini and Fanselow 2015). Rats showing high anxiety-like behaviours on either the OF task or EPM have reduced markers for neural activity in the PFC (Kalisch et al. 2004; Prinssen et al. 2012), which may reflect a reduction in dendritic complexity (Miller et al. 2012). Rats demonstrating enhanced measures of anxiety-like behaviour on the EPM also show reduced electrically evoked DA release in the PFC, VTA and amygdala (Homberg et al. 2002). Altered basal DA release in the VTA may underlie the observed differential effect of cocaine on DA release in the ventral striatum of trait-anxious rats. Since cocaine exposure was associated with reduced electrically evoked DA release in the NAc core of trait-anxious rats (Homberg et al. 2003), this may underlie the enhanced escalation of cocaine SA in these animals (Dilleen et al. 2012).

3.4 Incentive Salience Attribution

Previous studies have mapped the neural correlates of sign versus goal-tracking using cue-evoked c-fos expression. This work predominantly implicates enhanced activation of striatal circuits, midline thalamic nuclei, lateral habenula and the amygdala of sign-tracking behaviour (Dilleen et al. 2012; Flagel et al. 2011a; Yager et al. 2015). The degree of cue-induced c-fos activation was differentially correlated between sign- and goal-trackers. Thus, sign-tracking behaviour was correlated with activity between a medial thalamic nucleus, the paraventricular thalamus (PVT) and the ventral striatum, while goal-tracking behaviour was correlated with activation between the PFC and PVT (Flagel et al. 2011a). Further, the pattern of PVT c-fos activation was differentially expressed in sign- and goal-trackers, showing activation in neurons receiving inputs from the prelimbic cortex in goal-trackers and neurons receiving projections from the NAc in sign-trackers (Haight et al. 2017). This differential regulation of activity suggests that sign-tracking behaviour may be associated with predominately ‘bottom-up’ mechanisms, whereas goal-tracking behaviour may preferentially recruit ‘top-down’ frontal cortical mechanisms to maintain goal-directed behaviour.

Consistent with a bottom-up mechanism, DA release was increased in the NAc core of sign-tracking rats during CS presentation (Flagel et al. 2011b), possibly reflecting enhanced motivational attribution to the cue. Supporting this view, intra-NAc core infusions of the DA receptor antagonist α-flupenthixol attenuated cue-induced reinstatement of cocaine-seeking in sign- but not goal-tracking rats (Saunders et al. 2013). Enhanced cue-evoked DA release was coupled with faster DA reuptake (Singer et al. 2016) and reduced expression of D2 receptor transcript in the NAc core of sign-tracking (Flagel et al. 2008, 2011b). Implicating a broader circuitry, neural activity in the ventral pallidum, which receives input from both the NAc and VTA (Heimer and Wilson 1975), was also increased by drug-cue presentation in sign-tracking rats (Ahrens et al. 2016, 2018). In addition, the ventral hippocampus contributes to the expression of sign-tracking behaviour (Fitzpatrick et al. 2016), possibly by regulating DA release in the ventral striatum (Lipska et al. 2002).

The differential behaviour of sign- and goal-tracking rats may also be explained by cortically mediated attentional processes. Thus, sign-tracking rats showed impairments on a sustained attention task and reduced task-related acetylcholine efflux in the PFC compared with goal-trackers (Paolone et al. 2013). Such results are consistent with the idea that rats with a high propensity to attribute incentive salience to reward cues also exhibit relatively poor attentional control. This notion is supported by recent evidence that DA efflux was increased in the PFC of sign-trackers in response to a cue, which correlated with their level of interaction with the cue, while goal-trackers exhibited an increase in acetylcholine that was unrelated to the expression of conditioned approach (Pitchers et al. 2017). Beyond DA and acetylcholine, the sign-tracking phenotype also implicates 5-HT dysfunction in the PFC (e.g. Winstanley et al. 2004; Campus et al. 2016).

4 Implications for Neural Mechanisms of SUD Vulnerability

The review of the literature above reveals a striking convergence in the neural substrates of SUD vulnerability traits, which though distinct in their neural loci, broadly encompass abnormalities in DA-ergic transmission in various striatal sub-territories and the PFC (see Fig. 1). Indeed striatal DA biomarkers are common across all drug-associated behavioural endophenotypes, and this is especially true of D2 receptors, for which binding as measured by D2/D3 receptor availability, and expression is reduced in the majority of behavioural traits linked to SUD, serving as a vulnerability marker (Dalley et al. 2007; Nader et al. 2006; Hooks et al. 1994; Morgan et al. 2002) and a consequence of extended drug use (Volkow et al. 1993, 2002; Wang et al. 1997; Sevy et al. 2008; Okita et al. 2016). Supporting this view, molecular and pharmacological interventions that diminish D2 receptors in the midbrain, including transgenic approaches in mice (Bello et al. 2011), strongly influence drug motivation (de Jong et al. 2015) and relapse (Xue et al. 2011).

However, while the evidence is compelling that deficient striatal D2 receptor function facilitates the escalation of drug SA, the role of this receptor in the etiology of *compulsive* drug behaviours is less clear. For example, rats screened for compulsive-like methamphetamine SA show *enhanced* markers of D1 and D2 receptor expression in the NAc (Cadet et al. 2016), while D2 receptors were downregulated and D1 receptors upregulated in the dorsal striatum of rats showing compulsive alcohol-seeking (Jadhav et al. 2018). Furthermore, a reduction in D2 expression in the dorsal striatum was associated with compulsive-like, punishment-resistant, and food-seeking in rats (Johnson and Kenny 2010) and was accompanied by identical deficits in ventral striatal plasticity as rats responding compulsively for cocaine (Kasanetz et al. 2010; Brown et al. 2017).

Thus, reduced D2 receptor expression in the dorsal striatum of novelty-preferring rats (Hooks et al. 1994) may represent a vulnerability marker for the development of drug-related compulsivity. A greater understanding of the evident role of the dorsal striatum in compulsive drug SA is thus needed. In this context, inactivation of the dorsolateral striatum (DLS) disrupts the expression of punished cocaine-seeking behaviour in rats (Jonkman et al. 2012), a region acknowledged as important for mediating habitual control over drug-seeking (Zapata et al. 2010; Corbit et al. 2012).

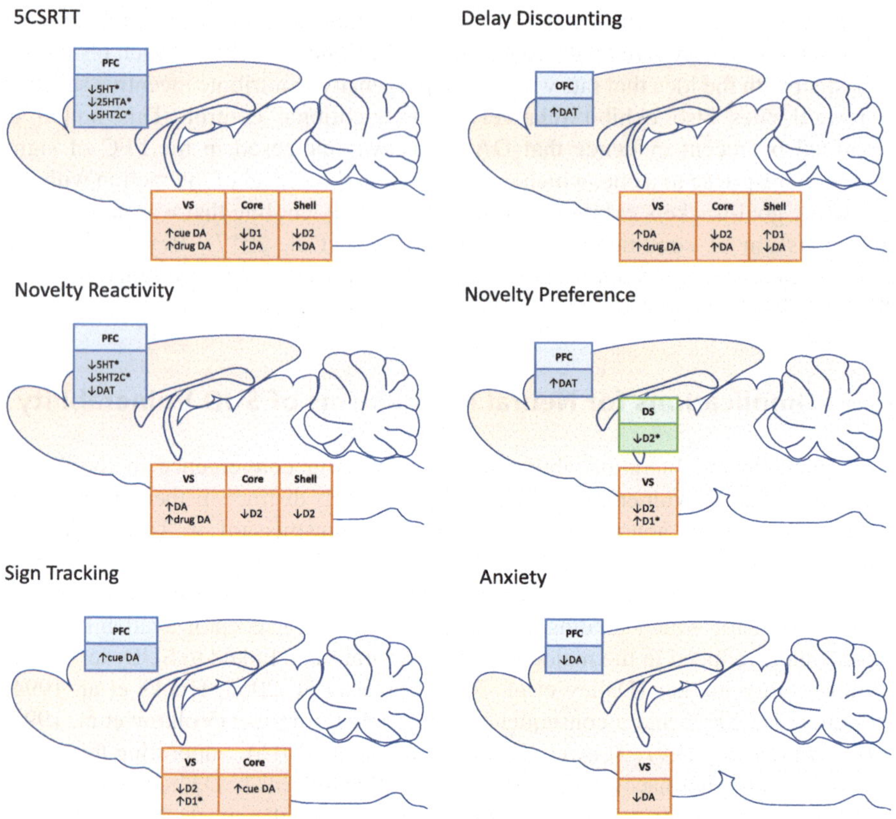

Fig. 1 Summary of the recognised neural biomarkers underlying individual variation in addictive-relevant behavioural endophenotypes. The recognised addiction endophenotypes all implicate abnormalities in serotonergic and/or dopaminergic function in the prefrontal cortex and ventral and dorsal striatum. However, the directionality and profile of these neurochemical biomarkers vary from one trait to the next. Some of these markers are additionally associated with compulsive drug-seeking behaviours (denoted by ∗), and to date only the 'traits' of high impulsivity in the 5CSRTT and high novelty preference predict the development of compulsive cocaine SA. ↓/↑ decreased/increased concentration, expression or function, *DA* dopamine, *5-HT* serotonin, *PFC* prefrontal cortex, *OFC* orbitofrontal cortex, *DS* dorsal striatum, *VS* ventral striatum, *Core* nucleus accumbens core, *Shell* nucleus accumbens shell

However, it has been reported that HI rats show a delay in the recruitment of the DLS over cocaine-seeking compared with LI rats (Murray et al. 2014). The reason for this unexpected delay may have been influenced by a pre-drug deficiency in D2/3 receptors in the NAc shell of HI rats. Indeed, only after protracted cocaine SA was a downregulation in D2 receptor transcript observed in the DLS of HI rats (Besson et al. 2013). By contrast, LI rats exhibited a reduction in D2 receptor expression after only a brief period of cocaine SA (Besson et al. 2013). A possible explanation for these puzzling results is that cocaine and other stimulant drugs regulate D2 receptors in the ventral striatum in a baseline-dependent manner (Caprioli et al. 2013, 2015).

Thus, the delay in the recruitment of DA-dependent mechanisms in the DLS development, subserving habitual instrumental control, may reflect a delayed correction of the initially low availability of D2 receptors in HI rats. Although this does not account for the apparent vulnerability of HI rats to develop compulsive cocaine SA, it suggests the *enhanced* D2 receptor expression in the NAc shell of novelty-reactive rats may offer resilience and thus be a protective factor against the emergence of compulsive drug-seeking (Bock et al. 2013).

Dysregulation 5-HT2C receptor function may also underlie risk for addiction-like behaviour in rodents. Thus, while no baseline differences were observed in 5-HT2C receptor transcript expression in the NAc of HI rats compared to LI rats, both short- and long-term cocaine SA reduced 5-HT2C expression in the NAc shell of HI rats (Besson et al. 2013). Since reduced 5-HT2C receptor function increases DA release in the NAc (e.g. Manvich et al. 2012; Filip and Cunningham 2002), this may be one explanation for the increased escalation of cocaine SA in HI rats (Dalley et al. 2007). However, it may also have relevance for the onset of compulsive drug SA since drugs that activate the 5-HT2C receptor (e.g. hallucinogens) have low addiction potential and even counteract the reinforcing effects of several classes of abused drug (Canal and Murnane 2017). This interaction is thought to involve the suppression of voltage- and calcium-gated potassium channels activated in medium spiny neurons of the NAc shell by cocaine (Imbrici et al. 2000; Mu et al. 2010). This may in turn underlie compulsive cocaine-seeking in rats associated with reduced 5-HT turnover in the NAc (Pelloux et al. 2012) and increased methylation and transcript expression of these potassium channels in rats responding compulsively for methamphetamine (Cadet et al. 2017). Thus, the effect of cocaine SA to reduce 5-HT2C expression in the NAc shell of HI rats may 'take the brake off' potassium channel sensitisation and affect neuronal excitability in this region. Importantly, one of these potassium channels, the small conductance calcium-activated potassium channel, is reported to promote the development of long-term depression (LTD) in the striatum (Hopf et al. 2010) and may represent a plausible mechanism underlying the impairment in LTD associated with compulsive drug-seeking (Kasanetz et al. 2010; Brown et al. 2017).

Compulsive drug-seeking is also hypothesised to involve a loss of top-down cognitive control over habitual behaviour, driving maladaptively enhanced habitual stimulus-response actions (Everitt and Robbins 2005, 2016). Indeed, there is significant evidence for impairments in frontal cortical networks in addiction (reviewed in Goldstein and Volkow 2011) and in mediating the expression of drug-related behaviours in rodents, including compulsive use (Kasanetz et al. 2010; Pelloux et al. 2012, 2015b; Chen et al. 2013). Further, the HI and novelty-reactive phenotypes are both associated with serotonergic dysfunction in the PFC (Besson et al. 2013; Dalley et al. 2002; Anastasio et al. 2014; Piazza et al. 1991; Antoniou et al. 2008), with postulated effects on PFC glutamatergic control over DA release in the midbrain and striatum, (Jackson et al. 2001; Katsidoni et al. 2011), in turn affecting relapse to cocaine-seeking (Pentkowski et al. 2010) and incubation of cocaine-cue craving (Swinford-Jackson et al. 2016). More specifically, 5-HT turnover is reduced in the PFC of rats resistant to the effect of punishment on cocaine-seeking (a compulsive phenotype), an effect mimicked by forebrain 5-HT depletion (Pelloux et al. 2012), and ameliorated by systemic administration of the 5-HT2C agonist mCPP (Pelloux et al. 2012).

There is also evidence to implicate alterations in dopaminergic activity in the PFC of addiction vulnerability endophenotypes, although the directionality of these effects varies with individual trait. Enhanced DA-ergic tone, reflecting enhanced function of the DA transporter, is associated with novelty reactivity (Marusich et al. 2011), while enhanced reward cue-induced DA release is present in sign-tracking animals (Pitchers et al. 2017). Conversely, there is a reduction in DA transporter efficacy in novelty-preferring animals (Yamamoto et al. 2013) and stimulated DA release in this region in anxious animals (Homberg et al. 2002). DA synaptic plasticity mechanisms in the PFC represent an important mechanism underling relapse to drug-seeking (reviewed in van den Oever et al. 2010). Indeed, both drug administration and withdrawal produce significant neuroadaptations within this region (e.g. Ben-Shahar et al. 2009; Tang et al. 2004), which affect the intrinsic excitability of these neurons (e.g. Ford et al. 2009). This altered excitability may in turn enhance the responsivity of these cells to cues and contexts associated with drug availability and driving relapse. Rapid alterations in plasticity mechanisms in the PFC are also observed following exposure to cues associated with drug availability (e.g. van den Oever et al. 2008). Additionally, synaptic plasticity mechanisms in the PFC are important for extinction learning (e.g. Busquet et al. 2008), which may also influence relapse behaviour. Tonic DA levels in the PFC have significant influence on induction of both long-term potentiation (LTP) and depression (LTD) in this region. As such, moderate elevations in tonic DA facilitate LTP induction, but this is impaired when DA levels are high. In contrast, in the absence, or under conditions of reduced tonic DA, LTD is favoured (Kolomiets et al. 2009). Thus, when considering the findings of perturbed prefrontal cortical DA-ergic function underlying addiction vulnerability traits, both enhanced and reduced DA-ergic tone may facilitate the development of plasticity mechanisms underlying relapse, driving the enhanced expression of this compulsive behaviour in vulnerable animals.

5 Conclusions

It is now accepted that differential vulnerability to addiction involves antecedent neurobiological risk factors, environmental variables and drug exposure, further influenced by inherent gender effects (Ait-Daoud et al. 2019), which together modulate the probabilistic outcome of an individual developing harmful drug use. While the precise aetiological mechanisms underlying the transition to addiction are unknown, there is overwhelming evidence to suggest that specific neurobehavioural endophenotypes contribute to this process, each in distinct ways that also depend on the class of abused drug. Studies in rodents have greatly accelerated the neural and psychological description of the transitions that lead to addiction and collectively form a key translational axis to facilitate the identification of novel brain mechanisms for therapeutic intervention.

Acknowledgements The author's research was funded by a Medical Research Council (MRC) Programme Grant (G1002231) and by a core award from the MRC (G1000183) and Wellcome Trust (093875/Z/10/Z) to the Behavioural and Clinical Neuroscience Institute at Cambridge University. BJ is supported by the MRC and recent fellowships from the AXA Research Fund, the National Health and MRC of Australia and the Cambridge Newton Trust. JJ was supported by an MRC Doctoral Training Programme grant at Cambridge University. JWD has received grants from Boehringer Ingelheim Pharma GmbH and GlaxoSmithKline. The remaining authors declare no competing interests.

References

Acevedo MB, Fabio MC, Fernandez MS, Pautassi RM (2016) Anxiety response and restraint-induced stress differentially affect ethanol intake in female adolescent rats. Neuroscience 334:259–274

Acewicz A, Mierzejewski P, Jastrzebska A, Korkosz I, Karas K, Sienkiewicz-Jarosz H et al (2014) Anxiety- and depressive-like traits in Warsaw alcohol high-preferring (WHP) and Warsaw alcohol low-preferring (WLP) rats. Pharmacol Biochem Behav 122:261–265

Adriani W, Caprioli A, Granstrem O, Carli M, Laviola G (2003) The spontaneously hypertensive-rat as an animal model of ADHD: evidence for impulsive and non-impulsive subpopulations. Neurosci Biobehav Rev 27:639–651

Ahrens AM, Meyer PJ, Ferguson LM, Robinson TE, Aldridge JW (2016) Neural activity in the ventral pallidum encodes variation in the incentive value of a reward cue. J Neurosci 36:7957–7970

Ahrens AM, Ferguson LM, Robinson TE, Aldridge JW (2018) Dynamic encoding of incentive salience in the ventral pallidum: dependence on the form of the reward cue. eNeuro 5. https://doi.org/10.1523/ENEURO.0328-17.2018

Ait-Daoud N, Blevins D, Khanna S, Sharma S, Holstege CP, Amin P (2019) Women and addiction: an update. Med Clin North Am 103:699–711

Ambrosio E, Goldberg SR, Elmer GI (1995) Behavior genetic investigation of the relationship between spontaneous locomotor activity and the acquisition of morphine self-administration behavior. Behav Pharmacol 6:229–237

Anastasio NC, Stutz SJ, Fox RG, Sears RM, Emeson RB, DiLeone RJ et al (2014) Functional status of the serotonin 5-HT2C receptor (5-HT2CR) drives interlocked phenotypes that precipitate relapse-like behaviors in cocaine dependence. Neuropsychopharmacology 39:370–382

Anderson RI, Spear LP (2011) Autoshaping in adolescence enhances sign-tracking behavior in adulthood: impact on ethanol consumption. Pharmacol Biochem Behav 98:250–260

Anthony JC, Tien AY, Petronis KR (1989) Epidemiologic evidence on cocaine use and panic attacks. Am J Epidemiol 129:543–549

Antoniou K, Papathanasiou G, Papalexi E, Hyphantis T, Nomikos GG, Spyraki C et al (2008) Individual responses to novelty are associated with differences in behavioral and neurochemical profiles. Behav Brain Res 187:462–472

Arenas MC, Aguilar MA, Montagud-Romero S, Mateos-Garcia A, Navarro-Frances CI, Minarro J et al (2016) Influence of the novelty-seeking endophenotype on the rewarding effects of psychostimulant drugs in animal models. Curr Neuropharmacol 14:87–100

Arnett J (1994) Sensation seeking: a new conceptualization and a new scale. Personal Individ Differ 16:289–296

Badiani A, Belin D, Epstein D, Calu D, Shaham Y (2011) Opiate versus psychostimulant addiction: the differences do matter. Nat Rev Neurosci 12:685–700

Barlow RL, Gorges M, Wearn A, Niessen HG, Kassubek J, Dalley JW et al (2018) Ventral striatal D2/3 receptor availability is associated with impulsive choice behavior as well as limbic corticostriatal connectivity. Int J Neuropsychopharmacol 21:705–715

Beck AT, Epstein N, Brown G, Steer RA (1988) An inventory for measuring clinical anxiety: psychometric properties. J Consult Clin Psychol 56:893–897

Beckmann JS, Marusich JA, Gipson CD, Bardo MT (2011) Novelty seeking, incentive salience and acquisition of cocaine self-administration in the rat. Behav Brain Res 216:159–165

Belin D, Deroche-Gamonet V (2012) Responses to novelty and vulnerability to cocaine addiction: contribution of a multi-symptomatic animal model. Cold Spring Harb Perspect Med 2:a011940

Belin D, Mar AC, Dalley JW, Robbins TW, Everitt BJ (2008) High impulsivity predicts the switch to compulsive cocaine-taking. Science 320:1352–1355

Belin D, Berson N, Balado E, Piazza PV, Deroche-Gamonet V (2011) High-novelty-preference rats are predisposed to compulsive cocaine self-administration. Neuropsychopharmacology 36:569–579

Belin-Rauscent A, Fouyssac M, Bonci A, Belin D (2016a) How preclinical models evolved to resemble the diagnostic criteria of drug addiction. Biol Psychiatry 79:39–46

Belin-Rauscent A, Daniel ML, Puaud M, Jupp B, Sawiak S, Howett D et al (2016b) From impulses to maladaptive actions: the insula is a neurobiological gate for the development of compulsive behavior. Mol Psychiatry 21:491–499

Bello EP, Mateo Y, Gelman DM, Noain D, Shin JH, Low MJ et al (2011) Cocaine supersensitivity and enhanced motivation for reward in mice lacking dopamine D2 autoreceptors. Nat Neurosci 14:1033–1038

Ben-Shahar O, Obara I, Ary AW, Ma N, Mangiardi MA, Medina RL et al (2009) Extended daily access to cocaine results in distinct alterations in Homer 1b/c and NMDA receptor subunit expression within the medial prefrontal cortex. Synapse 63:598–609

Besson M, Pelloux Y, Dilleen R, Theobald DE, Lyon A, Belin-Rauscent A et al (2013) Cocaine modulation of frontostriatal expression of Zif268, D2, and 5-HT2c receptors in high and low impulsive rats. Neuropsychopharmacology 38:1963–1973

Bickel WK, Jarmolowicz DP, Mueller ET, Koffarnus MN, Gatchalian KM (2012) Excessive discounting of delayed reinforcers as a trans-disease process contributing to addiction and other disease-related vulnerabilities: emerging evidence. Pharmacol Ther 134:287–297

Blanchard MM, Mendelsohn D, Stamp JA (2009) The HR/LR model: further evidence as an animal model of sensation seeking. Neurosci Biobehav Rev 33:1145–1154

Bock R, Shin JH, Kaplan AR, Dobi A, Markey E, Kramer PF et al (2013) Strengthening the accumbal indirect pathway promotes resilience to compulsive cocaine use. Nat Neurosci 16:632–638

Britton DR, Britton KT (1981) A sensitive open field measure of anxiolytic drug activity. Pharmacol Biochem Behav 15:577–582

Broos N, Diergaarde L, Schoffelmeer AN, Pattij T, de Vries TJ (2012) Trait impulsive choice predicts resistance to extinction and propensity to relapse to cocaine seeking: a bidirectional investigation. Neuropsychopharmacology 37:1377–1386

Brown PJ, Wolfe J (1994) Substance abuse and post-traumatic stress disorder comorbidity. Drug Alcohol Depend 35:51–59

Brown RM, Kupchik YM, Spencer S, Garcia-Keller C, Spanswick DC, Lawrence AJ et al (2017) Addiction-like synaptic impairments in diet-induced obesity. Biol Psychiatry 81:797–806

Buckholtz JW, Treadway MT, Cowan RL, Woodward ND, Benning SD, Li R et al (2010) Mesolimbic dopamine reward system hypersensitivity in individuals with psychopathic traits. Nat Neurosci 13:419–421

Busquet P, Hetzenauer A, Sinnegger-Brauns MJ, Striessnig J, Singewald N (2008) Role of L-type Ca2+ channel isoforms in the extinction of conditioned fear. Learn Mem 15:378–386

Cadet JL, Krasnova IN, Walther D, Brannock C, Ladenheim B, McCoy MT et al (2016) Increased expression of proenkephalin and prodynorphin mRNAs in the nucleus accumbens of compulsive methamphetamine taking rats. Sci Rep 6:37002

Cadet JL, Brannock C, Krasnova IN, Jayanthi S, Ladenheim B, McCoy MT et al (2017) Genome-wide DNA hydroxymethylation identifies potassium channels in the nucleus accumbens as discriminators of methamphetamine addiction and abstinence. Mol Psychiatry 22:1196–1204

Campus P, Accoto A, Maiolati M, Latagliata C, Orsini C (2016) Role of prefrontal 5-HT in the strain-dependent variation in sign-tracking behavior of C57BL/6 and DBA/2 mice. Psychopharmacology (Berl) 233:1157–1169

Canal CE, Murnane KS (2017) The serotonin 5-HT2C receptor and the non-addictive nature of classic hallucinogens. J Psychopharmacol 31:127–143

Caprioli D, Hong YT, Sawiak SJ, Ferrari V, Williamson DJ, Jupp B et al (2013) Baseline-dependent effects of cocaine pre-exposure on impulsivity and D2/3 receptor availability in the rat striatum: possible relevance to the attention-deficit hyperactivity syndrome. Neuropsychopharmacology 38:1460–1471

Caprioli D, Sawiak SJ, Merlo E, Theobald DE, Spoelder M, Jupp B et al (2014) Gamma aminobutyric acidergic and neuronal structural markers in the nucleus accumbens core underlie trait-like impulsive behavior. Biol Psychiatry 75:115–123

Caprioli D, Jupp B, Hong YT, Sawiak SJ, Ferrari V, Wharton L et al (2015) Dissociable rate-dependent effects of oral methylphenidate on impulsivity and D2/3 receptor availability in the striatum. J Neurosci 35:3747–3755

Cardona D, Lopez-Crespo G, Sanchez-Amate MC, Flores P, Sanchez-Santed F (2011) Impulsivity as long-term sequelae after chlorpyrifos intoxication: time course and individual differences. Neurotox Res 19:128–137

Chamberlain SR, Sahakian BJ (2007) The neuropsychiatry of impulsivity. Curr Opin Psychiatry 20:255–261

Chang SE, Smith KS (2016) An omission procedure reorganizes the microstructure of sign-tracking while preserving incentive salience. Learn Mem 23:151–155

Chappell AM, Carter E, McCool BA, Weiner JL (2013) Adolescent rearing conditions influence the relationship between initial anxiety-like behavior and ethanol drinking in male Long Evans rats. Alcohol Clin Exp Res 37(Suppl 1):E394–E403

Chefer VI, Zakharova I, Shippenberg TS (2003) Enhanced responsiveness to novelty and cocaine is associated with decreased basal dopamine uptake and release in the nucleus accumbens: quantitative microdialysis in rats under transient conditions. J Neurosci 23:3076–3084

Chen BT, Yau HJ, Hatch C, Kusumoto-Yoshida I, Cho SL, Hopf FW et al (2013) Rescuing cocaine-induced prefrontal cortex hypoactivity prevents compulsive cocaine seeking. Nature 496:359–362

Ciccocioppo R, Economidou D, Cippitelli A, Cucculelli M, Ubaldi M, Soverchia L et al (2006) Genetically selected Marchigian Sardinian alcohol-preferring (msP) rats: an animal model to study the neurobiology of alcoholism. Addict Biol 11:339–355

Colombo G, Agabio R, Lobina C, Reali R, Zocchi A, Fadda F et al (1995) Sardinian alcohol-preferring rats: a genetic animal model of anxiety. Physiol Behav 57:1181–1185

Corbit LH, Nie H, Janak PH (2012) Habitual alcohol seeking: time course and the contribution of subregions of the dorsal striatum. Biol Psychiatry 72:389–395

Dalley JW, Robbins TW (2017) Fractionating impulsivity: neuropsychiatric implications. Nat Rev Neurosci 18:158–171

Dalley JW, Theobald DE, Eagle DM, Passetti F, Robbins TW (2002) Deficits in impulse control associated with tonically-elevated serotonergic function in rat prefrontal cortex. Neuropsychopharmacology 26:716–728

Dalley JW, Fryer TD, Brichard L, Robinson ES, Theobald DE, Laane K et al (2007) Nucleus accumbens D2/3 receptors predict trait impulsivity and cocaine reinforcement. Science 315:1267–1270

Daruna J, Barnes P (1993) A neurodevelopmental view of impulsivity and its relationship to the superfactors of personality. In: McCown W, Johnson J, Shure M (eds) The impulsive client: theory, research and treatment. American Psychological Association, Washington

de Jong JW, Roelofs TJ, Mol FM, Hillen AE, Meijboom KE, Luijendijk MC et al (2015) Reducing ventral tegmental dopamine D2 receptor expression selectively boosts incentive motivation. Neuropsychopharmacology 40:2085–2095 de Wit H (2009) Impulsivity as a determinant and consequence of drug use: a review of underlying processes. Addict Biol 14:22–31

Deroche-Gamonet V, Belin D, Piazza PV (2004) Evidence for addiction-like behavior in the rat. Science 305:1014–1017

Dickson PE, McNaughton KA, Hou L, Anderson LC, Long KH, Chesler EJ (2015) Sex and strain influence attribution of incentive salience to reward cues in mice. Behav Brain Res 292:305–315

Diergaarde L, Pattij T, Poortvliet I, Hogenboom F, de Vries W, Schoffelmeer AN et al (2008) Impulsive choice and impulsive action predict vulnerability to distinct stages of nicotine seeking in rats. Biol Psychiatry 63:301–308

Dilleen R, Pelloux Y, Mar AC, Molander A, Robbins TW, Everitt BJ et al (2012) High anxiety is a predisposing endophenotype for loss of control over cocaine, but not heroin, self-administration in rats. Psychopharmacology (Berl) 222:89–97

Duclot F, Hollis F, Darcy MJ, Kabbaj M (2011) Individual differences in novelty-seeking behavior in rats as a model for psychosocial stress-related mood disorders. Physiol Behav 104:296–305

Eagle DM, Bari A, Robbins TW (2008) The neuropsychopharmacology of action inhibition: cross-species translation of the stop-signal and go/no-go tasks. Psychopharmacology (Berl) 199:439–456

Economidou D, Pelloux Y, Robbins TW, Dalley JW, Everitt BJ (2009) High impulsivity predicts relapse to cocaine-seeking after punishment-induced abstinence. Biol Psychiatry 65:851–856

Ersche KD, Turton AJ, Chamberlain SR, Muller U, Bullmore ET, Robbins TW (2012a) Cognitive dysfunction and anxious-impulsive personality traits are endophenotypes for drug dependence. Am J Psychiatry 169:926–936

Ersche KD, Jones PS, Williams GB, Smith DG, Bullmore ET, Robbins TW (2012b) Distinctive personality traits and neural correlates associated with stimulant drug use versus familial risk of stimulant dependence. Biol Psychiatry 74:137–144

Everitt BJ, Robbins TW (2005) Neural systems of reinforcement for drug addiction: from actions to habits to compulsion. Nat Neurosci 8:1481–1489

Everitt BJ, Robbins TW (2016) Drug addiction: updating actions to habits to compulsions ten years on. Annu Rev Psychol 67:23–50

Everitt BJ, Belin D, Economidou D, Pelloux Y, Dalley JW, Robbins TW (2008) Review. Neural mechanisms underlying the vulnerability to develop compulsive drug-seeking habits and addiction. Philos Trans R Soc Lond B Biol Sci 363:3125–3135

Fernandez MS, Baez B, Bordon A, Espinosa L, Martinez E, Pautassi RM (2017) Short-term selection for high and low ethanol intake yields differential sensitivity to ethanol's motivational effects and anxiety-like responses in adolescent Wistar rats. Prog Neuropsychopharmacol Biol Psychiatry 79:220–233

Field M, Cox WM (2008) Attentional bias in addictive behaviors: a review of its development, causes, and consequences. Drug Alcohol Depend 97:1–20

Filip M, Cunningham KA (2002) Serotonin 5-HT(2C) receptors in nucleus accumbens regulate expression of the hyperlocomotive and discriminative stimulus effects of cocaine. Pharmacol Biochem Behav 71:745–756

Fink LH, Anastasio NC, Fox RG, Rice KC, Moeller FG, Cunningham KA (2015) Individual differences in impulsive action reflect variation in the cortical serotonin 5-HT2A receptor system. Neuropsychopharmacology 40:1957–1968

Fitzpatrick CJ, Creeden JF, Perrine SA, Morrow JD (2016) Lesions of the ventral hippocampus attenuate the acquisition but not expression of sign-tracking behavior in rats. Hippocampus 26:1424–1434

Flagel SB, Watson SJ, Akil H, Robinson TE (2008) Individual differences in the attribution of incentive salience to a reward-related cue: influence on cocaine sensitization. Behav Brain Res 186:48–56

Flagel SB, Robinson TE, Clark JJ, Clinton SM, Watson SJ, Seeman P et al (2010) An animal model of genetic vulnerability to behavioral disinhibition and responsiveness to reward-related cues: implications for addiction. Neuropsychopharmacology 35:388–400

Flagel SB, Cameron CM, Pickup KN, Watson SJ, Akil H, Robinson TE (2011a) A food predictive cue must be attributed with incentive salience for it to induce c-fos mRNA expression in cortico-striatal-thalamic brain regions. Neuroscience 196:80–96

Flagel SB, Clark JJ, Robinson TE, Mayo L, Czuj A, Willuhn I et al (2011b) A selective role for dopamine in stimulus-reward learning. Nature 469:53–57

Flagel SB, Waselus M, Clinton SM, Watson SJ, Akil H (2014) Antecedents and consequences of drug abuse in rats selectively bred for high and low response to novelty. Neuropharmacology 76 (Pt B):425–436

Ford KA, Wolf ME, XT H (2009) Plasticity of L-type Ca2+ channels after cocaine withdrawal. Synapse 63:690–697

Garofalo S, di Pellegrino G (2015) Individual differences in the influence of task-irrelevant Pavlovian cues on human behavior. Front Behav Neurosci 9:163

Gerra G, Angioni L, Zaimovic A, Moi G, Bussandri M, Bertacca S et al (2004) Substance use among high-school students: relationships with temperament, personality traits, and parental care perception. Subst Use Misuse 39:345–367

Giorgi O, Piras G, Corda MG (2007) The psychogenetically selected Roman high- and low-avoidance rat lines: a model to study the individual vulnerability to drug addiction. Neurosci Biobehav Rev 31:148–163

Giuliano C, Pena-Oliver Y, Goodlett CR, Cardinal RN, Robbins TW, Bullmore ET et al (2018) Evidence for a long-lasting compulsive alcohol seeking phenotype in rats. Neuropsychopharmacology 43:728–738

Goldstein RZ, Volkow ND (2011) Dysfunction of the prefrontal cortex in addiction: neuroimaging findings and clinical implications. Nat Rev Neurosci 12:652–669

Goodwin RD, Fergusson DM, Horwood LJ (2004) Association between anxiety disorders and substance use disorders among young persons: results of a 21-year longitudinal study. J Psychiatr Res 38:295–304

Grant BF, Stinson FS, Dawson DA, Chou SP, Dufour MC, Compton W et al (2004) Prevalence and co-occurrence of substance use disorders and independent mood and anxiety disorders: results from the National Epidemiologic Survey on Alcohol and Related Conditions. Arch Gen Psychiatry 61:807–816

Haight JL, Fuller ZL, Fraser KM, Flagel SB (2017) A food-predictive cue attributed with incentive salience engages subcortical afferents and efferents of the paraventricular nucleus of the thalamus. Neuroscience 340:135–152

Hamilton KR, Mitchell MR, Wing VC, Balodis IM, Bickel WK, Fillmore M et al (2015) Choice impulsivity: definitions, measurement issues, and clinical implications. Pers Disord 6:182–198

Harro J (2018) Animals, anxiety, and anxiety disorders: How to measure anxiety in rodents and why. Behav Brain Res 352:81–93

Hayton SJ, Mahoney MK, Olmstead MC (2012) Behavioral traits predicting alcohol drinking in outbred rats: an investigation of anxiety, novelty seeking, and cognitive flexibility. Alcohol Clin Exp Res 36:594–603

Heimer L, Wilson R (1975) The subcortical projections of the allocortex: similarities in the neural associations of the hippocampus, the piriform cortex, and the neocortex. Raven Press, New York

Henniger MS, Spanagel R, Wigger A, Landgraf R, Holter SM (2002) Alcohol self-administration in two rat lines selectively bred for extremes in anxiety-related behavior. Neuropsychopharmacology 26:729–736

Hittner JB, Swickert R (2006) Sensation seeking and alcohol use: a meta-analytic review. Addict Behav 31:1383–1401

Holland PC (1979) Differential effects of omission contingencies on various components of Pavlovian appetitive conditioned responding in rats. J Exp Psychol Anim Behav Process 5:178–193

Homberg JR, van den Akker M, Raaso HS, Wardeh G, Binnekade R, Schoffelmeer AN et al (2002) Enhanced motivation to self-administer cocaine is predicted by self-grooming behaviour and relates to dopamine release in the rat medial prefrontal cortex and amygdala. Eur J Neurosci 15:1542–1550

Homberg JR, Wardeh G, Raaso HS, Schoffelmeer AN, De Vries TJ (2003) Neuroadaptive changes in mesocorticolimbic dopamine and acetylcholine neurons following cocaine or saline self-administration are dependent on pre-existing individual differences. Neuroscience 121:829–836

Hooks MS, Jones GH, Smith AD, Neill DB, Justice JB Jr (1991) Response to novelty predicts the locomotor and nucleus accumbens dopamine response to cocaine. Synapse 9:121–128

Hooks MS, Juncos JL, Justice JB Jr, Meiergerd SM, Povlock SL, Schenk JO et al (1994) Individual locomotor response to novelty predicts selective alterations in D1 and D2 receptors and mRNAs. J Neurosci 14:6144–6152

Hopf FW, Seif T, Mohamedi ML, Chen BT, Bonci A (2010) The small-conductance calcium-activated potassium channel is a key modulator of firing and long-term depression in the dorsal striatum. Eur J Neurosci 31:1946–1959

Hughes RN (1968) Effects of age on novelty reactions and exploration in rats. Q J Exp Psychol 20:189–192

Hughson AR, Horvath AP, Holl K, Palmer AA, Solberg Woods LC, Robinson TE et al (2019) Incentive salience attribution, "sensation-seeking" and "novelty-seeking" are independent traits in a large sample of male and female heterogeneous stock rats. Sci Rep 9:2351

Ibias J, Pellon R (2011) Schedule-induced polydipsia in the spontaneously hypertensive rat and its relation to impulsive behaviour. Behav Brain Res 223:58–69

Imbrici P, Tucker SJ, D'Adamo MC, Pessia M (2000) Role of receptor protein tyrosine phosphatase alpha (RPTPalpha) and tyrosine phosphorylation in the serotonergic inhibition of voltage-dependent potassium channels. Pflugers Arch 441:257–262

Jackson ME, Frost AS, Moghaddam B (2001) Stimulation of prefrontal cortex at physiologically relevant frequencies inhibits dopamine release in the nucleus accumbens. J Neurochem 78:920–923

Jadhav KS, Peterson VL, Halfon O, Ahern G, Fouhy F, Stanton C et al (2018) Gut microbiome correlates with altered striatal dopamine receptor expression in a model of compulsive alcohol seeking. Neuropharmacology 141:249–259

Johnson PM, Kenny PJ (2010) Dopamine D2 receptors in addiction-like reward dysfunction and compulsive eating in obese rats. Nat Neurosci 13:635–641

Johnson JG, Cohen P, Pine DS, Klein DF, Kasen S, Brook JS (2000) Association between cigarette smoking and anxiety disorders during adolescence and early adulthood. JAMA 284:2348–2351

Jonkman S, Pelloux Y, Everitt BJ (2012) Differential roles of the dorsolateral and midlateral striatum in punished cocaine seeking. J Neurosci 32:4645–4650

Jupp B, Dalley JW (2014) Behavioral endophenotypes of drug addiction: etiological insights from neuroimaging studies. Neuropharmacology 76(Pt B):487–497

Jupp B, Caprioli D, Saigal N, Reverte I, Shrestha S, Cumming P et al (2013) Dopaminergic and GABA-ergic markers of impulsivity in rats: evidence for anatomical localisation in ventral striatum and prefrontal cortex. Eur J Neurosci 37:1519–1528

Jupp B, Murray JE, Jordan ER, Xia J, Fluharty M, Shrestha S et al (2016) Social dominance in rats: effects on cocaine self-administration, novelty reactivity and dopamine receptor binding and content in the striatum. Psychopharmacology (Berl) 233:579–589

Kalisch R, Salome N, Platzer S, Wigger A, Czisch M, Sommer W et al (2004) High trait anxiety and hyporeactivity to stress of the dorsomedial prefrontal cortex: a combined phMRI and Fos study in rats. Neuroimage 23:382–391

Kalivas PW, Volkow ND (2005) The neural basis of addiction: a pathology of motivation and choice. Am J Psychiatry 162:1403–1413

Kasanetz F, Deroche-Gamonet V, Berson N, Balado E, Lafourcade M, Manzoni O et al (2010) Transition to addiction is associated with a persistent impairment in synaptic plasticity. Science 328:1709–1712

Katsidoni V, Apazoglou K, Panagis G (2011) Role of serotonin 5-HT2A and 5-HT2C receptors on brain stimulation reward and the reward-facilitating effect of cocaine. Psychopharmacology (Berl) 213:337–354

Kawa AB, Bentzley BS, Robinson TE (2016) Less is more: prolonged intermittent access cocaine self-administration produces incentive-sensitization and addiction-like behavior. Psychopharmacology (Berl) 233:3587–3602

Kayir H, Semenova S, Markou A (2014) Baseline impulsive choice predicts the effects of nicotine and nicotine withdrawal on impulsivity in rats. Prog Neuropsychopharmacol Biol Psychiatry 48:6–13

Kerman IA, Clinton SM, Bedrosian TA, Abraham AD, Rosenthal DT, Akil H et al (2011) High novelty-seeking predicts aggression and gene expression differences within defined serotonergic cell groups. Brain Res 1419:34–45

Kim S, Lee D (2011) Prefrontal cortex and impulsive decision making. Biol Psychiatry 69:1140–1146

Kolomiets B, Marzo A, Caboche J, Vanhoutte P, Otani S (2009) Background dopamine concentration dependently facilitates long-term potentiation in rat prefrontal cortex through postsynaptic activation of extracellular signal-regulated kinases. Cereb Cortex 19:2708–2718

Koob GF, Le Moal M (2001) Drug addiction, dysregulation of reward, and allostasis. Neuropsychopharmacology 24:97–129

Kreek MJ, Nielsen DA, Butelman ER, LaForge KS (2005) Genetic influences on impulsivity, risk taking, stress responsivity and vulnerability to drug abuse and addiction. Nat Neurosci 8:1450–1457

Kreek MJ, Levran O, Reed B, Schlussman SD, Zhou Y, Butelman ER (2012) Opiate addiction and cocaine addiction: underlying molecular neurobiology and genetics. J Clin Invest 122:3387–3393

Langen B, Fink H (2004) Anxiety as a predictor of alcohol preference in rats? Prog Neuropsychopharmacol Biol Psychiatry 28:961–968

Lipska BK, Halim ND, Segal PN, Weinberger DR (2002) Effects of reversible inactivation of the neonatal ventral hippocampus on behavior in the adult rat. J Neurosci 22:2835–2842

Logan GD, Cowan WB, Davis KA (1984) On the ability to inhibit simple and choice reaction time responses: a model and a method. J Exp Psychol Hum Percept Perform 10:276–291

Loos M, van der Sluis S, Bochdanovits Z, van Zutphen IJ, Pattij T, Stiedl O et al (2009) Activity and impulsive action are controlled by different genetic and environmental factors. Genes Brain Behav 8:817–828

Lovic V, Saunders BT, Yager LM, Robinson TE (2011) Rats prone to attribute incentive salience to reward cues are also prone to impulsive action. Behav Brain Res 223:255–261

Lukkes JL, Thompson BS, Freund N, Andersen SL (2016) The developmental inter-relationships between activity, novelty preferences, and delay discounting in male and female rats. Dev Psychobiol 58:231–242

Luscher C, Malenka RC (2011) Drug-evoked synaptic plasticity in addiction: from molecular changes to circuit remodeling. Neuron 69:650–663

Luthi A, Luscher C (2014) Pathological circuit function underlying addiction and anxiety disorders. Nat Neurosci 17:1635–1643

Mabrouk OS, Han JL, Wong JT, Akil H, Kennedy RT, Flagel SB (2018) The in vivo neurochemical profile of selectively bred high-responder and low-responder rats reveals baseline, cocaine-evoked, and novelty-evoked differences in monoaminergic systems. ACS Chem Nerosci 9:715–724

Mahler SV, de Wit H (2010) Cue-reactors: individual differences in cue-induced craving after food or smoking abstinence. PLoS One 5:e15475

Manvich DF, Kimmel HL, Howell LL (2012) Effects of serotonin 2C receptor agonists on the behavioral and neurochemical effects of cocaine in squirrel monkeys. J Pharmacol Exp Ther 341:424–434

Marinelli M, White FJ (2000) Enhanced vulnerability to cocaine self-administration is associated with elevated impulse activity of midbrain dopamine neurons. J Neurosci 20:8876–8885

Martin-Soelch C, Linthicum J, Ernst M (2007) Appetitive conditioning: neural bases and implications for psychopathology. Neurosci Biobehav Rev 31:426–440

Marusich JA, Bardo MT (2009) Differences in impulsivity on a delay-discounting task predict self-administration of a low unit dose of methylphenidate in rats. Behav Pharmacol 20:447–454

Marusich JA, Darna M, Charnigo RJ, Dwoskin LP, Bardo MT (2011) A multivariate assessment of individual differences in sensation seeking and impulsivity as predictors of amphetamine self-administration and prefrontal dopamine function in rats. Exp Clin Psychopharmacol 19:275–284

McLaughlin I, Dani JA, de Biasi M (2017) The medial habenula and interpeduncular nucleus circuitry is critical in addiction, anxiety, and mood regulation. J Neurochem 142(Suppl 2):130–143

McNamara R, Dalley JW, Robbins TW, Everitt BJ, Belin D (2010) Trait-like impulsivity does not predict escalation of heroin self-administration in the rat. Psychopharmacology (Berl) 212:453–464

Merikangas KR, Mehta RL, Molnar BE, Walters EE, Swendsen JD, Aguilar-Gaziola S et al (1998) Comorbidity of substance use disorders with mood and anxiety disorders: results of the International Consortium in Psychiatric Epidemiology. Addict Behav 23:893–907

Meyer PJ, Lovic V, Saunders BT, Yager LM, Flagel SB, Morrow JD et al (2012) Quantifying individual variation in the propensity to attribute incentive salience to reward cues. PLoS One 7: e38987

Miller MM, Morrison JH, McEwen BS (2012) Basal anxiety-like behavior predicts differences in dendritic morphology in the medial prefrontal cortex in two strains of rats. Behav Brain Res 229:280–288

Miller ML, Ren Y, Szutorisz H, Warren NA, Tessereau C, Egervari G et al (2018) Ventral striatal regulation of CREM mediates impulsive action and drug addiction vulnerability. Mol Psychiatry 23:1328–1335

Moeller FG, Dougherty DM, Barratt ES, Schmitz JM, Swann AC, Grabowski J (2001) The impact of impulsivity on cocaine use and retention in treatment. J Subst Abuse Treat 21:193–198

Molander AC, Mar A, Norbury A, Steventon S, Moreno M, Caprioli D et al (2011) High impulsivity predicting vulnerability to cocaine addiction in rats: some relationship with novelty preference but not novelty reactivity, anxiety or stress. Psychopharmacology (Berl) 215:721–731

Moreno M, Cardona D, Gomez MJ, Sanchez-Santed F, Tobena A, Fernandez-Teruel A et al (2010) Impulsivity characterization in the Roman high- and low-avoidance rat strains: behavioral and neurochemical differences. Neuropsychopharmacology 35:1198–1208

Moreno M, Gutierrez-Ferre VE, Ruedas L, Campa L, Sunol C, Flores P (2012) Poor inhibitory control and neurochemical differences in high compulsive drinker rats selected by schedule-induced polydipsia. Psychopharmacology (Berl) 219:661–672

Morgan D, Grant KA, Gage HD, Mach RH, Kaplan JR, Prioleau O et al (2002) Social dominance in monkeys: dopamine D2 receptors and cocaine self-administration. Nat Neurosci 5:169–174

Moschak TM, Carelli RM (2017) Impulsive rats exhibit blunted dopamine release dynamics during a delay discounting task independent of cocaine history. eNeuro 4

Mu P, Moyer JT, Ishikawa M, Zhang Y, Panksepp J, Sorg BA et al (2010) Exposure to cocaine dynamically regulates the intrinsic membrane excitability of nucleus accumbens neurons. J Neurosci 30:3689–3699

Muller SE, Weijers HG, Boning J, Wiesbeck GA (2008) Personality traits predict treatment outcome in alcohol-dependent patients. Neuropsychobiology 57:159–164

Murray JE, Dilleen R, Pelloux Y, Economidou D, Dalley JW, Belin D et al (2014) Increased impulsivity retards the transition to dorsolateral striatal dopamine control of cocaine seeking. Biol Psychiatry 76:15–22

Nadal R, Armario A, Janak PH (2002) Positive relationship between activity in a novel environment and operant ethanol self-administration in rats. Psychopharmacology (Berl) 162:333–338

Nader MA, Morgan D, Gage HD, Nader SH, Calhoun TL, Buchheimer N et al (2006) PET imaging of dopamine D2 receptors during chronic cocaine self-administration in monkeys. Nat Neurosci 9:1050–1056

Nader MA, Czoty PW, Gould RW, Riddick NV (2008) Review. Positron emission tomography imaging studies of dopamine receptors in primate models of addiction. Philos Trans R Soc Lond B Biol Sci 363:3223–3232

Nees F, Tzschoppe J, Patrick CJ, Vollstadt-Klein S, Steiner S, Poustka L et al (2012) Determinants of early alcohol use in healthy adolescents: the differential contribution of neuroimaging and psychological factors. Neuropsychopharmacology 37:986–995

Nestler EJ (2001) Molecular basis of long-term plasticity underlying addiction. Nat Rev Neurosci 2:119–128

Noel X, Brevers D, Bechara A, Hanak C, Kornreich C, Verbanck P et al (2011) Neurocognitive determinants of novelty and sensation-seeking in individuals with alcoholism. Alcohol Alcohol 46:407–415

Oberlin BG, Grahame NJ (2009) High-alcohol preferring mice are more impulsive than low-alcohol preferring mice as measured in the delay discounting task. Alcohol Clin Exp Res 33:1294–1303

Okita K, Mandelkern MA, London ED (2016) Cigarette use and striatal dopamine D2/3 receptors: possible role in the link between smoking and nicotine dependence. Int J Neuropsychopharmacol 19:pyw074

Paolone G, Mallory CS, Cherian AK, Miller TR, Blakely RD, Sarter M (2013) Monitoring cholinergic activity during attentional performance in mice heterozygous for the choline transporter: a model of cholinergic capacity limits. Neuropharmacology 75:274–285

Patkar AA, Murray HW, Mannelli P, Gottheil E, Weinstein SP, Vergare MJ (2004) Pre-treatment measures of impulsivity, aggression and sensation seeking are associated with treatment outcome for African-American cocaine-dependent patients. J Addict Dis 23:109–122

Pelloux Y, Dilleen R, Economidou D, Theobald D, Everitt BJ (2012) Reduced forebrain serotonin transmission is causally involved in the development of compulsive cocaine seeking in rats. Neuropsychopharmacology 37:2505–2514

Pelloux Y, Costentin J, Duterte-Boucher D (2015a) Differential involvement of anxiety and novelty preference levels on oral ethanol consumption in rats. Psychopharmacology (Berl) 232:2711–2721

Pelloux Y, Murray JE, Everitt BJ (2015b) Differential vulnerability to the punishment of cocaine related behaviours: effects of locus of punishment, cocaine taking history and alternative reinforcer availability. Psychopharmacology (Berl) 232:125–134

Pellow S, Chopin P, File SE, Briley M (1985) Validation of open:closed arm entries in an elevated plus-maze as a measure of anxiety in the rat. J Neurosci Methods 14:149–167

Pentkowski NS, Duke FD, Weber SM, Pockros LA, Teer AP, Hamilton EC et al (2010) Stimulation of medial prefrontal cortex serotonin 2C (5-HT(2C)) receptors attenuates cocaine-seeking behavior. Neuropsychopharmacology 35:2037–2048

Perry JL, Larson EB, German JP, Madden GJ, Carroll ME (2005) Impulsivity (delay discounting) as a predictor of acquisition of IV cocaine self-administration in female rats. Psychopharmacology (Berl) 178:193–201

Perusini JN, Fanselow MS (2015) Neurobehavioral perspectives on the distinction between fear and anxiety. Learn Mem 22:417–425

Piazza PV, Deminiere JM, Le Moal M, Simon H (1989) Factors that predict individual vulnerability to amphetamine self-administration. Science 245:1511–1513

Piazza PV, Deminiere JM, Maccari S, Mormede P, Le Moal M, Simon H (1990) Individual reactivity to novelty predicts probability of amphetamine self-administration. Behav Pharmacol 1:339–345

Piazza PV, Rouge-Pont F, Deminiere JM, Kharoubi M, Le Moal M, Simon H (1991) Dopaminergic activity is reduced in the prefrontal cortex and increased in the nucleus accumbens of rats predisposed to develop amphetamine self-administration. Brain Res 567:169–174
Pitchers KK, Kane LF, Kim Y, Robinson TE, Sarter M (2017) 'Hot' vs. 'cold' behavioural-cognitive styles: motivational-dopaminergic vs. cognitive-cholinergic processing of a Pavlovian cocaine cue in sign- and goal-tracking rats. Eur J Neurosci 46:2768–2781
Poulos CX, Le AD, Parker JL (1995) Impulsivity predicts individual susceptibility to high levels of alcohol self-administration. Behav Pharmacol 6:810–814
Prinssen EP, Nicolas LB, Klein S, Grundschober C, Lopez-Lopez C, Kessler MS et al (2012) Imaging trait anxiety in high anxiety F344 rats: focus on the dorsomedial prefrontal cortex. Eur Neuropsychopharmacol 22:441–451
Radwanska K, Kaczmarek L (2012) Characterization of an alcohol addiction-prone phenotype in mice. Addict Biol 17:601–612
Richards JB, Zhang L, Mitchell SH, de Wit H (1999) Delay or probability discounting in a model of impulsive behavior: effect of alcohol. J Exp Anal Behav 71:121–143
Robbins TW (2002) The 5-choice serial reaction time task: behavioural pharmacology and functional neurochemistry. Psychopharmacology (Berl) 163:362–380
Robinson TE, Berridge KC (2001) Incentive-sensitization and addiction. Addiction 96:103–114
Robinson TE, Flagel SB (2009) Dissociating the predictive and incentive motivational properties of reward-related cues through the study of individual differences. Biol Psychiatry 65:869–873
Robinson ES, Eagle DM, Economidou D, Theobald DE, Mar AC, Murphy ER et al (2009) Behavioural characterisation of high impulsivity on the 5-choice serial reaction time task: specific deficits in 'waiting' versus 'stopping'. Behav Brain Res 196:310–316
Sargent JD, Tanski S, Stoolmiller M, Hanewinkel R (2010) Using sensation seeking to target adolescents for substance use interventions. Addiction 105:506–514
Saunders BT, Robinson TE (2012) The role of dopamine in the accumbens core in the expression of Pavlovian-conditioned responses. Eur J Neurosci 36:2521–2532
Saunders BT, Yager LM, Robinson TE (2013) Cue-evoked cocaine "craving": role of dopamine in the accumbens core. J Neurosci 33:13989–14000
Sawiak SJ, Jupp B, Taylor T, Caprioli D, Carpenter TA, Dalley JW (2016) In vivo gamma-aminobutyric acid measurement in rats with spectral editing at 4.7T. J Magn Reson Imaging 43:1308–1312
Schellekens AF, de Jong CA, Buitelaar JK, Verkes RJ (2015) Co-morbid anxiety disorders predict early relapse after inpatient alcohol treatment. Eur Psychiatry 30:128–136
Schippers MC, Binnekade R, Schoffelmeer AN, Pattij T, de Vries TJ (2012) Unidirectional relationship between heroin self-administration and impulsive decision-making in rats. Psychopharmacology (Berl) 219:443–452
Schneider T, Bizarro L, Asherson PJ, Stolerman IP (2012) Hyperactivity, increased nicotine consumption and impaired performance in the five-choice serial reaction time task in adolescent rats prenatally exposed to nicotine. Psychopharmacology (Berl) 223:401–415
Seif T, Chang SJ, Simms JA, Gibb SL, Dadgar J, Chen BT et al (2013) Cortical activation of accumbens hyperpolarization-active NMDARs mediates aversion-resistant alcohol intake. Nat Neurosci 16:1094–1100
Sevy S, Smith GS, Ma Y, Dhawan V, Chaly T, Kingsley PB et al (2008) Cerebral glucose metabolism and D2/D3 receptor availability in young adults with cannabis dependence measured with positron emission tomography. Psychopharmacology (Berl) 197:549–556
Sherman JE, Zinser MC, Sideroff SI, Baker TB (1989) Subjective dimensions of heroin urges: influence of heroin-related and affectively negative stimuli. Addict Behav 14:611–623
Singer BF, Guptaroy B, Austin CJ, Wohl I, Lovic V, Seiler JL et al (2016) Individual variation in incentive salience attribution and accumbens dopamine transporter expression and function. Eur J Neurosci 43:662–670

Spanagel R, Montkowski A, Allingham K, Stohr T, Shoaib M, Holsboer F et al (1995) Anxiety: a potential predictor of vulnerability to the initiation of ethanol self-administration in rats. Psychopharmacology (Berl) 122:369–373

Spear LP (2000) The adolescent brain and age-related behavioral manifestations. Neurosci Biobehav Rev 24:417–463

Spillane NS, Muller CJ, Noonan C, Goins RT, Mitchell CM, Manson S (2012) Sensation-seeking predicts initiation of daily smoking behavior among American Indian high school students. Addict Behav 37:1303–1306

Stead JD, Clinton S, Neal C, Schneider J, Jama A, Miller S et al (2006) Selective breeding for divergence in novelty-seeking traits: heritability and enrichment in spontaneous anxiety-related behaviors. Behav Genet 36:697–712

Steimer T (2011) Animal models of anxiety disorders in rats and mice: some conceptual issues. Dialogues Clin Neurosci 13:495–506

Stein JS, Renda CR, Barker SM, Liston KJ, Shahan TA, Madden GJ (2015) Impulsive choice predicts anxiety-like behavior, but not alcohol or sucrose consumption, in male Long-Evans rats. Alcohol Clin Exp Res 39:932–940

Stephenson MT, Helme DW (2006) Authoritative parenting and sensation seeking as predictors of adolescent cigarette and marijuana use. J Drug Educ 36:247–270

Styn MA, Bovbjerg DH, Lipsky S, Erblich J (2013) Cue-induced cigarette and food craving: a common effect? Addict Behav 38:1840–1843

Suto N, Austin JD, Vezina P (2001) Locomotor response to novelty predicts a rat's propensity to self-administer nicotine. Psychopharmacology (Berl) 158:175–180

Swain Y, Muelken P, LeSage MG, Gewirtz JC, Harris AC (2018) Locomotor activity does not predict individual differences in morphine self-administration in rats. Pharmacol Biochem Behav 166:48–56

Swinford-Jackson SE, Anastasio NC, Fox RG, Stutz SJ, Cunningham KA (2016) Incubation of cocaine cue reactivity associates with neuroadaptations in the cortical serotonin (5-HT) 5-HT2C receptor (5-HT2CR) system. Neuroscience 324:50–61

Tang W, Wesley M, Freeman WM, Liang B, Hemby SE (2004) Alterations in ionotropic glutamate receptor subunits during binge cocaine self-administration and withdrawal in rats. J Neurochem 89:1021–1033

Tomie A, Aguado AS, Pohorecky LA, Benjamin D (1998) Ethanol induces impulsive-like responding in a delay-of-reward operant choice procedure: impulsivity predicts autoshaping. Psychopharmacology (Berl) 139:376–382

Tournier BB, Steimer T, Millet P, Moulin-Sallanon M, Vallet P, Ibanez V et al (2013) Innately low D2 receptor availability is associated with high novelty-seeking and enhanced behavioural sensitization to amphetamine. Int J Neuropsychopharmacol 16:1819–1834

Tunstall BJ, Kearns DN (2015) Sign-tracking predicts increased choice of cocaine over food in rats. Behav Brain Res 281:222–228

Tuominen K, Hilakivi LA, Paivarinta P, Korpi ER (1990) Behavior of alcohol-preferring AA and alcohol-avoiding ANA rat lines in tests of anxiety and aggression. Alcohol 7:349–353

Uhl GR (2006) Molecular genetics of addiction vulnerability. NeuroRx 3:295–301

van den Oever MC, Goriounova NA, Li KW, van der Schors RC, Binnekade R, Schoffelmeer AN et al (2008) Prefrontal cortex AMPA receptor plasticity is crucial for cue-induced relapse to heroin-seeking. Nat Neurosci 11:1053–1058

van den Oever MC, Spijker S, Smit AB, de Vries TJ (2010) Prefrontal cortex plasticity mechanisms in drug seeking and relapse. Neurosci Biobehav Rev 35:276–284

Verdejo-Garcia A, Lawrence AJ, Clark L (2008) Impulsivity as a vulnerability marker for substance-use disorders: review of findings from high-risk research, problem gamblers and genetic association studies. Neurosci Biobehav Rev 32:777–810

Versaggi CL, King CP, Meyer PJ (2016) The tendency to sign-track predicts cue-induced reinstatement during nicotine self-administration, and is enhanced by nicotine but not ethanol. Psychopharmacology (Berl) 233:2985–2997

Viglinskaya IV, Overstreet DH, Kashevskaya OP, Badishtov BA, Kampov-Polevoy AB, Seredenin SB et al (1995) To drink or not to drink: tests of anxiety and immobility in alcohol-preferring and alcohol-nonpreferring rat strains. Physiol Behav 57:937–941

Vogel JR, Beer B, Clody DE (1971) A simple and reliable conflict procedure for testing anti-anxiety agents. Psychopharmacologia 21:1–7

Volkow ND, Fowler JS, Wang GJ, Hitzemann R, Logan J, Schlyer DJ et al (1993) Decreased dopamine D2 receptor availability is associated with reduced frontal metabolism in cocaine abusers. Synapse 14:169–177

Volkow ND, Wang GJ, Maynard L, Fowler JS, Jayne B, Telang F et al (2002) Effects of alcohol detoxification on dopamine D2 receptors in alcoholics: a preliminary study. Psychiatry Res 116:163–172

Wang GJ, Volkow ND, Fowler JS, Logan J, Abumrad NN, Hitzemann RJ et al (1997) Dopamine D2 receptor availability in opiate-dependent subjects before and after naloxone-precipitated withdrawal. Neuropsychopharmacology 16:174–182

Wang T, Han W, Chitre AS, Polesskaya O, Solberg Woods LC, Palmer AA et al (2018) Social and anxiety-like behaviors contribute to nicotine self-administration in adolescent outbred rats. Sci Rep 8:18069

Watson P, de Wit S, Hommel B, Wiers RW (2012) Motivational mechanisms and outcome expectancies underlying the approach bias toward addictive substances. Front Psych 3:440

Whohlwill JF (1984) What are sensation seekers seeking? Behav Brain Sci 7:453

Winstanley CA (2011) The utility of rat models of impulsivity in developing pharmacotherapies for impulse control disorders. Br J Pharmacol 164:1301–1321

Winstanley CA, Dalley JW, Theobald DE, Robbins TW (2004) Fractionating impulsivity: contrasting effects of central 5-HT depletion on different measures of impulsive behavior. Neuropsychopharmacology 29:1331–1343

Winstanley CA, Olausson P, Taylor JR, Jentsch JD (2010) Insight into the relationship between impulsivity and substance abuse from studies using animal models. Alcohol Clin Exp Res 34:1306–1318

Wong CC, Schumann G (2008) Review. Genetics of addictions: strategies for addressing heterogeneity and polygenicity of substance use disorders. Philos Trans R Soc Lond B Biol Sci 363:3213–3222

Xue Y, Steketee JD, Rebec GV, Sun W (2011) Activation of D(2)-like receptors in rat ventral tegmental area inhibits cocaine-reinstated drug-seeking behavior. Eur J Neurosci 33:1291–1298

Yager LM, Robinson TE (2010) Cue-induced reinstatement of food seeking in rats that differ in their propensity to attribute incentive salience to food cues. Behav Brain Res 214:30–34

Yager LM, Pitchers KK, Flagel SB, Robinson TE (2015) Individual variation in the motivational and neurobiological effects of an opioid cue. Neuropsychopharmacology 40:1269–1277

Yamamoto DJ, Nelson AM, Mandt BH, Larson GA, Rorabaugh JM, Ng CM et al (2013) Rats classified as low or high cocaine locomotor responders: a unique model involving striatal dopamine transporters that predicts cocaine addiction-like behaviors. Neurosci Biobehav Rev 37:1738–1753

Zapata A, Minney VL, Shippenberg TS (2010) Shift from goal-directed to habitual cocaine seeking after prolonged experience in rats. J Neurosci 30:15457–15463

Zukerman M (1979) Sensation seeking: beyond the optimal level of arousal. Lawrence Erlbaum Associates, Hillsdale

Activity-Dependent Epigenetic Remodeling in Cocaine Use Disorder

Alberto J. López, Cody A. Siciliano, and Erin S. Calipari

Contents

1 Introduction 232
2 Synaptic Mechanisms of Substance Use Disorder 234
3 The Interface Between Neural Activity and Epigenetic Modifications in Substance Use Disorder 237
4 Epigenetic Regulation of Neural Plasticity 242
4.1 Histone Posttranslational Modifications, DNA Methylation, and Nucleosome Remodeling 242
4.2 Histone Acetylation 243
4.3 Histone Methylation 244
4.4 Nucleosome Remodeling 244
4.5 DNA Methylation [For More Detailed Review on DNA Methylation in Cocaine Use Disorders, See Vaillancourt et al. (2017)] 245
4.6 Histone Marks Do Not Occur in Isolation 245

A. J. López · C. A. Siciliano
Department of Pharmacology, Vanderbilt University School of Medicine, Nashville, TN, USA

Vanderbilt Center for Addiction Research, Vanderbilt University School of Medicine, Nashville, TN, USA

Vanderbilt Brain Institute, Vanderbilt University School of Medicine, Nashville, TN, USA

E. S. Calipari (✉)
Department of Pharmacology, Vanderbilt University School of Medicine, Nashville, TN, USA

Vanderbilt Center for Addiction Research, Vanderbilt University School of Medicine, Nashville, TN, USA

Vanderbilt Brain Institute, Vanderbilt University School of Medicine, Nashville, TN, USA

Department of Molecular Physiology and Biophysics, Vanderbilt Institute for Infection, Immunology, and Infection, Vanderbilt University School of Medicine, Nashville, TN, USA

Department of Psychiatry and Behavioral Sciences, Vanderbilt Institute for Infection, Immunology, and Infection, Vanderbilt University School of Medicine, Nashville, TN, USA
e-mail: erin.calipari@vanderbilt.edu

M. A. Nader, Y. L. Hurd (eds.), *Substance Use Disorders*,
Handbook of Experimental Pharmacology 258, https://doi.org/10.1007/164_2019_257

5 The Interplay Between Acute Drug Effects and Activity-Dependent Epigenetic Dysregulation in the Transition to Substance Use Disorder 246
6 Transient Changes as a Scaffold for Long-Term Epigenetic Changes 249
7 Causally Linking Epigenetic Modification to Substance Use Disorder 250
8 Linking Changes in Epigenome to Changes in Synaptic Function 252
9 Defining Causal Links Between Epigenetic Factors and Neural Activity in Substance Use Disorder 253
References 254

Abstract

Substance use disorder (SUD) is a behavioral disorder characterized by cycles of abstinence, drug seeking, and relapse. SUD is characterized by aberrant learning processes which develop after repeated exposure to drugs of abuse. At the core of this phenotype is the persistence of symptoms, such as craving and relapse to drug seeking, long after the cessation of drug use. The neural basis of these behavioral changes has been linked to dysfunction in neural circuits across the brain; however, the molecular drivers that allow for these changes to persist beyond the lifespan of any individual protein remain opaque. Epigenetic adaptations – where DNA is modified to increase or decrease the probability of gene expression at key genes – have been identified as a mechanism underlying the long-lasting nature of drug-seeking behavior. Thus, to understand SUD, it is critical to define the interplay between neuronal activation and longer-term changes in transcription and epigenetic remodeling and define their role in addictive behaviors. In this review, we discuss the current understanding of drug-induced changes to circuit function, recent discoveries in epigenetic mechanisms that mediate these changes, and, ultimately, how these adaptations drive the persistent nature of relapse, with emphasis on adaptations in models of cocaine use disorder. Understanding the complex interplay between epigenetic gene regulation and circuit activity will be critical in elucidating the neural mechanisms underlying SUD. This, with the advent of novel genetic-based techniques, will allow for the generation of novel therapeutic avenues to improve treatment outcomes in SUD.

Keywords

Circuitry · Dopamine · Epigenome · Genomics · Motivation · Plasticity

1 Introduction

Substance use disorder (SUD) is a chronic relapsing neuropsychiatric disease, characterized by high levels of drug consumption, inability to terminate drug consumption once started, heightened responsivity to drug-associated cues, drug seeking, craving, and relapse even after long periods of abstinence (Aguilar et al. 2009; Le Moal and Koob 2007). This wide range of symptoms, many of which are driven by deficits in learning and memory processes, are difficult to treat, and patients typically experience remittent symptoms for their entire lifetime. Indeed, one critical characteristic of this disorder is the persistence of symptoms long after the cessation of drug use. For example, there are high rates of relapse in individuals with SUD, even after years of successful abstinence (de Wit 1996; Jaffe et al. 1989). Yet, the long-lasting mechanisms that confer resilience or susceptibility to drug seeking and craving remain only partially identified. Thus, understanding the factors that confer these long-lasting behavioral deficits is critical to understand both the pathology of the disorder and to developing efficacious evidence-based therapies.

To this end, it is paramount to understand the molecular dysfunction that underlies the behavioral dysregulation in SUD. Preclinical models utilizing drug self-administration in animals have recapitulated many of the behavioral phenotypes associated with SUD, and a large body of work has focused on the molecular dysregulation that underlies these behaviors (White et al. 2016; Maze et al. 2010; Stipanovich et al. 2008; Malvaez et al. 2011; Smith et al. 2013). Cocaine-induced changes in neuronal gene expression, molecular and cell signaling, and plasticity have been implicated in driving the behavioral symptomatology of SUD (Beitner-Johnson and Nestler 1991; Kuhar et al. 1991; Anderson and Pierce 2005). However, while each of these factors has been causally linked to particular behavioral phenotypes, compiling these discoveries into a comprehensive framework has been lacking. The development of SUD is controlled by drug-induced alterations in neural circuit activity, which lead to complex changes in transcriptional and receptor-based signaling, which then drive persistent neural plasticity changes that change the brain's subsequent response to drugs and other environmental stimuli (Le Moal and Koob 2007; Hyman et al. 2006; Volkow et al. 2003; Campbell and Wood 2019; Calipari et al. 2019). Here we discuss the current literature and highlight the importance of understanding the bidirectional interaction between neural circuit activity, epigenetic/transcriptional mechanisms, and behavior.

The behavioral symptomology of SUD persists long beyond a transient drug-induced change in neural activity, and even past the turnover of many of the proteins that have been implicated in this disorder; however, our understanding of long-term mechanisms that could drive these seemingly indefinite changes are lacking. Recently, epigenetics has become an avenue of interest with regard to potential mechanisms underlying the long-lasting nature of SUD (Walker et al. 2015; Robison and Nestler 2011). Although historically defined as the heritable interaction between genes and gene products that generate cell fate, as the neuroepigenetic field has developed, the term now refers to changes in gene regulation independent of changes in the DNA sequence itself (Barrett and Wood 2008; Rudenko and Tsai 2014). Epigenetic factors allow for dynamic and stable regulation of gene expression and are emerging as key mechanisms underlying long-lasting changes in neural morphology and function in postmitotic neurons. Several drug-induced changes to neuronal function have been linked to recruitment of various epigenetic mechanisms, including changes in histone posttranslational modifications, nucleosome remodeling, and DNA methylation (White et al. 2016; López et al. 2018; Malvaez et al. 2018; Levine et al. 2011; Vaillancourt et al. 2017).

In this review, we will further assess the epigenetic and circuit-based changes that underlie the alterations in learning and motivation that characterize SUD. We further review the known adaptations that occur at the neural circuit, synaptic, cellular, and epigenetic levels and how these adaptations interface to drive relapse of cocaine-seeking behavior. The aforementioned avenues of research are often studied independently and in parallel of each other. While this strategy is effective in identifying mechanistic contributors, it fails to encapsulate the long-lasting nature of SUD. As such, SUD is unlikely caused by a single kinase, synapse, receptor, histone mark, or transcription factor. Likely, the resilience and long-lasting nature of drug-seeking behavior is a culmination of changes in synaptic function leading to changes in nuclear processes that ultimately provide a feedback loop to future changes in circuit activity and behavior. Interdisciplinary approaches to understanding the neural control of behavior – where molecular, circuit, and behavioral avenues intersect – will generate a more complete understanding of SUD. Lastly, we evaluate emerging molecular- and circuit-level technologies and their potential to re-commandeer endogenous mechanisms to reverse the drug-induced adaptations which leave individuals susceptible to relapse.

2 Synaptic Mechanisms of Substance Use Disorder

Drug-induced alterations in synaptic function have been the primary focus of neuroscience research into SUDs, and we now have an in-depth understanding of the synaptic changes that occur and how these changes relate to addictive behaviors (Ungless et al. 2001; Jones and Bonci 2005; Thomas et al. 2001; Wolf 2016) (Fig. 1). Perhaps the most studied circuit in this body of literature is the mesolimbic dopamine (DA) pathway, comprising of dopaminergic projections from the ventral midbrain to the ventral striatum [also known as the nucleus accumbens (NAc) (Siciliano et al. 2015; Ferris et al. 2013)]. After cocaine exposure, several groups have reported increased AMPA/NMDA ratios in dopaminergic neurons in the ventral tegmental area (VTA), as well as increased expression of high-conductance GluA2-lacking AMPA receptors in D1-expressing medium spiny neurons (MSNs) in the NAc (Ungless et al. 2001; Thomas et al. 2001; Conrad et al. 2008; Loweth et al. 2014). Paradoxically, while there is increased excitability of DA neurons, DA release probability measured at presynaptic terminals in the NAc is markedly decreased (Siciliano et al. 2015). Together, impaired dopaminergic modulation of postsynaptic activity combined with hyperexcitability of D1-expressing MSNs drives several aspects of addictive behaviors, most notably time-dependent increases in cocaine-conditioned reinforcement, whereby cocaine-associated cues trigger seeking behaviors which become more robust farther into abstinence from cocaine (Calipari et al. 2019; Wolf 2016; Childress et al. 1999).

This effect, termed "incubation of cocaine craving," becomes stronger through 30 days into withdrawal from cocaine and persists for a seemingly indefinite period of time (Grimm et al. 2001). Interesting, the synaptic alterations that underlie these effects persist far past the turnover half-life of any of the specific proteins involved (Calipari et al. 2019; Horikawa and Nawa 1998). These synaptic changes are cell-type specific, suggesting that the epigenetic factors driving these changes do not happen on a global scale (Pascoli et al. 2014; MacAskill et al. 2014), but can be different – even opposite – depending on the neural circuits being altered in these

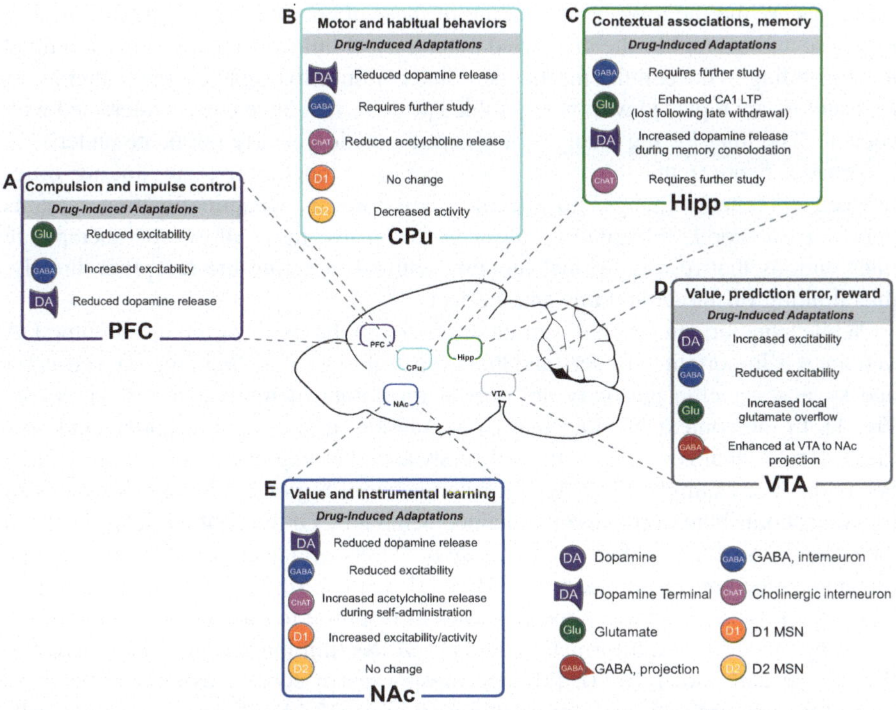

Fig. 1 Drug exposure drives long-lasting alterations in neural circuits in a cell-type-specific fashion. Drug-induced adaptations within defined brain regions are involved in a wide range of behavioral processes including executive control (PFC, **a**) (Sorg et al. 1997; Campanac and Hoffman 2013; Williams and Steketee 2005; Trantham et al. 2002; Cameron et al. 2019); habit formation (CPu, **b**) (Hurd et al. 1990; Park et al. 2013; Yager et al. 2015); drug-associated context and memory (Hipp, **c**) (Kutlu and Gould 2016; Kramar et al. 2014); reward prediction and value (VTA, **d**) (Bocklisch et al. 2013; Kalivas and Duffy 2002; Liu et al. 2005); and reward and contextual integration (NAc, **e**) (Smith et al. 2013; Siciliano et al. 2015; Mark et al. 1999, 2011). The cell-type-specific changes in activity that have been reported across the brain and are outlined in a region-specific fashion. Within each region, there is heterogeneity of cell types, each contributing differentially to behavioral outputs, making understanding the cell-type-specific epigenetic adaptations underlying these alterations critical. A single molecular change within a defined brain region may have opposite effects on behavior. For example, in the NAc, changes that increase the activity of D1 or D2 MSNs (*orange* and *yellow*, respectively), have opposite effects on reward-associated behaviors. Further, within this region, different molecular adaptations have been observed in cholinergic interneurons (*magenta*), D1 MSNs, D2 MSNs, and at dopamine terminals from the VTA – all of which have been implicated in cocaine-seeking behavior. The above circuitry only serves as an overview of the major circuitry linked to cocaine seeking. However, various other brain regions have been linked to the chronic nature of cocaine-associated behaviors, including the medial habenula (López et al. 2018, 2019; McCallum and Glick 2009), the ventral pallidum (Farrell et al. 2019; Mahler et al. 2014; Pardo-Garcia et al. 2019), and lateral hypothalamus (Ahmed et al. 2005; Zhou et al. 2008; Boutrel et al. 2005). Together, while the field has identified epigenetic and transcriptomic changes in these brain regions, it will be critical to characterize the epigenetic adaptations within specific cell types to understand how these changes are linked to the specific molecular changes that underlie the neural control of discrete aspects of motivated behaviors. *CPu*, caudate-putamen; *Hipp*, hippocampus; *MSN*, medium spiny neuron; *NAc*, nucleus accumbens; *PFC*, prefrontal cortex; *VTA*, ventral tegmental area

processes. While the long-lasting nature of these alterations are a hallmark of drug exposure and exemplify the protracted pathology of human SUD, we have a limited understanding of the cellular mechanisms that continue to propagate these alterations as receptors are replaced with newly folded proteins that have not yet interacted with cocaine. The long-lasting changes in synaptic function clearly implicate underlying epigenetic changes that alter receptor expression indefinitely, but linking drug-induced epigenetic changes to specific alterations in synaptic function remains poorly understood. Elucidating these mechanisms may allow for therapeutic interventions that restore normal function without targeting the receptors directly, thus limiting off-target and unwanted effects.

While synaptic remodeling is often discussed in the terms of the mesolimbic DA system, it is important to understand that even within a single brain region, cell-type- and synapse-specific plasticity are critical mediators of motivated behaviors (see Fig. 1). In the context of molecular dysregulation, it is critical to understand how these genetic changes in specific cell types alter the expression of reward-related behaviors. For example, the NAc is a heterogeneous region made up of various cell types that contribute to cocaine-maintained behaviors. Of the total number of cells in the rodent NAc, 95% of them are made up of MSNs, which contain D1 and D2 type dopamine receptors (Kupchik et al. 2015). D1 and D2 MSNs are virtually nonoverlapping cell types that have opposing roles in response to cocaine reward, with D1 encoding reward-based information, and D2 MSNs limiting reward-driven behavior (Le Moine and Bloch 1995). D1 MSN responses to cocaine-associated cues are critical to drug seeking, and optical stimulation of D2 MSNs reduces cocaine self-administration (Bachtell and Self 2008; Kravitz et al. 2012). Moreover, the molecular mechanisms and cocaine response within these two cell populations are often divergent, due to the contrasting effects of D1 vs D2 receptor activation. Specifically, D1- and D2-expressing MSNs have unique basal gene expression patterns that contribute to their respective genetic identity (Chandra et al. 2015). Moreover, acute cocaine and cocaine-associated cues increase activity in D1-expressing MSNs, while leading to hyperpolarization of D2-expressing MSNs (Calipari et al. 2016; Bertran-Gonzalez et al. 2008; Jordi et al. 2013). The downstream molecular adaptations to cocaine within these cell populations also diverge, including DARPP-32 phosphorylation and various CREB-dependent gene expression patterns (Chandra et al. 2015; Bateup et al. 2008).

In addition to these output neurons, there are also GABAergic and cholinergic interneurons that regulate both DA release from presynaptic DA terminals originating in the VTA and modulate the activity of MSNs (Fig. 1) (Collins et al. 2016). Until recently, technical limitations have prevented the identification and characterization of cocaine response in each of these cell types. However, the advent of cell-type-specific assays, such as fluorescence-activated cell sorting (FACS), translating ribosomal affinity purification (TRAP), single-cell RNA sequencing, and Cre-expressing mouse lines (Chandra et al. 2015; Finegersh and Homanics 2016), makes a more thorough assessment of each cell type's contribution to cocaine-seeking behavior possible. Because of the different, often opposing, roles of each of these cell types in drug-associated behavior, it is important to understand how epigenetic regulation of activity within each population can alter behavioral outputs.

3 The Interface Between Neural Activity and Epigenetic Modifications in Substance Use Disorder

As mentioned above, SUD research has focused on the neural circuit dysfunction induced by drugs of abuse. Pinpointing the interface between neural activity, transcription, and epigenetic processes has been difficult due to the complex technical nature of these studies. SUD is a learning disorder where particular actions and outcomes [i.e., taking drug and the associated high (Hyman et al. 2006; Itzhak and Martin 2002; Mews and Calipari 2017)] are associated with cues or contexts. Enhanced activation of brain reward systems by these cues is a key feature that drives relapse to drug use (MacNiven et al. 2018). Underlying this phenomenon is the ability to learn information about environmental stimuli which relies on experience-dependent plasticity, where experience with a stimulus changes subsequent neural responses to that stimulus. These neural changes need to be plastic, respond quickly to new information in the environment, and be long-lasting to maintain these memories over time (Mews and Calipari 2017). While learning induced by natural reinforcers is critical to survival in mammalian species, dysregulation of these processes by drugs of abuse drives addictive behaviors. Further, while not an emphasis of this review, it is important to consider that when evaluating the molecular and synaptic responses in cocaine-induced behaviors, the route, dose, and schedule of cocaine exposure are critical factors in the subsequent neural response and drug-induced maladaptation, thus adding a layer of complexity into defining the mechanisms driving drug-induced plasticity (Calipari et al. 2013, 2014, 2015; Calipari and Jones 2014; Kawa et al. 2019).

At the heart of experience-dependent plasticity lies the capacity of neural circuits to undergo activity-induced structural and functional changes. In SUD, this process happens in two phases: first, drugs activate or inhibit certain neural circuits which leads to the induction of epigenetic and transcriptional changes within defined neural populations. Second, these epigenetic modifications either serve as a scaffold for more long-lasting changes or act themselves to change the way that these cells respond to subsequent drug-associated stimuli (see Fig. 2). Here, we will primarily focus on the role of the second phase of this process in addictive behaviors. The maintenance of such permanent changes requires efficient posttranslational and transcriptional regulation. A large body of work has defined the importance of both changes in neural circuit dynamics and epigenetic regulation in the expression of reward-related behaviors (Russo et al. 2010; Russo and Nestler 2013; Dudai and Morris 2013). The ability of a cell to efficiently activate transcriptional processes in response to an incoming stimulus is controlled by epigenetic regulation, where the structure of and accessibility to DNA is modified to increase or decrease the probability of gene expression at key genes. This is executed by altering the interactions between the genome and regulatory mechanisms at the level of chromatin. Chromatin is the focal point of transcriptional gene regulation and is comprised

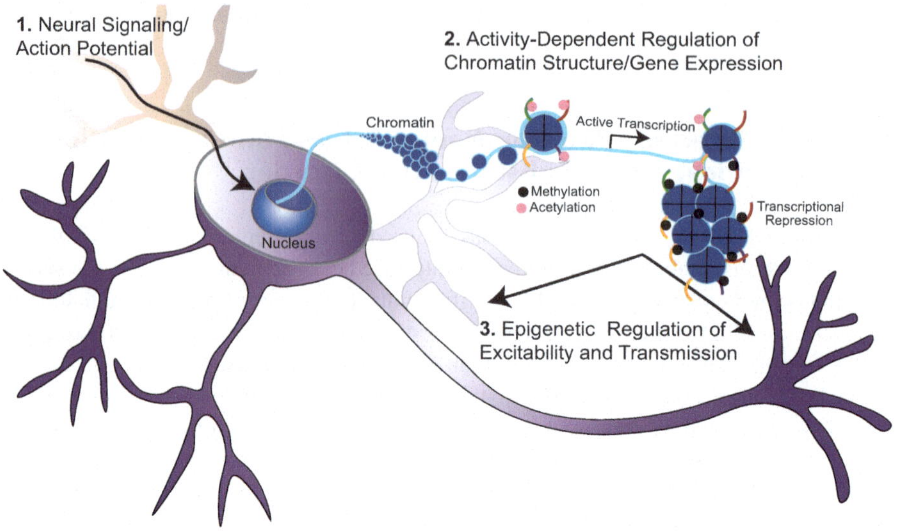

Fig. 2 The bidirectional interaction between epigenetic changes and synaptic function. Neurons are complex information processors that are capable of integrating various inputs to ultimately generate downstream signals. (1) Incoming signals are transmitted from and extracellular signal through receptors and channels and their associated intracellular effectors that converge at the nucleus. (2) These internal molecular cascades trigger activity-dependent changes in transcription within the nucleus. (3) In addition to the acute induction of immediate early genes that leads to stabilized signal processing (e.g., plasticity, LTP), DNA (*teal*) and histone proteins (*blue*) can be modified (*pink* and *black*) to alter future response to activity and drive long-lasting changes in neural excitability and signaling. In the case of drugs of abuse, such as cocaine, repeated drug exposure alters basal gene expression and circuit-specific excitability via widespread epigenetic changes

of a basic repeating unit: the nucleosome. The nucleosome consists of DNA wrapped around a protein octamer, assembled from two molecules each of histone H2A, H2B, H3, and H4 (Fig. 3a). Each histone has tails of amino acids that can be modified allowing for a complex mosaic of chemical modifications – i.e., epigenetic marks – that can dynamically regulate chromatin architecture and subsequent gene transcription (Barrett and Wood 2008; Rivera and Ren 2013). Together these processes are termed the epigenome and serve as the interface between the genome, cellular activity, and the environment.

While basic epigenetic mechanisms controlling transcription have been well described in recent years (see Table 1), how activity-dependent changes within defined cell types interface with epigenetic modifications to guide behaviors remains a major outstanding question in the field. In general, information is transmitted from a synaptic signal, in the form of an action potential or receptor activation, to the nucleus to trigger molecular machinery for epigenetic remodeling on a fast timescale (outlined in Fig. 2). This signal activates a number of immediate early genes as well as other transcriptional processes that alter DNA conformation in order to change the expression levels of key genes (Brami-Cherrier 2005; Ressler et al. 2002). In this

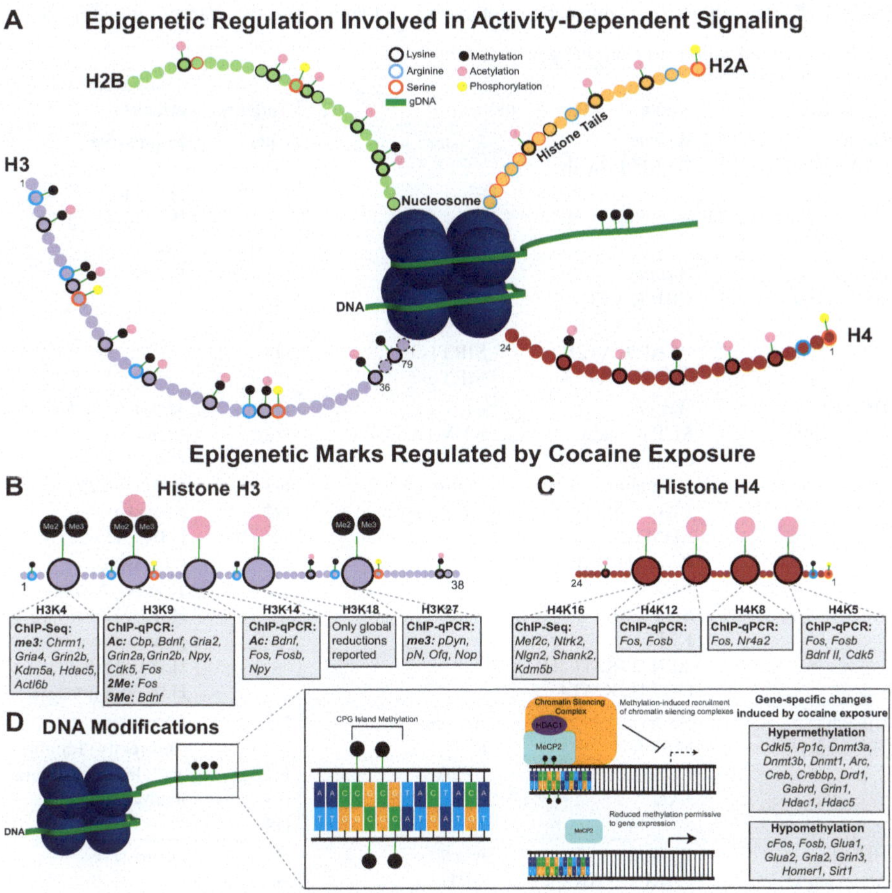

Fig. 3 Epigenetic modifications regulated by cocaine exposure. Cocaine-induced neuronal activation leads to rapid changes in chromatin structure. (**a**) The nucleosome, the functional subunit of chromatin, is composed of 147bp of DNA (*green*) spooled around a histone octamer core (*blue*). In addition to direct DNA methylation (*black*), each histone protein can be modified at stereotyped residues, such as lysine (K, *black circle*), arginine (R, *blue circle*), or serine (S, *red circle*), in an activity-dependent manner to regulate gene expression. Cocaine alters circuit function by generating a unique epigenetic environment at targeted gene loci. Recent work from the neuroepigenetic field has identified cocaine-induced modifications at histone H3 (**b**) (Jordi et al. 2013; Kumar et al. 2005; Wang et al. 2009; Renthal et al. 2009; Farris et al. 2015; Renthal and Nestler 2008; Maze et al. 2011; Feng et al. 2014; Freeman et al. 2008; Caputi et al. 2014), histone H4 (**c**) (Malvaez et al. 2011; Jordi et al. 2013; Kumar et al. 2005; Levine et al. 2005; Renthal et al. 2007, 2009; Rogge et al. 2013; Ferguson et al. 2015), the recruitment of DNA methylation machinery (**d**) (Vaillancourt et al. 2017; Wright et al. 2015; Anier et al. 2010; Massart et al. 2015; Carouge et al. 2010; Pol Bodetto et al. 2013; Baker-Andresen et al. 2013), and the synaptic and plasticity-related gene loci targets. It is critical to note that no single histone mark regulates cocaine-induced gene expression, but it is the overall epigenetic environment that can regulate the suppression or expression of a gene. Similar to neural activity, these various epigenetic modifications are integrated to generate an overall permissive or repressive gene expression environment. Understanding the combinatorial effects of these individual histone marks will be critical in studying the long-lasting nature of cocaine-induced changes to the epigenome, transcriptome, and, ultimately, circuit function. *Me2*, dimethylation; *Me3*, trimethylation

Table 1 Commonly studied epigenetic mechanisms and their respective transcriptional impact

Chromatin modifications in neuronal gene regulation				
Modification	Known regulatory enzyme(s)		Target(s)	Transcriptional effect(s)
DNA methylation	*Writers* DNMT1-3a,3b	*Erasers* TET1-3	CpG DNA	Repressive (proximal promoter) Permissive (gene body)
Histone acetylation	*Writers* CBP/KAT3A p300/KAT3B PCAF/KAT2B GCN5/KAT2A	*Erasers* HDAC1-3 HDAC8 SIRT1-3 SIRT6-7	H1 H2A H2B H3 H4	Permissive
Histone methylation	*Writers* SET-domain containing (14 members) KMT1C/G9a/EHMT2 KMT1D/GLP/EHMT1 SUV39H1/KMT1A ASH1L/KMT2H DOT1L/KMT4	*Erasers* KDM1A/LSD1 JmjC family (17 members, see Agger et al.)	H1 H2A H2B H3 H4	*Mono-methylation:* Permissive *Dimethylation:* H3K4, -K79 permissive H3K9, H3K27 repressive *Trimethylation:* H3K4, H3K79 permissive H3K9, H3K27, H3K79 repressive
Histone phosphorylation	*Writers* MSK1/2 ERK1/2 JAK2	*Erasers* PP1 PP2A	H1 H2A H2B H3 H4	Permissive (indirectly) (enables acetylation prevents methylation)
Histone ribosylation	*Writers* PARP1, PARP3/ARTD1, RTD3 SIRT2	*Erasers* ARH3 PARG	H1 H2A H2B H3 H4	Permissive
Histone serotonylation	*Writers* TGM2	*Erasers* Unknown	H3	Permissive
Histone SUMOylation	*Writers* SUMO1 SUMO2	*Erasers*[a] SENP2–3 SENP5–6	H1 H2A H2B H3 H4	Repressive
Histone ubiquitination	*Writers* RING1 UBE2D1 UBE2B RNF40 BARD1	*Erasers* USP2, USP3, USP7, USP12/46, USP16, USP21,USP22, USP36 BAP1	H1 H2A H2B H3 H4	*UBE2B, RNF40, USP family, BAP1* Permissive *RING1, BARD1* Repressive

(continued)

Table 1 (continued)

Chromatin modifications in neuronal gene regulation				
Modification	Known regulatory enzyme(s)		Target(s)	Transcriptional effect(s)
Nucleosome remodeling	*Complex*	*Relevant subunits*	H1 H2A H2B H3 H4 gDNA	Both repressive and permissive
	nBAF	*nBAF:* BAF53B/ ACTL6B CREST BAF45B/C		
	ISWI-containing complexes	*ISWI:* BAZ1A SMARCA1/ SNF2L, SMARCA2/ SNF2H		
	NuRD	*NuRD:* HDAC1/2 Mi-2a/b, MTA1/2/3 RbAp46/48		

Various epigenetic mechanisms have been identified as critical in neuronal gene expression and are highlighted above, including (1) DNA methylation (Vaillancourt et al. 2017), (2) histone acetylation (Gräff and Tsai 2013; Peixoto and Abel 2012; de Ruijter et al. 2003; Barnes et al. 2019; Fischle et al. 2002), (3) histone methylation (Agger et al. 2008; Roidl and Hacker 2014), (4) histone phosphorylation (Watson and Higgins 2016), (5) histone ribosylation (Messner and Hottiger 2011; Hassa et al. 2006), (6) histone serotonylation (Farrelly et al. 2019), (7) histone SUMOylation (Shiio and Eisenman 2003; Nathan et al. 2003), (8) histone ubiquitination (Cao and Yan 2012), and (9) nucleosome remodeling (López and Wood 2015; Sun et al. 2017; Goodwin and Picketts 2018). Each identified PTM is regulated by a unique family of enzymes, providing a unique profile of transcriptional regulation. See Zhao and Garcia (2015) for a catalog of discovered histone modifications (in neuronal and non-neuronal tissue) (Zhao and Garcia 2015)
[a]Indicates presumptive regulator

view, epigenetic regulation arbitrates acute and transient gene expression in response to upstream neural activity and changes in intrinsic cellular processes (Campbell and Wood 2019). Thus, repeated and sustained firing of cells in a circuit can trigger specific changes to denote the importance of that information. Circuit activity triggers intracellular signaling cascades such as the PKA or MAPK/ERK pathways that are activated by G protein-coupled receptors and calcium and therefore provides a means for information carried in circuit activity to be transmitted to the nucleus (Ménard et al. 2015). In the nucleus, epigenetic signatures demarcate and regulate genes associated with synaptic remodeling, associative processes, and memory formation (Dulac 2010; Sultan and Day 2011). These changes can alter the excitability of the cell and change its ability to respond to subsequent incoming signals. Remarkably, but not surprisingly, the plasticity mechanisms linked to drug addiction correspond to well-described neuronal and circuit plasticity in learning and memory (see Fig. 1). This process is the primary molecular mechanism underlying learning-related plasticity in postmitotic neurons. Thus, understanding how this process is dysregulated in SUD will shed light onto the basic process, its importance in behavioral control, and provide potential targets for treatment.

4 Epigenetic Regulation of Neural Plasticity

When studying activity-dependent transcription, the key regulators are often immediate early genes, which are activated shortly after stimulation of the cell. It is tempting to attempt to identify a single gene that controls the addictive phenotype; however, the complex nature of a disorder involving learning mechanisms makes it more likely that a complex network of interconnected genes regulates the connectivity of neurons across the brain. In fact, it is likely that many of the immediate early genes that are identified as key players in addictive behaviors are simply the first-in-line transcriptional responses that start a string of events that alters DNA accessibility and neural circuit function (Zhao et al. 2014). The behavioral, circuit, and morphology data point to one important adaptation in drug-addicted individuals. Specific synapses are strengthened, while others are weakened for long periods of time that last far beyond the lifespan of any individual protein (McPherson 2015). These long-lasting changes in synaptic strength are critical mediators of drug seeking and relapse; thus, understanding how they are maintained is of critical importance to our understanding of the brain and how it is dysregulated in SUD (Ungless et al. 2001; Thomas et al. 2001; Siciliano et al. 2015; Conrad et al. 2008; Loweth et al. 2014).

4.1 Histone Posttranslational Modifications, DNA Methylation, and Nucleosome Remodeling

Neurons continually adapt to a changing environment and thus require systems that quickly adjust chromatin structure, transcription, and subsequent cellular excitability. This is done via complex changes in receptor membrane expression, phosphorylation, and epigenetic changes that are transient, such as histone acetylation or phosphorylation, or more long-lived, such as specific histone methylation and DNA methylation, and both of these processes are dysregulated in SUD (Campbell and Wood 2019; Robison and Nestler 2011; Rudenko and Tsai 2014; Fass et al. 2013). Indeed, several types of epigenetic modifications have been associated with learning and memory, including DNA methylation, and posttranslational modification of histone proteins by acetylation, methylation, and phosphorylation (Dulac 2010; Alarcón et al. 2004; Gräff and Tsai 2013; Korzus et al. 2004; Levenson et al. 2004; Wood et al. 2006; Nelson and Monteggia 2011). Importantly, modification of the epigenetic landscape provides a mechanism by which the transcriptional response to stimuli can be permanently altered, thus providing a molecular route to lasting modifications of neuronal and circuit functions such as the expression of SUD.

As mentioned above, central to epigenetic regulation of gene expression is the nucleosome: a complex system upon which posttranslational modifications control rapid or sustained changes in DNA accessibility (Fig. 3). Each histone within the nucleosome core has tails of amino acids that can be modified (Rivera and Ren 2013) (see Fig. 3 and Table 1). The interaction between histone tails and DNA has a profound influence on gene accessibility and transcription. This interaction can be transiently modified via various posttranslational modifications (PTMs), including phosphorylation, acetylation, ubiquitination, serotonylation, methylation, or physical sliding of nucleosomes via nucleosome remodeling complexes (referred to as nucleosome remodeling) (Kouzarides 2007; Berger 2007; Farrelly et al. 2019). In addition, DNA itself can be directly modified through the addition and removal of methyl groups. Each of these modifications can provide a different regulation of gene accessibility, either restricting or enabling transcription to occur (see Table 1). Histone PTMs elicit structural and functional changes within chromatin and regulate various epigenetic processes. Acetylation, for instance, along with methylation, is the most extensively studied histone modification and has broad effects on chromatin function and nuclear signaling pathways (Roth et al. 2003; Shahbazian and Grunstein 2007; Berndsen and Denu 2008). Each of these epigenetic modifications, and their role in transcriptional regulation, is described below and in Table 1.

4.2 Histone Acetylation

Histone acetylation is one of the most extensively studied PTMs. Addition of acetyl groups to lysine residues on histone tails is generally considered to be permissive for gene expression through relaxation of the histone protein-DNA interaction. The reduced histone-DNA interaction is thought to allow access to subsequent transcriptional regulators (e.g., transcription factors, RNA polymerase II). Activity-dependent histone acetylation is known to be regulated by two competing families of epigenetic writers: histone deacetylases (HDACs) remove acetyl groups from lysine residues, while histone acetyltransferases (HATs) add acetyl groups to histone tails. Generally, HDACs are considered transcriptional repressors, functioning as molecular brake pads to gene expression, whereas HATs are viewed as transcriptional primers, priming transcriptional activity through permissive histone acetylation (Roth et al. 2003; Shahbazian and Grunstein 2007). Additionally, histone acetylation marks can be bound by small protein modules called bromodomains, often referred to as "readers." These domains are conserved within many chromatin-associated proteins – including HATs themselves – that regulate transcription-mediated biological processes (Bannister and Kouzarides 2011; Burdge and Lillycrop 2010; Filippakopoulos and Knapp 2014; De La Cruz et al. 2005). Histone acetylation in particular has spurred considerable interest and is most robustly associated with promoting associative learning and memory formation, which, as discussed previously, is one of the critical learning processes dysregulated in SUD.

4.3 Histone Methylation

Another extensively studied histone PTM critical in regulating gene accessibility is histone methylation. Histone methylation is concentrated on lysine residues of the histone tail (Zhang and Reinberg 2001), positively regulated by lysine methyltransferases (KMTs) and negatively regulated by lysine demethylases (KDMs). However, single residue methylation can occur in mono- (me), di- (me2), or tri-methylated (me3) stages (Kouzarides 2007). Moreover, these multiplexed methylation states are capable of exerting influence of gene expression and are regulated by independent enzymes. For example, G9a (renamed KMT1C) is able to lay mono- and dimethyl marks but appears unable to trimethylate histone residues. In addition, the mechanism by which histone methylation alters chromatin accessibility remains unclear, as methylation-state regulation of gene expression occurs in a residue specific manner. For example, H3K9me2/3 is generally considered to be a repressive mark, whereas H3K4me3 is often associated with gene activation (Santos-Rosa et al. 2002; Baylin and Ohm 2006).

4.4 Nucleosome Remodeling

Nucleosome remodeling is an often-overlooked posttranslational modification, in which large nucleosome remodeling complexes slide or evict nucleosomes to alter large-scale chromatin structure. As such, nucleosome remodeling can be considered both permissive and repressive epigenetic modifications, as nucleosome remodeling complexes (NRCs) can simultaneously increase accessibility of particular genes while decreasing accessibility of others. Neuronal Brg1-/hBrm-associated factor (nBAF) is the primary NRC in the brain and is composed of various proteins containing either nucleosome or DNA-dependent ATPase function (Table 1) (Staahl and Crabtree 2013; López and Wood 2015; Vogel-Ciernia and Wood 2014). While nBAF is the most extensively studied NRC, both ISWI and NuRD NRCs play key roles in neuronal gene regulation.

Critically, these epigenetic mechanisms do not occur in isolation and modify both transcriptional activity and the enzymatic function of other epigenetic modifiers. For example, the NuRD complex consists of HDAC1/HDAC2 and is capable of simultaneously deacetylating histone residues and remodeling nucleosome structure. Interestingly, subunits within nBAF have histone reading bromodomains, and subunits with ISWI complexes carry histone-interactive SANT domains, suggesting both nBAF and ISWI use histone modification states to further regulate gene accessibility. However, a complete understanding of these mechanisms in neuroscience remains lacking.

4.5 DNA Methylation [For More Detailed Review on DNA Methylation in Cocaine Use Disorders, See Vaillancourt et al. (2017)]

DNA methylation is the stable addition of a methyl group to a nucleotide, most often in the form of 5' methylated cytosine (5mC) (Bird 2002). 5mC is typically added by methyl-CpG-binding domain (MBDs) proteins, of which MECP2 has been most extensively studied, whereas demethylation is carried out via DNA methyltransferases (DNMTs). Previously believed to function purely as a gene repressor, the role of DNA methylation in transcriptional regulation has been further defined: when present in the gene promoter, DNA methylation typically represses genes through the recruitment of HDACs to deacetylate nearby histone tails while simultaneously preventing transcription factor binding; however, when present in the gene body, recent data suggests it may function as a gene activator (Jones 2012; Baubec and Schübeler 2014; Wolf et al. 2006).

4.6 Histone Marks Do Not Occur in Isolation

These various epigenetic mechanisms form a powerful system of regulating gene expression. While each modification is often studied in isolation and has been individually linked to changes in transcription, it is critical to be cognizant of the fact that these modifications, and their regulators, function in concert with each other. Similar to how individual neurons are able to integrate various, often conflicting, circuit inputs, the transcriptional machinery within the nucleus must be able to integrate a dynamic epigenetic landscape to ultimately drive or repress gene expression. As no single gene can be used as a readout for the activity and function of a neuron, no single epigenetic modification can provide an accurate readout for the transcriptional landscape for a given gene. As such, recent work has sought to identify specific patterns of histone modifications and the subsequent transcriptional effect at single gene loci (Tweedie-Cullen et al. 2012; Karch et al. 2013). Moving forward the addiction field should begin to link how these epigenetic marks collectively form an epigenetically permissive or repressive environment and how drugs of abuse mediate their transcriptional signatures through collective changes in histone modifications.

The various epigenetic writers and erasers often directly compete for influence, as they often share gene targets and residues for regulating PTMs and other epigenetic marks. More so, their role in activity-dependent gene expression has been extensively reviewed elsewhere and will not be a focus on this review (Barrett and Wood 2008; Sultan and Day 2011; Peixoto and Abel 2012). However, mounting evidence over the past two decades has provided key insights into how drugs of abuse, such as cocaine, are able to recruit or disengage these epigenetic writers to alter gene expression. Together, these epigenetic modifications can regulate various aspects of cellular function and, in neurons, are regulated by activity-dependent processes that alter the neuronal responses to subsequent stimuli. Their role in drug-dependent plasticity that leads to addictive behaviors is critical and underlies the long-lasting synaptic plasticity that is important in

SUD. As mentioned above, these marks allow for persistent upregulation or downregulation of genes involved in neural activity. However, as mentioned previously, at what genes these epigenetic marks occur and which cell types in which they occur are critical determinants in the role they have on behavior. Thus, increases in transcription in a reward-related brain region can alter behavior differentially depending on the cell type in which they are expressed. Understanding how epigenetic modifications that maintain this synaptic plasticity will be critical in understanding how these modifications occur and how they maintain synaptic changes that drive behavior.

5 The Interplay Between Acute Drug Effects and Activity-Dependent Epigenetic Dysregulation in the Transition to Substance Use Disorder

Within epigenetic marks it is important to consider how they were induced and what their ultimate role is on neural activity. Epigenetic modifications serve two major functions in differentiated neurons. First, they act to determine which genes are upregulated on a transient timescale upon cellular activation – for example, after acute drug exposure. Second, they act to control stable gene expression on a timescale that extends beyond the initial transient signal – i.e., changes that are seen during long-term withdrawal. The interplay between these two classes of epigenetic modifications is relatively unstudied. Thus, better insight into how drug-induced transient changes in chromatin structure lead to stable and long-lasting epigenetic regulation of gene expression is needed.

The interplay between quick temporally specific neuronal activation and longer-term changes in transcription is critical in the expression of appropriate, or in the case of SUD, inappropriate behaviors. The first step in drug-induced epigenetic remodeling relies on the actions of drugs on reward pathways within the brain. The reinforcing properties of drugs of abuse, such as cocaine, are attributed to their ability to induce changes in neural activity throughout the central nervous system. In particular, cocaine alters neuronal activity throughout the mesolimbic pathway by blocking the dopamine transporter and thus increasing DA levels (Chen et al. 2006). These acute drug effects are rapid and mediate the "high" induced by the drug and act to promote drug seeking in the future (Volkow et al. 1997). These drug-induced increases in neurotransmitter levels happen on the order of seconds and are faster than any specific transcriptional initiation event and, thus, are the first step in driving drug-induced transcriptional dysregulation (Yorgason et al. 2011). Transient increases in neural activity, neurotransmitter release, and signaling converge to subsequently drive the epigenetic remodeling that occurs following drug exposure. These transcriptional/epigenetic changes are induced by action potential and calcium- or G-protein-dependent signaling cascades. Neural activity signals can trigger chromatin remodeling via the calcium-/calmodulin-dependent kinase II (CaMKII), which becomes activated upon cellular depolarization and influx of calcium. CaMKII stimulates transcription of BDNF, a well-known neurotrophin involved in neuroplasticity, by phosphorylating and thus releasing the DNA methylation "reader" methyl CpG-binding protein 2 (MeCP2), a highly abundant chromosomal protein within the brain, from its promoter (Im et al. 2010; Nott et al. 2016; Zhou et al. 2006). This process has been shown to be highly involved in addictive behaviors (Bali et al. 2011). The activation of G protein-coupled receptors can induce similar effects via effectors such as cAMP signaling to set off a signaling cascade via the PKA pathway and members of the mitogen-activated protein kinases (MAPKs), which can directly phosphorylate histones to prompt further changes in chromatin structure (Gräff and Tsai 2013; Nestler 2016). This pathway has also been directly linked to cocaine-induced plasticity throughout the ventral midbrain and corticolimbic circuitry.

The acute epigenetic remodeling that occurs in response to cocaine exposure has been primarily studied in regions downstream of VTA dopaminergic projections. For example, acute cocaine exposure increases various acetylation marks throughout the dorsal striatum including increased acH3 and acH4 and increased acH4K5, acH4K8, acH4K12, and acH4K16 at *cFos* and *fosb* promoters (Jordi et al. 2013; Kumar et al. 2005). With regard to the ventral striatum, similar increases in acetylation at sites such as H3K14, H2BK12, and H4K5, H4K8, H4K12, and H4K16 in the NAc in response to acute cocaine have been observed (Malvaez et al. 2011; Levine et al. 2005). Extensive research in the role of striatal MSNs have provided evidence for the divergent roles in D1- and D2-expressing MSNs. Indeed, recent work has demonstrated a likewise divergent epigenetic response in these cell types in response to varying treatments of cocaine. Acute cocaine increases the combinatorial H3 phosphoacetylation in D1 MSNs of the NAc (Bertran-Gonzalez et al. 2008; Jordi et al. 2013), likely mediated by the D1-specific adaptations to DARPP-32 (Stipanovich et al. 2008; Nairn et al. 2004). Moreover, cocaine acutely increases H3K9me2 and H3K9me3 in both D1 and D2 MSNs (Jordi et al. 2013). Lastly, increased MECP2 has also been found throughout the NAc and caudate/putamen following acute cocaine exposure, suggesting induction of DNA methylation (Deng et al. 2011; Mao et al. 2012). However, the gene targets subject to presumptive DNA methylation remain unknown. As mentioned above, it is important to note that these observed changes in histone modifications do not occur in isolation. Any single epigenetic mark is unlikely to induce or repress gene expression on its own. Broad-scale epigenomic changes (such as global changes in acetylation or complete remodeling by nucleosome remodeling complexes) occur in concert with various marks, enzymes, and regulators. For example, cocaine-induced increases in acH3 (particularly at the H3S10 residue) recruit HATs and mediate increased H3K14ac (Jordi et al. 2013; Ciccarelli and Giustetto 2014). Moreover, acute cocaine recruits ARC to pH3S10-tagged transcripts, functioning as a potential feedback mechanism on neuronal gene expression (Salery et al. 2017). Recently, a potential mechanism for how histone modifiers (e.g., HDAC3) may interact with large-scale remodelers (such as nBAF) to regulate activity-dependent gene expression and plasticity has been proposed (Shu et al. 2018). Future work should further elucidate how these various epigenetic modifiers regulate gene expression in concert and in competition with one another.

Acute cocaine exposure recruits mechanisms critical to early phases of circuit plasticity and drug-seeking behavior. Typically, these changes to chromatin occur at and have been studied with regard to immediate early genes (such as *cFos*, *Bdnf*, *Arc*, and *Fosb*) (Zhao et al. 2014; Miller and Marshall 2005). However, repeated cocaine intake generates a novel epigenetic landscape at not only immediate early genes but also various gene targets linked to plasticity and synaptic function. These changes occur throughout the mesolimbic and mesocortical pathways and are believed to underlie the persistence of cocaine-seeking behavior. In the VTA, Schmidt et al. identified increased H3K9 and H3K14 acetylation at the *Bdnf I* promoter, coinciding with cocaine-induced increases in *Bdnf I* expression (Schmidt et al. 2012). Similarly, striatal BDNF transmission is known to increase the motivation to self-administer cocaine (Im et al. 2010; Graham et al. 2007, 2009; Grimm et al. 2003; Hall et al. 2003; Lu et al. 2004; Horger et al. 1999; Schoenbaum et al. 2007), and increases have been linked to the increased spine changes that are characteristic of cocaine exposure (Zhou et al. 2006). BDNF activates the enzyme nitric oxide synthase, leading to nitrosylation and dismissal of chromatin-bound HDAC2, thus ultimately increasing histone acetylation at genes involved in neural plasticity for LTP and learning (Nott et al. 2008). However, while these transient immediate early genes and growth factors are a critical component of synaptic plasticity induced by drugs, they are just the first step in a line of epigenetic modifications and synaptic remodeling that ultimately solidifies information about drugs and associated stimuli in the brain. Thus, it is important to understand how these initial changes lay the groundwork for the activity-dependent circuit remodeling that ultimately underlies addiction.

Yet, the major question is whether these changes are seen following repeated cocaine exposure and whether they are long-lasting. Whereas activity-induced gene expression and protein synthesis is transient, the circuit rewiring linked to associative learning and memory storage is long-lasting (Tonegawa et al. 2015). Notably, histone acetylation is known as a highly dynamic modification that rapidly turns over. Equally, even the extended half-life of channel proteins such as AMPA and NMDA receptors – whose expression is manipulated by drugs of abuse – is transitory when compared to timescales of pathological states of addiction, as drug relapse can occur even after years of abstinence and clinical intervention. Therefore, persistent changes in transcriptional regulation caused by drugs of abuse are likely maintained by the complex interplay of short-lived epigenetic marks – e.g., transient histone acetylation with dramatic effects on gene expression – that regulate synaptic and circuit strengths and permanent epigenetic aberrations that preserve transcriptional dysregulation in concert with alterations at the synapse and cell signaling. Recently, gene-specific enrichment of H3K4me3 was identified in the hippocampus of chronic cocaine users (Zhou et al. 2011). Yet, these changes to histone methylation did not correlate with changes in gene expression. Similarly, chronic cocaine self-administration induces long-lasting changes in acetylation states in the prefrontal cortex that correspond with increases in *Dot1l/Kmt4*, *Kdm5a*, *Kdm6a*, *Kdm6b*, and *Kdm7a* (Sadakierska-Chudy et al. 2017). However, despite these changes in KDM expression, no subsequent changes in global histone methylation state was observed, demonstrating that changes in any given histone mark are unable to dictate gene expression alone (and vice versa). However, it is possible that these changes to histone methylation (and its regulatory enzymes) do not alter baseline levels of particular genes but do leave the transcriptome in a permissive or repressive state for subsequent challenges (such as withdrawal and cue- and drug-induced relapse).

6 Transient Changes as a Scaffold for Long-Term Epigenetic Changes

All of the aforementioned mechanisms rely on acute changes that are transient in nature and are likely involved in quick and adaptive responses of cellular circuits to environmental information. But the question is how these precisely timed processes ultimately lead to permanently altered epigenetic landscapes that underlie dysregulated transcription in addiction. In addition to the long-lasting circuit changes induced by cocaine (see Fig. 2), cocaine exposure induces long-lasting changes in gene expression via targeted alterations in epigenetic structure. While there are various residues on histone tails susceptible to posttranslational modifications, it appears that cocaine induces stereotyped marks to generate long-lasting gene expression (Fig. 3). With regard to the striatum, repeated cocaine exposure drastically alters the epigenetic landscape. Both experimenter-administered chronic cocaine and repeated cocaine self-administration have led to increased acH3 and acH4 in the NAc (Malvaez et al. 2011; Wang et al. 2009; Renthal et al. 2007), particularly at plasticity-related genes, such as *Fosb*, *cFos*, *Bdnf I*, and *Cdk5*. These changes in histone marks are partially explained by cocaine's effects on various epigenetic writers, such as HDACs and KMTs. For example, chronic cocaine has been shown to cause export of HDAC5 from the nucleus in MSNs of the NAc (Renthal et al. 2007), alter HDAC expression (Renthal et al. 2009), and misregulate G9a/KMT1C function and subsequent histone methylation (Maze et al. 2010). Again, it is critical to emphasize that these epigenetic adaptations do not occur in isolation and are often competitive with one another. While previous studies have indicated simultaneous increases in H3 acetylation and methylation (Jordi et al. 2013), recent ChIP-seq studies identified gene-specific increases in both acH3 and acH4 in the NAc. Further, gene targets depleted with acH3/H4 correspond to gene targets which show enrichment for meH3 (Renthal et al. 2009; LaPlant and Nestler 2011). Moreover, gene-specific changes in nucleosome remodelers have been seen at the *Cdk5* promoter (Kumar et al. 2005), further suggesting the interaction between various epigenetic mechanisms to ultimately generate loci-specific transcription. Cocaine has been demonstrated to alter HDAC-mediated regulation of other histone modifiers – repeated cocaine disengages HDAC1 at KMT1C, leading to enhanced H3K9me2 in the NAc (Kennedy et al. 2013).

DNA methylation and several of its key regulatory enzymes appear sensitive to repeated cocaine exposure. Following self-administration, there is an increase in *Dnmt3a/b* expression and alterations of methylation at the *cFos* promoter (Wright et al. 2015) that persists following a period of withdrawal (Laplant et al. 2010). MECP2 levels have been demonstrated to increase in the striatum and hippocampus following self-administration (Im et al. 2010). Repeated cocaine is able to generate pervasive changes to the epigenome. These changes occur not only in a brain region-specific fashion but also in a cell-type-specific fashion. Accordingly, results support an emerging view that rapid changes in DNA methylation – traditionally viewed as a permanent and immutable mark in postmitotic cells – are involved in activity-dependent regulation of neuronal gene transcription. DNA methyltransferase, DNMT1, is highly expressed across the brain, and transient increases in DNMT1 expression are not only seen with Pavlovian learning but have been reported after administration of drugs of abuse (Goto et al. 1994; Numachi et al. 2007). In fact, following chronic exposure to drug, increases in DNA methylation in the striatum are persistent and evident even after extended periods of withdrawal (Mychasiuk et al. 2013). Notably, in the case of Pavlovian learning – a critical process involved in SUD – acquisition and extinction of memory have been linked to alterations in the methylation machinery in the prefrontal cortex, including changes to the TET family of enzymes, targeted DNA methylation, and recruitment of MECP2, suggesting that these DNA modifications are critical to the maintenance of long-term memories associated with addiction (Alaghband et al. 2016; Bredy et al. 2007; Bredy 2013; Li et al. 2014; Viola et al. 2016). These findings highlight the dynamic nature of the neuronal DNA methylome and suggest an important role for DNA methylation in the stabilization of epigenetic change that is instigated by drugs of abuse (Feng et al. 2015). In fact, both acute and chronic cocaine have been shown to cause hypomethylation of the *FosB* promoter in the striatum, linked to decreased binding of MeCP2 and upregulation of FosB expression (Anier et al. 2010). Thus, it is possible that acute histone changes allow for changes in DNA conformation and subsequent DNA methylation that stabilizes long-term memory and persistent changes in cellular function, as seen through the long-lasting nature of DNA methylation and targeted recruitment of DNA methylation in a gene-specific fashion following cocaine self-administration (Massart et al. 2015; Baker-Andresen et al. 2015).

As outlined earlier, the aforementioned changes in chromatin structure produce plasticity at the synaptic and circuit level, including alterations of the AMPA and NMDA receptor levels and their subunit composition. Just like with dendritic spines where thin spines serve as a scaffold to create more mature spines, transient epigenetic marks can set a series of events in place that help to consolidate information permanently only if the stimulus is incredibly salient or encountered repeatedly over long periods of time. This can serve as a gating mechanism, so that the long-term changes would only happen after repeated exposure.

7 Causally Linking Epigenetic Modification to Substance Use Disorder

Cocaine-associated behaviors have been linked with change in function of various epigenetic modifiers (Malvaez et al. 2011; Renthal et al. 2007; Kennedy et al. 2013; Rogge et al. 2013). For example, the associative processes that occur with cocaine exposure and cocaine-associated behaviors can be altered through targeting of specific epigenetic mechanisms. Bidirectional manipulation of histone acetylation in the NAc has profound effects on cocaine-associated behaviors. Genetic and pharmacological loss of HDAC3 function in the NAc enhances the acquisition of cocaine-conditioned place preference (CPP), with predictive increases to cocaine-induced acetylation (Rogge et al. 2013; Malvaez et al. 2013). However, this is unlikely through a mediation of the rewarding properties of cocaine but more likely regulating the associative processes, as HDAC3 inhibition during extinction not only accelerates extinction but also blunts cocaine-primed reinstatement of CPP. Cocaine-primed reinstatement has also been demonstrated to enhance H4K8Ac and alter HDAC3-dependent gene regulation in the medial habenula, an epithalamic region strongly linked to drug-seeking and drug-associated behaviors (López et al. 2018, 2019). Conversely, NAc-specific loss of CBP (a histone acetyltransferase) led to a hypoacetyl state in response to acute and chronic cocaine and blocked cocaine-induced CPP (Malvaez et al. 2011). Additionally, DARPP-32-mediated decreases in pH3S10 are also able to block cocaine-induced CPP (Stipanovich et al. 2008). Similarly, overexpression of KMT1C in the NAc led to increases in H3K9me2 which corresponded with decreased cocaine-CPP. Pharmacological inhibition of KMT1C was able to reverse the effects on H3K9me2 and enhance cocaine-CPP (Maze et al. 2010). Lastly, mutations to nBAF blunt cocaine-induced CPP that is restored through local overexpression of BDNF into the NAc (White et al. 2016; Alaghband et al. 2018). These epigenetic mechanisms have been demonstrated to play an important role in learning and memory and appear to mediate the associative properties of SUD.

Two major aspects in cocaine seeking are the reinforcing properties of the drug and the enhanced motivation to seek drug; each aspect is regulated by various molecular and circuit pathways. For example, recent work has characterized the formation of habitual cocaine seeking via the recruitment of MSNs in the dorsal lateral striatum (DLS) during long-access cocaine self-administration (Malvaez et al. 2018; Fouyssac et al. 2017; Murray et al. 2015). This DLS recruitment is mediated via disengagement of HDAC3 – pharmacological or genetic inhibition of HDAC3 in the DLS accelerated habit formation, whereas overexpression of HDAC3 in the DLS suppresses habit formation (Malvaez et al. 2018). Moreover, systemic HDAC inhibition suppresses acquisition of cocaine self-administration (Romieu et al. 2008). Similarly, HDAC3 inhibition enhanced extinction and blocked cue-induced reinstatement of cocaine seeking (Hitchcock et al. 2018). So while similar findings in CPP may not provide insights into HDAC-mediated regulation of reinforcing properties of cocaine, these findings in self-administration studies suggest HDACs may regulate motivational aspects of cocaine seeking as well as the changes that occur following repeated volitional exposure. This body of work demonstrates that HDACs function as molecular brake pads to not only acute gene expression but also recruitment of neural pathways in behavior. Drugs of abuse, such as cocaine, alter these molecular mechanisms leading to long-term alteration in circuit function.

While histone acetylation is a well-studied mechanism in the addiction field, recent work has further defined a role for KMT1C-mediated histone methylation in cocaine seeking. Overexpression of KMT1C in the NAc shell and subsequent increases in H3K9me2 enhance cocaine self-administration and generate increased susceptibility of stress-induced reinstatement (Anderson et al. 2017). Furthermore, while loss of nBAF function (through deletion of nBAF-specific subunit CREST) had no effect on the initial motivation to respond for cocaine, CREST deletions in the NAc slow the acquisition of cocaine self-administration and alter the acquisition of cocaine-associated memories (Alaghband et al. 2018). Overall, an elaborate interplay of epigenetic mechanisms regulates the various circuit and molecular mechanisms of drug seeking.

8 Linking Changes in Epigenome to Changes in Synaptic Function

To date, the field has identified various pathways, individual transcription factors, and altered epigenetic mechanisms engaged by cocaine exposure. But we, as a field, have yet to fully characterize how these individual levels of analysis combine to alter behavior. It is unlikely that any single gene, transcription factor, or epigenetic writer is responsible for the various aspects of SUD, nor will any single molecular mechanism provide an avenue for effective long-lasting therapeutics. Moreover, the heterogeneity that exists across cell types (e.g., D1 vs D2 MSNs) and brain regions (e.g., dorsal vs ventral striatum), although not fully elaborated or emphasized in this review, provides a further complication in understanding how the identified epigenetic changes ultimately lead to long-lasting changes in circuit function and behavior. Moving forward, it will be important to identify the mechanisms within defined cellular populations – based on genetic identity, circuit connectivity, or functional recruitment – that alter subsequent cocaine response and cocaine-associated behaviors.

Changes in the resting membrane potential, gene priming, and stable receptor expression levels can all alter the probability that a specific cell will fire and thus can increase the incorporation of these neurons into memory ensembles and strengthen synaptic connections. Maintenance of these tonic levels of neurotransmitter, changes in transporter function, and postsynaptic receptor content have been shown to be regulated by epigenetic modifications at the chromatin level. Specific methyl and acetyl marks can act to change stable expression levels of proteins involved in this process, such as AMPA and NMDA receptors, which can change the speed and efficiency with which new synapses can be formed and destabilized. This can also change the response magnitude of these cells and circuits to salient stimuli in the environment, thus driving maladaptive behaviors. These specific processes have been shown to be dysregulated in both human subjects with cocaine use disorder and rodent models of cocaine-associated behaviors (Volkow et al. 2003; Calipari et al. 2016; Breiter et al. 1997; Dackis and O'Brien 2005). (While the focus of this chapter has been specifically the cocaine-induced adaptations in plasticity, circuitry, and epigenetic mechanisms, other drugs of abuse are likewise able to induce unique molecular and neural circuit signatures to drive drug seeking as well). Thus, basal epigenetic regulation of membrane-associated proteins can alter the excitability of neurons and concomitant behavioral processes associated with addiction. For example, long-term potentiation induced by theta-burst stimulation is impaired as a result of nBAF loss of function in the NAc (White et al. 2016; Vogel-Ciernia et al. 2013). Maze et al. demonstrated altered synaptic pruning in the NAc following KMT1C overexpression (Maze et al. 2010). Moreover, HDAC inhibition or deletion leads to increased synaptic plasticity in both the hippocampus and NAc, likely mediated by enhanced expression of various immediate early genes, such as *Nr4a2*, *cFos*, and *Bdnf* (Malvaez et al. 2013; Barrett et al. 2011). Yet, how cocaine-induced changes in nuclear chromatin structure feed into altered circuits remains an elusive question. Nevertheless, while immediate early genes are critical in generating LTP, learning, memory, and various associative processes, it remains unclear how epigenetic adaptations at these loci ultimately generate differential function in neural circuits. Kennedy et al. linked changes in HDAC-mediated repression in histone methylation to altered expression of various GABA-receptor subunits, including *Gabra1* and *Gabra2* that is linked to altered synaptic function in the NAc (Kennedy et al. 2013). Altered acetylation at other various synaptic proteins have also been reported, including increased acH3 at *Gria2*, *Grin1*, and *Grin2b* in the NAc (Wang et al. 2009). Although increased AMPA/NMDA ratios are a hallmark feature of cocaine exposure, how epigenetic dysfunction at these individual gene loci are linked to altered NAc function is a key open question.

Conversely, repeated stimulation of strengthened synapses can result in activity-dependent epigenetic remodeling via calcium-dependent signaling (Nestler 2013). This increase in the activity level of neurons can lead to the activation of immediate early genes and concomitant wide-scale nuclear changes in the accessibility of DNA and transcriptional processes. In addition, these changes can lead to a feedforward loop in which activity-dependent epigenetic changes lead to enhanced sensitivity to subsequent inputs. If these inputs are in neuronal pathways driving reinforcement learning, this can act to increase self-administration and drug seeking. Thus, it is the communication between the nuclear changes in DNA conformation/transcription and the precise changes in membrane excitability that allows for the refinement of information at the level of each individual neuron. Inflexibility in both the behavioral adaptations and related neural circuitry is what underlies drug addiction in a way that results in the strong and stable storage and expression of drug-associated memories over all others.

9 Defining Causal Links Between Epigenetic Factors and Neural Activity in Substance Use Disorder

As discussed throughout this review, long-term cocaine exposure and cocaine-seeking behavior generate widespread changes to the epigenome, ultimately leading to not only targeted changes in single genes but recruitment of a cocaine-specific transcriptional network, in a cell-type- and circuit-specific manner. Moreover, cocaine-repressed genes provide an equally critical component to SUD as cocaine-induced transcripts and should not be overlooked. Moving forward, it will be crucial to generate an encompassing perspective on the full transcriptional and molecular adaptations induced by repeated cocaine. A full acknowledgment and understanding of how drugs of abuse engage these networks will provide a more promising avenue of success for treating such disorders. In line with this view, work from Walker et al. has identified a full gene network induced by repeated cocaine self-administration and reinstatement of cocaine seeking (Walker et al. 2018). Similarly, transcriptional dysregulations in the PFC over various periods of forced abstinence from repeated cocaine exposure have been identified (Li et al. 2017). However, the molecular mechanisms which regulate these transcriptional adaptations remain unknown. Moreover, how induction of the identified gene network leads to changes in circuit activity and behavior has not been defined. Yet, the advent of new viral and molecular strategies now allows researchers the ability to target these epigenetic modifications to particular loci within particular subsets of cell populations. For example, both engineered zinc-finger proteins (ZFPs) and CRISPR/dCas9 systems allow for gene-specific targeting of transcriptional regulators and have previously been used to selectively increase or decrease the expression of single genes. However, combined with novel viral and Cre-dependent approaches, these technologies can now be adapted to target specific epigenetic writers or erasers in cell-type-, pathway-, and gene-loci-specific manners (Savell et al. 2018; Heller et al. 2014, 2016; Kwapis et al. 2018). Paired with in vivo techniques for circuit monitoring [such as Miniscopes (Silva 2017), in vivo fiber photometry (Calipari et al. 2017), and fast scan cyclic voltammetry (Willuhn et al. 2014)], the field of neuroepigenetics now has the potential to directly link epigenetic regulation and circuit activity to behavioral outcomes. Ultimately, these insights will lead to the development of effective therapeutics for the varying aspects of SUD.

Acknowledgments A.J.L. is supported by NIH Grant K00 DA048436. C.A.S. is supported by NIH grant K99 DA045103 (NIDA) and a NARSAD Young Investigator Award from the Brain and Behavior Research Foundation. E.S.C is supported by NIH grants R00 DA042111 and DP1 DA048931 (NIDA), a NARSAD Young Investigator Award from the Brain and Behavior Research Foundation, and funding from the Whitehall Foundation and Edward Mallinckrodt Jr. Foundation.

References

Agger K, Christensen J, Cloos PA, Helin K (2008) The emerging functions of histone demethylases. Curr Opin Genet Dev 18:159–168

Aguilar MA, Rodríguez-Arias M, Miñarro J (2009) Neurobiological mechanisms of the reinstatement of drug-conditioned place preference. Brain Res Rev 59:253–277

Ahmed SH et al (2005) Gene expression evidence for remodeling of lateral hypothalamic circuitry in cocaine addiction. Proc Natl Acad Sci 102:11533–11538

Alaghband Y, Bredy TW, Wood MA (2016) The role of active DNA demethylation and Tet enzyme function in memory formation and cocaine action. Neurosci Lett. https://doi.org/10.1016/j.neulet.2016.01.023

Alaghband Y et al (2018) CREST in the nucleus accumbens core regulates cocaine conditioned place preference, cocaine-seeking behavior, and synaptic plasticity. J Neurosci 38:9514–9526

Alarcón JM et al (2004) Chromatin acetylation, memory, and LTP are impaired in CBP+/− mice: a model for the cognitive deficit in Rubinstein-Taybi syndrome and its amelioration. Neuron 42:947–959

Anderson SM, Pierce RC (2005) Cocaine-induced alterations in dopamine receptor signaling: implications for reinforcement and reinstatement. Pharmacol Ther 106:389–403

Anderson EM et al (2017) Overexpression of the histone dimethyltransferase G9a in nucleus accumbens shell increases cocaine self-administration, stress-induced reinstatement, and anxiety. J Neurosci 38:1657–1617

Anier K, Malinovskaja K, Aonurm-Helm A, Zharkovsky A, Kalda A (2010) DNA methylation regulates cocaine-induced behavioral sensitization in mice. Neuropsychopharmacology 35:2450

Bachtell RK, Self DW (2008) Renewed cocaine exposure produces transient alterations in nucleus accumbens AMPA receptor-mediated behavior. J Neurosci 28:12808–12814

Baker-Andresen D, Ratnu VS, Bredy TW (2013) Dynamic DNA methylation: a prime candidate for genomic metaplasticity and behavioral adaptation. Trends Neurosci 36:3–13

Baker-Andresen D et al (2015) Persistent variations in neuronal DNA methylation following cocaine self-administration and protracted abstinence in mice. Neuroepigenetics 4:1–11

Bali P, Im H-I, Kenny PJ (2011) Methylation, memory and addiction. Epigenetics 6:671–674

Bannister AJ, Kouzarides T (2011) Regulation of chromatin by histone modifications. Cell Res 21:381–395

Barnes CE, English DM, Cowley SM (2019) Acetylation & Co: an expanding repertoire of histone acylations regulates chromatin and transcription. Essays Biochem 63:97–107

Barrett RM, Wood MA (2008) Beyond transcription factors: the role of chromatin modifying enzymes in regulating transcription required for memory. Learn Mem 15:460–467

Barrett RM et al (2011) Hippocampal focal knockout of CBP affects specific histone modifications, long-term potentiation, and long-term memory. Neuropsychopharmacology 36:1545–1556

Bateup HS et al (2008) Cell type-specific regulation of DARPP-32 phosphorylation by psychostimulant and antipsychotic drugs. Nat Neurosci 11:932–939

Baubec T, Schübeler D (2014) Genomic patterns and context specific interpretation of DNA methylation. Curr Opin Genet Dev 25:85–92

Baylin SB, Ohm JE (2006) Epigenetic gene silencing in cancer – a mechanism for early oncogenic pathway addiction? Nat Rev Cancer 6:107–116

Beitner-Johnson D, Nestler EJ (1991) Morphine and cocaine exert common chronic actions on tyrosine hydroxylase in dopaminergic brain reward regions. J Neurochem 57:344–347

Berger SL (2007) The complex language of chromatin regulation during transcription. Nature 447:407

Berndsen CE, Denu JM (2008) Catalysis and substrate selection by histone/protein lysine acetyltransferases. Curr Opin Struct Biol 18:682–689

Bertran-Gonzalez J et al (2008) Opposing patterns of signaling activation in dopamine D1 and D2 receptor-expressing striatal neurons in response to cocaine and haloperidol. J Neurosci 28:5671–5685

Bird A (2002) DNA methylation patterns and epigenetic memory. Genes Dev 16(1):6–21. https://doi.org/10.1101/gad.947102.6

Bocklisch C et al (2013) Cocaine disinhibits dopamine neurons by potentiation of GABA transmission in the ventral tegmental area. Science 341:1521–1525

Boutrel B et al (2005) Role for hypocretin in mediating stress-induced reinstatement of cocaine-seeking behavior. Proc Natl Acad Sci U S A 102:19168–19173

Brami-Cherrier K (2005) Parsing molecular and behavioral effects of cocaine in mitogen- and stress-activated protein kinase-1-deficient mice. J Neurosci 25:11444–11454

Bredy T (2013) The 6Th base: TET3-mediated DNA hydroxymethylation regulates the formation of memory for fear extinction. Biol Psychiatry 73:5S

Bredy TW et al (2007) Histone modifications around individual BDNF gene promoters in prefrontal cortex are associated with extinction of conditioned fear. Learn Mem 14(4):268–276. https://doi.org/10.1101/lm.500907.lation

Breiter HC et al (1997) Acute effects of cocaine on human brain activity and emotion. Neuron 19:591–611

Burdge GC, Lillycrop KA (2010) Nutrition, epigenetics, and developmental plasticity: implications for understanding human disease. Annu Rev Nutr 30:315–339

Calipari ES, Ferris MJ, Zimmer BA, Roberts DC, Jones SR (2013) Temporal pattern of cocaine intake determines tolerance vs sensitization of cocaine effects at the dopamine transporter. Neuropsychopharmacology 38(12):2385–2392

Calipari ES, Jones SR (2014) Sensitized nucleus accumbens dopamine terminal responses to methylphenidate and dopamine transporter releasers after intermittent-access self-administration. Neuropharmacology 82:1–10

Calipari ES, Ferris MJ, Siciliano CA, Zimmer BA, Jones SR (2014) Intermittent cocaine self-administration produces sensitization of stimulant effects at the dopamine transporter. J Pharmacol Exp Ther 349(2):192–198

Calipari ES, Siciliano CA, Zimmer BA, Jones SR (2015) Brief intermittent cocaine self-administration and abstinence sensitizes cocaine effects on the dopamine transporter and increases drug seeking. Neuropsychopharmacology 40(3):728–735

Calipari ES et al (2016) In vivo imaging identifies temporal signature of D1 and D2 medium spiny neurons in cocaine reward. Proc Natl Acad Sci 113:2726–2731

Calipari ES et al (2017) Dopaminergic dynamics underlying sex-specific cocaine reward. Nat Commun 8:13877

Calipari ES et al (2019) Synaptic microtubule-associated protein EB3 and SRC phosphorylation mediate structural and behavioral adaptations during withdrawal from cocaine self-administration. J Neurosci. pii: 0024-19. https://doi.org/10.1523/JNEUROSCI.0024-19.2019

Cameron CM, Murugan M, Choi JY, Engel EA, Witten IB (2019) Increased cocaine motivation is associated with degraded spatial and temporal representations in IL-NAc neurons. Neuron. https://doi.org/10.1016/J.NEURON.2019.04.015

Campanac E, Hoffman DA (2013) Repeated cocaine exposure increases fast-spiking interneuron excitability in the rat medial prefrontal cortex. J Neurophysiol 109:2781–2792

Campbell RR, Wood MA (2019) How the epigenome integrates information and reshapes the synapse. Nat Rev Neurosci 20:133–147

Cao J, Yan Q (2012) Histone ubiquitination and deubiquitination in transcription, DNA damage response, and cancer. Front Oncol 2:1–9

Caputi FF et al (2014) Dynorphin/KOP and nociceptin/NOP gene expression and epigenetic changes by cocaine in rat striatum and nucleus accumbens. Prog Neuropsychopharmacol Biol Psychiatry 49:36–46

Carouge D, Host L, Aunis D, Zwiller J, Anglard P (2010) CDKL5 is a brain MeCP2 target gene regulated by DNA methylation. Neurobiol Dis 38:414–424

Chandra R et al (2015) Opposing role for Egr3 in nucleus accumbens cell subtypes in cocaine action. J Neurosci 35:7927–7937

Chen R et al (2006) Abolished cocaine reward in mice with a cocaine-insensitive dopamine transporter. Proc Natl Acad Sci 103:9333–9338

Childress AR et al (1999) Limbic activation during cue-induced cocaine craving. Am J Psychiatry 156:11–18

Ciccarelli A, Giustetto M (2014) Role of ERK signaling in activity-dependent modifications of histone proteins. Neuropharmacology 80:34–44

Collins AL, Aitken TJ, Greenfield VY, Ostlund SB, Wassum KM (2016) Nucleus accumbens acetylcholine receptors modulate dopamine and motivation. Neuropsychopharmacology 41:2830

Conrad KL et al (2008) Formation of accumbens GluR2-lacking AMPA receptors mediates incubation of cocaine craving. Nature 454:118–121

Dackis C, O'Brien C (2005) Neurobiology of addiction: treatment and public policy ramifications. Nat Neurosci 8:1431–1436

De La Cruz X, Lois S, Sánchez-Molina S, Martínez-Balbás MA (2005) Do protein motifs read the histone code? Bioessays 27:164–175

de Ruijter AJM, van Gennip AH, Caron HN, Kemp S, van Kuilenburg ABP (2003) Histone deacetylases (HDACs): characterization of the classical HDAC family. Biochem J 370:737–749

de Wit H (1996) Priming effects with drugs and other reinforcers. Exp Clin Psychopharmacol 4:5–10
Deng JV et al (2011) Behavioral responses to psychostimulants. Nat Neurosci 13:1128–1136
Dudai Y, Morris RGM (2013) Memorable trends. Neuron 80:742–750
Dulac C (2010) Brain function and chromatin plasticity. Nature 465:728–735
Farrell MR et al (2019) Ventral pallidum is essential for cocaine reinstatement after voluntary abstinence. bioRxiv:653741. https://doi.org/10.1101/653741
Farrelly LA et al (2019) Histone serotonylation is a permissive modification that enhances TFIID binding to H3K4me3. Nature 567:535–539
Farris SP, Harris RA, Ponomarev I (2015) Epigenetic modulation of brain gene networks for cocaine and alcohol abuse. Front Neurosci 9:1–10
Fass DM et al (2013) Crebinostat: a novel cognitive enhancer that inhibits histone deacetylase activity and modulates chromatin-mediated neuroplasticity. Neuropharmacology 64:81–96
Feng J et al (2014) Chronic cocaine-regulated epigenomic changes in mouse nucleus accumbens. Genome Biol 15:R65
Feng J et al (2015) Role of Tet1 and 5-hydroxymethylcytosine in cocaine action. Nat Neurosci 18:536–544
Ferguson D et al (2015) SIRT1-FOXO3a regulate cocaine actions in the nucleus accumbens. J Neurosci 35:3100–3111
Ferris MJ, Calipari ES, Yorgason JT, Jones SR (2013) Examining the complex regulation and drug-induced plasticity of dopamine release and uptake using voltammetry in brain slices. ACS Chem Nerosci 4:693–703
Filippakopoulos P, Knapp S (2014) Targeting bromodomains: epigenetic readers of lysine acetylation. Nat Rev Drug Discov 13:337–356
Finegersh A, Homanics GE (2016) Chromatin immunoprecipitation and gene expression analysis of neuronal subtypes after fluorescence activated cell sorting. J Neurosci Methods 263:81–88
Fischle W et al (2002) Enzymatic activity associated with class II HDACs is dependent on a multiprotein complex containing HDAC3 and SMRT/N-CoR. Mol Cell 9:45–57
Fouyssac M, Everitt BJ, Belin D (2017) Cellular basis of the intrastriatal functional shifts that underlie the development of habits: relevance for drug addiction. Curr Opin Behav Sci 13:144–151
Freeman WM et al (2008) Persistent alterations in mesolimbic gene expression with abstinence from cocaine self-administration. Neuropsychopharmacology 33:1807–1817
Goodwin LR, Picketts DJ (2018) The role of ISWI chromatin remodeling complexes in brain development and neurodevelopmental disorders. Mol Cell Neurosci. https://doi.org/10.1016/j.mcn.2017.10.008
Goto K et al (1994) Expression of DNA methyltransferase gene in mature and immature neurons as well as proliferating cells in mice. Differentiation 56:39–44
Gräff J, Tsai L-H (2013) Histone acetylation: molecular mnemonics on the chromatin. Nat Rev Neurosci 14:97
Graham DL et al (2007) Dynamic BDNF activity in nucleus accumbens with cocaine use increases self-administration and relapse. Nat Neurosci 10:1029–1037
Graham DL et al (2009) Tropomyosin-related kinase B in the mesolimbic dopamine system: region-specific effects on cocaine reward. Biol Psychiatry 65:696–701
Grimm JW, Hope BT, Wise RA, Shaham Y (2001) Incubation of cocaine craving after withdrawal. Nature 412:141–142
Grimm JW et al (2003) Time-dependent increases in brain-derived neurotrophic factor protein levels within the mesolimbic dopamine system after withdrawal from cocaine: implications for incubation of cocaine craving. J Neurosci 23:742–747
Hall FS, Drgonova J, Goeb M, Uhl GR (2003) Reduced behavioral effects of cocaine in heterozygous brain-derived neurotrophic factor (BDNF) knockout mice. Neuropsychopharmacology 28:1485
Hassa PO, Haenni SS, Elser M, Hottiger MO (2006) Nuclear ADP-ribosylation reactions in mammalian cells: where are we today and where are we going? Microbiol Mol Biol Rev 70:789–829

Heller EA et al (2014) Locus-specific epigenetic remodeling controls addiction- and depression-related behaviors. Nat Neurosci 17:1720–1727
Heller EA et al (2016) Targeted epigenetic remodeling of the Cdk5 gene in nucleus accumbens regulates cocaine- and stress-evoked behavior. J Neurosci 36:4690–4697
Hitchcock LN, Raybuck JD, Wood MA, Lattal KM (2018) Effects of a histone deacetylase 3 inhibitor on extinction and reinstatement of cocaine self-administration in rats. Psychopharmacology (Berl). 3. doi: https://doi.org/10.1007/s00213-018-5122-2
Horger BA et al (1999) Enhancement of locomotor activity and conditioned reward to cocaine by brain-derived neurotrophic factor. J Neurosci 19:4110–4122
Horikawa HPM, Nawa H (1998) Turnover rates of the AMPA-type glutamate receptor GluR1 measured by transient gene expression. J Neurosci Methods 84:173–179
Hurd YL, Weiss F, Koob G, Ungerstedt U (1990) The influence of cocaine self-administration on in vivo dopamine and acetylcholine neurotransmission in rat caudate-putamen. Neurosci Lett 109:227–233
Hyman SE, Malenka RC, Nestler EJ (2006) Neural mechanisms of addiction: the role of reward-related learning and memory. Annu Rev Neurosci 29:565–598
Im HI, Hollander JA, Bali P, Kenny PJ (2010) MeCP2 controls BDNF expression and cocaine intake through homeostatic interactions with microRNA-212. Nat Neurosci 13:1120–1127
Itzhak Y, Martin JL (2002) Cocaine-induced conditioned place preference in mice: Induction, extinction and reinstatement by related psychostimulants. Neuropsychopharmacology 26:130–134
Jaffe JH, Cascella NG, Kumor KM, Sherer MA (1989) Jaffe_COC_Craving_Psychopharm_1989.pdf
Jones PA (2012) Functions of DNA methylation: Islands, start sites, gene bodies and beyond. Nat Rev Genet 13:484–492
Jones S, Bonci A (2005) Synaptic plasticity and drug addiction. Curr Opin Pharmacol 5:20–25
Jordi E et al (2013) Differential effects of cocaine on histone posttranslational modifications in identified populations of striatal neurons. Proc Natl Acad Sci U S A 110:9511–9516
Kalivas PW, Duffy P (2002) Repeated cocaine administration alters extracellular glutamate in the ventral tegmental area. J Neurochem 70:1497–1502
Karch KR, DeNizio JE, Black BE, Garcia BA (2013) Identification and interrogation of combinatorial histone modifications. Front Genet 4:1–15
Kawa AB, Allain F, Robinson TE, Samaha AN (2019) The transition to cocaine addiction: the importance of pharmacokinetics for preclinical models. Psychopharmacology (Berl). https://doi.org/10.1007/s00213-019-5164-0
Kennedy PJ et al (2013) Class i HDAC inhibition blocks cocaine-induced plasticity by targeted changes in histone methylation. Nat Neurosci 16:434–440
Korzus E, Rosenfeld MG, Mayford M (2004) CBP histone acetyltransferase activity is a critical component of memory consolidation. Neuron 42:961–972
Kouzarides T (2007) Chromatin modifications and their function. Cell 128:693–705
Kramar CP, Chefer VI, Wise RA, Medina JH, Barbano MF (2014) Dopamine in the dorsal hippocampus impairs the late consolidation of cocaine-associated memory. Neuropsychopharmacology 39:1645–1653
Kravitz AV, Tye LD, Kreitzer AC (2012) Distinct roles for direct and indirect pathway striatal neurons in reinforcement. Nat Neurosci 15:816–818
Kuhar MJ, Ritz MC, Boja JW (1991) The dopamine hypothesis of the reinforcing properties of cocaine. Trends Neurosci 14:299–302
Kumar A et al (2005) Chromatin remodeling is a key mechanism underlying cocaine-induced plasticity in striatum. Neuron 48:303–314
Kupchik YM et al (2015) Coding the direct/indirect pathways by D1 and D2 receptors is not valid for accumbens projections. Nat Neurosci 18:1230–1232

Kutlu MG, Gould TJ (2016) Effects of drugs of abuse on hippocampal plasticity and hippocampus-dependent learning and memory: contributions to development and maintenance of addiction. Learn Mem 23:515–533

Kwapis JL et al (2018) Epigenetic regulation of the circadian gene Per1 contributes to age-related changes in hippocampal memory. Nat Commun 9

LaPlant Q, Nestler EJ (2011) CRACKing the histone code: cocaine's effects on chromatin structure and function. Horm Behav 59:321–330

Laplant Q et al (2010) Dnmt3a regulates emotional behavior and spine plasticity in the nucleus accumbens. Nat Neurosci 13:1137–1143

Le Moal M, Koob GF (2007) Drug addiction: pathways to the disease and pathophysiological perspectives. Eur Neuropsychopharmacol 17:377–393

Le Moine C, Bloch B (1995) D1 and D2 dopamine receptor gene expression in the rat striatum: sensitive cRNA probes demonstrate prominent segregation of D1 and D2 mRNAS in distinct neuronal populations of the dorsal and ventral striatum. J Comp Neurol 355:418–426

Levenson JM et al (2004) Regulation of histone acetylation during memory formation in the hippocampus. J Biol Chem 279:40545–40559

Levine AA et al (2005) CREB-binding protein controls response to cocaine by acetylating histones at the fosB promoter in the mouse striatum. Proc Natl Acad Sci U S A 102:19186–19191

Levine A et al (2011) Molecular mechanism for a gateway drug: epigenetic changes initiated by nicotine prime gene expression by cocaine. Sci Transl Med 3:107ra109

Li X et al (2014) Neocortical Tet3-mediated accumulation of 5-hydroxymethylcytosine promotes rapid behavioral adaptation. Proc Natl Acad Sci U S A 111:7120–7125

Li M et al (2017) Dynamic expression changes in the transcriptome of the prefrontal cortex after repeated exposure to cocaine in mice. Front Pharmacol 8:1–10

Liu Q, Pu L, Poo M (2005) Repeated cocaine exposure in vivo facilitates LTP induction in midbrain dopamine neurons. Nature 437:1027

López AJ, Wood MA (2015) Role of nucleosome remodeling in neurodevelopmental and intellectual disability disorders. Front Behav Neurosci 9:1–10

López AJ et al (2018) Medial habenula cholinergic signaling regulates cocaine-associated relapse-like behavior. Addict Biol. https://doi.org/10.1111/adb.12605

López AJ et al (2019) Epigenetic regulation of immediate-early gene Nr4a2/Nurr1 in the medial habenula during reinstatement of cocaine-associated behavior. Neuropharmacology 153:13–19

Loweth JA et al (2014) Synaptic depression via mGluR1 positive allosteric modulation suppresses cue-induced cocaine craving. Nat Neurosci 17:73–80

Lu L, Dempsey J, Liu SY, Bossert JM, Shaham Y (2004) A single infusion of brain-derived neurotrophic factor into the ventral tegmental area induces long-lasting potentiation of cocaine seeking after withdrawal. J Neurosci 24:1604–1611

MacAskill AF, Cassel JM, Carter AG (2014) Cocaine exposure reorganizes cell type- and input-specific connectivity in the nucleus accumbens. Nat Neurosci 17:1198–1207

MacNiven KH et al (2018) Association of neural responses to drug cues with subsequent relapse to stimulant use. JAMA Netw Open 1:e186466

Mahler SV et al (2014) Designer receptors show role for ventral pallidum input to ventral tegmental area in cocaine seeking. Nat Neurosci 17(4):577–585. https://doi.org/10.1038/nn.3664

Malvaez M, Mhillaj E, Matheos DP, Palmery M, Wood MA (2011) CBP in the nucleus accumbens regulates cocaine-induced histone acetylation and is critical for cocaine-associated behaviors. J Neurosci 31:16941–16948

Malvaez M et al (2013) HDAC3-selective inhibitor enhances extinction of cocaine-seeking behavior in a persistent manner. Proc Natl Acad Sci U S A 110:2647–2652

Malvaez M et al (2018) Habits are negatively regulated by histone deacetylase 3 in the dorsal striatum. Biol Psychiatry 84(5):383–392. https://doi.org/10.1016/j.biopsych.2018.01.025

Mao L et al (2012) In vivo: a differential role of NMDA receptors. Neurochem Int 59:610–617

Mark GP, Hajnal A, Kinney AE, Keys AS (1999) Self-administration of cocaine increases the release of acetylcholine to a greater extent than response-independent cocaine in the nucleus accumbens of rats. Psychopharmacology (Berl) 143:47–53
Mark GP, Shabani S, Dobbs LK, Hansen ST (2011) Cholinergic modulation of mesolimbic dopamine function and reward. Physiol Behav 104:76–81
Massart R et al (2015) Role of DNA methylation in the nucleus accumbens in incubation of cocaine craving. J Neurosci 35:8042–8058
Maze I et al (2010) Essential role of the histone methyltransferase G9a in cocaine-induced plasticity. Science 327:213–216
Maze I et al (2011) Cocaine dynamically regulates heterochromatin and repetitive element unsilencing in nucleus accumbens. Proc Natl Acad Sci U S A 108:3035–3040
McCallum SE, Glick SD (2009) 18-Methoxycoronaridine blocks acquisition but enhances reinstatement of a cocaine place preference. Neurosci Lett 458:57–59
McPherson PS (2015) Eating locally: microautophagy and protein turnover at the synapse. Neuron 88:619–621
Ménard C, Gaudreau P, Quirion R (2015) Signaling pathways relevant to cognition-enhancing drug targets. J Dement Care 13:59–98
Messner S, Hottiger MO (2011) Histone ADP-ribosylation in DNA repair, replication and transcription. Trends Cell Biol 21:534–542
Mews P, Calipari ES (2017) Cross-talk between the epigenome and neural circuits in drug addiction. Prog Brain Res 235:19–63
Miller CA, Marshall JF (2005) Altered Fos expression in neural pathways underlying cue-elicited drug seeking in the rat. Eur J Neurosci 21:1385–1393
Murray JE et al (2015) Basolateral and central amygdala differentially recruit and maintain dorsolateral striatum dependent cocaine-seeking habits. Nat Commun 6:1–9
Mychasiuk R, Muhammad A, Ilnytskyy S, Kolb B (2013) Persistent gene expression changes in NAc, mPFC, and OFC associated with previous nicotine or amphetamine exposure. Behav Brain Res 256:655–661
Nairn AC et al (2004) The role of DARPP-32 in the actions of drugs of abuse. Neuropharmacology 47:14–23
Nathan D, Sterner DE, Berger SL (2003) Histone modifications: now summoning sumoylation. Proc Natl Acad Sci 100:13118–13120
Nelson ED, Monteggia LM (2011) Epigenetics in the mature mammalian brain: effects on behavior and synaptic transmission. Neurobiol Learn Mem 96:53–60
Nestler EJ (2013) Cellular basis of memory for addiction. Dialogues Clin Neurosci 15:431–443
Nestler EJ (2016) Reflections on: "A general role for adaptations in G-Proteins and the cyclic AMP system in mediating the chronic actions of morphine and cocaine on neuronal function". Brain Res 1645:71–74
Nott A, Watson PM, Robinson JD, Crepaldi L, Riccio A (2008) S-nitrosylation of histone deacetylase 2 induces chromatin remodelling in neurons. Nature 455:411
Nott A et al (2016) Histone deacetylase 3 associates with MeCP2 to regulate FOXO and social behavior. Nat Neurosci 19:1497
Numachi Y et al (2007) Methamphetamine-induced hyperthermia and lethal toxicity: role of the dopamine and serotonin transporters. Eur J Pharmacol 572:120–128
Pardo-Garcia TR et al (2019) Ventral pallidum is the primary target for accumbens D1 projections driving cocaine seeking. J Neurosci 39:2041–2051
Park K, Volkow ND, Pan Y, Du C (2013) Chronic cocaine dampens dopamine signaling during cocaine intoxication and unbalances D1 over D2 receptor signaling. J Neurosci 33:15827–15836
Pascoli V et al (2014) Contrasting forms of cocaine-evoked plasticity control components of relapse. Nature 509:459
Peixoto L, Abel T (2012) The role of histone acetylation in memory formation and cognitive impairments. Neuropsychopharmacology 38:62–76

Pol Bodetto S et al (2013) Cocaine represses protein phosphatase-1Cβ through DNA methylation and methyl-CpG binding protein-2 recruitment in adult rat brain. Neuropharmacology 73:31–40
Renthal W, Nestler EJ (2008) Epigenetic mechanisms in drug addiction. Trends Mol Med 14:341–350
Renthal W et al (2007) Histone deacetylase 5 epigenetically controls behavioral adaptations to chronic emotional stimuli. Neuron 56:517–529
Renthal W et al (2009) Genome-wide analysis of chromatin regulation by cocaine reveals a role for sirtuins. Neuron 62:335–348
Ressler KJ, Paschall G, Zhou X, Davis M (2002) Regulation of synaptic plasticity genes during consolidation of fear conditioning. J Neurosci 22:7892–7902
Rivera CM, Ren B (2013) Mapping human epigenomes. Cell 155:39–55
Robison AJ, Nestler EJ (2011) Transcriptional and epigenetic mechanisms of addiction. Nat Rev Neurosci 12:623–637
Rogge GA, Singh H, Dang R, Wood MA (2013) HDAC3 is a negative regulator of cocaine-context-associated memory formation. J Neurosci 33:6623–6632
Roidl D, Hacker C (2014) Histone methylation during neural development. Cell Tissue Res 356:539–552
Romieu P et al (2008) Histone deacetylase inhibitors decrease cocaine but not sucrose self-administration in rats. J Neurosci 28:9342–9348
Roth SY, Denu JM, Allis CD (2003) Histone acetyltransferases. Annu Rev Biochem 70:81–120
Rudenko A, Tsai L-H (2014) Epigenetic modifications in the nervous system and their impact upon cognitive impairments. Neuropharmacology 80:70–82
Russo SJ, Nestler EJ (2013) The brain reward circuitry in mood disorders. Nat Rev Neurosci 14:609–625
Russo SJ et al (2010) The addicted synapse: mechanisms of synaptic and structural plasticity in nucleus accumbens. Trends Neurosci 33:267–276
Sadakierska-Chudy A et al (2017) Cocaine administration and its withdrawal enhance the expression of genes encoding histone-modifying enzymes and histone acetylation in the rat prefrontal cortex. Neurotox Res 32:141–150
Salery M et al (2017) Activity-regulated cytoskeleton-associated protein accumulates in the nucleus in response to cocaine and acts as a brake on chromatin remodeling and long-term behavioral alterations. Biol Psychiatry. https://doi.org/10.1016/j.biopsych.2016.05.025
Santos-Rosa H et al (2002) Active genes are tri-methylated at K4 of histone H3. Nature 419:407–411
Savell KE et al (2018) A neuron-optimized CRISPR/dCas9 activation system for robust and specific gene regulation. bioRxiv:371500. https://doi.org/10.1101/371500
Schmidt HD et al (2012) Increased brain-derived neurotrophic factor (BDNF) expression in the ventral tegmental area during cocaine abstinence is associated with increased histone acetylation at BDNF exon I-containing promoters. J Neurochem 120:202–209
Schoenbaum G, Stalnaker TA, Shaham Y (2007) A role for BDNF in cocaine reward and relapse. Nat Neurosci 10:935–936
Shahbazian MD, Grunstein M (2007) Functions of site-specific histone acetylation and deacetylation. Annu Rev Biochem 76:75–100
Shiio Y, Eisenman RN (2003) Histone sumoylation is associated with transcriptional repression. Proc Natl Acad Sci 100:13225–13230
Shu G et al (2018) Deleting HDAC3 rescues long-term memory impairments induced by disruption of the neuron-specific chromatin remodeling subunit BAF53b. Learn Mem 25(3):109–115. https://doi.org/10.1101/lm.046920.117.25
Siciliano CA, Calipari ES, Ferris MJ, Jones SR (2015) Adaptations of presynaptic dopamine terminals induced by psychostimulant self-administration. ACS Chem Nerosci 6:27–36
Silva AJ (2017) Miniaturized two-photon microscope: seeing clearer and deeper into the brain. Light Sci Appl 6:e17104

Smith RJ, Lobo MK, Spencer S, Kalivas PW (2013) Cocaine-induced adaptations in D1 and D2 accumbens projection neurons (a dichotomy not necessarily synonymous with direct and indirect pathways). Curr Opin Neurobiol 23:546–552

Sorg BA, Davidson DL, Kalivas PW, Prasad BM (1997) Repeated daily cocaine alters subsequent cocaine-induced increase of extracellular dopamine in the medial prefrontal cortex. J Pharmacol Exp Ther 281:54–61

Staahl BT, Crabtree GR (2013) Creating a neural specific chromatin landscape by npBAF and nBAF complexes. Curr Opin Neurobiol 23:903–913

Stipanovich A et al (2008) A phosphatase cascade by which rewarding stimuli control nucleosomal response. Nature 453:879–884

Sultan FA, Day JJ (2011) Epigenetic mechanisms in memory and synaptic function. Epigenomics 3:157–181

Sun HS et al (2017) Regulation of BAZ1A and nucleosome positioning in the nucleus accumbens in response to cocaine. Neuroscience 353:1–6

Thomas MJ, Beurrier C, Bonci A, Malenka RC (2001) Long-term depression in the nucleus accumbens: a neural correlate of behavioral sensitization to cocaine. Nat Neurosci 4:1217–1223

Tonegawa S, Pignatelli M, Roy DS, Ryan TJ (2015) Memory engram storage and retrieval. Curr Opin Neurobiol 35:101–109

Trantham H, Szumlinski KK, McFarland K, Kalivas PW, Lavin A (2002) Repeated cocaine administration alters the electrophysiological properties of prefrontal cortical neurons. Neuroscience 113:749–753

Tweedie-Cullen RY et al (2012) Identification of combinatorial patterns of post-translational modifications on individual histones in the mouse brain. PLoS One 7:e36980

Ungless MA, Whistler JL, Malenka RC, Bonci A (2001) Single cocaine exposure in vivo induces long-term potentiation in dopamine neurons. Nature 411:583–587

Vaillancourt K, Ernst C, Mash D, Turecki G (2017) DNA methylation dynamics and cocaine in the brain: progress and prospects. Genes (Basel) 8(5). pii: E138. doi: https://doi.org/10.3390/genes8050138

Viola TW et al (2016) Increased cocaine-induced conditioned place preference during periadolescence in maternally separated male BALB/c mice: the role of cortical BDNF, microRNA-212, and MeCP2. Psychopharmacology (Berl) 233:3279–3288

Vogel-Ciernia A, Wood MA (2014) Neuron-specific chromatin remodeling: a missing link in epigenetic mechanisms underlying synaptic plasticity, memory, and intellectual disability disorders. Neuropharmacology 80:18–27

Vogel-Ciernia A et al (2013) The neuron-specific chromatin regulatory subunit BAF53b is necessary for synaptic plasticity and memory. Nat Neurosci 16:552–561

Volkow ND et al (1997) Relationship between subjective effects of cocaine and dopamine transporter occupancy. Nature 386:827

Volkow ND, Fowler JS, Wang G-J (2003) The addicted brain: insights from imaging studies. J Clin Invest 111(p):1444–1451

Walker DM, Cates HM, Heller EA, Nestler EJ (2015) Regulation of chromatin states by drugs of abuse. Curr Opin Neurobiol 30:112–121

Walker DM et al (2018) Cocaine self-administration alters transcriptome-wide responses in the brain's reward circuitry. Biol Psychiatry. https://doi.org/10.1016/j.biopsych.2018.04.009

Wang L et al (2009) Chronic cocaine-induced H3 acetylation and transcriptional activation of CaMKII a in the nucleus accumbens is critical for motivation for drug reinforcement. Neuropsychopharmacology 35:913–928

Watson NA, Higgins JMG (2016) Histone kinases and phosphatases. Chromatin Signal Dis:75–94. https://doi.org/10.1016/B978-0-12-802389-1.00004-6

White AOAO et al (2016) BDNF rescues BAF53b-dependent synaptic plasticity and cocaine-associated memory in the nucleus accumbens. Nat Commun 7:11725

Williams JM, Steketee JD (2005) Effects of repeated cocaine on the release and clearance of dopamine within the rat medial prefrontal cortex. Synapse 55:98–109

Willuhn I, Burgeno LM, Groblewski PA, Phillips PE (2014) Excessive cocaine use results from decreased phasic dopamine signaling in the striatum. Nat Neurosci 17(5):704–709. https://doi.org/10.1038/nn.3694

Wolf ME (2016) Synaptic mechanisms underlying persistent cocaine craving. Nat Rev Neurosci 17:351–365

Wolf SF, Jolly DJ, Lunnen KD, Friedmann T, Migeon BR (2006) Methylation of the hypoxanthine phosphoribosyltransferase locus on the human X chromosome: implications for X-chromosome inactivation. Proc Natl Acad Sci 81:2806–2810

Wood MA, Hawk JD, Abel T (2006) Combinatorial chromatin modifications and memory storage: a code for memory? Learn Mem 13:241–244

Wright KN et al (2015) Methyl supplementation attenuates cocaine-seeking behaviors and cocaine-induced c-Fos activation in a DNA methylation-dependent manner. J Neurosci 35:8948–8958

Yager LM, Garcia AF, Wunsch AM, Ferguson SM (2015) The ins and outs of the striatum: role in drug addiction. Neuroscience 301:529–541

Yorgason JT, Jones SR, España RA (2011) Low and high affinity dopamine transporter inhibitors block dopamine uptake within 5 sec of intravenous injection. Neuroscience 182:125–132

Zhang Y, Reinberg D (2001) Transcription regulation by histone methylation: interplay between different covalent modifications of the core histone tails. Genes Dev 15(18):2343–2360. https://doi.org/10.1101/gad.927301.vcalcd

Zhao Y, Garcia BA (2015) Comprehensive catalog of currently documented histone modifications. Cold Spring Harb Perspect Biol 7

Zhao C, Eisinger BE, Driessen TM, Gammie SC (2014) Addiction and reward-related genes show altered expression in the postpartum nucleus accumbens. Front Behav Neurosci 8:388

Zhou Z et al (2006) Brain-specific phosphorylation of MeCP2 regulates activity-dependent Bdnf transcription, dendritic growth, and spine maturation. Neuron 52:255–269

Zhou Y et al (2008) Effects of cocaine place conditioning, chronic escalating-dose "binge" pattern cocaine administration and acute withdrawal on orexin/hypocretin and preprodynorphin gene expressions in lateral hypothalamus of Fischer and Sprague–Dawley rats. Neuroscience 153:1225–1234

Zhou Z, Yuan Q, Mash DC, Goldman D (2011) Substance-specific and shared transcription and epigenetic changes in the human hippocampus chronically exposed to cocaine and alcohol. Proc Natl Acad Sci 108:6626–6631

Molecular Mechanisms of Amphetamines

Maarten E. A. Reith and Margaret E. Gnegy

Contents

1 Introduction 266
2 Amphetamine and Dopamine (DA) Uptake, Efflux, and Storage 267
2.1 Amphetamine as a Substrate for Uptake at the DA Transporter (DAT) 267
2.2 Role of Na^+ and Transporter Conformation 268
2.3 DA Synthesis and VMAT2 270
2.4 Organic Cation 3 Transporter (OCT3) 272
3 Requirements for Amphetamine Stimulation of Outward Transport of DA 273
3.1 Intracellular Calcium 273
3.2 PKC Activity 273
3.3 CaMKII Activity 277
3.4 ERK Activity 278
4 Effects of Modifiers of Presynaptic Amphetamine Action on Behavior and Therapeutic Possibilities Directed at Amphetamine Abuse 279
4.1 DAT Blockers/Substrates 279
4.2 VMAT2 Blockers/Substrates 281
4.3 PKC Inhibitors 282
4.4 CaMKII Inhibitors 285
4.5 OCT3 Inhibitors 285
5 Concluding Remarks 286
References 286

M. E. A. Reith (✉)
Department of Psychiatry, New York University School of Medicine, New York, NY, USA
e-mail: Maarten.Reith@nyulangone.org; maarten.reith@nyumc.org

M. E. Gnegy
Department of Pharmacology, University of Michigan School of Medicine, Ann Arbor, MI, USA
e-mail: pgnegy@umich.edu

M. A. Nader, Y. L. Hurd (eds.), *Substance Use Disorders*,
Handbook of Experimental Pharmacology 258, https://doi.org/10.1007/164_2019_251

Abstract

There is a plethora of amphetamine derivatives exerting stimulant, euphoric, anti-fatigue, and hallucinogenic effects; all structural properties allowing these effects are contained within the amphetamine structure. In the first part of this review, the interaction of amphetamine with the dopamine transporter (DAT), crucially involved in its behavioral effects, is covered, as well as the role of dopamine synthesis, the vesicular monoamine transporter VMAT2, and organic cation 3 transporter (OCT3). The second part deals with requirements in amphetamine's effect on the kinases PKC, CaMKII, and ERK, whereas the third part focuses on where we are in developing anti-amphetamine therapeutics. Thus, treatments are discussed that target DAT, VMAT2, PKC, CaMKII, and OCT3. As is generally true for the development of therapeutics for substance use disorder, there are multiple preclinically promising specific compounds against (meth)amphetamine, for which further development and clinical trials are badly needed.

Keywords

Amphetamine use disorder · Catecholamine · Dopamine · Monoamine transporter · Neurotransmitter release · Protein kinase

1 Introduction

As psychoactive substances, amphetamines exert stimulant, euphoric, and anti-fatigue effects. Their structures derive from the β-phenylethylamine core structure. Human use of natural amphetamines dates back millennia. Thus, *Catha edulis* (Khat) is an evergreen plant in Africa and the Arabian Peninsula; chewing its fresh leaves increases energy levels, alertness, self-esteem, and elation. The effects of Khat are attributed mostly to one active component, cathinone, i.e., amphetamine with a keto functional group in the aliphatic chain (see Carvalho et al. 2012). The plant *Ephedra sinica* in the family Ephedraceae is known in China as Ma huang ("looking for trouble"), and its major active component was identified in 1887 as ephedrine (see Sulzer et al. 2005). As contained by the herb, ephedrine was originally used for treating asthma and upper respiratory infections. Over-the-counter ephedrine was a popular appetite suppressant and performance booster until it was banned from use as dietary supplement by the FDA in 2004. Ephedrine is amphetamine with an aliphatic hydroxyl substitution and an extra nitrogen-methyl group. Synthetic amphetamine was invented in 1887. After its introduction commercially in 1932 as Benzedrine, it became highly popular as an alertness enhancer and a treatment for asthma. Since 1939 amphetamine is only available by prescription for weight control, narcolepsy, and attention deficit disorder, in several formulations, among which Adderall is well-known as a mixture of d- and l-amphetamine (see Sulzer 2011).

Substitutions at the aromatic ring of amphetamine, at the α and β carbons of the aliphatic chain, and at the amine terminal yield a wide range of amphetamines (see Carvalho et al. 2012). Aromatic ring substitutions along with *N*-substitutions can give hallucinogenic activity, with 2,5-dimethoxyphenylisopropylamine (DMA) and 2,5-dimethoxy-4-methylamphetamine (DOM) as prominent examples. Both hallucinogenic and stimulant actions are seen with methylenedioxy substitutions on the phenyl ring (3,4-methylenedioxyamphetamine (MDA) and 3,4-methylenedioxymethamphetamine (MDMA)). Additionally, there is a whole new series of amphetamines based on the cathinone structure on the market, in many cases, disguised as "bath salts," with slight modifications of the parent drugs in order to circumvent drug laws (Mayer et al. 2017).

All structural properties allowing the above pharmacological effects are, in essence, contained within the amphetamine structure. Substitutions can enhance a certain effect; for example, only high doses of amphetamine, well above what are considered therapeutic doses, are needed for psychotic effects such as delusions, paranoia, and hallucinations (Wallis et al. 1949; Herman and Nagler 1954; Johnson and Milner 1966). This review focuses on amphetamine as the prototype of the plethora of amphetamine-like structures. The overall focus is on presynaptic mechanisms of action of amphetamine and on the use of mechanistic knowledge for developing anti-amphetamine therapeutics.

2 Amphetamine and Dopamine (DA) Uptake, Efflux, and Storage

2.1 Amphetamine as a Substrate for Uptake at the DA Transporter (DAT)

Although the capability of monoamine transporters to transport nonphenolic phenethylamines such as amphetamine is a universally accepted dogma, most initial experiments failed to demonstrate active uptake of these amines into noradrenergic neurons (Ross and Renyi 1966; Thoenen et al. 1968; Baldessarini and Vogt 1971). Evidence for the substrate character of amphetamine came from the work by the group of De Souza (Zaczek et al. 1991), demonstrating active uptake of [^{3}H]amphetamine into striatal synaptosomes that was saturable, of high affinity, and ouabain-sensitive and temperature-dependent. Some skepticism could be advanced regarding these results because of the highly lipophilic nature of amphetamine, causing substantial background signal from nonspecifically accumulated [^{3}H]amphetamine. Any lingering doubts were dispelled by subsequent patch-clamp experiments with systems heterologously expressing hDAT (human DAT) which demonstrated inward current associated with active amphetamine uptake along with determination of accumulated amphetamine by HPLC (Sonders et al. 1997; Sitte et al. 1998). The same approach that uncovered [^{3}H]amphetamine uptake into striatal synaptosomes did not enable measuring [^{3}H]amphetamine uptake into cortical synaptosomes (Zaczek et al. 1991), even though [^{3}H]norepinephrine (NE) or [^{3}H]serotonin (5-HT) uptake is routinely measured into such synaptosomes. Regarding uptake by the 5-HT transporter (SERT), current data show the affinity of amphetamine to be low (Rothman et al. 2001). As far as uptake by the NE transporter (NET) in the cortex, it is likely that the transport rate for amphetamine is not high enough for detection with [^{3}H]substrate. This is very possible, as different substrates for a given transporter can have different translocation rates. Indeed, whereas transport of [^{3}H]DA by DAT in striatal synaptosomes displays a V_{max} between 25 and 125 pmol/mg protein/min) (Holz and Coyle 1974; Zimanyi et al. 1989; Xu et al. 1995), that of [^{3}H]amphetamine has a V_{max} of only ~0.03 pmol/mg protein/min (as calculated from the value based on mg tissue in the work of Zaczek et al. (1991)). If the V_{max} of amphetamine for uptake by NET is also much lower than that of NE, this would undoubtedly produce a nondetectable signal in the standard tritiated ligand uptake assays. Convincing demonstration of amphetamine's substrate property in the case of the NE transporter (NET) comes from the work of the Rudnick lab (Wall et al. 1995). In LLC porcine kidney 1 cells (LLC-PK1) transfected with NET (LLC-NET cells), amphetamine induced efflux of preloaded [^{3}H]MPP$^+$ (1-methyl-4-phenylpyridinium) through a process of exchange which requires amphetamine uptake. A concentration of amphetamine that inhibited uptake of the [^{3}H]substrate used for preloading by 80% caused a similar amount of efflux from LLC-DAT cells as compared with NET cells, but very little efflux from LLC-SERT cells. This work, as well as that of Rothman et al. (2001), reports on amphetamine and a number of its derivatives in uptake and efflux experiments with DAT, NET, and SERT; the results indicate varying relative potencies toward uptake and efflux, indicating that inhibitory potency and the ability to stimulate efflux are independent properties for amphetamine-like compounds.

It is important to keep in mind that in addition to amphetamine uptake into cells or nerve terminals by the DAT (or NET), there is passive diffusion of amphetamine into the cell interior based on its appreciable lipophilicity (Lentzen and Philippu 1981). The diffusion process brings in amphetamine rapidly until the inside and outside concentrations are equal. In parental HEK cells (without the hDAT enabling active amphetamine uptake), the diffusion of amphetamine reaches its plateau in 1 min; this accumulated amphetamine is only a fraction of what is observed after 1 min of amphetamine uptake by HEK-hDAT cells (Sitte et al. 1998).

2.2 Role of Na$^+$ and Transporter Conformation

It is well-known that the binding of many DAT blockers is stimulated by Na$^+$ (Li and Reith 1999; Corera et al. 2000), but the role of Na$^+$ in the first recognition step for substrates (initiating uptake) for DAT has been debated for some time (see Corera et al. 2000). In the case of substrates, the measuring tool is substrate-induced inhibition of binding of a radiolabeled blocker to DAT, and to see the effect of Na$^+$, one needs a Na$^+$-free buffer which in turn hinders measurable binding of a Na$^+$-dependent radiolabeled blocker. For SERT, the Rudnick group (Humphreys et al. 1994) could take advantage of [^{125}I]RTI-55 (a phenyltropane analog of cocaine) binding in the absence of Na$^+$, and they were able to show that 5-HT binding was stimulated by Na$^+$. In our work on substrate binding to DAT (Li and Reith 1999, 2000), we were finally able to truly measure the effect of Na$^+$ on substrate binding in a Na^+-free buffer that still allowed the detection of sufficient [^{3}H]WIN 35,428 binding (Li et al. 2002). This approach showed that the binding of amphetamine, as that of DA, tyramine, and octopamine, in cell-free membrane preparations, does not require Na^+ and is not stimulated by Na^+. In contrast to the situation with cell-free preparations, Na^+ stimulates the binding of DA in cells, pointing to the importance of the intracellular ion environment and membrane potential in the interaction of DA with the DAT and the integration of Na^+ in this interaction (Chen et al. 2003; Chen and Reith 2004).

Although Na^+ is not strictly required for amphetamine binding to DAT per se, Na^+ plays an important role regarding the availability of the proper DAT conformation that substrates, including amphetamine, can access. In order for amphetamine to be taken up by DAT, it first needs to bind to the outward-facing state of the transporter, which is the ion/substrate-free (apo) state in which the transporter is open to the extracellular environment. This is the start of each substrate translocation cycle that describes the movement of substrate through the transporter, with the different conformations originally depicted in cartoon-style (Rudnick and Clark 1993) before the advent of actual structures; currently, these conformations are specified by crystal structures for the DAT-like transporters LeuT (Yamashita et al. 2005) and dDAT (Penmatsa et al. 2015). In the following, some references describe equivalent LeuT or dDAT conformations. Na^+ binding prepares the DAT for amphetamine binding by stabilizing the transporter in the fully outward-facing state, with the extracellular gate entirely open and Na^+ (and also Cl^-) bound (Singh et al. 2008). Prior to the structural work, the capability of Na^+ to promote outward-facing DAT conformations became clear (Chen et al. 2004b). After stabilization of the outward conformation by Na^+, the translocation cycle continues by amphetamine binding to the primary S1 binding site, which induces closure of the extracellular gate, giving the occluded conformation (Na^+, Cl^-, substrate bound) (Singh et al. 2007; Zhou et al. 2007). If the equivocal two-site model of the Javitch/Weinstein group for substrate (Shi et al. 2008) is applied to amphetamine, a second amphetamine molecule binds to the secondary S2 site in the extracellular vestibule of DAT, facilitating transition to a conformation open to the cytosol, the full inward-facing state (Krishnamurthy and Gouaux 2012). Ion and substrate then dissociate from S1, generating the apo inward-facing state. A detailed mechanism for release of Na^+ from the second Na^+ site has been proposed by Malinauskaite et al. (2014) based on structures of MhsT, a *Bacillus halodurans* transporter in the same family as DAT and LeuT. Finally, the DAT reorients itself to the outward-facing apo state, a step that is rate-limiting in the overall translocation process (Zimanyi et al. 1989; Chen et al. 2001; Erreger et al. 2008). An allosteric interaction network that links Na^+ binding with conformational changes during transport is conserved between the bacterial LeuT and human DAT (Stolzenberg et al. 2015).

It can be seen that in the above cycle, the uptake of amphetamine is stoichiometrically coupled to that of Na^+. The dDAT structure bound with amphetamine to its central binding site is partially occluded, as with DA; in contrast, inhibitors such as cocaine hold the transporter in an outward-open conformation (Wang et al. 2015). The LeuT does not provide information about Cl^- transport, but DAT requires external Cl^- for activity, and the classical cotransport model postulates uptake of DA (or amphetamine) along with Cl^- (Rudnick and Clark 1993). In contrast to this cotransport model, ion substitution in whole-hDAT-cell patch-clamp experiments suggests that both extracellular and intracellular Cl^- facilitate transporter turnover (Erreger et al. 2008).

Amphetamine's lipophilicity allows it to be taken up into the cell interior, but in order for its intracellular concentration to rise above that present externally, it needs to be actively taken up by DAT (Jones et al. 1999). Active uptake of substrate by DAT is driven by the Na^+ gradient, with high Na^+ levels extraneuronally and low Na^+ levels intraneuronally; the Na^+ gradient is maintained by Na^+, K^+-ATPase (see Rudnick and Clark 1993). With each substrate molecule, two Na^+ ions are translocated inwardly in accordance with the outward-directed Na^+ gradient. Indeed, increasing Na^+ permeability by veratridine or batrachotoxin is inhibitory to DA uptake by striatal synaptosomes (Holz and Coyle 1974). Reducing the outward Na^+ gradient not only decreased DA uptake (Holz and Coyle 1974; Liang and Rutledge 1982), but had a profound effect on DA efflux by DAT in the reversed mode. Thus, inhibition of Na^+, K^+-ATPase by ouabain caused efflux of preloaded [^{3}H]DA in striatal slices and potentiated amphetamine-induced [^{3}H]DA release. Liang and Rutledge (1982) conclude that amphetamine-induced efflux of [^{3}H]DA is regulated not only by the [^{3}H]DA gradient and the availability of the transporter at the inside of the membrane but also by the outward-directed Na^+ gradient.

Transport of one molecule of positively charged substrate, two molecules of Na^+, and one Cl^- is electrogenic (Berfield et al. 1999), raising the expectation that both uptake and efflux are dependent upon membrane potential. Although uptake was clearly found to be dependent on membrane potential (Sonders et al. 1997), for a long time DA efflux through DAT in the reversed mode was thought to be membrane potential-independent (see Leviel 2011). With the advent of patch-clamping combined with amperometry on cells expressing hDAT, Khoshbouei et al. (2003) were able to demonstrate that amphetamine-induced DA efflux is not only regulated by intracellular Na^+ but is also dependent upon membrane potential with DA efflux being electrogenic; essential to amphetamine's activation of DA efflux is its ability to increase intracellular Na^+ as measured by intracellular Na^+ fluorescence from Sodium Green.

2.3 DA Synthesis and VMAT2

Despite the knowledge that amphetamine is a substrate for the DAT and NET, questions still remain as to the physiological mechanism of amphetamine action. As a competitive substrate for the monoamine transporters, amphetamine will block uptake and elicit reverse transport (Liang and Rutledge 1982). In many mechanistic respects, amphetamine acts differently from pure reuptake blockers (Carlsson et al. 1966; Heikkila et al. 1975). For instance, the pattern of DA metabolites is entirely different for amphetamine versus a blocker like cocaine. Administration of amphetamine but not uptake blockers results in a rapid decline in dihydroxyphenylacetic acid (DOPAC) (Butcher et al. 1988; Hurd and Ungerstedt 1989; Nomikos et al. 1990), a metabolite of a newly synthesized pool of DA (Zetterstrom et al. 1988).

At lower doses, amphetamine preferentially releases a newly synthesized pool of DA. Administration of the tyrosine hydroxylase inhibitor α-methyl-*para*-tyrosine (AMPT) simultaneously with amphetamine blocks the DA-releasing effect of amphetamine (Smith 1963; Weissman et al. 1966; Chiueh and Moore 1975; Butcher et al. 1988). In the in vivo study of Chiueh and Moore (1975), perfusion of AMPT into cat ventricles 10 min prior to amphetamine blocked the accumulation of [^{3}H]DA that was newly synthesized from perfused [^{3}H]tyrosine. DA stores will not be depleted by the AMPT in these short time frames, leading to the conclusion that newly synthesized DA is a principal substrate for amphetamine-stimulated DA efflux. DAT-mediated DA efflux is distinguished from exocytosis and the effect of DAT blockers in that extracellular Ca^{2+} is not required for amphetamine-stimulated reverse transport (Raiteri et al. 1976; Arnold et al. 1977).

In addition to the plasmalemmal transporter, DAT, amphetamine acts at the vesicular monoamine transporter, VMAT2. For an excellent historical account of the interaction of amphetamine and vesicles, see Sulzer et al. (2005). Amphetamine binds directly to VMAT2 (Gonzalez et al. 1994; Peter et al. 1994; Teng et al. 1998; Partilla et al. 2006) and can elicit efflux of [^{3}H]DA from vesicles by carrier-mediated exchange (Peter et al. 1994; Partilla et al. 2006). At higher concentrations, amphetamine elicits release of DA from vesicles through an uptake-independent pathway (Floor and Meng 1996) and, acting as a weak base, disrupts the proton gradient needed to retain intravesicular DA (Sulzer et al. 1995; Floor and Meng 1996). Controversy has surrounded the role of VMAT2 and synaptic vesicles in the mechanism of amphetamine action. Initial studies found that depleting DA stores with reserpine either in vivo or in vitro in slices either had no effect or actually increased amphetamine-stimulated DA efflux (Chiueh and Moore 1975; Niddam et al. 1985; Ofori et al. 1986; Parker and Cubeddu 1986). Reserpine is more effective in reducing DA efflux and locomotor behavior elicited by higher doses of amphetamine than by lower doses (0.5–1 mg/kg) (Cadoni et al. 1995; Sabol and Seiden 1998). A caveat in interpreting the effect of reserpine is that by depleting DA it will increase tyrosine hydroxylase activity (German et al. 1981).

Undoubtedly vesicles contribute strongly to the maximal DA released by amphetamine, although VMAT2 is not absolutely required for amphetamine to release DA from nerve terminals (Pifl et al. 1995; Fon et al. 1997; Wang et al. 1997; Patel et al. 2003). Egana et al. (2009) used pull-down assays to identify a functional interaction between DAT and the synaptic vesicle protein synaptogyrin. A recent study, using the VMAT2 inhibitor (+)-CYY477, a highly selective congener of tetrabenazine, found that the drug blocked locomotion stimulated by 3.0 mg/kg amphetamine in mice but had no effect on cocaine-stimulated locomotor activity (Freyberg et al. 2016). Unlike with reserpine pretreatment, the DA stores were likely intact following (+)-CYY477. Using sophisticated genetic and optical approaches in *Drosophila melanogaster*, Freyberg et al. (2016) determined that amphetamine requires both DAT and VMAT2 and, moreover, that amphetamine must be taken up by VMAT2 into the vesicle. Two very important conclusions arose from these studies. First, it was clear from their experiments that amphetamine was acting as a "releaser" at DAT, not an uptake blocker. If amphetamine were only acting to block reuptake at DAT, (+)-CYY477, which is very selective for VMAT2, would not block amphetamine actions. Second, their data contradicted the notion that amphetamine blocks DA sequestration into vesicles by VMAT2, thereby making more DA available for efflux by DAT. If this were true, VMAT2 blockers would mimic or enhance the effect of amphetamine. (+)-CYY477 did not deplete vesicular stores, yet blocked the effect of amphetamine. However, reserpine, another VMAT2 blocker, depletes vesicular DA and can enhance the DA-releasing and locomotor action of amphetamine (Smith 1963; Chiueh and Moore 1975). It is evident that more needs to be learned concerning amphetamine and drug effects to reconcile potentially disparate results with alpha-MPT and VMAT blockers such as reserpine, tetrabenazine, and (+)-CYY477.

If amphetamine depletes vesicles of DA, one might expect that amphetamine would reduce exocytotic DA release. A number of studies reported reductions in stimulation-dependent DA release (Kuhr et al. 1985; Jones et al. 1998). However, the interaction between amphetamine action and stimulation-induced exocytotic DA release appears to be quite complex, depending on the dose of amphetamine, the preparation used, the degree of stimulation, and activation of presynaptic DA autoreceptors (Wieczorek and Kruk 1994; Schmitz et al. 2001; Siciliano et al. 2014). Recently, a new model of amphetamine action has been formulated that proposes that amphetamine elevates tonic DA (non-exocytotic) signaling through reverse transport and depleting vesicular stores, but activates phasic DA signaling by enhancing vesicular DA release from the readily releasable pool (Covey et al. 2013). These conclusions were drawn from experiments using fast-scan cyclic voltammetry in either freely moving or anesthetized rats (Avelar et al. 2013; Daberkow et al. 2013). Again, one must strongly consider the dose of amphetamine in interpretation of these actions (Calipari and Ferris 2013).

2.4 Organic Cation 3 Transporter (OCT3)

Of late, compelling evidence has been presented for the participation of OCT3 (SLC22A3) in amphetamine-stimulated DA efflux and behavior. OCT3 is a candidate for "uptake 2," a low-affinity, Na^+- and Cl^--independent, high-capacity uptake system for monoamines (Lightman and Iversen 1969). OCT3 is present in the periphery and the CNS and is present in glia and neurons including DA neurons (Gasser 2019). OCT3 transports monoamines, including DA, norepinephrine, and serotonin, but does not bind amphetamine or cocaine (Zhu et al. 2010). OCT3 is sensitively inhibited by corticosterone and decynium 22 (D22) but insensitive to cocaine (Gasser 2019). In a recent study on the role of OCT3 in amphetamine action (Mayer et al. 2018), D22 inhibited amphetamine-stimulated DA release, assessed using in vivo high-speed chronoamperometry, and locomotor behavior in OCT3$^{+/+}$ but not OCT3$^{-/-}$ mice. Amphetamine-stimulated efflux of [^{3}H]MPP$^+$ from superior cervical ganglia (a model for neurons carrying OCT3 and NET) was relatively insensitive to cocaine, but highly sensitive to D22 and corticosterone. Most notably, despite not being a substrate for OCT3, amphetamine elicited the release of [^{3}H] MPP^+ from YFP-hOCT3 HEK293 cells. These results strongly suggest that amphetamine is able to passively diffuse across the cell membrane and stimulate release of catecholamines through OCT3.

3 Requirements for Amphetamine Stimulation of Outward Transport of DA

3.1 Intracellular Calcium

Although amphetamine-stimulated outward transport of DA does not require extracellular Ca^{2+} (Raiteri et al. 1976; Arnold et al. 1977), intracellular Ca^{2+} is required. Amphetamine-induced increases in intracellular Ca^{2+} were reported in bovine chromaffin cells (Mundorf et al. 1999) and rat PC12 cells (Kantor et al. 2001) both of which contain the NET and in hDAT-HEK293 cells (Gnegy et al. 2004; Sambo et al. 2017). Chelation of intracellular Ca^{2+} with the cell-permeant Ca^{2+} chelator BAPTA-AM blocked the amphetamine-stimulated release of DA from PC12 and rat striatal slices (Kantor et al. 2001; Gnegy et al. 2004). The source of the intracellular Ca^{2+} spikes stimulated by 10 μM amphetamine in bovine chromaffin cells was apparently synaptic vesicles because blockade of the Ca^{2+} pumps in the endoplasmic reticulum and mitochondria did not affect the calcium spikes. Moreover, the content of vesicular Ca^{2+} was decreased after amphetamine treatment. However, the study in rat PC12 cells and hDAT-HEK293 cells demonstrated some involvement of extracellular Ca^{2+} (effect of nisoxetine or removal of extracellular Ca^{2+}) and as well as of Ca^{2+} stores in the endoplasmic reticulum (blockade by thapsigargin) (Gnegy et al. 2004). Giambalvo (2004) postulated that an increase in intracellular pH in response to amphetamine coupled with the increased Na^+ resulting from amphetamine transport would increase intracellular Ca^{2+} through enhanced Na/Ca exchange. The DAT-dependent depolarization elicited by amphetamine increases activity of voltage-gated ion channels, such as L-type Ca^{2+} channels (Cameron et al. 2015) and Ca^{2+}-activated potassium channels (Lin et al. 2016).

The increase in intracellular Ca^{2+} stimulated by amphetamine activates two major modulators of amphetamine action: protein kinase C (PKC) and Ca^{2+} and calmodulin-stimulated protein kinase II (CaMKII).

3.2 PKC Activity

In 1992, Giambalvo (1992a) first published a collection of papers that identified a distinct role for PKC in the amphetamine-stimulated reverse transport of DA. She demonstrated both in vivo and in vitro that low concentrations of amphetamine (0.1 mg/kg or $\leq 10^{-8}$ M) inhibited particulate PKC activity, while higher concentrations of amphetamine ($\geq$0.3 mg/kg or $>10^{-7}$ M) activated particulate

PKC activity, with opposing effects on soluble PKC activity. The activation or inhibition of PKC was kinetically due to increases or decreases, respectfully, in the affinity for Ca^{2+} (Giambalvo 1992a, b) which automatically ascribed the effect to a conventional, Ca^{2+}-sensitive PKC isozyme. Moreover, there was a direct correlation between the IC_{50} for inhibition of particulate PKC and IC_{50} for inhibition of amphetamine-stimulated DA efflux by the PKC inhibitors in vitro (Giambalvo 1992b). Studies in striatal synaptoneurosomes demonstrated that some, but not all, of the PKC activity increased by amphetamine was due to occupation of DA receptors (Giambalvo 2003). The activation of PKC by amphetamine was inhibited by treatment of the synaptoneurosomes with BAPTA-AM or AMPT or by DAT blockers. Induction of reverse transport with low extracellular sodium or with the Na^+ K^+ ATPase inhibitor ouabain also increased particulate PKC activity. Thus outward transport through DAT had a stimulatory effect on PKC activity (Giambalvo 2003).

A parallel series of experiments explored the effects of acute and repeated amphetamine on the phosphorylation of the calmodulin-binding growth-associated protein-43, (GAP-43), to assess if changes in phosphorylation of this protein correlated with synaptic plasticity elicited by repeated amphetamine. In addition to binding calmodulin (in the absence of Ca^{2+}), GAP-43 is phosphorylated by PKC at one specific site, ser^{41} (Apel et al. 1990). Availability of a specific antibody permits $phosphoser^{41}$-GAP-43 to be a readout for PKC activity (Meiri et al. 1991). In a study in rat synaptosomes, Iwata et al. (1997) demonstrated that amphetamine dose-dependently increased the phosphorylation of GAP-43. The activation was maximal at 2 min, was blocked by the PKC inhibitor R31-8220, and required access of amphetamine to DAT. Interestingly, the amphetamine-stimulated phosphorylation was only partially dependent on Ca^{2+} and was not affected by either a DA D1 or D2 receptor blocker. The most parsimonious explanation for the activation of PKC in response to amphetamine is the amphetamine-stimulated elevation of cytosolic Ca^{2+} in the nerve terminal. Further, amphetamine elevates phospholipase C activity which would increase the diacylglycerol required for activation of conventional PKC isozymes (Giambalvo 2004).

The Ca^{2+}- and diacylglycerol-requiring β isozyme of PKC binds to DAT and contributes to amphetamine-stimulated DA efflux (Johnson et al. 2005b; Hadlock et al. 2011). Either select inhibitors of PKCβ or genetic deletion inhibits DAT-mediated efflux of DA in response to amphetamine (Kantor and Gnegy 1998; Chen et al. 2009; Zestos et al. 2016). Further studies involving inhibitors of PKCβ will be described below (Sect. 4.3).

Numerous studies show that activation of PKC influences trafficking of DAT but the results have been seemingly disparate. Incubation with high doses of a phorbol ester, phorbol myristate acetate (PMA), or amphetamine elicits internalization of DAT from the plasmalemmal membrane. The PKC-mediated reduction in DA uptake can be relatively rapid within 5 min (Gulley and Zahniser 2003) and consists of two phases, an initial desensitization of inward transport followed by an internalization of the transporter (Richards and Zahniser 2009). There are numerous excellent reviews describing the amphetamine- and PKC-stimulated internalization of DAT

(Zahniser and Sorkin 2009; Schmitt and Reith 2010; Ramamoorthy et al. 2011; Rastedt et al. 2017).

PKCβ also plays a role in DAT trafficking; activation of PKCβ rapidly inserts DAT into the plasmalemmal membrane (Johnson et al. 2005a; Furman et al. 2009). Studies using total internal reflection fluorescent microscopy demonstrated that activation of GFP-hDAT-mouse neuroblastoma N2a cells by amphetamine or DA increases surface DAT within 10 s. The substrate-induced increase in surface DAT was dose- and DAT-dependent and reversed upon removal of substrate. The increase was not dependent on D2 DA receptors but was blocked by inhibitors of PKCβ (Furman et al. 2009). These data appear to conflict with the internalization studies described above, but a clearer understanding of the reverse transport cycle and action of amphetamine might supply a unifying explanation.

With knowledge that the DAT was responsible for uptake of DA and seemingly the efflux of DA in response to amphetamine, Fischer and Cho (1979) conducted seminal experiments in support of a model of exchange diffusion through the transporter; that is, the movement of substrate from compartment one facilitates the movement of the same or another substrate into compartment two (Jardetzky 1966). In this way amphetamine movement through the transporter as a substrate would elicit the reverse transport of DA. This simple explanation was called into question following the discovery that substrates elicit currents through the neurotransmitter transporters (Sonders et al. 1997). As discussed above, transport through DAT is electrogenic. Three different currents pass through the DAT: a current coupled with substrate movement, a current uncoupled to the movement of substrate through the transporter, and a leak current, which represents the movement of ions down their electrochemical gradient independent of substrate (Sonders et al. 1997). Using heterologous hDAT-HEK293 cells, Sitte et al. (1998) found that uptake and releasing rates for DAT substrates did not form a perfect correlation; rather, the releasing action correlated with the ionic currents. In other words, there is asymmetry between uptake and outward transport instead of the symmetry expected in the exchange diffusion model. Further, in addition to the facilitated reverse transport through DAT, amphetamine can release DA through a channel-like mode, at a rate similar to exocytosis albeit with much less frequency than the regular transport mode (Kahlig et al. 2005). Thus amphetamine-stimulated DA efflux mediated by DAT is dependent on voltage and intracellular sodium and elicits depolarization (Khoshbouei et al. 2003; Carvelli et al. 2004; Meinild et al. 2004).

If the transporter is operating with a single pathway for substrates and uncoupled ion movement, then it is unlikely that inward and outward transport could occur simultaneously. Thus PKC activation could temper influx while promoting efflux, explaining how PKC activation initially desensitizes the uptake process but promotes release of DA. However, DAT exists in oligomers (Hastrup et al. 2001; Sorkina et al. 2003) which opens the possibility that one monomer can participate in influx, while another is mediating reverse transport. This is suggested by the clever studies of Seidel et al. (2005) who transfected cells with a concatemer consisting of a GABA transporter and a serotonin transporter. Treatment with amphetamine, which binds to the serotonin but not the GABA transporter, reduced GABA influx and enhanced GABA efflux. These data strongly suggest that amphetamine can act at dimers and that influx and efflux occur through separate but coupled monomers (Sitte and Freissmuth 2010, 2015). Moreover, the amphetamine-stimulated efflux of GABA was reduced by inhibitors of PKC indicating that activation of PKC by amphetamine would affect one unit of the dimer to enhance the outward transport (Seidel et al. 2005). The asymmetry of amphetamine uptake and stimulated efflux is reinforced by the fact that inhibition of PKC does not block uptake of DAT substrates but does reduce amphetamine-stimulated DA efflux (Kantor and Gnegy 1998; Johnson et al. 2005b; Zestos et al. 2016). One other way that DAT oligomerization has been linked with amphetamine action is related to transporter trafficking. The capability of amphetamine to reduce surface DAT has been linked with its ability to dissociate DAT oligomers at the cell surface, enabling monomers to be endocytosed (Chen and Reith 2008; Li et al. 2010).

Several studies strongly suggest that the substrate for the potentiating action of PKC on amphetamine-stimulated outward transport is DAT. The N-terminus of the DAT is a rich substrate for phosphorylation by several different protein kinases, notably PKC, CaMKII, and ERK (Foster and Vaughan 2017). Vaughan et al. (1997) originally demonstrated that phosphorylation of the DAT was elevated by incubation of synaptosomes with a PKC activator or with the phosphatase inhibitor, okadaic acid. The phosphorylation of DAT occurs only on the N-terminal serines and threonines (Foster et al. 2002). Amphetamine, but not uptake blockers, stimulated the phosphorylation of DAT which was blocked by inhibitors of PKC (Cervinski et al. 2005). Although amphetamine-stimulated phosphorylation of DAT was followed by a downregulation of the transporter, the latter event does not depend on N-terminus phosphorylation. Either deletion or mutation of known phosphorylation sites within the first 21 amino acids blocks phosphorylation of DAT but not DAT downregulation (Granas et al. 2003; Cervinski et al. 2005). N-terminus phosphorylation of DAT is important for amphetamine-induced DA efflux (Khoshbouei et al. 2004), however. Deletion of the first 22 amino acids of DAT ablated DA efflux elicited by amphetamine but had no effect on DA uptake. Mutation of serines 2, 4, 7, 12, and 13 to non-phosphorylatable alanine significantly reduced amphetamine action (Khoshbouei et al. 2004; Wang et al. 2016; Karam et al. 2017; Rastedt et al. 2017). Through the use of phospho-specific antibodies, Karam et al. (2017) found that PKC activation by PMA, AMPH, and okadaic acid increased the phosphorylation of DAT at serine 7 and serine 12 in hDAT-HEK293-derived Em4 cells. Phosphorylation induced by amphetamine and okadaic acid was reduced by inhibition of either PKC or CaMKII. The requirement of this phosphorylation for amphetamine-stimulated locomotion has been demonstrated in *Drosophila melanogaster* larvae; amphetamine stimulates a DAT-dependent increase in crawling behavior in those larvae. Human DAT rescues the behavior in *dDAT* null *Drosophila* larvae. Addition of an hDAT mutant where 5 N-terminal serines were mutated to phosphate-mimicking aspartate (hDAT-StoD) but not to alanine (hDAT-StoA) restored amphetamine sensitivity (Pizzo et al. 2013; Karam et al. 2017). These studies further demonstrated that the membrane raft protein flotillin is required for amphetamine-stimulated behaviors. Therefore the AMPH-stimulated phosphorylation of DAT in the N-terminus does not actually mediate efflux, but it may induce a conformation and membrane localization that permits reverse transport.

Studies in rat pheochromocytoma (PC12) cells, which contain the norepinephrine transporter (NET), raise the question of the importance in N-terminal serines for inhibition of amphetamine-stimulated DA efflux by PKC inhibitors. In a PC12 cell line that released DA but contained NET but not DAT, AMPH-stimulated DA efflux was mimicked by PKC activation and blocked by PKC inhibitors (Kantor et al. 2001). The AMPH-stimulated DA efflux required intracellular but not extracellular Ca^{2+} and was not altered by reserpine pretreatment. These results mirror those found for DAT in rat striatum (Kantor and Gnegy 1998). However, there are no N-terminal serines in NET; three threonines are present in positions 19, 30, and 58; they are not involved in PKC-mediated downregulation of NET (Ramamoorthy et al. 2011). The main phosphorylation sites for PKC-induced internalization of NET are T258 and S259, but conversion of those sites to alanine abolishes only 60% of phosphorylation. So PKC phosphorylation of an N-terminus threonine that is permissive for amphetamine-induced DA efflux is possible (Ramamoorthy et al. 2011).

3.3 CaMKII Activity

A role for calmodulin (CaM) and CaM kinase II in the release of DA and behaviors stimulated by amphetamine began with investigations into the molecular mechanisms responsible for amphetamine sensitization. Humans and laboratory animals exhibit enhanced behavioral effects to amphetamine upon withdrawal from repeated ($\geq$2 times) amphetamine treatment (Robinson and Becker 1986). Concomitant with the enhanced behavior is an increase in amphetamine-stimulated DA efflux greater than that achieved following saline pretreatment. The "sensitized" amphetamine-sensitive DA efflux exhibits a very different characteristic from that in naïve animals: extracellular Ca^{2+} and CaMKII are required (Kantor et al. 1999). The same was true in animals sensitized to cocaine (Pierce and Kalivas 1997). Using anti-phosphoser^{41}-GAP-43 and anti-3 phosphosynapsin I, Iwata et al. (1996) detected enhanced phosphorylation of both the PKC substrate GAP-43 and the CaMKII substrate synapsin I in striatum from rats that received a sensitizing regimen of amphetamine as compared to drug-naïve controls. Notably there was no effect of amphetamine on the phosphorylation of synapsin I in controls. Although amphetamine did not increase phosphorylation of synapsin I in vivo in control rats, potential effects of amphetamine on the CaMKII substrate site of synapsin were investigated in striatal synaptosomes (Iwata et al. 1997). Treatment of the synaptosomes with amphetamine increased the phosphorylation of synapsin I but at very low concentrations, from 1 to 100 nM; phosphorylation by amphetamine was maximal at 1 min and was inhibited by the DAT blocker, nomifensine.

Further explorations into the role of CaMKII revealed striking parallels to the findings with PKC. Fog et al. (2006) used the C-terminus of hDAT to identify the α isoform of CaMKII (αCaMKII) as a binding protein of DAT. Activation of CaMKII increased the amphetamine-stimulated release of DA in heterologous cells and cultured mouse midbrain DA neurons, while inhibition of CaMKII inhibited DA release by amphetamine in heterologous cells, mouse midbrain DA neurons, and mouse striatal slices. The binding site for αCaMKII was the C-terminus, but CaMKII stimulated phosphorylation of an N-terminus peptide. The conclusion from their study is that αCaMKII stimulates reversed DA transport by binding to the C-terminus of DAT and thereby phosphorylating N-terminal serines. αCaMKII also co-immunoprecipitated with DAT in mouse striatal synaptosomes, and mice lacking αCaMKII display reduced amphetamine-induced DA efflux which is mimicked in mice with reduced αCaMKII activity as part of the Angelman syndrome (Steinkellner et al. 2012). Both in vitro and in vivo application of membrane-permeable C terminal DAT peptides attenuates amphetamine-induced DA release, indicating the importance of DAT C terminal protein-protein interactions in this process (Rickhag et al. 2013). The involvement of αCaMKII in the in vivo action of amphetamine was investigated in αCaMKII-deficient mice by Steinkellner et al. (2012). DA efflux induced by amphetamine in the striatum was reduced as measured by microdialysis, as was the acute locomotor response to amphetamine. While the rewarding effect of amphetamine in the conditioned place preference test was preserved in the CaMKII knockout mice, the sensitization of locomotor activity was markedly reduced. Thus, for amphetamine to exert most of its in vivo effects, the presence of αCaMKII is required, not only in acute but also chronic exposure paradigms. The conflicting results concerning the lack of effect of CaMKII inhibitors in reducing amphetamine-stimulated DA release in control rats (Iwata et al. 1996; Kantor et al. 1999) versus the obvious inhibitory effects in mouse (Fog et al. 2006) and *Drosophila* (Karam et al. 2017) are not yet explained but may simply be due to species differences.

3.4 ERK Activity

Another prominent N-terminus phosphorylation site in DAT that affects, but may not be required for, amphetamine-stimulated DA efflux is threonine 53 (T53), which is proximal to transmembrane domain 1. In an investigation of protein kinases that phosphorylate the N-terminus of DAT, p53 was revealed as a prominent substrate of the extracellular receptor kinase (ERK) (Foster et al. 2002). Foster et al. (2012) found that this site was important for both DA uptake and amphetamine-stimulated DA efflux. The direction of the change in influx/efflux differed depending on the methods used for analysis (Foster et al. 2002; Challasivakanaka et al. 2017), but, notably, both influx and efflux were affected and in the same direction.

4 Effects of Modifiers of Presynaptic Amphetamine Action on Behavior and Therapeutic Possibilities Directed at Amphetamine Abuse

The reinforcing effects of amphetamine depend on dopaminergic transmission (Wise and Bozarth 1985; Vezina et al. 2002; Iversen 2006). There is no approved drug for treating amphetamine abuse, and no drug tested thus far has shown sufficient efficacy to merit clinical use (Lee et al. 2018a). Limited benefit in treating amphetamine abuse has been demonstrated for methylphenidate, buprenorphine, modafinil, and naltrexone (Lee et al. 2018a); DAT substrates show efficacy in preclinical assays of stimulant dependence (Howell and Negus 2014). However, methylphenidate, buprenorphine, and DAT substrates have a significant abuse liability. A preferred treatment, of course, would be one that has no abuse liability.

4.1 DAT Blockers/Substrates

DAT inhibitors, of course, continue to be important tools in studying effects of amphetamine. Thus, if a given effect can be blocked by a DAT inhibitor, a role for amphetamine uptake by DAT is indicated. In this way it can be distinguished from an effect resulting from passive diffusion of amphetamine into the cell interior based on its lipophilicity (see Sect. 2.1). However, the more interesting question is whether DAT inhibitors (or substrates) can be used to attenuate amphetamine effects without themselves exerting untoward effects. Theoretically, because forward transport (uptake) and reverse transport (release) are separate and mechanistically different processes (see Sects. 2.1 and 3.2), it should be possible to target each one individually. Proof of principle comes from the demonstration that interfering with the binding of PIP2 to the N-terminus of DAT (by the peptide pal-HRQKHFEKRR) impairs amphetamine-induced DA efflux without affecting uptake (Hamilton et al. 2014). Developments in the last decade point to a number of promising compounds or leads.

Bupropion is clinically used as an antidepressant and as a smoking cessation agent (Malcolm et al. 2015). It is also being investigated as a candidate agonist medication for methamphetamine addiction (Brensilver et al. 2013). Bupropion, along with benztropine and GBR 12935, falls in the category of atypical DAT inhibitors with a preference for more inward-facing DAT conformations and surprising lack of behaviorally stimulatory action (Katz et al. 1999; Schmitt et al. 2008; Schmitt and Reith 2011; Loland et al. 2012) (see also below). Preclinically, bupropion as well as its *S*- and *R*-hydroxy metabolites produced full methamphetamine-like effects in a drug discrimination test (Banks et al. 2016). Unfortunately, recent clinical trials have not been able to uncover efficacy against methamphetamine in humans (Carson and Taylor 2014; Heinzerling et al. 2014; Anderson et al. 2015). High rates of medication nonadherence and placebo response rates weakening statistical power remain important obstacles in interpreting stimulant dependence pharmacotherapy trials.

Phenmetrazine is a stimulant that has been used clinically as an appetite suppressant before it was withdrawn from the market. Its abuse potential can be mitigated by giving its prodrug, phendimetrazine, a schedule III controlled drug used as appetite suppressant. Preclinical studies show phendimetrazine, as amphetamine, attenuates cocaine self-administration (Banks et al. 2013a, b; Czoty et al. 2016). Phendimetrazine itself functions as a DAT inhibitor, which can also interfere with the substrate property of its metabolite phenmetrazine (Solis et al. 2016), thereby somewhat mitigating its amphetamine-like DA-releasing effect. It would be of great interest to test phendimetrazine's effect on the action of amphetamine.

Other anti-amphetamine agents in preclinical research are the "partial substrates" also called "partial releasers." In a large series of phenethylamine structures, Blough and colleagues (see Reith et al. 2015) observed that upon increasing size, substrate releaser activity converted to uptake inhibition; as the increasing size of the phenethylamine structure nears the edge of the pharmacophore, the releasing potency weakens even before the compound becomes an uptake inhibitor. It is in this structural border region where we find the partial releasers. Thus, PAL-1045 (*N*-ethyl-naphtylaminopropane or ENAP) and PAL-193 (3,4-methylenedioxy-*N*-ethylamphetamine), rather than being substrates with full releasing capability, released no more than 78% and 61%, respectively, of preloaded [^{3}H]MPP$^+$ from rat synaptosomes (Rothman et al. 2012; Reith et al. 2015). PAL-1045, as bupropion, stabilizes inward conformations of monoamine transporters but, unlike bupropion, is still a substrate (Bhat et al. 2017 and see below final paragraph of this section). Whereas the full releaser 2-naphthyl analog of amphetamine, NAP, dose-dependently increased accumbal dialysate DA, PAL-1045 showed a low-efficacy flat dose-response curve (Rothman et al. 2012) in accordance with its partial releasing character. Within a structurally different family of diphenylmethyl-containing compounds, SoRI-9804 and SoRI-20040 only partially inhibited amphetamine-induced release of [^{3}H]DA or [^{3}H]MPP$^+$ from rat striatal synaptosomes at concentrations that themselves did not evoke release (SoRI-20040, in contrast to SoRI-9804, caused some release but not at concentrations up to 50 μM). In the presence of a fixed concentration of either compound, the amphetamine concentration efflux curve had a lower plateau than in their absence but was shifted to the right only minimally compared with the presence of an uptake blocker (cocaine or indatraline) (Rothman et al. 2009). Another difference was that a pure uptake blocker did not lower the efflux plateau of amphetamine (only shifted the amphetamine concentration curve to the right). In a previous study, the Rothman group had shown that SoRI-9804 and SoRI-20040 also only partially inhibited DA uptake by rat striatal synaptosomes (Pariser et al. 2008). The in vitro pharmacology is intriguing, and it needs to be assessed how consequential these effects will be in in vivo behavioral assays.

Finally, because inward-facing conformations of DAT are deficient in mediating DA efflux as exemplified by inward-facing D345N DAT (Chen et al. 2004a), one would speculate that amphetamine-induced efflux ought to be attenuated by inhibitors or substrates that increase the proportion of DAT residing in an inward-facing conformation. As detailed above, bupropion is such an inhibitor and was being considered as an anti-amphetamine treatment agent (Brensilver et al. 2013). Intriguingly, this property of bupropion also appears to underlie its in vitro pharmacochaperoning capability in rescuing folding-defective mutant DA transporters that occur in patients with infantile/juvenile dystonia/Parkinsonism (Beerepoot et al. 2016). In this context, it is relevant that noribogaine (the major metabolite of ibogaine, a compound useful in opioid detoxification based on anecdotal (Alper et al. 2008) and clinical/observational (Brown and Alper 2018) evidence) has the same chaperoning capability. Noribogaine and ibogaine stabilize inward SERT as well as DAT albeit with lower affinity for the latter (Jacobs et al. 2007; Bulling et al. 2012). A recent, very detailed biochemical and electrophysiological study on SERT shows PAL-1045 to be able to pharmacochaperone almost as well as noribogaine, with the two compounds apparently binding to the same site with the difference that PAL-1045 is still a substrate, while noribogaine is a non-(or almost?)-transported inhibitor (Bhat et al. 2017). This is an encouraging result because the binding site for ibogaine may well be outside the commonly considered binding sites for inhibitors and substrates. Bulling et al. (2012) rule out as binding sites for ibogaine the S1 site, the S2 site, and sites within the cytoplasmic pathway (to hold the transporter inward-open). The location is at present unknown, but its likely absence from the permeation pathway would allow forward substrate translocation. All evidence taken together so far indicate a potential for PAL-1045 to be an agonist treatment agent against amphetamine stimulant use disorder. As a side note, there is no evidence to suggest that the stabilizing effects of ibogaine on SERT and DAT are involved in its opioid detoxifying capability.

4.2 VMAT2 Blockers/Substrates

As detailed in Sect. 2.3, one component of amphetamine's action is the redistribution of DA from monoaminergic storage vesicles to the cytosol, by amphetamine acting as a substrate for the vesicular monoamine transporter (which in the brain is of the VMAT2 isoform) rather than a blocker of DA uptake into vesicles (Freyberg et al. 2016). As pointed out in Sect. 2.3, more work is needed to fully reconcile this role of vesicular redistributed DA serving as substrate for reverse transport by DAT with older results pointing to a preferential role of newly synthesized DA for amphetamine-induced release. Evidence as detailed below has been collected in the last two decades that point to VMAT2 as a relevant target for anti-amphetamine medication development, which adds weight to the scenario of vesicular redistributed DA being involved in behavioral effects of amphetamine.

Lobeline is the principal alkaloid of the plant *Lobelia inflata* LINN., the leaves of which were chewed for their central nicotine-like effects (Dwoskin and Crooks 2002). However, in contrast to nicotine, lobeline is not avidly self-administered, does not stimulate locomotion, and does not produce conditioned place preference (Fudala and Iwamoto 1986; Stolerman et al. 1995; Harrod et al. 2001, 2003). Clinically, lobeline has been used as a short-acting respiratory stimulant and to treat bronchitic asthma (King et al. 1928). With the advent of other, more effective medications, and due to some untoward side effects of lobeline, its clinical use has come to a halt (see Dwoskin and Crooks 2002). However, an intriguing observation suggested that its chemical structure contains properties that make lobeline an important starting point for developing anti-amphetamine: Lobeline inhibited amphetamine-induced overflow of DA from striatal slices (Dwoskin and Crooks 2002). Lobeline also inhibited [^{3}H]DA uptake into vesicles and promoted spontaneous [^{3}H]DA efflux from vesicles; the uptake inhibition was found to involve the tetrabenazine binding site on the vesicular VMAT2, but tetrabenazine itself did not enable spontaneous [^{3}H]DA efflux. In order to explain the ability of lobeline to interfere with the action of amphetamine or methamphetamine in enhancing cytosolic DA (which with the caveats mentioned above leads to DAT reversal and DA release extraneuronally), it was proposed that lobeline redistributes vesicular DA into a pool in cytosol that is not available to undergo reverse transport by DAT (Dwoskin and Crooks 2002). Much effort since these original observations has gone into developing lobeline analogs that are more selective for VMAT2 in comparison with DAT, SERT, and nicotine receptors. Through defunctionalization of lobeline to lobelane, and further dihydroxypropylation of the nitrogen in the central piperidine ring, GZ-793A was developed and found to attenuate methamphetamine self-administration in an oral formulation (Nickell et al. 2014). A recent study showed that GZ-793A decreased methamphetamine self-administration without altering food-maintained responding (Kangiser et al. 2018); the same group used a new scaffold to develop GZ-11610, which is highly selective for VMAT2 and specifically attenuates methamphetamine-induced hyperactivity (Lee et al. 2018b). Another promising series of lobeline-derived compounds consist of lobelane derivatives in which the central piperidine ring is replaced by a more conformationally restricted pyrrolidine ring (Nickell et al. 2014). Their biochemical in vitro profiles are encouraging for further preclinical work in behavioral assays. So far, all derivatives, as lobeline and lobelane themselves, inhibit vesicular [^{3}H]DA uptake at much lower concentrations than the binding of [^{3}H]tetrabenazine, a hallmark of a substrate property of the compounds. How important this is mechanistically is not clear, as pure VMAT2 inhibitors such as tetrabenazine itself and the more VMAT2-selective (+)-CYY477 are also capable of attenuating amphetamine's behavioral effects (Meyer et al. 2011; Freyberg et al. 2016). Although methamphetamine and amphetamine are known to exert various effects that differ (Goodwin et al. 2009), their similar actions in redistributing DA from vesicles into cytosol and enabling reverse transport through DAT (Eshleman et al. 1994; Jones et al. 1998; Rothman et al. 2001) make it likely that treatment compounds that have been tested in behavioral assays with methamphetamine will be equally effective in combatting amphetamine effects.

4.3 PKC Inhibitors

It is possible that protein kinase inhibitors which inhibit reverse but not forward transport through the DAT could be efficacious. Inhibitors of PKC and CaMKII have been tested in preclinical models of stimulant abuse and shown some efficacy (Lee and Messing 2008; Garcia-Pardo et al. 2016). Our focus in the rest of this article will be on the effects of PKC and CaMKII inhibitors on amphetamine-stimulated behaviors.

The report demonstrating a direct correlation between the IC_{50} for inhibition of particulate PKC and IC_{50} for inhibition of amphetamine-stimulated DA efflux by PKC inhibitors (Giambalvo 1992b) sparked further research on the effect of PKC inhibitors on amphetamine-stimulated activities (Gnegy 2003). General PKC inhibitors reduce amphetamine-stimulated DA efflux in rat striatum and nucleus accumbens (Giambalvo 1992a, b; Kantor and Gnegy 1998; Loweth et al. 2009) as do inhibitors more specific for PKCβ (Kantor et al. 1999; Johnson et al. 2005b; Zestos et al. 2016). Mice containing homozygous deletions for PKCβ had reduced DA influx and efflux in response to amphetamine as compared to wild type (Chen et al. 2009). A reduction in surface DAT in the PKCβ knockout mice was attributable to altered trafficking of the transporter (Chen et al. 2009). Nonselective or β isoform-selective PKC inhibitors reduced hyperlocomotion in rats stimulated by amphetamine, mirroring the effects on amphetamine-induced DA efflux (Browman et al. 1998; Zestos et al. 2016). As compared to wild type, amphetamine-stimulated locomotor activity was reduced in PKCβ knockout mice (Chen et al. 2009). In a microdialysis study where DA efflux and locomotor behavior were simultaneously monitored, perfusion of the selective PKCβ inhibitor, ruboxistaurin, into rat nucleus accumbens reduced DA efflux and locomotor behavior in response to amphetamine given intraperitoneally (Zestos et al. 2016). Ruboxistaurin had no effect on basal levels of DA, norepinephrine, glutamate, or GABA as shown by a stable isotope label retrodialysis procedure. Intracerebral injection of a structurally similar drug with specificity for PKCβ, enzastaurin, into rats shifted the dose-response curve for amphetamine-stimulated locomotor activity to the right. Interestingly, intracerebral enzastaurin decreased amphetamine-maintained responding in a fixed ratio 5 schedule of reinforcement with no effect on responding for sucrose (Altshuler et al. 2016).

In addition to reducing amphetamine-stimulated efflux, PKC activation inhibits (Cubeddu et al. 1989; Nimitvilai et al. 2013) and PKC inhibitors enhance the activity of DA autoreceptors (Luderman et al. 2015). The D2-like agonist, quinpirole, was more effective in inhibiting DA release in rat striatal synaptosomes from PKCβ knockout mice than from wild type (Luderman et al. 2015). Further, selective PKCβ inhibitors enhanced the D2 autoreceptor-stimulated decrease in DA release following both chemical and electrical stimulation. Because PKCβ activation internalizes D2 receptors (Namkung and Sibley 2004), inhibition of PKCβ led to retention of surface D2-like receptors in striatal synaptosomes and thus greater autoreceptor activity.

Based on these results, one could posit that inhibition of PKC would reduce the rise in extracellular DA following amphetamine treatment in two ways: by reducing reverse transport of DA through DAT and by enhancing DA autoreceptor activity. Yet in microdialysis experiments that simultaneously measured DA overflow in rat nucleus accumbens and locomotor behavior, blockade of DA autoreceptors had no effect on amphetamine stimulation of these activities (Zestos et al. 2019). Similarly, autoreceptor blockade did not affect inhibition of the amphetamine-stimulated activities by the PKCβ inhibitor, ruboxistaurin. The results were the opposite for cocaine, however. As with amphetamine, ruboxistaurin inhibited cocaine-stimulated DA overflow and locomotor activity. However, after pretreatment of the nucleus accumbens with the DA D2-like receptor blocker, raclopride, ruboxistaurin had no effect on cocaine-stimulated activities. These results indicate that inhibition of PKCβ reduces amphetamine-stimulated DA overflow and locomotor activity by diminishing DAT reverse transport, but blocks cocaine-stimulated effects by decreasing internalization of DA autoreceptors (Zestos et al. 2019).

One problem with considering a therapeutic use for PKC inhibitors in the brain is their poor absorption into the brain (Chico et al. 2009) and the possibility of deleterious effects from nonspecific and global inhibition of PKC. The assumption of generalized deleterious effects is not necessarily true; enzastaurin accesses the CNS and was well tolerated in human trials (Schwartzberg et al. 2014). PKC is implicated in CNS disorders, such as bipolar disorder (Zarate and Manji 2009) and drug abuse disorder, and PKC inhibitors have been considered as therapeutics (Zarate and Manji 2009; Garcia-Pardo et al. 2016). Tamoxifen has been used to successfully treat bipolar mania (Zarate and Manji 2009), and its effect has been attributed to its inhibition of PKC (Einat et al. 2007; Mikelman et al. 2017a). Although best known as a selective estrogen receptor modulator (SERM) at low doses, tamoxifen inhibits PKC at higher doses (O'Brian et al. 1985) and crosses the blood-brain barrier (Lien et al. 1991). Notably, tamoxifen does not simply bind to the ATP substrate site of PKC; it competitively inhibits the binding to the phosphatidylserine binding site on the C2 regulatory subunit (Su et al. 1985). Moreover, it has greater potency for inhibition of conventional Ca^{2+} and diacylglycerol-activated PKC isoforms (Edashige et al. 1991; Gundimeda et al. 1996). Tamoxifen inhibits amphetamine-stimulated DA efflux in rat striatal synaptosomes and in heterologous hDAT-N2A cells (Mikelman et al. 2017b, 2018). Tamoxifen itself is not ideal, however, because the SERM activity would elicit a variety of unwanted effects (Shelly et al. 2008). An analog of tamoxifen, named 6c, was synthesized and proved highly potent in the inhibition of PKC but not in binding to estrogen receptors (Carpenter et al. 2016). 6c is CNS permeant and inhibits amphetamine-stimulated DA overflow when given directly into the rat nucleus accumbens or intraperitoneally (Carpenter et al. 2017). The drug inhibits hyperactivity to amphetamine but also reduces the more motivationally relevant behavior of amphetamine self-stimulation. As with enzastaurin, 6c significantly inhibited AMPH self-administration but not food administration. The drug did not bind to DAT or affect its trafficking. Notably, 6c exhibited selectivity in inhibition of PKC substrates; the drug inhibited the formation of phosphoser^{41}-GAP-43 with an IC_{50} of 30 nM, while the IC_{50} for inhibition of phosphoser$^{152/156}$-myristoylated alanine-rich C-kinase substrate (MARCKS) was 189 nM. Thus 6c holds therapeutic promise because it is potent and CNS permeant, exhibits substrate selectivity, and blocks amphetamine neurochemical and behavioral actions.

4.4 CaMKII Inhibitors

Issues to consider in developing CaMKII therapeutics are (1) the type of amphetamine exposure (acute vs. repeated) and (2) global deleterious effects from impacting CaMKII pathways needed for a multitude of functions unrelated to drug use disorder. Regarding the mode of drug exposure, in the rat, as opposed to mice, the effects of either CaMKII activation or inhibition on amphetamine actions are apparent only after repeated amphetamine treatments. Repeated, intermittent amphetamine leads to a sensitization resulting in enhanced amphetamine-induced DA efflux, enhanced locomotor activity, and enhanced motivation to take amphetamine (Robinson and Becker 1986; Vezina 2004). Either CaMKII inhibitors or viral silencing of CaMKII with a dominant negative mutant reduces the enhancement in amphetamine-stimulated DA efflux (Kantor et al. 1999), locomotor behavior (Pierce et al. 1998), and self-administration of amphetamine (Loweth et al. 2008) but only to levels seen in saline-pretreated rats. Inhibition of CaMKII in the rat had no effect on acute amphctamine treatment. Conversely, transient overexpression of CaMKII in the nucleus accumbens led to a long-lasting increase in amphetamine-stimulated locomotion and self-administration (Loweth et al. 2010). This effect was likely postsynaptic to DA neurons because no enhancement was found when CaMKII was overexpressed in the DA cell bodies in the ventral tegmental area.

Regarding the likely global deleterious effect of CaMKII inhibitors, one could, for now only preclinically, consider regional selectivity. Thus, the role of CaMKII specifically in DA neurons was demonstrated elegantly in *Drosophila melanogaster*. Expression of CaMKIINtide, a specific inhibitor of CaMKII, in the *Drosophila* DA neurons inhibited hyperlocomotion stimulated by amphetamine but not the uptake blocker methylphenidate (Pizzo et al. 2014). Amphetamine-induced hyperlocomotion in *Drosophila* was dependent on phosphorylation of the N-terminal serines which appears to localize the DAT in membrane rafts (Karam et al. 2017). In addition, it appears possible to limit the global effects of kinase inhibitors by administering them only for a short period of time needed to interfere with memory reconsolidation of drug effects of learned associations between the rewarding properties of drugs and environmental cues associated with their consumption (Garcia-Pardo et al. 2016). Thus, kinase inhibitors may need to be taken for only a short time, until drug-related memories are disrupted. For now CaMKII remains a viable target for drug development for treatment of psychostimulant (including amphetamine) use disorder.

4.5 OCT3 Inhibitors

As detailed in Sect. 2.4, OCT3 can play an important role in outward transport of DA and therefore is a relevant, new target for amphetamine therapeutics. Work on D-22, an OCT3 inhibitor, points to its antidepressant-like action in increasing extracellular 5-HT, opening up a new line of investigation of potential antidepressants acting at OCT3 (Horton et al. 2013). This new line of compounds to be developed in the context of depression treatment may well be beneficial as well for the treatment of amphetamine use disorder.

5 Concluding Remarks

As is clear from the amphetamine literature, our knowledge base regarding amphetamine action is extensive and goes back more than half a century. Although we increasingly understand in more detail the molecular mechanisms underlying effects of amphetamine, it is also clear that we are still not able to fit all pieces of the puzzle into a coherent story. However, it is gratifying to see that the acquired knowledge has led us closer to treatment options for amphetamine use disorder. The molecular knowledge has led to promising lead compounds (DAT blockers/substrates, VMAT2 substrates, PKC inhibitors) or promising novel targets (CaMKII, OCT3). A search for treatment compounds not only will be beneficial in the area of abuse of amphetamines (methamphetamine or Adderall) but will likely overlap considerably into treatment for misuse of other psychostimulants such as cocaine or into treatment of depression.

Acknowledgments The most recent work by the authors described in this review was supported by NIH DA 019676 (MEAR) and R01DA011697 (MEG). We are grateful for the input given on Sect. 4.1 by Kyle C. Schmitt.

References

Alper KR, Lotsof HS, Kaplan CD (2008) The ibogaine medical subculture. J Ethnopharmacol 115:9–24

Altshuler R, Gnegy M, Jutkiewicz E (2016) The protein kinase Cbeta inhibitor, enzastaurin, decreases amphetamine-stimulated behaviors in rats. FASEB J 30:1183–1188

Anderson AL, Li SH, Markova D, Holmes TH, Chiang N, Kahn R, Campbell J, Dickerson DL, Galloway GP, Haning W, Roache JD, Stock C, Elkashef AM (2015) Bupropion for the treatment of methamphetamine dependence in non-daily users: a randomized, double-blind, placebo-controlled trial. Drug Alcohol Depend 150:170–174

Apel ED, Byford MF, Au D, Walsh KA, Storm DR (1990) Identification of the protein kinase C phosphorylation site in neuromodulin. Biochemistry 29:2330–2335

Arnold EB, Molinoff PB, Rutledge CO (1977) The release of endogenous norepinephrine and dopamine from cerebral cortex by amphetamine. J Pharmacol Exp Ther 202:544–557

Avelar AJ, Juliano SA, Garris PA (2013) Amphetamine augments vesicular dopamine release in the dorsal and ventral striatum through different mechanisms. J Neurochem 125:373–385

Baldessarini RJ, Vogt M (1971) The uptake and subcellular distribution of aromatic amines in the brain of the rat. J Neurochem 18:2519–2533

Banks ML, Blough BE, Fennell TR, Snyder RW, Negus SS (2013a) Effects of phendimetrazine treatment on cocaine vs food choice and extended-access cocaine consumption in rhesus monkeys. Neuropsychopharmacology 38:2698–2707

Banks ML, Blough BE, Negus SS (2013b) Interaction between behavioral and pharmacological treatment strategies to decrease cocaine choice in rhesus monkeys. Neuropsychopharmacology 38:395–404

Banks ML, Smith DA, Blough BE (2016) Methamphetamine-like discriminative stimulus effects of bupropion and its two hydroxy metabolites in male rhesus monkeys. Behav Pharmacol 27:196–203

Beerepoot P, Lam VM, Salahpour A (2016) Pharmacological chaperones of the dopamine transporter rescue dopamine transporter deficiency syndrome mutations in heterologous cells. J Biol Chem 291:22053–22062

Berfield JL, Wang LC, Reith ME (1999) Which form of dopamine is the substrate for the human dopamine transporter: the cationic or the uncharged species? J Biol Chem 274:4876–4882

Bhat S, Hasenhuetl PS, Kasture A, El-Kasaby A, Baumann MH, Blough BE, Sucic S, Sandtner W, Freissmuth M (2017) Conformational state interactions provide clues to the pharmacochaperone potential of serotonin transporter partial substrates. J Biol Chem 292:16773–16786

Brensilver M, Heinzerling KG, Shoptaw S (2013) Pharmacotherapy of amphetamine-type stimulant dependence: an update. Drug Alcohol Rev 32:449–460

Browman KE, Kantor L, Richardson S, Badiani A, Robinson TE, Gnegy ME (1998) Injection of the protein kinase C inhibitor Ro31-8220 into the nucleus accumbens attenuates the acute response to amphetamine: tissue and behavioral studies. Brain Res 814:112–119

Brown TK, Alper K (2018) Treatment of opioid use disorder with ibogaine: detoxification and drug use outcomes. Am J Drug Alcohol Abuse 44:24–36

Bulling S, Schicker K, Zhang YW, Steinkellner T, Stockner T, Gruber CW, Boehm S, Freissmuth M, Rudnick G, Sitte HH, Sandtner W (2012) The mechanistic basis for noncompetitive ibogaine inhibition of serotonin and dopamine transporters. J Biol Chem 287:18524–18534

Butcher SP, Fairbrother IS, Kelly JS, Arbuthnott GW (1988) Amphetamine-induced dopamine release in the rat striatum: an in vivo microdialysis study. J Neurochem 50:346–355

Cadoni C, Pinna A, Russi G, Consolo S, Di Chiara G (1995) Role of vesicular dopamine in the in vivo stimulation of striatal dopamine transmission by amphetamine: evidence from microdialysis and Fos immunohistochemistry. Neuroscience 65:1027–1039

Calipari ES, Ferris MJ (2013) Amphetamine mechanisms and actions at the dopamine terminal revisited. J Neurosci 33:8923–8925

Cameron KN, Solis E Jr, Ruchala I, De Felice LJ, Eltit JM (2015) Amphetamine activates calcium channels through dopamine transporter-mediated depolarization. Cell Calcium 58:457–466

Carlsson A, Fuxe K, Hamberger B, Lindqvist M (1966) Biochemical and histochemical studies on the effects of imipramine-like drugs and (+)-amphetamine on central and peripheral catecholamine neurons. Acta Physiol Scand 67:481–497

Carpenter C, Sorenson RJ, Jin Y, Klossowski S, Cierpicki T, Gnegy M, Showalter HD (2016) Design and synthesis of triarylacrylonitrile analogues of tamoxifen with improved binding selectivity to protein kinase C. Bioorg Med Chem 24:5495–5504

Carpenter C, Zestos AG, Altshuler R, Sorenson RJ, Guptaroy B, Showalter HD, Kennedy RT, Jutkiewicz E, Gnegy ME (2017) Direct and systemic administration of a CNS-permeant tamoxifen analog reduces amphetamine-induced dopamine release and reinforcing effects. Neuropsychopharmacology 42:1940–1949

Carson DS, Taylor ER (2014) Commentary on Heinzerling et al. (2014): a growing methamphetamine dependence therapeutics graveyard. Addiction 109:1887–1888

Carvalho M, Carmo H, Costa VM, Capela JP, Pontes H, Remiao F, Carvalho F, Bastos Mde L (2012) Toxicity of amphetamines: an update. Arch Toxicol 86:1167–1231

Carvelli L, McDonald PW, Blakely RD, DeFelice LJ (2004) Dopamine transporters depolarize neurons by a channel mechanism. Proc Natl Acad Sci U S A 101:16046–16051

Cervinski MA, Foster JD, Vaughan RA (2005) Psychoactive substrates stimulate dopamine transporter phosphorylation and down-regulation by cocaine-sensitive and protein kinase C-dependent mechanisms. J Biol Chem 280:40442–40449

Challasivakanaka S, Zhen J, Smith ME, Reith MEA, Foster JD, Vaughan RA (2017) Dopamine transporter phosphorylation site threonine 53 is stimulated by amphetamines and regulates dopamine transport, efflux, and cocaine analog binding. J Biol Chem 292:19066–19075

Chen N, Reith ME (2004) Interaction between dopamine and its transporter: role of intracellular sodium ions and membrane potential. J Neurochem 89:750–765
Chen N, Reith ME (2008) Substrates dissociate dopamine transporter oligomers. J Neurochem 105:910–920
Chen N, Vaughan RA, Reith ME (2001) The role of conserved tryptophan and acidic residues in the human dopamine transporter as characterized by site-directed mutagenesis. J Neurochem 77:1116–1127
Chen N, Rickey J, Reith ME (2003) Na+ stimulates binding of dopamine to the dopamine transporter in cells but not in cell-free preparations. J Neurochem 86:678–686
Chen N, Rickey J, Berfield JL, Reith ME (2004a) Aspartate 345 of the dopamine transporter is critical for conformational changes in substrate translocation and cocaine binding. J Biol Chem 279:5508–5519
Chen N, Zhen J, Reith ME (2004b) Mutation of Trp84 and Asp313 of the dopamine transporter reveals similar mode of binding interaction for GBR12909 and benztropine as opposed to cocaine. J Neurochem 89:853–864
Chen R, Furman CA, Zhang M, Kim MN, RWt G, Leitges M, Gnegy ME (2009) Protein kinase Cbeta is a critical regulator of dopamine transporter trafficking and regulates the behavioral response to amphetamine in mice. J Pharmacol Exp Ther 328:912–920
Chico LK, van Eldik LJ, Watterson DM (2009) Targeting protein kinases in central nervous system disorders. Nat Rev Drug Discov 8:892–909
Chiueh CC, Moore KE (1975) D-amphetamine-induced release of "newly synthesized" and "stored" dopamine from the caudate nucleus in vivo. J Pharmacol Exp Ther 192:642–653
Corera AT, Costentin J, Bonnet JJ (2000) Binding of uptake blockers to the neuronal dopamine transporter: further investigation about cationic and anionic requirements. Naunyn Schmiedeberg's Arch Pharmacol 362:213–221
Covey DP, Juliano SA, Garris PA (2013) Amphetamine elicits opposing actions on readily releasable and reserve pools for dopamine. PLoS One 8:e60763
Cubeddu LX, Lovenberg TW, Hoffman IS, Talmaciu RK (1989) Phorbol esters and D2-dopamine receptors. J Pharmacol Exp Ther 251:687–693
Czoty PW, Blough BE, Fennell TR, Snyder RW, Nader MA (2016) Attenuation of cocaine self-administration by chronic oral phendimetrazine in rhesus monkeys. Neuroscience 324:367–376
Daberkow DP, Brown HD, Bunner KD, Kraniotis SA, Doellman MA, Ragozzino ME, Garris PA, Roitman MF (2013) Amphetamine paradoxically augments exocytotic dopamine release and phasic dopamine signals. J Neurosci 33:452–463
Dwoskin LP, Crooks PA (2002) A novel mechanism of action and potential use for lobeline as a treatment for psychostimulant abuse. Biochem Pharmacol 63:89–98
Edashige K, Sato EF, Akimaru K, Yoshioka T, Utsumi K (1991) Nonsteroidal antiestrogen suppresses protein kinase C – its inhibitory effect on interaction of substrate protein with membrane. Cell Struct Funct 16:273–281
Egana LA, Cuevas RA, Baust TB, Parra LA, Leak RK, Hochendoner S, Pena K, Quiroz M, Hong WC, Dorostkar MM, Janz R, Sitte HH, Torres GE (2009) Physical and functional interaction between the dopamine transporter and the synaptic vesicle protein synaptogyrin-3. J Neurosci 29:4592–4604
Einat H, Yuan P, Szabo ST, Dogra S, Manji HK (2007) Protein kinase C inhibition by tamoxifen antagonizes manic-like behavior in rats: implications for the development of novel therapeutics for bipolar disorder. Neuropsychobiology 55:123–131
Erreger K, Grewer C, Javitch JA, Galli A (2008) Currents in response to rapid concentration jumps of amphetamine uncover novel aspects of human dopamine transporter function. J Neurosci 28:976–989
Eshleman AJ, Henningsen RA, Neve KA, Janowsky A (1994) Release of dopamine via the human transporter. Mol Pharmacol 45:312–316
Fischer JF, Cho AK (1979) Chemical release of dopamine from striatal homogenates: evidence for an exchange diffusion model. J Pharmacol Exp Ther 208:203–209

Floor E, Meng L (1996) Amphetamine releases dopamine from synaptic vesicles by dual mechanisms. Neurosci Lett 215:53–56

Fog JU, Khoshbouei H, Holy M, Owens WA, Vaegter CB, Sen N, Nikandrova Y, Bowton E, McMahon DG, Colbran RJ, Daws LC, Sitte HH, Javitch JA, Galli A, Gether U (2006) Calmodulin kinase II interacts with the dopamine transporter C terminus to regulate amphetamine-induced reverse transport. Neuron 51:417–429

Fon EA, Pothos EN, Sun BC, Killeen N, Sulzer D, Edwards RH (1997) Vesicular transport regulates monoamine storage and release but is not essential for amphetamine action. Neuron 19:1271–1283

Foster JD, Vaughan RA (2017) Phosphorylation mechanisms in dopamine transporter regulation. J Chem Neuroanat 83-84:10–18

Foster JD, Pananusorn B, Vaughan RA (2002) Dopamine transporters are phosphorylated on N-terminal serines in rat striatum. J Biol Chem 277:25178–25186

Foster JD, Yang JW, Moritz AE, Challasivakanaka S, Smith MA, Holy M, Wilebski K, Sitte HH, Vaughan RA (2012) Dopamine transporter phosphorylation site threonine 53 regulates substrate reuptake and amphetamine-stimulated efflux. J Biol Chem 287:29702–29712

Freyberg Z, Sonders MS, Aguilar JI, Hiranita T, Karam CS, Flores J, Pizzo AB, Zhang Y, Farino ZJ, Chen A, Martin CA, Kopajtic TA, Fei H, Hu G, Lin YY, Mosharov EV, McCabe BD, Freyberg R, Wimalasena K, Hsin LW, Sames D, Krantz DE, Katz JL, Sulzer D, Javitch JA (2016) Mechanisms of amphetamine action illuminated through optical monitoring of dopamine synaptic vesicles in Drosophila brain. Nat Commun 7:10652

Fudala PJ, Iwamoto ET (1986) Further studies on nicotine-induced conditioned place preference in the rat. Pharmacol Biochem Behav 25:1041–1049

Furman CA, Chen R, Guptaroy B, Zhang M, Holz RW, Gnegy M (2009) Dopamine and amphetamine rapidly increase dopamine transporter trafficking to the surface: live-cell imaging using total internal reflection fluorescence microscopy. J Neurosci 29:3328–3336

Garcia-Pardo MP, Roger-Sanchez C, Rodriguez-Arias M, Minarro J, Aguilar MA (2016) Pharmacological modulation of protein kinases as a new approach to treat addiction to cocaine and opiates. Eur J Pharmacol 781:10–24

Gasser PJ (2019) Roles for the uptake2 transporter OCT3 in regulation of dopaminergic neurotransmission and behavior. Neurochem Int 123:46–49

German DC, McMillen BA, Sanghera MK, Saffer SI, Shore PA (1981) Effects of severe dopamine depletion on dopamine neuronal impulse flow and on tyrosine hydroxylase regulation. Brain Res Bull 6:131–134

Giambalvo CT (1992a) Protein kinase C and dopamine transport – 1. Effects of amphetamine in vivo. Neuropharmacology 31:1201–1210

Giambalvo CT (1992b) Protein kinase C and dopamine transport – 2. Effects of amphetamine in vitro. Neuropharmacology 31:1211–1222

Giambalvo CT (2003) Differential effects of amphetamine transport vs. dopamine reverse transport on particulate PKC activity in striatal synaptoneurosomes. Synapse 49:125–133

Giambalvo CT (2004) Mechanisms underlying the effects of amphetamine on particulate PKC activity. Synapse 51:128–139

Gnegy ME (2003) The effect of phosphorylation on amphetamine-mediated outward transport. Eur J Pharmacol 479:83–91

Gnegy ME, Khoshbouei H, Berg KA, Javitch JA, Clarke WP, Zhang M, Galli A (2004) Intracellular Ca2+ regulates amphetamine-induced dopamine efflux and currents mediated by the human dopamine transporter. Mol Pharmacol 66:137–143

Gonzalez AM, Walther D, Pazos A, Uhl GR (1994) Synaptic vesicular monoamine transporter expression: distribution and pharmacologic profile. Brain Res Mol Brain Res 22:219–226

Goodwin JS, Larson GA, Swant J, Sen N, Javitch JA, Zahniser NR, De Felice LJ, Khoshbouei H (2009) Amphetamine and methamphetamine differentially affect dopamine transporters in vitro and in vivo. J Biol Chem 284:2978–2989

Granas C, Ferrer J, Loland CJ, Javitch JA, Gether U (2003) N-terminal truncation of the dopamine transporter abolishes phorbol ester- and substance P receptor-stimulated phosphorylation without impairing transporter internalization. J Biol Chem 278:4990–5000

Gulley JM, Zahniser NR (2003) Rapid regulation of dopamine transporter function by substrates, blockers and presynaptic receptor ligands. Eur J Pharmacol 479:139–152

Gundimeda U, Chen Z-H, Gopalakrishna R (1996) Tamoxifen modulates protein kinase C via oxidative stress in estrogen receptor-negative breast cancer cells. J Biol Chem 271:13504–13514

Hadlock GC, Nelson CC, Baucum AJ 2nd, Hanson GR, Fleckenstein AE (2011) Ex vivo identification of protein-protein interactions involving the dopamine transporter. J Neurosci Methods 196:303–307

Hamilton PJ, Belovich AN, Khelashvili G, Saunders C, Erreger K, Javitch JA, Sitte HH, Weinstein H, Matthies HJG, Galli A (2014) PIP2 regulates psychostimulant behaviors through its interaction with a membrane protein. Nat Chem Biol 10:582–589

Harrod SB, Dwoskin LP, Crooks PA, Klebaur JE, Bardo MT (2001) Lobeline attenuates d-methamphetamine self-administration in rats. J Pharmacol Exp Ther 298:172–179

Harrod SB, Dwoskin LP, Green TA, Gehrke BJ, Bardo MT (2003) Lobeline does not serve as a reinforcer in rats. Psychopharmacology 165:397–404

Hastrup H, Karlin A, Javitch JA (2001) Symmetrical dimer of the human dopamine transporter revealed by cross-linking Cys-306 at the extracellular end of the sixth transmembrane segment. Proc Natl Acad Sci U S A 98:10055–10060

Heikkila RE, Orlansky H, Cohen G (1975) Studies on the distinction between uptake inhibition and release of (3H)dopamine in rat brain tissue slices. Biochem Pharmacol 24:847–852

Heinzerling KG, Swanson AN, Hall TM, Yi Y, Wu Y, Shoptaw SJ (2014) Randomized, placebo-controlled trial of bupropion in methamphetamine-dependent participants with less than daily methamphetamine use. Addiction 109:1878–1886

Herman M, Nagler SH (1954) Psychoses due to amphetamine. J Nerv Ment Dis 120:268–272

Holz RW, Coyle JT (1974) The effects of various salts, temperature, and the alkaloids veratridine and batrachotoxin on the uptake of [3H] dopamine into synaptosomes from rat striatum. Mol Pharmacol 10:746–758

Horton RE, Apple DM, Owens WA, Baganz NL, Cano S, Mitchell NC, Vitela M, Gould GG, Koek W, Daws LC (2013) Decynium-22 enhances SSRI-induced antidepressant-like effects in mice: uncovering novel targets to treat depression. J Neurosci 33:10534–10543

Howell LL, Negus SS (2014) Monoamine transporter inhibitors and substrates as treatments for stimulant abuse. Adv Pharmacol 69:129–176

Humphreys CJ, Wall SC, Rudnick G (1994) Ligand binding to the serotonin transporter: equilibria, kinetics, and ion dependence. Biochemistry 33:9118–9125

Hurd YL, Ungerstedt U (1989) In vivo neurochemical profile of dopamine uptake inhibitors and releasers in rat caudate-putamen. Eur J Pharmacol 166:251–260

Iversen L (2006) Neurotransmitter transporters and their impact on the development of psychopharmacology. Br J Pharmacol 147(Suppl 1):S82–S88

Iwata S, Hewlett GH, Ferrell ST, Czernik AJ, Meiri KF, Gnegy ME (1996) Increased in vivo phosphorylation state of neuromodulin and synapsin I in striatum from rats treated with repeated amphetamine. J Pharmacol Exp Ther 278:1428–1434

Iwata S, Hewlett GH, Gnegy ME (1997) Amphetamine increases the phosphorylation of neuromodulin and synapsin I in rat striatal synaptosomes. Synapse 26:281–291

Jacobs MT, Zhang YW, Campbell SD, Rudnick G (2007) Ibogaine, a noncompetitive inhibitor of serotonin transport, acts by stabilizing the cytoplasm-facing state of the transporter. J Biol Chem 282:29441–29447

Jardetzky O (1966) Simple allosteric model for membrane pumps. Nature 211:969–970

Johnson J, Milner G (1966) Psychiatric complications of amphetamine substances. Acta Psychiatr Scand 42:252–263

Johnson LA, Furman CA, Zhang M, Guptaroy B, Gnegy ME (2005a) Rapid delivery of the dopamine transporter to the plasmalemmal membrane upon amphetamine stimulation. Neuropharmacology 49:750–758

Johnson LA, Guptaroy B, Lund D, Shamban S, Gnegy ME (2005b) Regulation of amphetamine-stimulated dopamine efflux by protein kinase C beta. J Biol Chem 280:10914–10919

Jones SR, Gainetdinov RR, Wightman RM, Caron MG (1998) Mechanisms of amphetamine action revealed in mice lacking the dopamine transporter. J Neurosci 18:1979–1986

Jones SR, Joseph JD, Barak LS, Caron MG, Wightman RM (1999) Dopamine neuronal transport kinetics and effects of amphetamine. J Neurochem 73:2406–2414

Kahlig KM, Binda F, Khoshbouei H, Blakely RD, McMahon DG, Javitch JA, Galli A (2005) Amphetamine induces dopamine efflux through a dopamine transporter channel. Proc Natl Acad Sci U S A 102:3495–3500

Kangiser MM, Dwoskin LP, Zheng G, Crooks PA, Stairs DJ (2018) Varenicline and GZ-793A differentially decrease methamphetamine self-administration under a multiple schedule of reinforcement in rats. Behav Pharmacol 29:87–97

Kantor L, Gnegy ME (1998) Protein kinase C inhibitors block amphetamine-mediated dopamine release in rat striatal slices. J Pharmacol Exp Ther 284:592–598

Kantor L, Hewlett GH, Gnegy ME (1999) Enhanced amphetamine- and K+-mediated dopamine release in rat striatum after repeated amphetamine: differential requirements for Ca2+- and calmodulin-dependent phosphorylation and synaptic vesicles. J Neurosci 19:3801–3808

Kantor L, Hewlett GH, Park YH, Richardson-Burns SM, Mellon MJ, Gnegy ME (2001) Protein kinase C and intracellular calcium are required for amphetamine-mediated dopamine release via the norepinephrine transporter in undifferentiated PC12 cells. J Pharmacol Exp Ther 297:1016–1024

Karam CS, Sen N, Javitch JA (2017) Phospho-specific antibodies targeting the amino terminus of the human dopamine transporter. J Chem Neuroanat 83-84:91–98

Katz JL, Izenwasser S, Kline RH, Allen AC, Newman AH (1999) Novel 3alpha-diphenylmethoxytropane analogs: selective dopamine uptake inhibitors with behavioral effects distinct from those of cocaine. J Pharmacol Exp Ther 288:302–315

Khoshbouei H, Wang H, Lechleiter JD, Javitch JA, Galli A (2003) Amphetamine-induced dopamine efflux. A voltage-sensitive and intracellular Na+-dependent mechanism. J Biol Chem 278:12070–12077

Khoshbouei H, Sen N, Guptaroy B, Johnson L, Lund D, Gnegy ME, Galli A, Javitch JA (2004) N-terminal phosphorylation of the dopamine transporter is required for amphetamine-induced efflux. PLoS Biol 2:E78

King M, Hosmer H, Dresbach M (1928) Physiological reactions induced by alpha-lobeline. I. Intravenous injections during anesthesia and certain other forms of depression. J Pharmacol Exp Ther 32:241–272

Krishnamurthy H, Gouaux E (2012) X-ray structures of LeuT in substrate-free outward-open and apo inward-open states. Nature 481:469–474

Kuhr WG, Ewing AG, Near JA, Wightman RM (1985) Amphetamine attenuates the stimulated release of dopamine in vivo. J Pharmacol Exp Ther 232:388–394

Lee AM, Messing RO (2008) Protein kinases and addiction. Ann N Y Acad Sci 1141:22–57

Lee NK, Jenner L, Harney A, Cameron J (2018a) Pharmacotherapy for amphetamine dependence: a systematic review. Drug Alcohol Depend 191:309–337

Lee NR, Zheng G, Crooks PA, Bardo MT, Dwoskin LP (2018b) New scaffold for lead compounds to treat methamphetamine use disorders. AAPS J 20:29

Lentzen H, Philippu A (1981) Physico-chemical properties of phenethylamines and their uptake into synaptic vesicles of the caudate nucleus. Biochem Pharmacol 30:1759–1764

Leviel V (2011) Dopamine release mediated by the dopamine transporter, facts and consequences. J Neurochem 118:475–489

Li LB, Reith ME (1999) Modeling of the interaction of Na+ and K+ with the binding of dopamine and [3H]WIN 35,428 to the human dopamine transporter. J Neurochem 72:1095–1109

Li LB, Reith ME (2000) Interaction of Na+, K+, and Cl- with the binding of amphetamine, octopamine, and tyramine to the human dopamine transporter. J Neurochem 74:1538–1552

Li LB, Cui XN, Reith MA (2002) Is Na(+) required for the binding of dopamine, amphetamine, tyramine, and octopamine to the human dopamine transporter? Naunyn Schmiedeberg's Arch Pharmacol 365:303–311
Li Y, Cheng SY, Chen N, Reith ME (2010) Interrelation of dopamine transporter oligomerization and surface presence as studied with mutant transporter proteins and amphetamine. J Neurochem 114:873–885
Liang NY, Rutledge CO (1982) Evidence for carrier-mediated efflux of dopamine from corpus striatum. Biochem Pharmacol 31:2479–2484
Lien EA, Solheim E, Ueland PM (1991) Distribution of tamoxifen and its metabolites in rat and human tissues during steady-state treatment. Cancer Res 51:4837–4844
Lightman SL, Iversen LL (1969) The role of uptake2 in the extraneuronal metabolism of catecholamines in the isolated rat heart. Br J Pharmacol 37:638–649
Lin M, Sambo D, Khoshbouei H (2016) Methamphetamine regulation of firing activity of dopamine neurons. J Neurosci 36:10376–10391
Loland CJ, Mereu M, Okunola OM, Cao J, Prisinzano TE, Mazier S, Kopajtic T, Shi L, Katz JL, Tanda G, Newman AH (2012) R-modafinil (armodafinil): a unique dopamine uptake inhibitor and potential medication for psychostimulant abuse. Biol Psychiatry 72:405–413
Loweth JA, Baker LK, Guptaa T, Guillory AM, Vezina P (2008) Inhibition of CaMKII in the nucleus accumbens shell decreases enhanced amphetamine intake in sensitized rats. Neurosci Lett 444:157–160
Loweth JA, Svoboda R, Austin JD, Guillory AM, Vezina P (2009) The PKC inhibitor Ro31-8220 blocks acute amphetamine-induced dopamine overflow in the nucleus accumbens. Neurosci Lett 455:88–92
Loweth JA, Singer BF, Baker LK, Wilke G, Inamine H, Bubula N, Alexander JK, Carlezon WA Jr, Neve RL, Vezina P (2010) Transient overexpression of alpha-Ca2+/calmodulin-dependent protein kinase II in the nucleus accumbens shell enhances behavioral responding to amphetamine. J Neurosci 30:939–949
Luderman KD, Chen R, Ferris MJ, Jones SR, Gnegy ME (2015) Protein kinase C beta regulates the D(2)-like dopamine autoreceptor. Neuropharmacology 89:335–341
Malcolm E, Carroll FI, Blough B, Damaj MI, Shoaib M (2015) Examination of the metabolite hydroxybupropion in the reinforcing and aversive stimulus effects of nicotine in rats. Psychopharmacology 232:2763–2771
Malinauskaite L, Quick M, Reinhard L, Lyons JA, Yano H, Javitch JA, Nissen P (2014) A mechanism for intracellular release of Na+ by neurotransmitter/sodium symporters. Nat Struct Mol Biol 21:1006–1012
Mayer FP, Luf A, Nagy C, Holy M, Schmid R, Freissmuth M, Sitte HH (2017) Application of a combined approach to identify new psychoactive street drugs and decipher their mechanisms at monoamine transporters. Curr Top Behav Neurosci 32:333–350
Mayer FP, Schmid D, Owens WA, Gould GG, Apuschkin M, Kudlacek O, Salzer I, Boehm S, Chiba P, Williams PH, Wu HH, Gether U, Koek W, Daws LC, Sitte HH (2018) An unsuspected role for organic cation transporter 3 in the actions of amphetamine. Neuropsychopharmacology 43:2408–2417
Meinild AK, Sitte HH, Gether U (2004) Zinc potentiates an uncoupled anion conductance associated with the dopamine transporter. J Biol Chem 279:49671–49679
Meiri KF, Bickerstaff LE, Schwob JE (1991) Monoclonal antibodies show that kinase C phosphorylation of GAP-43 during axonogenesis is both spatially and temporally restricted in vivo. J Cell Biol 112:991–1005
Meyer AC, Horton DB, Neugebauer NM, Wooters TE, Nickell JR, Dwoskin LP, Bardo MT (2011) Tetrabenazine inhibition of monoamine uptake and methamphetamine behavioral effects: locomotor activity, drug discrimination and self-administration. Neuropharmacology 61:849–856
Mikelman S, Mardirossian N, Gnegy ME (2017a) Tamoxifen and amphetamine abuse: are there therapeutic possibilities? J Chem Neuroanat 83-84:50–58
Mikelman SR, Guptaroy B, Gnegy ME (2017b) Tamoxifen and its active metabolites inhibit dopamine transporter function independently of the estrogen receptors. J Neurochem 141:31–36

Mikelman SR, Guptaroy B, Schmitt KC, Jones KT, Zhen J, Reith MEA, Gnegy ME (2018) Tamoxifen directly interacts with the dopamine transporter. J Pharmacol Exp Ther 367:119–128
Mundorf ML, Hochstetler SE, Wightman RM (1999) Amine weak bases disrupt vesicular storage and promote exocytosis in chromaffin cells. J Neurochem 73:2397–2405
Namkung Y, Sibley DR (2004) Protein kinase C mediates phosphorylation, desensitization, and trafficking of the D2 dopamine receptor. J Biol Chem 279:49533–49541
Nickell JR, Siripurapu KB, Vartak A, Crooks PA, Dwoskin LP (2014) The vesicular monoamine transporter-2: an important pharmacological target for the discovery of novel therapeutics to treat methamphetamine abuse. Adv Pharmacol 69:71–106
Niddam R, Arbilla S, Scatton B, Dennis T, Langer SZ (1985) Amphetamine induced release of endogenous dopamine in vitro is not reduced following pretreatment with reserpine. Naunyn Schmiedeberg's Arch Pharmacol 329:123–127
Nimitvilai S, McElvain MA, Brodie MS (2013) Reversal of dopamine D2 agonist-induced inhibition of ventral tegmental area neurons by Gq-linked neurotransmitters is dependent on protein kinase C, G protein-coupled receptor kinase, and dynamin. J Pharmacol Exp Ther 344:253–263
Nomikos GG, Damsma G, Wenkstern D, Fibiger HC (1990) In vivo characterization of locally applied dopamine uptake inhibitors by striatal microdialysis. Synapse 6:106–112
O'Brian CA, Liskamp RM, Solomon DH, Weinstein IB (1985) Inhibition of protein kinase C by tamoxifen. Cancer Res 45:2462–2465
Ofori S, Bretton C, Hof P, Schorderet M (1986) Investigation of dopamine content, synthesis, and release in the rabbit retina in vitro: I. Effects of dopamine precursors, reserpine, amphetamine, and L-DOPA decarboxylase and monoamine oxidase inhibitors. J Neurochem 47:1199–1206
Pariser JJ, Partilla JS, Dersch CM, Ananthan S, Rothman RB (2008) Studies of the biogenic amine transporters. 12. Identification of novel partial inhibitors of amphetamine-induced dopamine release. J Pharmacol Exp Ther 326:286–295
Parker EM, Cubeddu LX (1986) Effects of d-amphetamine and dopamine synthesis inhibitors on dopamine and acetylcholine neurotransmission in the striatum. I. Release in the absence of vesicular transmitter stores. J Pharmacol Exp Ther 237:179–192
Partilla JS, Dempsey AG, Nagpal AS, Blough BE, Baumann MH, Rothman RB (2006) Interaction of amphetamines and related compounds at the vesicular monoamine transporter. J Pharmacol Exp Ther 319:237–246
Patel J, Mooslehner KA, Chan PM, Emson PC, Stamford JA (2003) Presynaptic control of striatal dopamine neurotransmission in adult vesicular monoamine transporter 2 (VMAT2) mutant mice. J Neurochem 85:898–910
Penmatsa A, Wang KH, Gouaux E (2015) X-ray structures of Drosophila dopamine transporter in complex with nisoxetine and reboxetine. Nat Struct Mol Biol 22:506–508
Peter D, Jimenez J, Liu Y, Kim J, Edwards RH (1994) The chromaffin granule and synaptic vesicle amine transporters differ in substrate recognition and sensitivity to inhibitors. J Biol Chem 269:7231–7237
Pierce RC, Kalivas PW (1997) Repeated cocaine modifies the mechanism by which amphetamine releases dopamine. J Neurosci 17:3254–3261
Pierce RC, Quick EA, Reeder DC, Morgan ZR, Kalivas PW (1998) Calcium-mediated second messengers modulate the expression of behavioral sensitization to cocaine. J Pharmacol Exp Ther 286:1171–1176
Pifl C, Drobny H, Reither H, Hornykiewicz O, Singer EA (1995) Mechanism of the dopamine-releasing actions of amphetamine and cocaine: plasmalemmal dopamine transporter versus vesicular monoamine transporter. Mol Pharmacol 47:368–373
Pizzo AB, Karam CS, Zhang Y, Yano H, Freyberg RJ, Karam DS, Freyberg Z, Yamamoto A, McCabe BD, Javitch JA (2013) The membrane raft protein Flotillin-1 is essential in dopamine neurons for amphetamine-induced behavior in Drosophila. Mol Psychiatry 18:824–833
Pizzo AB, Karam CS, Zhang Y, Ma CL, McCabe BD, Javitch JA (2014) Amphetamine-induced behavior requires CaMKII-dependent dopamine transporter phosphorylation. Mol Psychiatry 19:279–281

Raiteri M, Bertollini A, del Carmine R, Levi G (1976) Release of biogenic amines from isolated nerve endings. Adv Exp Med Biol 69:319–335

Ramamoorthy S, Shippenberg TS, Jayanthi LD (2011) Regulation of monoamine transporters: role of transporter phosphorylation. Pharmacol Ther 129:220–238

Rastedt DE, Vaughan RA, Foster JD (2017) Palmitoylation mechanisms in dopamine transporter regulation. J Chem Neuroanat 83-84:3–9

Reith ME, Blough BE, Hong WC, Jones KT, Schmitt KC, Baumann MH, Partilla JS, Rothman RB, Katz JL (2015) Behavioral, biological, and chemical perspectives on atypical agents targeting the dopamine transporter. Drug Alcohol Depend 147:1–19

Richards TL, Zahniser NR (2009) Rapid substrate-induced down-regulation in function and surface localization of dopamine transporters: rat dorsal striatum versus nucleus accumbens. J Neurochem 108:1575–1584

Rickhag M, Owens WA, Winkler MT, Strandfelt KN, Rathje M, Sorensen G, Andresen B, Madsen KL, Jorgensen TN, Wortwein G, Woldbye DP, Sitte H, Daws LC, Gether U (2013) Membrane-permeable C-terminal dopamine transporter peptides attenuate amphetamine-evoked dopamine release. J Biol Chem 288:27534–27544

Robinson TE, Becker JB (1986) Enduring changes in brain and behavior produced by chronic amphetamine administration: a review and evaluation of animal models of amphetamine psychosis. Brain Res 396:157–198

Ross SB, Renyi AL (1966) Uptake of tritiated tyramine and (+) amphetamine by mouse heart slices. J Pharm Pharmacol 18:756–757

Rothman RB, Baumann MH, Dersch CM, Romero DV, Rice KC, Carroll FI, Partilla JS (2001) Amphetamine-type central nervous system stimulants release norepinephrine more potently than they release dopamine and serotonin. Synapse 39:32–41

Rothman RB, Dersch CM, Ananthan S, Partilla JS (2009) Studies of the biogenic amine transporters. 13. Identification of "agonist" and "antagonist" allosteric modulators of amphetamine-induced dopamine release. J Pharmacol Exp Ther 329:718–728

Rothman RB, Partilla JS, Baumann MH, Lightfoot-Siordia C, Blough BE (2012) Studies of the biogenic amine transporters. 14. Identification of low-efficacy "partial" substrates for the biogenic amine transporters. J Pharmacol Exp Ther 341:251–262

Rudnick G, Clark J (1993) From synapse to vesicle: the reuptake and storage of biogenic amine neurotransmitters. Biochim Biophys Acta 1144:249–263

Sabol KE, Seiden LS (1998) Reserpine attenuates D-amphetamine and MDMA-induced transmitter release in vivo: a consideration of dose, core temperature and dopamine synthesis. Brain Res 806:69–78

Sambo DO, Lin M, Owens A, Lebowitz JJ, Richardson B, Jagnarine DA, Shetty M, Rodriquez M, Alonge T, Ali M, Katz J, Yan L, Febo M, Henry LK, Bruijnzeel AW, Daws L, Khoshbouei H (2017) The sigma-1 receptor modulates methamphetamine dysregulation of dopamine neurotransmission. Nat Commun 8:2228

Schmitt KC, Reith ME (2010) Regulation of the dopamine transporter: aspects relevant to psychostimulant drugs of abuse. Ann N Y Acad Sci 1187:316–340

Schmitt KC, Reith ME (2011) The atypical stimulant and nootropic modafinil interacts with the dopamine transporter in a different manner than classical cocaine-like inhibitors. PLoS One 6: e25790

Schmitt KC, Zhen J, Kharkar P, Mishra M, Chen N, Dutta AK, Reith ME (2008) Interaction of cocaine-, benztropine-, and GBR12909-like compounds with wild-type and mutant human dopamine transporters: molecular features that differentially determine antagonist-binding properties. J Neurochem 107:928–940

Schmitz Y, Lee CJ, Schmauss C, Gonon F, Sulzer D (2001) Amphetamine distorts stimulation-dependent dopamine overflow: effects on D2 autoreceptors, transporters, and synaptic vesicle stores. J Neurosci 21:5916–5924

Schwartzberg L, Hermann R, Flinn I, Flora D, Hsi ED, Hamid O, Shi P, Lin BK, Myrand SP, Nguyen TS, Dreyling M (2014) Open-label, single-arm, phase II study of enzastaurin in patients with follicular lymphoma. Br J Haematol 166:91–97

Seidel S, Singer EA, Just H, Farhan H, Scholze P, Kudlacek O, Holy M, Koppatz K, Krivanek P, Freissmuth M, Sitte HH (2005) Amphetamines take two to tango: an oligomer-based counter-transport model of neurotransmitter transport explores the amphetamine action. Mol Pharmacol 67:140–151
Shelly W, Draper MW, Krishnan V, Wong M, Jaffe RB (2008) Selective estrogen receptor modulators: an update on recent clinical findings. Obstet Gynecol Surv 63:163–181
Shi L, Quick M, Zhao Y, Weinstein H, Javitch JA (2008) The mechanism of a neurotransmitter: sodium symporter – inward release of Na+ and substrate is triggered by substrate in a second binding site. Mol Cell 30:667–677
Siciliano CA, Calipari ES, Ferris MJ, Jones SR (2014) Biphasic mechanisms of amphetamine action at the dopamine terminal. J Neurosci 34:5575–5582
Singh SK, Yamashita A, Gouaux E (2007) Antidepressant binding site in a bacterial homologue of neurotransmitter transporters. Nature 448:952–956
Singh SK, Piscitelli CL, Yamashita A, Gouaux E (2008) A competitive inhibitor traps LeuT in an open-to-out conformation. Science 322:1655–1661
Sitte HH, Freissmuth M (2010) The reverse operation of Na(+)/Cl(-)-coupled neurotransmitter transporters – why amphetamines take two to tango. J Neurochem 112:340–355
Sitte HH, Freissmuth M (2015) Amphetamines, new psychoactive drugs and the monoamine transporter cycle. Trends Pharmacol Sci 36:41–50
Sitte HH, Huck S, Reither H, Boehm S, Singer EA, Pifl C (1998) Carrier-mediated release, transport rates, and charge transfer induced by amphetamine, tyramine, and dopamine in mammalian cells transfected with the human dopamine transporter. J Neurochem 71:1289–1297
Smith CB (1963) Enhancement by reserpine and alpha-methyl dopa of the effects of D-amphetamine upon the locomotor activity of mice. J Pharmacol Exp Ther 142:343–350
Solis E Jr, Suyama JA, Lazenka MF, DeFelice LJ, Negus SS, Blough BE, Banks ML (2016) Dissociable effects of the prodrug phendimetrazine and its metabolite phenmetrazine at dopamine transporters. Sci Rep 6:31385
Sonders MS, Zhu SJ, Zahniser NR, Kavanaugh MP, Amara SG (1997) Multiple ionic conductances of the human dopamine transporter: the actions of dopamine and psychostimulants. J Neurosci 17:960–974
Sorkina T, Doolen S, Galperin E, Zahniser NR, Sorkin A (2003) Oligomerization of dopamine transporters visualized in living cells by fluorescence resonance energy transfer microscopy. J Biol Chem 278:28274–28283
Steinkellner T, Yang JW, Montgomery TR, Chen WQ, Winkler MT, Sucic S, Lubec G, Freissmuth M, Elgersma Y, Sitte HH, Kudlacek O (2012) Ca(2+)/calmodulin-dependent protein kinase IIalpha (alphaCaMKII) controls the activity of the dopamine transporter: implications for Angelman syndrome. J Biol Chem 287:29627–29635
Stolerman IP, Garcha HS, Mirza NR (1995) Dissociations between the locomotor stimulant and depressant effects of nicotinic agonists in rats. Psychopharmacology 117:430–437
Stolzenberg S, Quick M, Zhao C, Gotfryd K, Khelashvili G, Gether U, Loland CJ, Javitch JA, Noskov S, Weinstein H, Shi L (2015) Mechanism of the association between Na+ binding and conformations at the intracellular gate in neurotransmitter: sodium symporters. J Biol Chem 290:13992–14003
Su HD, Mazzei GJ, Vogler WR, Kuo JF (1985) Effect of tamoxifen, a nonsteroidal antiestrogen, on phospholipid/calcium-dependent protein kinase and phosphorylation of its endogenous substrate proteins from the rat brain and ovary. Biochem Pharmacol 34:3649–3653
Sulzer D (2011) How addictive drugs disrupt presynaptic dopamine neurotransmission. Neuron 69:628–649
Sulzer D, Chen TK, Lau YY, Kristensen H, Rayport S, Ewing A (1995) Amphetamine redistributes dopamine from synaptic vesicles to the cytosol and promotes reverse transport. J Neurosci 15:4102–4108
Sulzer D, Sonders MS, Poulsen NW, Galli A (2005) Mechanisms of neurotransmitter release by amphetamines: a review. Prog Neurobiol 75:406–433

Teng L, Crooks PA, Dwoskin LP (1998) Lobeline displaces [3H]dihydrotetrabenazine binding and releases [3H]dopamine from rat striatal synaptic vesicles: comparison with d-amphetamine. J Neurochem 71:258–265

Thoenen H, Hurlimann A, Haefely W (1968) Mechanism of amphetamine accumulation in the isolated perfused heart of the rat. J Pharm Pharmacol 20:1–11

Vaughan RA, Huff RA, Uhl GR, Kuhar MJ (1997) Protein kinase C-mediated phosphorylation and functional regulation of dopamine transporters in striatal synaptosomes. J Biol Chem 272:15541–15546

Vezina P (2004) Sensitization of midbrain dopamine neuron reactivity and the self-administration of psychomotor stimulant drugs. Neurosci Biobehav Rev 27:827–839

Vezina P, Lorrain DS, Arnold GM, Austin JD, Suto N (2002) Sensitization of midbrain dopamine neuron reactivity promotes the pursuit of amphetamine. J Neurosci 22:4654–4662

Wall SC, Gu H, Rudnick G (1995) Biogenic amine flux mediated by cloned transporters stably expressed in cultured cell lines: amphetamine specificity for inhibition and efflux. Mol Pharmacol 47:544–550

Wallis GG, Mc HJ, Scott OC (1949) Acute psychosis caused by dextro-amphetamine. Br Med J 2:1394

Wang YM, Gainetdinov RR, Fumagalli F, Xu F, Jones SR, Bock CB, Miller GW, Wightman RM, Caron MG (1997) Knockout of the vesicular monoamine transporter 2 gene results in neonatal death and supersensitivity to cocaine and amphetamine. Neuron 19:1285–1296

Wang KH, Penmatsa A, Gouaux E (2015) Neurotransmitter and psychostimulant recognition by the dopamine transporter. Nature 521:322–327

Wang Q, Bubula N, Brown J, Wang Y, Kondev V, Vezina P (2016) PKC phosphorylates residues in the N-terminal of the DA transporter to regulate amphetamine-induced DA efflux. Neurosci Lett 622:78–82

Weissman A, Koe BK, Tenen SS (1966) Antiamphetamine effects following inhibition of tyrosine hydroxylase. J Pharmacol Exp Ther 151:339–352

Wieczorek WJ, Kruk ZL (1994) Differential action of (+)-amphetamine on electrically evoked dopamine overflow in rat brain slices containing corpus striatum and nucleus accumbens. Br J Pharmacol 111:829–836

Wise RA, Bozarth MA (1985) Brain mechanisms of drug reward and euphoria. Psychiatr Med 3:445–460

Xu C, Coffey LL, Reith ME (1995) Translocation of dopamine and binding of 2 beta-carbomethoxy-3 beta-(4-fluorophenyl) tropane (WIN 35,428) measured under identical conditions in rat striatal synaptosomal preparations. Inhibition by various blockers. Biochem Pharmacol 49:339–350

Yamashita A, Singh SK, Kawate T, Jin Y, Gouaux E (2005) Crystal structure of a bacterial homologue of Na+/Cl−-dependent neurotransmitter transporters. Nature 437:215–223

Zaczek R, Culp S, De Souza EB (1991) Interactions of [3H]amphetamine with rat brain synaptosomes. II. Active transport. J Pharmacol Exp Ther 257:830–835

Zahniser NR, Sorkin A (2009) Trafficking of dopamine transporters in psychostimulant actions. Semin Cell Dev Biol 20:411–417

Zarate CA, Manji HK (2009) Protein kinase C inhibitors: rationale for use and potential in the treatment of bipolar disorder. CNS Drugs 23:569–582

Zestos AG, Mikelman SR, Kennedy RT, Gnegy ME (2016) PKCbeta inhibitors attenuate amphetamine-stimulated dopamine efflux. ACS Chem Neurosci 7:757–766

Zestos AG, Carpenter C, Kim Y, Low MJ, Kennedy RT, Gnegy ME (2019) Ruboxistaurin reduces cocaine-stimulated increases in extracellular dopamine by modifying dopamine-autoreceptor activity. ACS Chem Neurosci 10:1960–1969

Zetterstrom T, Sharp T, Collin AK, Ungerstedt U (1988) In vivo measurement of extracellular dopamine and DOPAC in rat striatum after various dopamine-releasing drugs; implications for the origin of extracellular DOPAC. Eur J Pharmacol 148:327–334

Zhou Z, Zhen J, Karpowich NK, Goetz RM, Law CJ, Reith ME, Wang DN (2007) LeuT-desipramine structure reveals how antidepressants block neurotransmitter reuptake. Science 317:1390–1393

Zhu HJ, Appel DI, Grundemann D, Markowitz JS (2010) Interaction of organic cation transporter 3 (SLC22A3) and amphetamine. J Neurochem 114:142–149

Zimanyi I, Lajtha A, Reith ME (1989) Comparison of characteristics of dopamine uptake and mazindol binding in mouse striatum. Naunyn Schmiedeberg's Arch Pharmacol 340:626–632

Clinical Trials for Stimulant Use Disorders: Addressing Heterogeneities That May Undermine Treatment Outcomes

Paul S. Regier, Kyle M. Kampman, and Anna Rose Childress

Contents

1 Cocaine Use on the Rise (Again) 300
2 The Challenges of Translation 301
3 Tonic and Phasic Dopamine Changes with Stimulant Administration 302
3.1 Enhancing Tonic Dopamine 302
3.2 Reducing Phasic Dopamine 304
3.3 Combination Pharmacotherapies: Addressing Both Tonic and Phasic Dopamine ... 306
4 Interindividual Phenotypic Heterogeneity 306
4.1 Sex Differences 307
4.2 Pharmacogenetics 308
4.3 Cue-Vulnerable Phenotypes 308
4.4 Stress-Related Phenotypes 309
4.5 Interaction of Cue-Vulnerability and Stress-Related Pathologies (Prior Adversity) ... 309
4.6 Poor Frontal Function Endophenotype 309
4.7 Drug Use Severity 310
5 Conclusions and Future Directions 311
References 311

Abstract

In recent years, use of cocaine and amphetamines and deaths associated with stimulants have been on the rise, and there are still no FDA-approved medications for stimulant use disorders. One contributing factor may involve heterogeneity. At the neurobiological level, dual dopamine dysfunction may be undermining medication efficacy, suggesting a need for combination pharmacotherapies. At the population level, individual variability is expressed in a number of ways and, if left unaddressed, may interfere with medication efficacy. This chapter reviews studies investigating medications to address dopamine dysfunction, and it also

P. S. Regier (✉) · K. M. Kampman · A. R. Childress
Department of Psychiatry, Perelman School of Medicine, Center for Studies of Addiction, University of Pennsylvania, Philadelphia, PA, USA
e-mail: pregier@pennmedicine.upenn.edu

M. A. Nader, Y. L. Hurd (eds.), *Substance Use Disorders*,
Handbook of Experimental Pharmacology 258, https://doi.org/10.1007/164_2019_303

identifies several prominent heterogeneities associated with stimulant (and other substance) use disorders. The chapter has implications for improving interventions to treat stimulant use disorders, and the theme of individual heterogeneity may have broader application across substance use disorders.

Keywords
Amphetamines · Cocaine · Heterogeneity · Medication-assisted treatment · Relapse

1 Cocaine Use on the Rise (Again)

Stimulant use disorder is a worldwide problem. After a 30-year national epidemic in the United States and a sharp decline from the early 2000s to 2010, occurrence of stimulant use is on the rise again. In 2017, more than 2.5 million Americans had a stimulant (cocaine, methamphetamines, prescription stimulants) use disorder (SAMHSA 2018). Of increasing concern, the number of users of stimulants (and misuse of prescription stimulants), new initiates of stimulants, and overdose deaths associated with stimulants have all been escalating since 2010 (Fig. 1). As a result of rising rates of cocaine and methamphetamines use, as well as increased prescription stimulant misuse (SAMHSA 2018), new illicit users of all stimulants actually surpassed those of opioids in 2017 (stimulants, 2.4 million; opioids, 2 million; NETI 2018). These alarming new trends have prompted the National Emerging Threats Initiative to identify stimulants as an urgent and developing problem in the United States (NETI 2018).

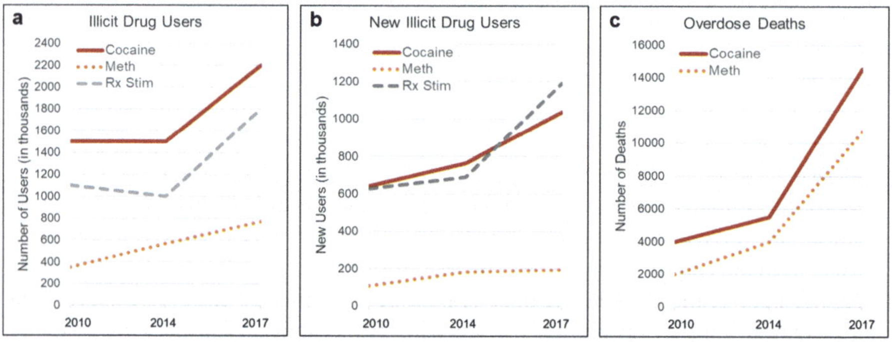

Fig. 1 Numbers reflect changes from 2010 to 2017. (**a**) The number of cocaine users (solid red line) has increased by 47%, number of methamphetamine users (orange dotted line) has increased by 119%, and nonmedical users (i.e., misusers) of prescription stimulants (gray dashed line) increased by 63%. (**b**) New initiates (first time users) of cocaine (solid red line) increased by 61%, new users of methamphetamines (orange dotted line) increased by 82%, and new initiates (misusers) of nonmedical prescription stimulants (gray dashed line) increased by 90%. (**c**) Overdose deaths associated with cocaine (solid red line) have sharply increased by 369%, and overdose deaths associated with methamphetamines (orange dotted line) have also drastically increased by 536%. (Data from SAMHSA and Center for Disease Control)

The World Drug Report for 2018 (UNODC 2018) indicates similar and alarming trends for the rest of the world. For example, in Canada, there was a sharp decline of stimulant use in the early 2000s, but that number has been increasing. In Europe, rates of stimulant use in 2015 were low; however, similar to the United States, increased trafficking of cocaine hints at signs of expansion. In South America, rates of cocaine use were also on the rise from 2010 to 2012. Brazil has become one of the largest consumer markets in the world for cocaine, where as many as 4.4 million individuals were users of smoked cocaine in 2013 (Abdalla et al. 2014). Methamphetamine use continues to be problematic in Mexico, China, and Thailand, and it has also increased in popularity in regions in the Middle East and South Asia as well (Chomchai and Chomchai 2015).

2 The Challenges of Translation

The Federal Drug Administration has yet to approve a single medication for the treatment of stimulant use disorders. Years of preclinical studies have revealed several compounds that show promise in current animal models of stimulant use disorders; however few have translated to success in human clinical trials. Success of studies can be measured in various ways; however for this review, we will refer to "effectiveness" in preclinical studies as measured by a reduction in drug-seeking behaviors, such as cue-triggered reinstatement and conditioned place preference, whereas "effectiveness" in clinical studies will be demonstrated by the reduction of self-reported drug use verified by negative urine toxicology. There are already several excellent reviews on clinical medication trials of stimulant use disorders and the various successes and failures (e.g., Dackis and O'Brien 2003; Anderson et al. 2009; Penberthy et al. 2010; Kampman 2010; Nuijten et al. 2011; Shorter and Kosten 2011; Mariani and Levin 2012; Stoops and Rush 2014; Siniscalchi et al. 2015; Shorter et al. 2015; Negus and Henningfield 2015). For this review, we will instead focus on issues of translation toward improving future medication trials. Therefore, the review will be limited in scope in two ways. First, there are many culprits for poor translation of medication treatment efficacy from preclinical studies to clinical trials. These include the lack of dose response and medication plasma levels in clinical trials, possible species differences, and failure to take heterogeneity (e.g., underlying brain states, phenotypes, pharmacogenetics) into account. A second limitation in scope is the interventions discussed. Across the lengthy stimulant epidemic, multiple preclinical targets of promise have been identified, but clinical trials for many of these are either early [e.g., glutamate modulators (e.g., Kalivas et al. 2003); calcium channel blockers (e.g., Anderson et al. 2008); vaccines (e.g., Heekin et al. 2017); and transcranial magnetic stimulation (e.g., Hanlon et al. 2015; Diana et al. 2017)] or still in the planning stage [e.g., corticotropin-releasing factor antagonists (e.g., Logrip et al. 2011); dynorphins/kappa agents (e.g., Carey et al. 2007; Redila and Chavkin 2008; Al-Hasani et al. 2013); orexins (e.g., James et al. 2018); 5HT-2C modulators (Bubar and Cunningham 2006); and deep brain stimulation (e.g., Luigjes et al. 2012)]. For this review, we focus on a strategy that has generated multiple clinical trials – agents that modulate (tonic vs. phasic) dopaminergic transmission – and that offers a useful opportunity to discuss the challenges in preclinical translation.

3 Tonic and Phasic Dopamine Changes with Stimulant Administration

Chronic administration of stimulants is associated with, at least, two types of dopamine dysfunction. The first of these is low, *tonic* dopamine, a feature of early cocaine cessation (Martinez et al. 2009, 2011; Ashok et al. 2017) and sometimes accompanied by symptoms of low energy and low mood/anhedonia. The second dysfunction is enhanced *phasic* dopamine release in response to drugs and drug-related cues (Berridge and Robinson 1998; Willuhn et al. 2014), a potential motivational trigger for relapse (Li et al. 2015; Courtney et al. 2016; Moeller and Paulus 2018; MacNiven et al. 2018) – a vulnerability that can persist several months after observable cessation symptoms (Wang et al. 2013; Parvaz et al. 2016). Analogous to preclinical findings of increased phasic dopamine are imaging data in humans demonstrating a cue-triggered mesolimbic activation (Childress et al. 1999; Kühn and Gallinat 2011; Chase et al. 2011; Young et al. 2014) and dopamine release (Volkow et al. 2006; Wong et al. 2006; Fotros et al. 2013). Based on this information, it may be necessary for medication-assisted treatment of stimulant use disorders to address both types of dopamine dysfunction in order to be effective. The framework for the current review is to examine medications intended to address either of these dysfunctions. One conclusion from the chapter is that it may currently be difficult to address both dysfunctions with a single medication and that a combination approach may be more feasible.

3.1 Enhancing Tonic Dopamine

Preclinical research has demonstrated that chronic stimulant administration is associated with abnormally low tonic dopamine (Segal and Kuczenski 1992a, b; Kalivas and Duffy 1993a, b; Di Chiara and Bassareo 2007), stimulating clinical research studies focused on improving dopamine tone (Dackis and Gold 1985; Ashok et al. 2017) – usually by administration of a dopamine agonist. These agonists have included medications that increase dopamine release [e.g., amphetamines enhance dopamine by three different mechanisms (Calipari and Ferris 2013)], block the dopamine transporter (e.g., modafinil, methylphenidate), or increase dopamine synthesis (e.g., levodopa).

3.1.1 Short-Acting Dopamine Enhancers

Short-acting dopamine transporter reuptake inhibitors have been useful for attenuating the subjective effects of stimulants in laboratory and clinical studies (Dackis et al. 2003; Hart et al. 2008; Verrico et al. 2014) and demonstrated a reduction of cocaine use in early observations and follow-up clinical pilot studies (Khantzian et al. 1984; Levin et al. 1998; Dackis et al. 2003, 2005). Unfortunately, several follow-up double-blind, placebo-controlled trials found no main effect on cocaine use (Schubiner et al. 2002; Anderson et al. 2009; Schmitz et al. 2012; Dackis et al. 2012). However, recent secondary analyses from large studies have renewed interest. For example, it was found that modafinil increased consecutive days of abstinence (Kampman et al. 2015) and reduced the number of cocaine-positive urines, due to the mediating effect of modafinil improving sleep (Morgan et al. 2016). Early studies of cocaine use disorder and the dysregulation of dopamine in chronic users found that *levodopa* (half-life of 1.5 h) reduced withdrawal symptoms (Wolfsohn and Angrist 1990), but these effects were unable to be replicated (Wolfsohn et al. 1993). Follow-up studies also found no main effect of levodopa on cocaine use (Shoptaw et al. 2005; Mooney et al. 2007). However, Schmitz et al. (2008) tested levodopa in the context of different behavioral treatments and found that levodopa was effective when paired with a more intense psychosocial treatment (e.g., contingency management). Encouragingly, a follow-up study found a similar result (Schmitz et al. 2010). The short half-life of levodopa, requiring multiple daily doses (Espay et al. 2017), may help to account for the mixed clinical results in substance use disorder populations, where medication compliance is a significant challenge.

3.1.2 Long-Acting Dopamine Enhancers

The potential abuse liability of short-acting dopamine agonists encouraged preclinical testing of chronically administered (Chiodo et al. 2008; Czoty et al. 2010) and/or longer-acting formulations (Czoty et al. 2016). These studies have provided some support (though see Czoty et al. 2013) for human studies with longer-acting (extended release) stimulants. An early study found that *d-amphetamine* had a tendency to reduce cocaine (but not opiate) use at the highest dose tested (Grabowski et al. 2001) and this was followed by a second study with similarly results (Grabowski et al. 2004). However, a study conducted around the same time found no difference of drug use (measured by urine analyses) between cocaine patients treated with d-amphetamine and controls, even though self-report of cocaine use and craving was lower in the treatment group (Shearer et al. 2003). More recently, a laboratory study found that d-amphetamine reduced cocaine (but not hydromorphone) self-administration in humans (Greenwald et al. 2010), and two clinical trials using extended-release amphetamines to treat cocaine use disorder with other comorbid disorders found a significant reduction of cocaine use compared to placebo (Levin et al. 2015; Nuijten et al. 2016).

3.1.3 Summary: Enhancing Tonic Dopamine

While clinical trials with extended-release dopamine enhancers have provided more positive drug use outcome results, in general, trials utilizing tonic dopamine enhancers as treatment have produced mixed results. This may reflect the challenge of "dual" dopamine dysfunctions: though dopamine agonists can help restore normal tonic levels of dopamine that have been disrupted by chronic stimulant use, if phasic dopamine is still enhanced in response to drug cues, an individual may still remain vulnerable to cue-triggered relapse (Sinha et al. 2005; Kosten et al. 2006). Having a single medication that could both increase tonic dopamine and reduce phasic dopamine events (e.g., a dopamine partial agonist) would be very appealing, but these are still in early development. Until such "dual-acting" agents are available for clinical trials, medications shown to inhibit phasic dopamine could be used in combination with tonic dopamine enhancers to treat both aspects of dopamine dysfunction, described next.

3.2 Reducing Phasic Dopamine

GABAergic drugs can modulate dopamine action, including the phasic response to drugs or drug-related stimuli. Preclinical studies have investigated the action of GABAergic drugs on drug-induced dopamine release and have found several candidates that decrease phasic dopamine response in the striatum. Clinical studies describing three different medications that enhance GABA are described below.

3.2.1 Gamma-Vinyl GABA (GVG)

GVG is an irreversible inhibitor of GABA transaminase (catabolic enzyme for GABA), eliciting an increase of GABA available at the synapse. Several preclinical studies demonstrated that GVG reduced phasic dopamine in response to drugs and drug-related cues (Dewey et al. 1992; Morgan and Dewey 1998; Kushner et al. 1999; Gerasimov et al. 2001; Schiffer et al. 2001a), offering compelling proof of mechanism. In clinical trials, Brodie et al. (2003, 2005) tested the efficacy of GVG for stimulant use disorders in humans, and the initial clinical studies were very encouraging. Two double-blind, placebo-controlled trials followed, the first of which reported a main effect of treatment with GVG significantly increased abstinence from cocaine and (although not a primary outcome measure) alcohol (Brodie et al. 2009). The second trial failed to replicate the first (Somoza et al. 2013); the authors discussed several factors that differed between the two studies, including lower medication compliance (approximately 40%) in the negative trial. Though long-term, high-dose use of GVG (e.g., in treatment-resistant pediatric epilepsy) can result in irreversible visual field deficits (Maguire et al. 2010; Clayton et al. 2013), a newer and reportedly safer version (CPP-115) has been developed and is currently being tested (Prescot et al. 2018; Juncosa et al. 2018).

3.2.2 Baclofen

Preclinical studies have found that baclofen, a GABA B receptor agonist, reduces stimulant-induced dopamine in the ventral striatum in animals (Fadda et al. 2003; Pitman et al. 2014) and blunts cue-induced limbic activation in humans (Young et al. 2014). Baclofen has also shown effectiveness at reducing cocaine-seeking and attenuating reinstatement in animals (Roberts et al. 1996; Campbell et al. 1999; Brebner et al. 2000a, b; Di Ciano and Everitt 2003; Weerts et al. 2007). The preclinical data suggest that baclofen would work best as an *anti-relapse* medication, as it was generally more effective in blocking reinstatement than in reducing ongoing drug use. Clinical translation of baclofen's efficacy has been challenging, despite early promise (Ling et al. 1998; Shoptaw et al. 2003). One of the primary difficulties is baclofen's short half-life (2–4 h), posing a problem for medication compliance in outpatient treatment, requiring 3–4 times daily dosing. Compounding this pharmacokinetic problem, recent studies in humans have shown that baclofen plasma levels can vary widely for the *same* oral dose (Marsot et al. 2014) and that GABA B receptor genetics may significantly impact clinical efficacy (Morley et al. 2018). Given these translational challenges, it is perhaps unsurprising that the early NIDA baclofen trial (Kahn et al. 2009) conducted with the short-acting formulation, in a cohort of actively using cocaine patients, and without knowledge of either plasma levels or genetics was unable to demonstrate overall clinical benefit. Fortunately, there are now ongoing efforts to improve GABA B agonists, either with a longer-acting, prodrug formulation (Lal et al. 2009; Veenstra-VanderWeele et al. 2017) or with positive allosteric modulators of the GABA B receptor that may have better pharmacokinetics and minimal side effects (Hwa et al. 2014; Augier et al. 2017).

3.2.3 Topiramate

Topiramate enhances GABA and decreases glutamate activity; both neurotransmitters have previously been shown to play important roles in drug seeking and relapse (Cornish and Kalivas 2000; McFarland and Kalivas 2001). This dual action has the effect of reducing drug-induced dopamine release (Dewey et al. 1992; Schiffer et al. 2001b) and cocaine administration (Kushner et al. 1999). Encouraged by these preclinical studies, Kampman et al. (2004) tested topiramate for treatment of cocaine use disorders and found that abstinence was significantly higher in the topiramate group after titration up to 200 mg was achieved (week 9). Two follow-up studies found positive results: one demonstrated main effects of topiramate on the reduction of cocaine use and craving (Johnson et al. 2013), and the other showed a significant increase in cocaine abstinence during the last 3 weeks of a 12-week trial (Kampman et al. 2013). More recently, another clinical study found mixed results, reporting that topiramate significantly reduced drug use, but the differences between topiramate vs. placebo groups were not present after the first 4 weeks of treatment (Baldaçara et al. 2016). Topiramate's very gradual induction to reach therapeutic levels (9 weeks; minimizes side effect profile; for review, see Shinn and Greenfield 2010) may undermine detection of efficacy in short trials and in populations with early attrition, common in patients with substance use disorders.

3.2.4 Summary: Reducing Phasic Dopamine

To date, topiramate has provided the most consistent and positive results for treating stimulant use disorders with a GABAergic drug. However, when used alone, GABA medications may address only one aspect of dual dopamine dysfunction (i.e., abnormally high phasic dopamine release in response to drugs and drug-related cues). This may help explain mixed results in other clinical trials investigating GABA medications. Combining medications that both enhance tonic dopamine *and* blunt phasic dopamine release might be an effective strategy, described below.

3.3 Combination Pharmacotherapies: Addressing Both Tonic and Phasic Dopamine

Results from preclinical studies demonstrated that combining dopamine agonists with other medications could effectively reduce cocaine administration in rats (Karkhanis et al. 2016) but combination medications in a handful of clinical trials have had mixed results (Stoops and Rush 2014). Encouragingly, in two recent trials, combination therapy with a dopamine enhancer and a GABA (and glutamate) modulator has shown promise for treatment of stimulant use disorders.

Researchers chose two medications, extended-release mixed amphetamine salts and topiramate, based on their more consistent and positive outcome results (relative to other dopamine and GABA medications) as well as the dual action of these medications on dopamine dysfunction. Results from recent trials involving the combination of extended-release amphetamines and topiramate are just beginning to be disseminated; however, early results are very encouraging. Mariani and Levin (2012) found, in a sample of 81 patients, that the combination medication condition was associated with better 3-week abstinence outcomes compared to placebo, particularly for cocaine patients that had used cocaine on 9 or more days during the previous 28 days prior to the study. Encouragingly, a recent follow-up study with 127 patients replicated this significant result (Levin et al. 2020).

3.3.1 Summary: Combination Pharmacotherapies

From a mechanistic standpoint, combination medication treatment with dopamine and GABA enhancers should address both aspects of dual dopamine dysfunction associated with chronic stimulant use. As a proof of concept for addressing multiple factors associated with dopamine dysfunction, the results from trials investigating the combination of extended-release amphetamines and topiramate suggest a viable path forward. However, treatment with topiramate has its hurdles, as the induction onto the full dose can take up to 9 weeks, and it also has side effects that are associated with high dropout rates. Newer GABAergic medications such as positive allosteric modulators – gaining increasing attention as a potential therapeutic strategy for treating substance use disorders (Agabio and Colombo 2014; Filip et al. 2015; Maccioni and Colombo 2019) – may provide an additional option for augmenting dopamine agonist treatment. Compared to topiramate, these agents may be easier to use and have an induction time to full dose that is much shorter.

4 Interindividual Phenotypic Heterogeneity

As discussed, the heterogeneity of underlying brain states among patients with stimulant use disorders (e.g., dual dysfunctions in dopamine transmission) may have undermined outcomes in prior medication trials. However, there exists another type of heterogeneity that can impact clinical trial outcomes, and that is *individual variability* within the population with substance use disorders. Phenotypic heterogeneity can be shaped by a wide variety of genetic and epigenetic/environmental variables (e.g., severity of the disorder, presence of comorbid disorders or other substance disorders, prior adversity, etc.). *Endo*phenotypes are particularly welcome for medication development, as their underlying biological substrate(s) may be intervention targets. But even when phenotype is complex, and/or its underlying determinants are not yet known (or even malleable), it may be very useful in the design of medication trials, as an initial stratification variable, or as a splitting variable/covariate in posttrial analyses. This section will discuss several heterogeneities that, if addressed, may improve the interpretability of intervention trials for stimulant use disorders – and for medication development across the addictions.

4.1 Sex Differences

Research has revealed sex differences in relation to drug-seeking behavior in animals and substance use disorders in humans. For example, in self-administration experiments, female rats display faster acquisition of drugs, have higher motivation to take drugs, experience more severe withdrawal symptoms, and exhibit greater cue- and drug-induced reinstatement compared to male rats (for review, see Becker 2016). In human research, data shows women are more vulnerable to substance use disorders (e.g., more rapid transition from recreational to compulsive use, heightened cue response, more relapse) compared to men, which may be mediated by menstrual cycle hormones (for review, see Bobzean et al. 2014). Research has also shown that some medication is not as effective for women compared to men [e.g., nicotine replacement for smoking cessation (Cepeda-Benito et al. 2004)]. Preliminary research for stimulants suggests gender differences may depend on medication category: early literature showed no differences between men and women for treatment of cocaine use disorders with desipramine or lithium treatment (Kosten et al. 1993). However, more recent studies demonstrated that disulfiram and naltrexone were less effective in women for treating alcohol use disorder (DeVito et al. 2014) and comorbid alcohol and cocaine use disorders (Pettinati et al. 2008; Suh et al. 2008), respectively. In addition, studies have shown sex differences related to the expression and treatment of stress-related pathologies. For example, compared to men, women have exhibited a heightened physiological response to yohimbine, an alpha-2 adrenergic *antagonist* (Moran-Santa Maria et al. 2014), and have also had better clinical outcomes with guanfacine, an alpha-2 adrenergic *agonist* (Fox et al. 2014). Finally, given the impact of estradiol on dopamine transmission (Becker 1990, 1999; Bazzett and Becker 1994), it may be especially important to take sex into account for the medications reviewed in this chapter intended to modulate both tonic and phasic dopamine.

4.2 Pharmacogenetics

An important source of heterogeneity in medication response is pharmacogenetics: some individuals are medication "responders" or "non-responders" due to their genetic variation. The addition of genotyping to clinical trials for addiction has enabled several preliminary demonstrations of the future potential for this approach (Jones et al. 2015). For example, cigarette smokers with genetic variants conferring "fast" nicotine metabolism respond poorly to nicotine replacement therapies but may respond well to alternative treatments (Chenoweth and Tyndale 2017). Opioid patients carrying a specific polymorphism of the delta opioid receptor have a better clinical response (reduced drug use) to buprenorphine treatment (Crist et al. 2013, 2018), and individual genetic variation has also been linked to treatment response in alcoholism for more than one medication category [e.g., naltrexone (Heilig et al. 2011); topiramate (Kranzler et al. 2014); baclofen (Morley et al. 2018)]. Fewer cocaine trials have made use of pharmacogenetics (Shorter et al. 2013; Jones et al. 2015), but known polymorphisms for several appealing medication targets already discussed [e.g., the dopamine transporter (Franklin et al. 2008); dopamine receptors (Savitz et al. 2013); the GABA B agonist baclofen (Morley et al. 2018)] strongly encourage the explicit use of genetic tools. Data-driven, genome-wide approaches can also be used to parse the heterogeneity in medication response (Kranzler et al. 2009), guiding and complementing the examination of hypothesis-driven polymorphisms.

4.3 Cue-Vulnerable Phenotypes

Studies have demonstrated interindividual variability in the response to drug- and reward-related cues (e.g., Robinson and Berridge 2001; Flagel et al. 2010; Regier et al. 2016); the elevated (mesolimbic) response to drug cues is a marker of vulnerability to drug-seeking in animals (Flagel et al. 2009) and is associated with differences in treatment efficacy (Mann et al. 2014). In humans, brain imaging (BOLD fMRI) during drug-cue exposure has been successfully used to characterize the relative vulnerability to drug cues, across a wide range of substance use disorders (Childress et al. 1999; Wexler et al. 2001; Bonson et al. 2002; Franklin et al. 2007; Langleben et al. 2008; Goldman et al. 2013; Jasinska et al. 2014; Kober et al. 2016). Importantly, the brain response to drug cues in substance users has demonstrated relapse-relevance (Li et al. 2015; Courtney et al. 2016; Moeller and Paulus 2018; MacNiven et al. 2018). This relapse link means that the brain response to drug cues can be used to help determine the general promise of a candidate medication for modulating mesolimbic circuitry and thus for preventing relapse in "cue-vulnerable" individuals. In the future, this approach could also be used to select individuals who most likely benefit from a "cue-targeted" medication.

4.4 Stress-Related Phenotypes

Substance use disorders have many overlapping features with other "stress-related" pathologies (e.g., cumulative lifetime stress, childhood abuse, trauma, anxiety, chronic stress; Sinha 2001, 2008, 2009; Goeders 2003; Hyman et al. 2008; Viola et al. 2014). Thus, addressing factors in individuals with comorbid stimulant use disorders and stress-related pathologies may enhance treatment efficacy. For example, Fox and Sinha (2014) discuss the ability of guanfacine, an alpha2-adrenergic agonist, in attenuating stress-induced responses (e.g., cue-induced craving) and reducing stress-related phenomena (e.g., anxiety), as well as enhancing cognitive control. A recent review identified the most promising medications for treating stress-related pathologies, which include kappa-opioid antagonists and noradrenergic agents (Greenwald 2018). Preclinical research has demonstrated the interaction of early-life stress and kappa-opioid receptor dysfunction, leading to more drug use, but that this effect could be mitigated by kappa-opioid receptor antagonist (Karkhanis et al. 2016).

4.5 Interaction of Cue-Vulnerability and Stress-Related Pathologies (Prior Adversity)

Not only are the described individual phenotypes (e.g., cue- and stress-vulnerable) a source of outcome heterogeneity, they may also interact in unexpected and important ways. For example, a prominent and concerning source of heterogeneity within the substance use disordered population is prior adversity, which is overrepresented in individuals with substance use disorders (e.g., Felitti et al. 1998; Rice et al. 2001; Medrano et al. 2002; Charney et al. 2007; Hyman et al. 2007). Preclinical studies have shown that early-life stress in animals is associated with increased vulnerabilities to drug self-administration and to cues signaling drug reward (for review, see Sinha 2001). Translating these findings to clinical research, Regier et al. (2016) recently demonstrated that individuals with prior adversity (e.g., emotional, physical, and/or sexual abuse) have a heightened mesolimbic response to cocaine reward cues. These findings highlight the significant interaction of appetitive and aversive motivational systems and their associated phenotypic vulnerabilities.

4.6 Poor Frontal Function Endophenotype

Preclinical studies show that chronic stimulant exposure can erode frontal inhibitory functions (Jentsch and Taylor 1999) and that animals with poorer baseline frontal function are more severely impacted by stimulant exposure (Ferland and Winstanley 2017). This interaction between pre-existing frontal function and stimulant exposure may account for the heterogeneity in frontal deficits found in clinical cohorts, with some patients demonstrating significant deficits in several executive functions (Goldstein and Volkow 2002, 2011; Hester and Garavan 2004), while others with similar histories of drug use may be less impaired (Carroll et al. 2011). As the brain's frontal circuitry is responsible for regulating downstream appetitive and aversive motivational systems, dysfunctions in this circuit would exacerbate the vulnerabilities described earlier (i.e., cue-triggered or stress-related pathologies). Encouragingly, cocaine patients with extended abstinence can show recovery of inhibitory function (Connolly et al. 2012), suggesting the "poor frontal function" endophenotype may be a reasonable target for intervention. Dopamine agonists (as previously discussed for improving dopamine tone) have been used to treat frontal dysfunction in cocaine patients with and without attention deficit hyperactivity disorder (Hester et al. 2010; Li et al. 2010; Dean et al. 2011). Although frontal symptoms are sometimes improved, this has not always translated into a reduction in cocaine use (Carpentier and Levin 2017). Thus, similar to the issue above with treating both aspects of dual dopamine dysfunction, non-stimulant medications [e.g., atomoxetine (Levin et al. 2009)] or combination medications (e.g., cognitive enhancers + GABA modulators) may offer a better alternative than monotherapies.

4.7 Drug Use Severity

Even though patients entering clinical trials usually carry the same diagnosis (e.g., "cocaine use disorder"), they vary in baseline urine status. Some patients are beginning to submit cocaine-free urines *even before formal treatment begins*, while others continue to use drugs up to, and beyond, treatment entry. Positive drug screens at treatment entry are widely recognized as a strong predictor of poor clinical outcome (Ehrman et al. 2001; Kampman et al. 2002; Patkar et al. 2002; Ahmadi et al. 2009); thus, baseline urine status is an important stratification variable in medication trials. A recent imaging study (Lam et al. 2013) revealed brain underpinnings for this phenotype, offering a possible medication target.

Though clinical research studies usually focus on patients with "severe" substance use disorder, it is worth noting that preclinical models often include a range of "severities," with only 15–20% of drug-taking animals displaying the "addiction-like" characteristics of clinical samples (Ahmed and Koob 1998; Deroche-Gamonet et al. 2004; Ahmed 2010). This "mismatch" between drug use severity in preclinical vs. clinical models may account, in part, for the poor translation of medication findings in animal studies (Cao et al. 2016). Relaxing eligibility criteria in some clinical research studies to allow individuals with mild and/or moderate substance use disorder may not only afford better translation from preclinical research but would also enable examination of medication efficacy according to the phenotype of drug use severity. This broadened recruitment strategy may reveal medications (e.g., agents with efficacy in less severe phenotypes) that would otherwise go undiscovered and that may, in turn, inform the search for medications effective against severe drug use. To better match clinical trials, preclinical studies might include more polysubstance use models, as the majority of individuals with substance use disorders often have more than one.

5 Conclusions and Future Directions

This chapter has examined medication trials in stimulant use disorders from the perspective of both heterogeneity of underlying brain states (using "dual dopamine dysfunction" as an example) and heterogeneity of individual phenotypes. Both types of heterogeneity can undermine clinical results. However, if acknowledged and addressed, these same heterogeneities can actually become useful tools for parsing medication outcomes for existing agents and for developing medications for novel targets.

Despite the prior challenges, future medication development for stimulant use disorders promises acceleration, by wider incorporation of brain information in human studies. Most clinical medication trials for stimulant use disorders have been conducted without any direct information about "target engagement," i.e., whether the candidate medication indeed reached the intended brain circuits by functional magnetic resonance imaging (fMRI) or receptors by positron emission tomography (PET). Information provided by these brain tools is helpful for determining the promise of a candidate medication *even before* proceeding to a clinical trial. If collected *concurrently* within a clinical trial, the brain-level information is valuable for parsing and interpreting the medication response. Even when conducted *after* a failed clinical trial (Le Foll et al. 2016), PET can offer valuable information for understanding why the trial may have failed. Fueling the wider use of brain information, new in silico techniques (Jones and Lin 2017) will speed the development of both tracers and medications, enabling highly specific compounds for long-pursued, addiction-relevant brain targets (e.g., the dopamine D3 receptor, Heidbreder and Newman 2010; Chien et al. 2010; Mach et al. 2011). These advances, especially when combined with readily available measures (e.g., medication plasma levels, genotyping, phenotyping, baseline drug use/severity), will not only speed medication discovery but will enable a critical matching of medication(s) to our patients' unique heterogeneities.

References

Abdalla RR, Madruga CS, Ribeiro M et al (2014) Prevalence of cocaine use in Brazil: data from the II Brazilian national alcohol and drugs survey (BNADS). Addict Behav 39:297–301

Agabio R, Colombo G (2014) GABAB receptor ligands for the treatment of alcohol use disorder: preclinical and clinical evidence. Front Neurosci 8:140. https://doi.org/10.3389/fnins.2014.00140

Ahmadi J, Kampman KM, Oslin DM et al (2009) Predictors of treatment outcome in outpatient cocaine and alcohol dependence treatment. Am J Addict 18:81–86. https://doi.org/10.1080/10550490802545174

Ahmed SH (2010) Validation crisis in animal models of drug addiction: beyond non-disordered drug use toward drug addiction. Neurosci Biobehav Rev 35:172–184. https://doi.org/10.1016/j.neubiorev.2010.04.005

Ahmed SH, Koob GF (1998) Transition from moderate to excessive drug intake: change in hedonic set point. Science 282:298–300. https://doi.org/10.1126/science.282.5387.298

Al-Hasani R, McCall JG, Foshage AM, Bruchas MR (2013) Locus coeruleus kappa-opioid receptors modulate reinstatement of cocaine place preference through a noradrenergic mechanism. Neuropsychopharmacology 38:2484–2497. https://doi.org/10.1038/npp.2013.151

Anderson SM, Famous KR, Sadri-Vakili G et al (2008) CaMKII: a biochemical bridge linking accumbens dopamine and glutamate systems in cocaine seeking. Nat Neurosci 11:344–353. https://doi.org/10.1038/nn2054

Anderson AL, Reid MS, Li S-H et al (2009) Modafinil for the treatment of cocaine dependence. Drug Alcohol Depend 104:133–139. https://doi.org/10.1016/j.drugalcdep.2009.04.015

Ashok AH, Mizuno Y, Volkow ND, Howes OD (2017) Association of stimulant use with dopaminergic alterations in users of cocaine, amphetamine, or methamphetamine: a systematic review and meta-analysis. JAMA Psychiat 74:511–519. https://doi.org/10.1001/jamapsychiatry.2017.0135

Augier E, Dulman RS, Damadzic R et al (2017) The GABAB positive allosteric modulator ADX71441 attenuates alcohol self-administration and relapse to alcohol seeking in rats. Neuropsychopharmacology 42:1789–1799. https://doi.org/10.1038/npp.2017.53

Baldaçara L, Cogo-Moreira H, Parreira BL et al (2016) Efficacy of topiramate in the treatment of crack cocaine dependence: a double-blind, randomized, placebo-controlled trial. J Clin Psychiatry 77:398–406. https://doi.org/10.4088/JCP.14m09377

Bazzett TJ, Becker JB (1994) Sex differences in the rapid and acute effects of estrogen on striatal D2 dopamine receptor binding. Brain Res 637:163–172. https://doi.org/10.1016/0006-8993(94)91229-7

Becker JB (1990) Direct effect of 17 beta-estradiol on striatum: sex differences in dopamine release. Synapse 5:157–164. https://doi.org/10.1002/syn.890050211

Becker JB (1999) Gender differences in dopaminergic function in striatum and nucleus accumbens. Pharmacol Biochem Behav 64:803–812. https://doi.org/10.1016/s0091-3057(99)00168-9

Becker JB (2016) Sex differences in addiction. Dialogues Clin Neurosci 18:395–402

Berridge KC, Robinson TE (1998) What is the role of dopamine in reward: hedonic impact, reward learning, or incentive salience? Brain Res Rev 28:309–369. https://doi.org/10.1016/S0165-0173(98)00019-8

Bobzean SAM, DeNobrega AK, Perrotti LI (2014) Sex differences in the neurobiology of drug addiction. Exp Neurol 259:64–74. https://doi.org/10.1016/j.expneurol.2014.01.022

Bonson KR, Grant SJ, Contoreggi CS et al (2002) Neural systems and cue-induced cocaine craving. Neuropsychopharmacology 26:376–386. https://doi.org/10.1016/S0893-133X(01)00371-2

Brebner K, Phelan R, Roberts DC (2000a) Effect of baclofen on cocaine self-administration in rats reinforced under fixed-ratio 1 and progressive-ratio schedules. Psychopharmacology (Berl) 148:314–321

Brebner K, Phelan R, Roberts DC (2000b) Intra-VTA baclofen attenuates cocaine self-administration on a progressive ratio schedule of reinforcement. Pharmacol Biochem Behav 66:857–862

Brodie JD, Figueroa E, Dewey SL (2003) Treating cocaine addiction: from preclinical to clinical trial experience with gamma-vinyl GABA. Synapse 50:261–265. https://doi.org/10.1002/syn.10278

Brodie JD, Figueroa E, Laska EM, Dewey SL (2005) Safety and efficacy of γ-vinyl GABA (GVG) for the treatment of methamphetamine and/or cocaine addiction. Synapse 55:122–125. https://doi.org/10.1002/syn.20097

Brodie JD, Case BG, Figueroa E et al (2009) Randomized, double-blind, placebo-controlled trial of vigabatrin for the treatment of cocaine dependence in Mexican parolees. Am J Psychiatry 166:1269–1277. https://doi.org/10.1176/appi.ajp.2009.08121811

Bubar MJ, Cunningham KA (2006) Serotonin 5-HT2A and 5-HT2C receptors as potential targets for modulation of psychostimulant use and dependence. Curr Top Med Chem 6:1971–1985

Calipari ES, Ferris MJ (2013) Amphetamine mechanisms and actions at the dopamine terminal revisited. J Neurosci 33:8923–8925. https://doi.org/10.1523/JNEUROSCI.1033-13.2013

Campbell UC, Lac ST, Carroll ME (1999) Effects of baclofen on maintenance and reinstatement of intravenous cocaine self-administration in rats. Psychopharmacology (Berl) 143:209–214

Cao D-N, Shi J-J, Hao W et al (2016) Advances and challenges in pharmacotherapeutics for amphetamine-type stimulants addiction. Eur J Pharmacol 780:129–135. https://doi.org/10.1016/j.ejphar.2016.03.040

Carey AN, Borozny K, Aldrich JV, McLaughlin JP (2007) Reinstatement of cocaine place-conditioning prevented by the peptide kappa-opioid receptor antagonist arodyn. Eur J Pharmacol 569:84–89. https://doi.org/10.1016/j.ejphar.2007.05.007

Carpentier P-J, Levin FR (2017) Pharmacological treatment of ADHD in addicted patients: what does the literature tell us? Harv Rev Psychiatry 25:50–64. https://doi.org/10.1097/HRP.0000000000000122

Carroll KM, Kiluk BD, Nich C et al (2011) Cognitive function and treatment response in a randomized clinical trial of computer-based training in cognitive-behavioral therapy. Subst Use Misuse 46:23–34. https://doi.org/10.3109/10826084.2011.521069

Cepeda-Benito A, Reynoso JT, Erath S (2004) Meta-analysis of the efficacy of nicotine replacement therapy for smoking cessation: differences between men and women. J Consult Clin Psychol 72:712–722. https://doi.org/10.1037/0022-006X.72.4.712

Charney DA, Palacios-Boix J, Gill KJ (2007) Sexual abuse and the outcome of addiction treatment. Am J Addict 16:93–100. https://doi.org/10.1080/10550490601184225

Chase HW, Eickhoff SB, Laird AR, Hogarth L (2011) The neural basis of drug stimulus processing and craving: an activation likelihood estimation meta-analysis. Biol Psychiatry 70:785–793. https://doi.org/10.1016/j.biopsych.2011.05.025

Chenoweth MJ, Tyndale RF (2017) Pharmacogenetic optimization of smoking cessation treatment. Trends Pharmacol Sci 38:55–66. https://doi.org/10.1016/j.tips.2016.09.006

Chien EYT, Liu W, Zhao Q et al (2010) Structure of the human dopamine D3 receptor in complex with a D2/D3 selective antagonist. Science 330:1091–1095. https://doi.org/10.1126/science.1197410

Childress AR, Mozley PD, McElgin W et al (1999) Limbic activation during cue-induced cocaine craving. Am J Psychiatry 156:11–18. https://doi.org/10.1176/ajp.156.1.11

Chiodo KA, Läck CM, Roberts DCS (2008) Cocaine self-administration reinforced on a progressive ratio schedule decreases with continuous D-amphetamine treatment in rats. Psychopharmacology (Berl) 200:465–473. https://doi.org/10.1007/s00213-008-1222-8

Chomchai C, Chomchai S (2015) Global patterns of methamphetamine use. Curr Opin Psychiatry 28:269. https://doi.org/10.1097/YCO.0000000000000168

Clayton LM, Stern WM, Newman WD et al (2013) Evolution of visual field loss over ten years in individuals taking vigabatrin. Epilepsy Res 105:262–271. https://doi.org/10.1016/j.eplepsyres.2013.02.014

Connolly CG, Foxe JJ, Nierenberg J et al (2012) The neurobiology of cognitive control in successful cocaine abstinence. Drug Alcohol Depend 121:45–53. https://doi.org/10.1016/j.drugalcdep.2011.08.007

Cornish JL, Kalivas PW (2000) Glutamate transmission in the nucleus accumbens mediates relapse in cocaine addiction. J Neurosci 20:RC89. https://doi.org/10.1523/JNEUROSCI.20-15-j0006.2000

Courtney KE, Schacht JP, Hutchison K et al (2016) Neural substrates of cue reactivity: association with treatment outcomes and relapse. Addict Biol 21:3–22. https://doi.org/10.1111/adb.12314

Crist RC, Clarke T-K, Ang A et al (2013) An intronic variant in OPRD1 predicts treatment outcome for opioid dependence in African-Americans. Neuropsychopharmacology 38:2003–2010. https://doi.org/10.1038/npp.2013.99

Crist RC, Doyle GA, Nelson EC et al (2018) A polymorphism in the OPRM1 3′ untranslated region is associated with methadone efficacy in treating opioid dependence. Pharmacogenomics J 18:173–179. https://doi.org/10.1038/tpj.2016.89

Czoty PW, Martelle JL, Nader MA (2010) Effects of chronic d-amphetamine administration on the reinforcing strength of cocaine in rhesus monkeys. Psychopharmacology (Berl) 209:375–382. https://doi.org/10.1007/s00213-010-1807-x

Czoty PW, Martelle SE, Gould RW, Nader MA (2013) Effects of chronic methylphenidate on cocaine self-administration under a progressive-ratio schedule of reinforcement in rhesus monkeys. J Pharmacol Exp Ther 345:374–382. https://doi.org/10.1124/jpet.113.204321

Czoty PW, Blough BE, Fennell TR et al (2016) Attenuation of cocaine self-administration by chronic oral phendimetrazine in rhesus monkeys. Neuroscience 324:367–376. https://doi.org/10.1016/j.neuroscience.2016.03.002

Dackis CA, Gold MS (1985) New concepts in cocaine addiction: the dopamine depletion hypothesis. Neurosci Biobehav Rev 9:469–477. https://doi.org/10.1016/0149-7634(85)90022-3

Dackis C, O'Brien C (2003) Glutamatergic agents for cocaine dependence. Ann N Y Acad Sci 1003:328–345

Dackis CA, Lynch KG, Yu E et al (2003) Modafinil and cocaine: a double-blind, placebo-controlled drug interaction study. Drug Alcohol Depend 70:29–37. https://doi.org/10.1016/S0376-8716(02)00335-6

Dackis CA, Kampman KM, Lynch KG et al (2005) A double-blind, placebo-controlled trial of modafinil for cocaine dependence. Neuropsychopharmacology 30:205–211. https://doi.org/10.1038/sj.npp.1300600

Dackis CA, Kampman KM, Lynch KG et al (2012) A double-blind, placebo-controlled trial of modafinil for cocaine dependence. J Subst Abuse Treat 43:303–312. https://doi.org/10.1016/j.jsat.2011.12.014

Dean AC, Sevak RJ, Monterosso JR et al (2011) Acute modafinil effects on attention and inhibitory control in methamphetamine-dependent humans. J Stud Alcohol Drugs 72:943–953

Deroche-Gamonet V, Belin D, Piazza PV (2004) Evidence for addiction-like behavior in the rat. Science 305:1014–1017. https://doi.org/10.1126/science.1099020

DeVito EE, Babuscio TA, Nich C et al (2014) Gender differences in clinical outcomes for cocaine dependence: randomized clinical trials of behavioral therapy and disulfiram. Drug Alcohol Depend 145:156–167. https://doi.org/10.1016/j.drugalcdep.2014.10.007

Dewey SL, Smith GS, Logan J et al (1992) GABAergic inhibition of endogenous dopamine release measured in vivo with 11C-raclopride and positron emission tomography. J Neurosci 12:3773–3780. https://doi.org/10.1523/JNEUROSCI.12-10-03773.1992

Di Chiara G, Bassareo V (2007) Reward system and addiction: what dopamine does and doesn't do. Curr Opin Pharmacol 7:69–76. https://doi.org/10.1016/j.coph.2006.11.003

Di Ciano P, Everitt BJ (2003) The GABA(B) receptor agonist baclofen attenuates cocaine- and heroin-seeking behavior by rats. Neuropsychopharmacology 28:510–518. https://doi.org/10.1038/sj.npp.1300088

Diana M, Raij T, Melis M et al (2017) Rehabilitating the addicted brain with transcranial magnetic stimulation. Nat Rev Neurosci 18:685–693. https://doi.org/10.1038/nrn.2017.113

Ehrman RN, Robbins SJ, Cornish JW (2001) Results of a baseline urine test predict levels of cocaine use during treatment. Drug Alcohol Depend 62:1–7

Espay AJ, Pagan FL, Walter BL et al (2017) Optimizing extended-release carbidopa/levodopa in Parkinson disease: consensus on conversion from standard therapy. Neurol Clin Pract 7:86–93. https://doi.org/10.1212/CPJ.0000000000000316

Fadda P, Scherma M, Fresu A et al (2003) Baclofen antagonizes nicotine-, cocaine-, and morphine-induced dopamine release in the nucleus accumbens of rat. Synapse 50:1–6. https://doi.org/10.1002/syn.10238

Felitti VJ, Anda RF, Nordenberg D et al (1998) Relationship of childhood abuse and household dysfunction to many of the leading causes of death in adults. Am J Prev Med 14:245–258. https://doi.org/10.1016/S0749-3797(98)00017-8

Ferland J-MN, Winstanley CA (2017) Risk-preferring rats make worse decisions and show increased incubation of craving after cocaine self-administration. Addict Biol 22:991–1001. https://doi.org/10.1111/adb.12388

Filip M, Frankowska M, Sadakierska-Chudy A et al (2015) GABAB receptors as a therapeutic strategy in substance use disorders: focus on positive allosteric modulators. Neuropharmacology 88:36–47. https://doi.org/10.1016/j.neuropharm.2014.06.016

Flagel SB, Akil H, Robinson TE (2009) Individual differences in the attribution of incentive salience to reward-related cues: implications for addiction. Neuropharmacology 56(Suppl 1):139–148. https://doi.org/10.1016/j.neuropharm.2008.06.027

Flagel SB, Robinson TE, Clark JJ et al (2010) An animal model of genetic vulnerability to behavioral disinhibition and responsiveness to reward-related cues: implications for addiction. Neuropsychopharmacology 35:388–400. https://doi.org/10.1038/npp.2009.142

Fotros A, Casey KF, Larcher K et al (2013) Cocaine cue-induced dopamine release in amygdala and hippocampus: a high-resolution PET [18F]fallypride study in cocaine dependent participants. Neuropsychopharmacology 38:1780–1788. https://doi.org/10.1038/npp.2013.77

Fox H, Sinha R (2014) The role of guanfacine as a therapeutic agent to address stress-related pathophysiology in cocaine-dependent individuals. Adv Pharmacol 69:217–265. https://doi.org/10.1016/B978-0-12-420118-7.00006-8

Fox HC, Morgan PT, Sinha R (2014) Sex differences in guanfacine effects on drug craving and stress arousal in cocaine-dependent individuals. Neuropsychopharmacology 39:1527–1537. https://doi.org/10.1038/npp.2014.1

Franklin TR, Wang Z, Wang J et al (2007) Limbic activation to cigarette smoking cues independent of nicotine withdrawal: a perfusion fMRI study. Neuropsychopharmacology 32:2301–2309. https://doi.org/10.1038/sj.npp.1301371

Franklin TR, Lohoff FW, Wang Z et al (2008) DAT genotype modulates brain and behavioral responses elicited by cigarette cues. Neuropsychopharmacology 34:717–728. https://doi.org/10.1038/npp.2008.124

Gerasimov MR, Schiffer WK, Gardner EL et al (2001) GABAergic blockade of cocaine-associated cue-induced increases in nucleus accumbens dopamine. Eur J Pharmacol 414:205–209

Goeders NE (2003) The impact of stress on addiction. Eur Neuropsychopharmacol 13:435–441. https://doi.org/10.1016/j.euroneuro.2003.08.004

Goldman M, Szucs-Reed RP, Jagannathan K et al (2013) Reward-related brain response and craving correlates of marijuana cue exposure: a preliminary study in treatment-seeking marijuana-dependent subjects. J Addict Med 7:8–16. https://doi.org/10.1097/ADM.0b013e318273863a

Goldstein RZ, Volkow ND (2002) Drug addiction and its underlying neurobiological basis: neuroimaging evidence for the involvement of the frontal cortex. Am J Psychiatry 159:1642–1652

Goldstein RZ, Volkow ND (2011) Dysfunction of the prefrontal cortex in addiction: neuroimaging findings and clinical implications. Nat Rev Neurosci 12:652–669. https://doi.org/10.1038/nrn3119

Grabowski J, Rhoades H, Schmitz J et al (2001) Dextroamphetamine for cocaine-dependence treatment: a double-blind randomized clinical trial. J Clin Psychopharmacol 21:522

Grabowski J, Rhoades H, Stotts A et al (2004) Agonist-like or antagonist-like treatment for cocaine dependence with methadone for heroin dependence: two double-blind randomized clinical trials. Neuropsychopharmacology 29:969–981. https://doi.org/10.1038/sj.npp.1300392

Greenwald MK (2018) Anti-stress neuropharmacological mechanisms and targets for addiction treatment: a translational framework. Neurobiol Stress 9:84–104. https://doi.org/10.1016/j.ynstr.2018.08.003

Greenwald MK, Lundahl LH, Steinmiller CL (2010) Sustained release *d*-amphetamine reduces cocaine but not 'speedball'-seeking in buprenorphine-maintained volunteers: a test of dual-agonist pharmacotherapy for cocaine/heroin polydrug abusers. Neuropsychopharmacology 35:2624–2637. https://doi.org/10.1038/npp.2010.175

Hanlon CA, Dowdle LT, Austelle CW et al (2015) What goes up, can come down: novel brain stimulation paradigms may attenuate craving and craving-related neural circuitry in substance dependent individuals. Brain Res 1628:199–209. https://doi.org/10.1016/j.brainres.2015.02.053

Hart CL, Haney M, Vosburg SK et al (2008) Smoked cocaine self-administration is decreased by modafinil. Neuropsychopharmacology 33:761–768. https://doi.org/10.1038/sj.npp.1301472

Heekin RD, Shorter D, Kosten TR (2017) Current status and future prospects for the development of substance abuse vaccines. Expert Rev Vaccines 16:1067–1077. https://doi.org/10.1080/14760584.2017.1378577

Heidbreder CA, Newman AH (2010) Current perspectives on selective dopamine D3 receptor antagonists as pharmacotherapeutics for addictions and related disorders. Ann N Y Acad Sci 1187:4–34. https://doi.org/10.1111/j.1749-6632.2009.05149.x

Heilig M, Goldman D, Berrettini W, O'Brien CP (2011) Pharmacogenetic approaches to the treatment of alcohol addiction. Nat Rev Neurosci 12:670–684. https://doi.org/10.1038/nrn3110

Hester R, Garavan H (2004) Executive dysfunction in cocaine addiction: evidence for discordant frontal, cingulate, and cerebellar activity. J Neurosci 24:11017–11022. https://doi.org/10.1523/JNEUROSCI.3321-04.2004

Hester R, Lee N, Pennay A et al (2010) The effects of modafinil treatment on neuropsychological and attentional bias performance during 7-day inpatient withdrawal from methamphetamine dependence. Exp Clin Psychopharmacol 18:489–497. https://doi.org/10.1037/a0021791

Hwa LS, Kalinichev M, Haddouk H et al (2014) Reduction of excessive alcohol drinking by a novel GABAB receptor positive allosteric modulator ADX71441 in mice. Psychopharmacology (Berl) 231:333–343. https://doi.org/10.1007/s00213-013-3245-z

Hyman SM, Paliwal P, Sinha R (2007) Childhood maltreatment, perceived stress, and stress-related coping in recently abstinent cocaine dependent adults. Psychol Addict Behav 21:233. https://doi.org/10.1037/0893-164X.21.2.233

Hyman SM, Paliwal P, Chaplin TM et al (2008) Severity of childhood trauma is predictive of cocaine relapse outcomes in women but not men. Drug Alcohol Depend 92:208–216. https://doi.org/10.1016/j.drugalcdep.2007.08.006

James MH, Stopper CM, Zimmer BA et al (2018) Increased number and activity of a lateral subpopulation of hypothalamic orexin/hypocretin neurons underlies the expression of an addicted state in rats. Biol Psychiatry 85(11):925–935. https://doi.org/10.1016/j.biopsych.2018.07.022

Jasinska AJ, Stein EA, Kaiser J et al (2014) Factors modulating neural reactivity to drug cues in addiction: a survey of human neuroimaging studies. Neurosci Biobehav Rev 38:1–16. https://doi.org/10.1016/j.neubiorev.2013.10.013

Jentsch JD, Taylor JR (1999) Impulsivity resulting from frontostriatal dysfunction in drug abuse: implications for the control of behavior by reward-related stimuli. Psychopharmacology (Berl) 146:373–390. https://doi.org/10.1007/PL00005483

Johnson BA, Ait-Daoud N, Wang X-Q et al (2013) Topiramate for the treatment of cocaine addiction: a randomized clinical trial. JAMA Psychiat 70:1338–1346. https://doi.org/10.1001/jamapsychiatry.2013.2295

Jones L, Lin L (2017) An in silico study on the isomers of pentacene: the case for air-stable and alternative C22H14 acenes for organic electronics. J Phys Chem A 121:2804–2813. https://doi.org/10.1021/acs.jpca.6b11770

Jones JD, Comer SD, Kranzler HR (2015) The pharmacogenetics of alcohol use disorder. Alcohol Clin Exp Res 39:391–402. https://doi.org/10.1111/acer.12643

Juncosa JI, Takaya K, Le HV et al (2018) Design and mechanism of (S)-3-amino-4-(difluoromethylenyl)cyclopent-1-ene-1-carboxylic acid, a highly potent γ-aminobutyric acid aminotransferase inactivator for the treatment of addiction. J Am Chem Soc 140:2151–2164. https://doi.org/10.1021/jacs.7b10965

Kahn R, Biswas K, Childress A-R et al (2009) Multi-center trial of baclofen for abstinence initiation in severe cocaine-dependent individuals. Drug Alcohol Depend 103:59–64. https://doi.org/10.1016/j.drugalcdep.2009.03.011

Kalivas PW, Duffy P (1993a) Time course of extracellular dopamine and behavioral sensitization to cocaine. I. Dopamine axon terminals. J Neurosci 13:266–275. https://doi.org/10.1523/JNEUROSCI.13-01-00266.1993

Kalivas PW, Duffy P (1993b) Time course of extracellular dopamine and behavioral sensitization to cocaine. II. Dopamine perikarya. J Neurosci 13:276–284. https://doi.org/10.1523/JNEUROSCI.13-01-00276.1993

Kalivas PW, McFarland K, Bowers S et al (2003) Glutamate transmission and addiction to cocaine. Ann N Y Acad Sci 1003:169–175. https://doi.org/10.1196/annals.1300.009

Kampman KM (2010) What's new in the treatment of cocaine addiction? Curr Psychiatry Rep 12:441–447. https://doi.org/10.1007/s11920-010-0143-5

Kampman KM, Volpicelli JR, Mulvaney F et al (2002) Cocaine withdrawal severity and urine toxicology results from treatment entry predict outcome in medication trials for cocaine dependence. Addict Behav 27:251–260

Kampman KM, Pettinati H, Lynch KG et al (2004) A pilot trial of topiramate for the treatment of cocaine dependence. Drug Alcohol Depend 75:233–240. https://doi.org/10.1016/j.drugalcdep.2004.03.008

Kampman KM, Pettinati HM, Lynch KG et al (2013) A double-blind, placebo-controlled trial of topiramate for the treatment of comorbid cocaine and alcohol dependence. Drug Alcohol Depend 133:94–99. https://doi.org/10.1016/j.drugalcdep.2013.05.026

Kampman KM, Lynch KG, Pettinati HM et al (2015) A double blind, placebo controlled trial of modafinil for the treatment of cocaine dependence without co-morbid alcohol dependence. Drug Alcohol Depend 155:105–110. https://doi.org/10.1016/j.drugalcdep.2015.08.005

Karkhanis AN, Beveridge TJR, Blough BE et al (2016) The individual and combined effects of phenmetrazine and mgluR2/3 agonist LY379268 on the motivation to self-administer cocaine. Drug Alcohol Depend 166:51–60. https://doi.org/10.1016/j.drugalcdep.2016.06.020

Khantzian EJ, Gawin F, Kleber HD, Riordan CE (1984) Methylphenidate (Ritalin®) treatment of cocaine dependence – a preliminary report. J Subst Abuse Treat 1:107–112. https://doi.org/10.1016/0740-5472(84)90033-3

Kober H, Lacadie CM, Wexler BE et al (2016) Brain activity during cocaine craving and gambling urges: an fMRI study. Neuropsychopharmacology 41:628–637. https://doi.org/10.1038/npp.2015.193

Kosten TA, Gawin FH, Kosten TR, Rounsaville BJ (1993) Gender differences in cocaine use and treatment response. J Subst Abuse Treat 10:63–66

Kosten TR, Scanley BE, Tucker KA et al (2006) Cue-induced brain activity changes and relapse in cocaine-dependent patients. Neuropsychopharmacology 31:644–650. https://doi.org/10.1038/sj.npp.1300851

Kranzler HR, Gelernter J, Anton RF et al (2009) Association of markers in the 3′ region of the GluR5 kainate receptor subunit gene to alcohol dependence. Alcohol Clin Exp Res 33:925–930. https://doi.org/10.1111/j.1530-0277.2009.00913.x

Kranzler HR, Wetherill R, Feinn R et al (2014) Posttreatment effects of topiramate treatment for heavy drinking. Alcohol Clin Exp Res 38:3017–3023. https://doi.org/10.1111/acer.12578

Kühn S, Gallinat J (2011) Common biology of craving across legal and illegal drugs – a quantitative meta-analysis of cue-reactivity brain response. Eur J Neurosci 33:1318–1326. https://doi.org/10.1111/j.1460-9568.2010.07590.x

Kushner SA, Dewey SL, Kornetsky C (1999) The irreversible γ-aminobutyric acid (GABA) transaminase inhibitor γ-vinyl-GABA blocks cocaine self-administration in rats. J Pharmacol Exp Ther 290:797–802

Lal R, Sukbuntherng J, Tai EHL et al (2009) Arbaclofen placarbil, a novel r-baclofen prodrug: improved absorption, distribution, metabolism, and elimination properties compared with R-baclofen. J Pharmacol Exp Ther 330:911–921. https://doi.org/10.1124/jpet.108.149773

Lam SCB, Wang Z, Li Y et al (2013) Wavelet-transformed temporal cerebral blood flow signals during attempted inhibition of cue-induced cocaine craving distinguish prognostic phenotypes. Drug Alcohol Depend 128:140–147. https://doi.org/10.1016/j.drugalcdep.2012.08.018

Langleben DD, Ruparel K, Elman I et al (2008) Acute effect of methadone maintenance dose on brain fMRI response to heroin-related cues. Am J Psychiatry 165:390–394. https://doi.org/10.1176/appi.ajp.2007.07010070

Le Foll B, Payer D, Di Ciano P et al (2016) Occupancy of dopamine D_3 and D_2 receptors by buspirone: a [^{11}C]-(+)-PHNO PET study in humans. Neuropsychopharmacology 41:529–537. https://doi.org/10.1038/npp.2015.177

Levin FR, Evans SM, McDowell DM, Kleber HD (1998) Methylphenidate treatment for cocaine abusers with adult attention-deficit/hyperactivity disorder: a pilot study. J Clin Psychiatry 59:300–305

Levin FR, Mariani JJ, Secora A et al (2009) Atomoxetine treatment for cocaine abuse and adult attention-deficit hyperactivity disorder (ADHD): a preliminary open trial. J Dual Diagn 5:41–56. https://doi.org/10.1080/15504260802628767

Levin FR, Mariani JJ, Specker S et al (2015) Extended-release mixed amphetamine salts vs placebo for comorbid adult attention-deficit/hyperactivity disorder and cocaine use disorder. JAMA Psychiat 72:593–602. https://doi.org/10.1001/jamapsychiatry.2015.41

Levin FR, Mariani JJ, Pavlicova M, Choi CJ, Mahony AL, Brooks DJ, Bisaga A, Dakwar E, Carpenter KM, Naqvi N, Nunes EV, Kampman K (2020) Extended release mixed amphetamine salts and topiramate for cocaine dependence: A randomized clinical replication trial with frequent users. Drug Alcohol Depend 206:107700

Li CR, Morgan PT, Matuskey D et al (2010) Biological markers of the effects of intravenous methylphenidate on improving inhibitory control in cocaine-dependent patients. Proc Natl Acad Sci U S A 107:14455–14459. https://doi.org/10.1073/pnas.1002467107

Li Q, Li W, Wang H et al (2015) Predicting subsequent relapse by drug-related cue-induced brain activation in heroin addiction: an event-related functional magnetic resonance imaging study. Addict Biol 20:968–978. https://doi.org/10.1111/adb.12182

Ling W, Shoptaw S, Majewska D (1998) Baclofen as a cocaine anti-craving medication: a preliminary clinical study. Neuropsychopharmacology 18:403–404. https://doi.org/10.1016/S0893-133X(97)00128-0

Logrip ML, Koob GF, Zorrilla EP (2011) Role of corticotropin-releasing factor in drug addiction: potential for pharmacological intervention. CNS Drugs 25:271–287. https://doi.org/10.2165/11587790-000000000-00000

Luigjes J, van den Brink W, Feenstra M et al (2012) Deep brain stimulation in addiction: a review of potential brain targets. Mol Psychiatry 17:572–583. https://doi.org/10.1038/mp.2011.114

Maccioni P, Colombo G (2019) Potential of GABAB receptor positive allosteric modulators in the treatment of alcohol use disorder. CNS Drugs 33:107–123. https://doi.org/10.1007/s40263-018-0596-3

Mach RH, Tu Z, Xu J et al (2011) Endogenous dopamine competes with the binding of a radiolabeled D3 receptor partial agonist in vivo: a positron emission tomography study. Synapse 65:724–732. https://doi.org/10.1002/syn.20891

MacNiven KH, Jensen ELS, Borg N et al (2018) Association of neural responses to drug cues with subsequent relapse to stimulant use. JAMA Netw Open 1:e186466. https://doi.org/10.1001/jamanetworkopen.2018.6466

Maguire MJ, Hemming K, Wild JM et al (2010) Prevalence of visual field loss following exposure to vigabatrin therapy: a systematic review. Epilepsia 51:2423–2431. https://doi.org/10.1111/j.1528-1167.2010.02772.x

Mann K, Vollstädt-Klein S, Reinhard I et al (2014) Predicting naltrexone response in alcohol-dependent patients: the contribution of functional magnetic resonance imaging. Alcohol Clin Exp Res 38:2754–2762. https://doi.org/10.1111/acer.12546

Mariani JJ, Levin FR (2012) Psychostimulant treatment of cocaine dependence. Psychiatr Clin North Am 35:425–439. https://doi.org/10.1016/j.psc.2012.03.012

Marsot A, Imbert B, Alvarez J-C et al (2014) High variability in the exposure of baclofen in alcohol-dependent patients. Alcohol Clin Exp Res 38:316–321. https://doi.org/10.1111/acer.12235

Martinez D, Greene K, Broft A et al (2009) Lower level of endogenous dopamine in patients with cocaine dependence: findings from PET imaging of D 2/D 3 receptors following acute dopamine depletion. Am J Psychiatry 166:1170–1177. https://doi.org/10.1176/appi.ajp.2009.08121801

Martinez D, Carpenter KM, Liu F et al (2011) Imaging dopamine transmission in cocaine dependence: link between neurochemistry and response to treatment. Am J Psychiatry 168:634–641. https://doi.org/10.1176/appi.ajp.2010.10050748

McFarland K, Kalivas PW (2001) The circuitry mediating cocaine-induced reinstatement of drug-seeking behavior. J Neurosci 21:8655–8663. https://doi.org/10.1523/JNEUROSCI.21-21-08655.2001

Medrano MA, Hatch JP, Zule WA, Desmond DP (2002) Psychological distress in childhood trauma survivors who abuse drugs. Am J Drug Alcohol Abuse 28:1–13

Moeller SJ, Paulus MP (2018) Toward biomarkers of the addicted human brain: using neuroimaging to predict relapse and sustained abstinence in substance use disorder. Prog Neuropsychopharmacol Biol Psychiatry 80:143–154. https://doi.org/10.1016/j.pnpbp.2017.03.003

Mooney ME, Schmitz JM, Moeller FG, Grabowski J (2007) Safety, tolerability and efficacy of levodopa–carbidopa treatment for cocaine dependence: two double-blind, randomized, clinical trials. Drug Alcohol Depend 88:214–223. https://doi.org/10.1016/j.drugalcdep.2006.10.011

Moran-Santa Maria MM, McRae-Clark A, Baker NL, Ramakrishnan V, Brady KT (2014) Yohimbine administration and cue-reactivity in cocaine-dependent individuals. Psychopharmacology (Berl) 231:4157–4165

Morgan AE, Dewey SL (1998) Effects of pharmacologic increases in brain GABA levels on cocaine-induced changes in extracellular dopamine. Synapse 28:60–65. https://doi.org/10.1002/(SICI)1098-2396(199801)28:1<60::AID-SYN7>3.0.CO;2-A

Morgan PT, Angarita GA, Canavan S et al (2016) Modafinil and sleep architecture in an inpatient–outpatient treatment study of cocaine dependence. Drug Alcohol Depend 160:49–56. https://doi.org/10.1016/j.drugalcdep.2015.12.004

Morley KC, Luquin N, Baillie A et al (2018) Moderation of baclofen response by a GABAB receptor polymorphism: results from the BacALD randomized controlled trial. Addiction 113:2205–2213. https://doi.org/10.1111/add.14373

Negus SS, Henningfield J (2015) Agonist medications for the treatment of cocaine use disorder. Neuropsychopharmacology 40:1815–1825. https://doi.org/10.1038/npp.2014.322

NETI (2018) Emerging threats report 2018: status and factors affecting the United States. National Drug Control Policy, High Intensity Drug Trafficking Areas, National Emerging Threats Initiative, Washington

Nuijten M, Blanken P, van den Brink W, Hendriks V (2011) Cocaine addiction treatments to improve control and reduce harm (CATCH): new pharmacological treatment options for crack-cocaine dependence in the Netherlands. BMC Psychiatry 11:135. https://doi.org/10.1186/1471-244X-11-135

Nuijten M, Blanken P, van de Wetering B et al (2016) Sustained-release dexamfetamine in the treatment of chronic cocaine-dependent patients on heroin-assisted treatment: a randomised, double-blind, placebo-controlled trial. Lancet 387:2226–2234. https://doi.org/10.1016/S0140-6736(16)00205-1

Parvaz MA, Moeller SJ, Goldstein RZ (2016) Incubation of cue-induced craving in adults addicted to cocaine measured by electroencephalography. JAMA Psychiat 73:1127–1134. https://doi.org/10.1001/jamapsychiatry.2016.2181

Patkar AA, Thornton CC, Berrettini WH et al (2002) Predicting treatment-outcome in cocaine dependence from admission urine drug screen and peripheral serotonergic measures. J Subst Abuse Treat 23:33–40

Penberthy JK, Ait-Daoud N, Vaughan M, Fanning T (2010) Review of treatment for cocaine dependence. Curr Drug Abuse Rev 3:49–62

Pettinati HM, Kampman KM, Lynch KG et al (2008) Gender differences with high-dose naltrexone in patients with co-occurring cocaine and alcohol dependence. J Subst Abuse Treat 34:378–390. https://doi.org/10.1016/j.jsat.2007.05.011

Pitman KA, Puil E, Borgland SL (2014) GABAB modulation of dopamine release in the nucleus accumbens core. Eur J Neurosci 40:3472–3480. https://doi.org/10.1111/ejn.12733

Prescot AP, Miller SR, Ingenito G et al (2018) In vivo detection of CPP-115 target engagement in human brain. Neuropsychopharmacology 43:646–654. https://doi.org/10.1038/npp.2017.156

Redila VA, Chavkin C (2008) Stress-induced reinstatement of cocaine seeking is mediated by the kappa opioid system. Psychopharmacology (Berl) 200:59–70. https://doi.org/10.1007/s00213-008-1122-y

Regier PS, Monge ZA, Franklin TR et al (2016) Emotional, physical and sexual abuse are associated with a heightened limbic response to cocaine cues. Addict Biol 22(6):1768–1777. https://doi.org/10.1111/adb.12445

Rice C, Mohr CD, Del Boca FK et al (2001) Self-reports of physical, sexual and emotional abuse in an alcoholism treatment sample. J Stud Alcohol 62:114–123

Roberts DC, Andrews MM, Vickers GJ (1996) Baclofen attenuates the reinforcing effects of cocaine in rats. Neuropsychopharmacology 15:417–423. https://doi.org/10.1016/0893-133X(96)00002-4

Robinson TE, Berridge KC (2001) Incentive-sensitization and addiction. Addiction 96:103–114. https://doi.org/10.1046/j.1360-0443.2001.9611038.x

SAMHSA (2018) Key substance use and mental health indicators in the United States: results from the 2017 National Survey on Drug Use and Health. Center for Behavioral Health Statistics and Quality, Substance Abuse and Mental Health Services Administration, Rockville

Savitz J, Hodgkinson CA, Martin-Soelch C et al (2013) DRD2/ANKK1 Taq1A polymorphism (rs1800497) has opposing effects on D2/3 receptor binding in healthy controls and patients with major depressive disorder. Int J Neuropsychopharmacol 16:2095–2101. https://doi.org/10.1017/S146114571300045X

Schiffer WK, Gerasimov M, Hofmann L et al (2001a) Gamma vinyl-GABA differentially modulates NMDA antagonist-induced increases in mesocortical versus mesolimbic DA transmission. Neuropsychopharmacology 25:704–712. https://doi.org/10.1016/S0893-133X(01)00268-8

Schiffer WK, Gerasimov MR, Marsteller DA et al (2001b) Topiramate selectively attenuates nicotine-induced increases in monoamine release. Synapse 42:196–198. https://doi.org/10.1002/syn.10000

Schmitz JM, Mooney ME, Moeller FG et al (2008) Levodopa pharmacotherapy for cocaine dependence: choosing the optimal behavioral therapy platform. Drug Alcohol Depend 94:142–150. https://doi.org/10.1016/j.drugalcdep.2007.11.004

Schmitz JM, Lindsay JA, Stotts AL et al (2010) Contingency management and levodopa-carbidopa for cocaine treatment: a comparison of three behavioral targets. Exp Clin Psychopharmacol 18:238–244. https://doi.org/10.1037/a0019195

Schmitz JM, Rathnayaka N, Green CE et al (2012) Combination of modafinil and d-amphetamine for the treatment of cocaine dependence: a preliminary investigation. Front Psychiatry 3:77. https://doi.org/10.3389/fpsyt.2012.00077

Schubiner H, Saules KK, Arfken CL et al (2002) Double-blind placebo-controlled trial of methylphenidate in the treatment of adult ADHD patients with comorbid cocaine dependence. Exp Clin Psychopharmacol 10:286–294

Segal DS, Kuczenski R (1992a) In vivo microdialysis reveals a diminished amphetamine-induced DA response corresponding to behavioral sensitization produced by repeated amphetamine pretreatment. Brain Res 571:330–337

Segal DS, Kuczenski R (1992b) Repeated cocaine administration induces behavioral sensitization and corresponding decreased extracellular dopamine responses in caudate and accumbens. Brain Res 577:351–355

Shearer J, Wodak A, Beek IV et al (2003) Pilot randomized double blind placebo-controlled study of dexamphetamine for cocaine dependence. Addiction 98:1137–1141. https://doi.org/10.1046/j.1360-0443.2003.00447.x

Shinn AK, Greenfield SF (2010) Topiramate in the treatment of substance related disorders: a critical review of the literature. J Clin Psychiatry 71:634–648. https://doi.org/10.4088/JCP.08r04062gry

Shoptaw S, Yang X, Rotheram-Fuller EJ et al (2003) Randomized placebo-controlled trial of baclofen for cocaine dependence: preliminary effects for individuals with chronic patterns of cocaine use. J Clin Psychiatry 64:1440–1448

Shoptaw S, Watson DW, Reiber C et al (2005) Randomized controlled pilot trial of cabergoline, hydergine and levodopa/carbidopa: Los Angeles Cocaine Rapid Efficacy Screening Trial (CREST). Addiction 100(Suppl 1):78–90. https://doi.org/10.1111/j.1360-0443.2005.00991.x

Shorter D, Kosten TR (2011) Novel pharmacotherapeutic treatments for cocaine addiction. BMC Med 9:119. https://doi.org/10.1186/1741-7015-9-119

Shorter D, Nielsen DA, Huang W et al (2013) Pharmacogenetic randomized trial for cocaine abuse: disulfiram and α1A-adrenoceptor gene variation. Eur Neuropsychopharmacol 23(11):1401–1407. https://doi.org/10.1016/j.euroneuro.2013.05.014

Shorter D, Domingo CB, Kosten TR (2015) Emerging drugs for the treatment of cocaine use disorder: a review of neurobiological targets and pharmacotherapy. Expert Opin Emerg Drugs 20:15–29. https://doi.org/10.1517/14728214.2015.985203

Sinha R (2001) How does stress increase risk of drug abuse and relapse? Psychopharmacology (Berl) 158:343–359. https://doi.org/10.1007/s002130100917

Sinha R (2008) Chronic stress, drug use, and vulnerability to addiction. Ann N Y Acad Sci 1141:105–130. https://doi.org/10.1196/annals.1441.030

Sinha R, Lacadie C, Skudlarski P et al (2005) Neural activity associated with stress-induced cocaine craving: a functional magnetic resonance imaging study. Psychopharmacology (Berl) 183:171–180. https://doi.org/10.1007/s00213-005-0147-8

Sinha R, Fox HC, Hong KA et al (2009) Enhanced negative emotion and alcohol craving, and altered physiological responses following stress and cue exposure in alcohol dependent individuals. Neuropsychopharmacology 34:1198–1208. https://doi.org/10.1038/npp.2008.78

Siniscalchi A, Bonci A, Biagio Mercuri N et al (2015) The role of topiramate in the management of cocaine addiction: a possible therapeutic option. Curr Neuropharmacol 13:815–818

Somoza EC, Winship D, Gorodetzky CW et al (2013) A multisite, double-blind, placebo-controlled clinical trial to evaluate the safety and efficacy of vigabatrin for treating cocaine dependence. JAMA Psychiat 70:630–637. https://doi.org/10.1001/jamapsychiatry.2013.872

Stoops WW, Rush CR (2014) Combination pharmacotherapies for stimulant use disorder: a review of clinical findings and recommendations for future research. Expert Rev Clin Pharmacol 7:363–374. https://doi.org/10.1586/17512433.2014.909283

Suh JJ, Pettinati HM, Kampman KM, O'Brien CP (2008) Gender differences in predictors of treatment attrition with high dose naltrexone in cocaine and alcohol dependence. Am J Addict 17:463–468. https://doi.org/10.1080/10550490802409074

UNODC (2018) World drug report 2018. United Nations Office on Drugs and Crime, Vienna

Veenstra-VanderWeele J, Cook EH, King BH et al (2017) Arbaclofen in children and adolescents with autism spectrum disorder: a randomized, controlled, phase 2 trial. Neuropsychopharmacology 42:1390–1398. https://doi.org/10.1038/npp.2016.237

Verrico CD, Haile CN, Mahoney JJ et al (2014) Treatment with modafinil and escitalopram, alone and in combination, on cocaine-induced effects: a randomized, double blind, placebo-controlled human laboratory study. Drug Alcohol Depend 141:72–78. https://doi.org/10.1016/j.drugalcdep.2014.05.008

Viola TW, Tractenberg SG, Levandowski ML et al (2014) Neurotrophic factors in women with crack cocaine dependence during early abstinence: the role of early life stress. J Psychiatry Neurosci 39:206–214. https://doi.org/10.1503/jpn.130027

Volkow ND, Wang G-J, Telang F et al (2006) Cocaine cues and dopamine in dorsal striatum: mechanism of craving in cocaine addiction. J Neurosci 26:6583–6588. https://doi.org/10.1523/JNEUROSCI.1544-06.2006

Wang G, Shi J, Chen N et al (2013) Effects of length of abstinence on decision-making and craving in methamphetamine abusers. PLoS One 8:e68791. https://doi.org/10.1371/journal.pone.0068791

Weerts EM, Froestl W, Kaminski BJ, Griffiths RR (2007) Attenuation of cocaine-seeking by GABA B receptor agonists baclofen and CGP44532 but not the GABA reuptake inhibitor tiagabine in baboons. Drug Alcohol Depend 89:206–213. https://doi.org/10.1016/j.drugalcdep.2006.12.023

Wexler BE, Gottschalk CH, Fulbright RK et al (2001) Functional magnetic resonance imaging of cocaine craving. Am J Psychiatry 158:86–95. https://doi.org/10.1176/appi.ajp.158.1.86

Willuhn I, Burgeno LM, Groblewski PA, Phillips PEM (2014) Excessive cocaine use results from decreased phasic dopamine signaling in the striatum. Nat Neurosci 17:704–709. https://doi.org/10.1038/nn.3694

Wolfsohn R, Angrist B (1990) A pilot trial of levodopa/carbidopa in early cocaine abstinence. J Clin Psychopharmacol 10:440–442

Wolfsohn R, Sanfilipo M, Angrist B (1993) A placebo-controlled trial of L-dopa/carbidopa in early cocaine abstinence. Neuropsychopharmacology 9:49–53. https://doi.org/10.1038/npp.1993.42

Wong DF, Kuwabara H, Schretlen DJ et al (2006) Increased occupancy of dopamine receptors in human striatum during cue-elicited cocaine craving. Neuropsychopharmacology 31:2716–2727. https://doi.org/10.1038/sj.npp.1301194

Young KA, Franklin TR, Roberts DCS et al (2014) Nipping cue reactivity in the bud: baclofen prevents limbic activation elicited by subliminal drug cues. J Neurosci 34:5038–5043. https://doi.org/10.1523/JNEUROSCI.4977-13.2014

Molecular Mechanism and Cannabinoid Pharmacology

Lesley D. Schurman, Dai Lu, Debra A. Kendall, Allyn C. Howlett, and Aron H. Lichtman

Contents

1 A Historical Perspective of, and Introduction to, Cannabinoids 324
1.1 Phytocannabinoids 326
1.2 Synthetic Cannabinoids 326
1.3 Endocannabinoids 327
2 Cannabinoid Receptor Discovery and Function 328
2.1 CB_1 Receptor In Vitro Evidence 328
2.2 CB_1 Receptor In Vivo Evidence 331
2.3 CB_1 Receptor Allosteric Modulation 332
2.4 CB_1 Receptor Functional Selectivity (Biased Agonism) 334
2.5 CB_2 Receptors 335
3 The Endocannabinoids and Their Enzymatic Regulation 335
3.1 *N*-Arachidonylethanolamine (Anandamide) 336
3.2 2-Arachidonoylglycerol (2-AG) 337
3.3 Other Endocannabinoids, Hemopressins, and Related Lipids 338
4 Drug Interactions 338

L. D. Schurman
Department of Pharmacology and Toxicology, Virginia Commonwealth University, Richmond, VA, USA

D. Lu
Rangel College of Pharmacy, Health Science Center, Texas A&M University, Kingsville, TX, USA

D. A. Kendall
Department of Pharmaceutical Sciences, University of Connecticut, Storrs, CT, USA

A. C. Howlett
Department of Physiology and Pharmacology and Center for Research on Substance Use and Addiction, Wake Forest School of Medicine, Winston-Salem, NC, USA

A. H. Lichtman (✉)
Department of Pharmacology and Toxicology, Virginia Commonwealth University, Richmond, VA, USA

Department of Medicinal Chemistry, Virginia Commonwealth University, Richmond, VA, USA
e-mail: aron.lichtman@vcuhealth.org

M. A. Nader, Y. L. Hurd (eds.), *Substance Use Disorders*,
Handbook of Experimental Pharmacology 258, https://doi.org/10.1007/164_2019_298

4.1 Opioid-Sparing Effects ... 339
4.2 Cytochrome P450 Enzymes ... 340
5 Conclusions ... 341
References ... 341

Abstract

Since antiquity, *Cannabis* has provoked enormous intrigue for its potential medicinal properties as well as for its unique pharmacological effects. The elucidation of its major cannabinoid constituents, Δ^9-tetrahydrocannabinol (THC) and cannabidiol (CBD), led to the synthesis of new cannabinoids (termed synthetic cannabinoids) to understand the mechanisms underlying the pharmacology of *Cannabis*. These pharmacological tools were instrumental in the ultimate discovery of the endogenous cannabinoid system, which consists of CB_1 and CB_2 cannabinoid receptors and endogenously produced ligands (endocannabinoids), which bind and activate both cannabinoid receptors. CB_1 receptors mediate the cannabimimetic effects of THC and are highly expressed on presynaptic neurons in the nervous system, where they modulate neurotransmitter release. In contrast, CB_2 receptors are primarily expressed on immune cells. The endocannabinoids are tightly regulated by biosynthetic and hydrolytic enzymes. Accordingly, the endocannabinoid system plays a modulatory role in many physiological processes, thereby generating many promising therapeutic targets. An unintended consequence of this research was the emergence of synthetic cannabinoids sold for human consumption to circumvent federal laws banning *Cannabis* use. Here, we describe research that led to the discovery of the endogenous cannabinoid system and show how knowledge of this system benefitted as well as unintentionally harmed human health.

Keywords

Allosteric modulation · Cannabinoid · *Cannabis* Use Disorder · CB_1/CB_2 receptor · CBD · Endocannabinoid · Opioid-sparing effects · Phytocannabinoid · Synthetic cannabinoid · THC

1 A Historical Perspective of, and Introduction to, Cannabinoids

Paleobotanical studies indicate that the *Cannabis* plant was present as long as 11,400 years ago during the Holocene epoch around Central Asia (Tarasov et al. 2007; Clarke and Merlin 2013). The earliest evidence of *Cannabis* use dates back 10,000 years to the end of the Ice Age in Japan (Okazaki et al. 2011), as well as 4,000 years BCE in China as recorded in the ancient Pharmacopoeia text "Shen Nung Pen Ts'ao Ching" (Jiang et al. 2006). Originally grown for its use as a fiber, food, and medicinal plant by shamans, *Cannabis* spread across the world due to human domestication and its adaptability to a wide range of climates (for an extensive account of the archeobotanical evidence for *Cannabis* use, see Pisanti and Bifulco 2019). The use of *Cannabis* as a recreational drug eventually became widespread, with an early description found in an 1857 article by *The Hasheesh Eater* (Lee 2013). *Cannabis* now represents the most commonly used psychoactive drug in the world after alcohol and tobacco.

Discussions surrounding the legal, ethical, and societal implications of *Cannabis* use have been ongoing for at least a century. The last several decades have seen an increasing rise in the frequency of physician-prescribed *Cannabis* for the treatment of various medical conditions such as chronic pain and psychiatric problems across a growing number of states in the United States (Whiting et al. 2015). The current renaissance of the medical employment of *Cannabis* as well as the changing legal landscape in twenty-first-century United States has forced issues associated with the safe use of *Cannabis* to a now higher prominence. These include routes of administration, content identification and labelling, drug interactions, dispensing, safety and untoward side effects, contraindications, and use or unintended exposure in specialty populations (the young and the elderly), to name but a few. The inclusion of *Cannabis* Use Disorder into the third edition of the *Diagnostic and Statistical Manual of Mental Disorders* (DSMIII) in 1980 makes discussion of its safe use pertinent given the reinforcing value of this ancient plant and as such the potential that exists for dependence. As of 2010, global reports of *Cannabis* Use Disorder prevalence estimated that 0.2% or 13.1 million people met diagnostic criteria (Degenhardt et al. 2013), compared to the US general population where a prevalence of 1.5% was reported in a 2015 National Survey of Drug Use and Health (Hasin et al. 2016; SAMHSA 2017). While *Cannabis* use is a necessary condition to develop *Cannabis* Use Disorder, not all users develop this disorder; therefore, use alone is not a sufficient predictor. The etiology of *Cannabis* Use Disorder is thus clearly complex.

Studying the reinforcing and rewarding effects of cannabinoids in preclinical settings remains a challenge. The most widely used preclinical investigative tool, murine species, do not show reliable or robust intravenous or oral self-administration of Δ^9-tetrahydrocannabinol (THC), the primary psychoactive constituent of *Cannabis* (Lefever et al. 2014; Wakeford et al. 2017; Barrus et al. 2018). Rat intracerebroventricular self-administration of THC (Braida et al. 2001; Zangen et al. 2006), as well as intravenous self-administration of the synthetic cannabinoid WIN 55,212-2 (Fattore et al. 2001; Mendizabal et al. 2006), has been reported. Whereas squirrel monkeys readily self-administer THC (Justinova et al. 2003), this phytocannabinoid functioned as a reinforcer in only half of rhesus and cynomolgus monkeys (John et al. 2017). Other behavioral measures have also been employed to assess the rewarding effects of THC, such as conditioned place preference and intracranial self-stimulation, with inconsistent results (Braida et al. 2004; Hempel et al. 2016; Tanda 2016). As such, the limited success of modeling the rewarding effects of *Cannabis* in research model organisms remains a considerable barrier to preclinical research investigating the neurobiology underlying the abuse liability of cannabinoids as well as assessing drugable targets to treat *Cannabis* Use Disorder.

The chemicals collectively termed cannabinoids can be organized into three broad classes or categories: phytocannabinoids (plant based; the individual molecular constituents of the *Cannabis* plant), synthetic cannabinoids (man-made cannabinoids), and endocannabinoids (cannabinoids produced by and within the body).

1.1 Phytocannabinoids

The *Cannabis* plant contains hundreds of phytochemicals, which include phytocannabinoids, terpenes, and phenolic compounds. To date, more than 560 chemicals have been identified in *Cannabis*, with approximately 120 of these constituents described as terpenophenolic cannabinoids or phytocannabinoids, primarily produced in the glandular trichomes of the plant (ElSohly et al. 2017). Phytocannabinoids are a broad group of closely related chemicals but with diverse structure as well as pharmacological actions. The availability of novel spectrometric methods in the 1960s facilitated the isolation of the primary psychoactive constituent of *Cannabis* Δ^9-THC (Gaoni and Mechoulam 1964) as well cannabidiol (CBD) (Mechoulam and Shvo 1963). For a full review of the chemical elucidation of phytocannabinoids through the 1970s, see Mechoulam et al. (1976). The elucidation of these structures sparked an enormous amount of basic research that revealed the effects of these drugs in the brain and body. Moreover, the FDA approved THC (referred to as dronabinol) to treat nausea and emesis associated with cancer chemotherapy, as well as AIDS-related cachexia as an appetite stimulant. The FDA recently approved CBD to treat severe forms of pediatric epilepsy. Although THC and CBD represent the best known phytocannabinoids, other predominant constituents include cannabigerol (CBG), cannabichromene (CBC), and tetrahydrocannabivarin (THCV). The phytocannabinoids exist as acids (e.g., THCA-A, CBD-A), which are nonenzymatically decarboxylated to their corresponding neutral forms (e.g., THC, CBD). This decarboxylation begins to occur after the plant is harvested during the drying process over time and/or the application of heat (Flores-Sanchez and Verpoorte 2008). Pharmacokinetic studies of cannabinoids have most often focused on THC. This phytocannabinoid is hydroxylated to the psychoactive metabolite 11-hydroxy-Δ^9-THC and then oxidized to the non-psychoactive Δ^9-THC-11-oic acid. THC and its metabolites remain sequestered in cell membranes and adipose tissues and are slowly released, which is why *Cannabis* use can be detected in urine long after use.

1.2 Synthetic Cannabinoids

Upon elucidation of the primary phytocannabinoids, medicinal chemists modified the structure of THC to understand the mechanisms underlying its pharmacological actions. Structurally diverse compounds that included bicyclic cannabinoids (Compton et al. 1992b) and aminoalkylindoles (Compton et al. 1992a; Wiley et al. 1998; Huffman et al. 2005) served as important tools that contributed to the eventual discoveries of cannabinoid receptors (Devane et al. 1988; Munro et al. 1993; see

Sect. 2) and the endocannabinoids (Devane et al. 1992; Mechoulam et al. 1995; Sugiura et al. 1995; see Sect. 3.3). Pharmaceutical companies also developed synthetic cannabinoids as potential medications. For example, the FDA approved nabilone, which is structurally similar to THC, for the treatment of nausea and vomiting associated with cancer chemotherapy.

An unforeseen consequence in studies publishing the synthesis and characterization of the synthetic cannabinoids in scientific journals was their diversion to recreational use and abuse (for full reviews, see Ford et al. 2017; Wiley et al. 2017). As these compounds elicit even greater intoxicating effects as THC but would not be detected in common drug screening tests, their use circumvents the law and drug testing of *Cannabis*. The first generation of synthetic cannabinoids, such as JWH018 (Huffman et al. 2005), were added to plant material and sold over the Internet and in convenience stores under various names such as "Spice" and "K-2" as marketing ploys. Administration of JWH018 and other synthetic cannabinoids has been linked to physiological toxicity (Freeman et al. 2013) and psychological complications (Celofiga et al. 2014). The first wave of synthetic cannabinoids were designated Schedule I drugs in 2011, and the United States also made them illegal. Since then, other synthetic cannabinoids emerged in a "cat-and-mouse" game between clandestine laboratories and law enforcement. One such example is the highly potent fubinaca, a Pfizer synthetic cannabinoid made Schedule I in 2014. Illicit synthetic cannabinoids frequently pose a greater public safety threat than *Cannabis*/THC as they have sparked a large increase in emergency room visits and often life-threatening consequences (Gerostamoulos et al. 2015). The adverse effects of recreationally used synthetic cannabinoids are likely a result of their higher efficacy and potency at cannabinoid receptors as well as other non-cannabinoid receptor sites of action (Grim et al. 2016).

1.3 Endocannabinoids

The endocannabinoid system refers collectively to cannabinoid receptors (CB_1 and CB_2) that are acted upon by endogenously produced cannabinoid ligands: the endocannabinoids (as well as by THC, other phytocannabinoids, and synthetic cannabinoids) and their biosynthetic and degradative enzymes (Blankman et al. 2007). The two most extensively studied endogenous ligands of cannabinoid receptors are arachidonylethanolamine (anandamide or AEA) and 2-arachidonoylglycerol (2-AG) (Devane et al. 1992; Mechoulam et al. 1995; Sugiura et al. 1995). The synthesis and degradation of these endocannabinoids are enzymatically regulated (Blankman and Cravatt 2013). The enzymes that regulate AEA and 2-AG are described below in Sects. 3.1 and 3.2. Other endogenous cannabinoid ligands have also been described (for a full review, see Pertwee 2015). The majority of these ligands are lipids and include 2-arachidonyl glyceryl ether (noladin ether) (Hanus et al. 2001), *N*-arachidonoyl dopamine (NADA) (Bisogno et al. 2000), and virodhamine (Porter et al. 2002).

2 Cannabinoid Receptor Discovery and Function

A major impetus for research geared toward understanding the molecular targets of cannabinoids included the identification of THC as the chief psychoactive constituent of *Cannabis*. Additionally, extensive efforts in medicinal chemistry provided useful tools to bind and activate specific cannabinoid receptor binding sites in biological tissues. The development of highly selective antagonists for each of these receptors (Rinaldi-Carmona et al. 1994, 1998) has greatly aided the investigation of cannabinoid receptor pharmacology as well as provided insight into the function of the endogenous cannabinoid system. The creation of mutant mice in which the CB_1 receptor (Ledent et al. 1999; Zimmer et al. 1999) or CB_2 receptor (Buckley et al. 2000) was genetically deleted provided a powerful complementary tool to distinguish receptor targets of cannabinoid agonists and reveal potential functions of the endogenous cannabinoid system. Below we describe research leading to the discovery of the CB_1 and CB_2 receptors.

2.1 CB_1 Receptor In Vitro Evidence

2.1.1 G Proteins and Adenylyl Cyclase

The history of cannabinoid receptors and their phytocannabinoid, endocannabinoid ligands, and analogs has recently been reviewed by authors who have made major discoveries in cannabinoid pharmacology (Mechoulam et al. 2014; Ligresti et al. 2016). A highly comprehensive review of the CB_1 and CB_2 cannabinoid receptors was submitted by the Cannabinoid Receptor Subcommittee of the International Union of Basic and Clinical Pharmacology (IUPHAR) (Howlett et al. 2002), followed by an evaluation of other targets for the endocannabinoids anandamide and 2-AG (Pertwee et al. 2010). Cellular signaling evoked by the CB_1 receptor has been comprehensively reviewed (McAllister and Glass 2002; Turu and Hunyady 2010; Console-Bram et al. 2012; Howlett and Abood 2017).

Cannabinoid receptors were initially identified and pharmacologically characterized based upon the ability of THC and antinociceptive analogs developed by Pfizer Central Research to attenuate cAMP accumulation in the neuronal cells and brain (Howlett et al. 1988). The N18TG2 mouse neuroblastoma cell line played an essential role in the discovery and function of CB_1 cannabinoid receptors. Based on the observation that pertussis toxin, which eliminates $G_{i/o}$ coupling, abrogated the inhibitory effect on cAMP accumulation, the CB_1 receptor was determined to be a G protein-coupled receptor (GPCR) (Howlett et al. 1986; Houston and Howlett 1993). Immunoprecipitation studies indicated that CB_1 receptors are pre-coupled to $G_{i/o}$ proteins in membrane preparations without the addition of exogenous agonists (Mukhopadhyay et al. 2000; Mukhopadhyay and Howlett 2001, 2005). These studies demonstrated that agonists promote dissociation of the G protein from the CB_1 receptor, whereas antagonist/inverse agonists maintain the CB_1 receptor-G_i protein interaction in a more stable form. We now know from antibody-capture scintillation proximity assays for [^{35}S]GTPγS binding that members of the $G_{i/o}$

family constitute about 75% of the G-protein activation by the high-efficacy receptor agonist CP55,940 (Eldeeb et al. 2016, 2017). G_s, $G_{q/11}$, G_{12}, and G_{13} each contributed 5–10% of the total activation under those assay conditions (Eldeeb et al. 2017). G_z, G_s, and $G_{q/11}$ were not found to be pre-associated with the CB_1 receptor in 3-[(3-cholamidopropyl)dimethylammonio]-1-propanesulfonate (CHAPS)-solubilized immunoprecipitation protocols (Mukhopadhyay et al. 2000). Specifically, pertussis toxin pre-treatment did not lead to increased G_s activation (Eldeeb et al. 2016). Evidence for agonist-selective regulation of various G proteins has come from G-protein activation studies (Glass and Northup 1999; Prather et al. 2000). Immunoprecipitation studies indicated that full agonists could activate all $G_{i/o}$ subtypes, whereas "partial agonists" only activate certain G_i subtypes and act as inverse agonists at other subtypes (Mukhopadhyay and Howlett 2005). These studies at the level of G-protein activation suggest that agonists may select differing signal pathways depending upon the G-protein availability in the environment of the CB_1 receptor.

Numerous reviews have identified the role of neuronal CB_1 receptor signal transduction based upon Gβγ protein release and $G_{\alpha i}$-mediated reduction of cAMP in the regulation of neurotransmission (Kano 2014; Lu and Mackie 2016), neurodevelopment (Diaz-Alonso et al. 2012; Gaffuri et al. 2012; Maccarrone et al. 2014), and synaptic plasticity (Garcia et al. 2016; Araque et al. 2017). Following $G_{i/o}$ activation and dissociation, CB_1 receptors can be phosphorylated by G-protein receptor kinases (GRKs), leading to interactions with β-arrestins 1 or 2 (Breivogel et al. 2013; Chen et al. 2014). β-arrestins are scaffolding proteins that internalize the CB_1 receptors from the plasma membrane and/or regulate CB_1 receptor-mediated signal transduction that is not related to G proteins (Nogueras-Ortiz and Yudowski 2016). For example, extracellular signal-regulated kinase (ERK)1 and 2 phosphorylation and activation can be regulated both by CB_1-mediated Gβγ release with diminished cAMP and PKA signaling and an extended phase mediated by β-arrestins (Rubino et al. 2006; Daigle et al. 2008; Dalton and Howlett 2012; Franklin et al. 2013; Mahavadi et al. 2014).

2.1.2 Radioligand Binding and Cloning of Cannabinoid Receptors in the CNS

The biological activity of Δ^9-THC and analogs being attributed to cannabinoid receptors was first identified using radioligand binding to a Pfizer analog $[^3H]$CP55,940 (Devane et al. 1988). Using this assay, brain cannabinoid receptors were demonstrated to be among the most abundant GPCRs, being highly expressed in the cortex, hippocampus, basal ganglia, and cerebellum consistent with cannabinoid effects on cognition, memory, hypoactivity, and sedation (Herkenham et al. 1990; Glass et al. 1997; Tsou et al. 1998).

An orphan 7-transmembrane receptor from rat appeared to exhibit neuroanatomical localization similar to that identified as the brain cannabinoid receptor, and using the $[^3H]$CP55,940 radioligand binding assay was subsequently identified to be what we now refer to as the CB_1 cannabinoid receptor (Matsuda et al. 1990). Based upon this rat clone, the human CB_1 receptor was shown to have 97% amino acid sequence identity but was shorter by one residue (Gerard et al. 1991). The mouse and rat exhibit identical amino acid sequences (Chakrabarti et al. 1995; Ho and Zhao 1996; Abood et al. 1997). Although there appears to be very similar pharmacological properties between human and rodent CB_1 receptors, some variation in ligand binding has been noted (McPartland et al. 2007).

The first reported splice variant of the human hCB_1 receptor, referred to as hCB_{1a}, is reduced by 167 base pairs in the coding region, thereby reducing the N-terminal extracellular domain by 61 residues and changing 28 residues in the remaining sequence (Shire et al. 1995). The second reported splice variant, hCB_{1b}, was the result of removal of 99 base pairs from the human mRNA, eliminating 33 residues in the N-terminal domain (Ryberg et al. 2005). It should be noted that these variants are not possible in rodents due to a sequence difference (Bonner 1996). An investigation of the pharmacological profile for the hCB_{1a} variant compared with hCB_1 expressed in CHO cells found that agonist ligands and the antagonist SR141716 bound to the receptor with threefold lower affinity; however, the cellular signaling via cAMP and ERK phosphorylation was not appreciably different (Rinaldi-Carmona et al. 1996; Xiao et al. 2008). CB_{1a} and CB_{1b} variants expressed in HEK293 cells exhibited no significant difference compared with CB_1 receptors in receptor binding affinity for Δ^9-THC, CP55,940, WIN55,212-2, HU210, or SR141716 and 2- to 3-fold lower affinity for 2-AG, but 200-fold lower affinity for anandamide (Ryberg et al. 2005). Both variants exhibited [^{35}S]GTPγS activation EC_{50} values and efficacies similar to CB_1 receptors; however, 2-AG acted as an inverse agonist in the [^{35}S]GTPγS activation assay (Ryberg et al. 2005). When expressed in $CB_1-/-$ mouse hippocampal neurons, hCB_{1a} and hCB_{1b} were less efficacious than CB_1 in producing depolarization-induced suppression of excitation (Straiker et al. 2012). These hCB_{1a} and hCB_{1b} mRNAs are expressed in low abundance, $<5\%$ of that of CB_1 (Shire et al. 1995; Ryberg et al. 2005; Xiao et al. 2008). However, the protein levels of splice variants were immuno-detectable in human and macaque brains (Bagher et al. 2013). Thus, the relevance of these splice variants to human cannabinoid receptor function is not readily apparent.

CB_1 receptors in the CNS function at the presynaptic terminals of neurons to curtail release of neurotransmitters, particularly in GABAergic more so than glutamatergic neurons (Katona et al. 1999; Szabo and Schlicker 2005; Puighermanal et al. 2009). However, CB_1 receptors are indeed present across all plasma membrane components including lipid rafts (Bari et al. 2005; Barnett-Norris et al. 2005) and intracellularly in endosomes and mitochondria (Benard et al. 2012). In addition to neurons, CB_1 receptors are expressed by astrocytes (Han et al. 2012; Oliveira da Cruz et al. 2016), oligodendrocytes and their precursors (Ilyasov et al. 2018), and perhaps other glial subtypes (Stella 2010). It should also be noted that the CB_1 receptor can be expressed in tissues outside the nervous systems, including the heart, lung, prostate, liver, uterus, ovary, testis, vas deferens, and bone (Galiegue et al. 1995). As such, peripheral CB_1 receptors mediate physiological processes such as gastrointestinal motility and energy balance, reproduction and fertility, pain, and skeletal muscle energy metabolism.

2.2 CB_1 Receptor In Vivo Evidence

The elucidation of the structures of the many phytocannabinoids present in *Cannabis* (e.g., THC, CBD, CBG, CBC, THCV) led to a great deal of studies investigating their pharmacological actions. The tremendous breadth of pharmacological actions of these compounds was initially hypothesized to reflect nonspecific or specific interactions (as reviewed in Martin 1986). The well-described effects of cannabinoids in inhibiting cAMP accumulation through GPCR-dependent mechanisms (see Sect. 2.1 above) provided strong evidence supporting specific mechanisms. However, given the extremely hydrophobic nature of THC and other cannabinoids, their much higher affinity for cell membranes than for aqueous media is not surprising. Accordingly, early studies hypothesized that cell membrane perturbation mediated the pharmacological effects of THC (Hillard et al. 1985, 1990). This perturbation of neuronal cell membranes was also proposed for the intoxicating effects of ethanol (Lyon et al. 1981) and volatile anesthetics (Seeman 1972). In assays using cholesterol liposomes, THC and other psychoactive cannabinoids elicited perturbation, while CBD elicited stabilizing effects in this artificial membrane system (Lawrence and Gill 1975). However, structure-activity relationship (SAR) studies did not bear out a correlation between membrane fluidization and intoxicating effects of cannabinoids (for a full review, see Martin 1986). It should be noted that the high concentration of THC necessary to disrupt membrane fluidity far exceeds typical physiological relevant concentrations. Finally, the n-octanol/water partition coefficients of a series of naturally occurring and synthetic cannabinoids did not correlate with their behavioral activity in measures of spontaneous activity, rectal temperature, tail-flick response, and ring immobility, suggesting that lipophilicity may represent a component, but not a primary determinant in driving the pharmacological activity of the cannabinoids (Thomas et al. 1990).

SAR studies investigating common in vivo pharmacological effects of cannabinoids demonstrated stereoselectivity in rodents, dogs, and nonhuman primates (Martin 1986), which strongly supported a receptor mechanism of action. Early studies reported that dogs displayed particular sensitivity to the ataxic effects of *Cannabis* extracts (Walton et al. 1938). Accordingly, the dog static ataxia test offered utility to investigate the SAR of synthetic cannabinoids (Adams et al. 1948a, b; Martin et al. 1975, 1984; Pars et al. 1976; Beardsley et al. 1987; Little et al. 1989; Compton and Martin 1990) and was also used to examine in vivo cannabimimetic effects of anandamide (Lichtman et al. 1998) prior to the knowledge of its rapid metabolism by FAAH. Over time, employment of the dog static ataxia assay gave way to rodent high-throughput screening and drug discrimination assays.

A high-throughput screening, developed by the late Professor Billy Martin for SAR studies and eventually coined the "tetrad test," evaluates the occurrence of decreased spontaneous activity, hypothermia, catalepsy, and thermal antinociception (Little et al. 1988). Whereas non-cannabinoid drugs produce one or a subset of pharmacological actions in this series of tests (Wiley and Martin 2003), THC (Little et al. 1988), potent synthetic THC analogs (Little et al. 1989), synthetic bicyclic cannabinoid analogs (Little et al. 1988; Compton et al. 1992b), synthetic aminoalkylindole analogs (Compton et al. 1992a), and synthetic anandamide analogs (Thomas et al. 1996) produce the entire constellation of tetrad effects in a stereoselective manor. Indeed, the pharmacological effects of synthetic cannabinoids in the tetrad assay highly correlate with binding affinity to the CB_1 receptor (Compton et al. 1993). Additionally, this assay can be used to estimate pA_2 and pK_B values of cannabinoids (Grim et al. 2017), as well as be modified to determine efficacy, which yields values of efficacy that highly correlate with agonist-stimulated $[^{35}S]GTP\gamma S$ binding (Grim et al. 2016).

In contrast to the tetrad assay, the drug discrimination paradigm offers a high degree of specificity in capturing the subjective effects of CB_1 receptor agonists (for a full review see Wiley et al. 2018). In this assay, laboratory animals are trained in an operant food-motivated task to discriminate between the subjective effects of a psychoactive drug and vehicle (Solinas et al. 2006). A large body of drug discrimination studies examining drugs from a multitude of classes demonstrate its tremendous utility and its exquisite sensitivity and specificity. Specifically, drugs that fully substitute for the training drug act through a similar mechanism of action. In a career spanning over 40 years beginning in the 1970s, Järbe and colleagues pioneered the drug discrimination paradigm to investigate cannabinoids (Järbe and Henriksson 1973, 1974; Henriksson et al. 1975; Jarbe et al. 1977). This work was particularly useful in identifying synthetic cannabinoids with cannabimimetic activity (Järbe and Gifford 2014; Järbe et al. 2016a, b). Studies employing CB_1 receptor antagonists confirm that this receptor mediates the discriminative stimulus of THC, synthetic cannabinoids, and MAGL inhibitors (Wiley et al. 1995; Owens et al. 2017). Moreover, other pharmacological agents leading to CB_1 receptor activation substitute for these training drugs. Finally, Jarbe and colleagues demonstrated that drug discrimination can determine efficacy of CB_1 receptors agonists (Järbe et al. 2014).

2.3 CB₁ Receptor Allosteric Modulation

The CB_1 cannabinoid receptor has been suggested as a therapeutic target for a number of disorders including chemotherapy-induced nausea, wasting syndrome associated with cancer and AIDS, pain, obesity, neurodegenerative disorders, and substance use disorders (Mackie 2006a; Pacher et al. 2006). Traditionally, therapeutic manipulation of the function of the CB_1 cannabinoid receptor is mainly achieved through the application of exogenous compounds that bind to the CB_1 receptor orthosteric site where the endogenous cannabinoids such as anandamide and 2-AG bind. Most endogenous compounds bind the orthosteric site, which is the main active site of the receptor. However, agonists or antagonists targeting the orthosteric sites of CB_1 receptors have been found with either psychotropic (Grotenhermen and Muller-Vahl 2012) or psychiatric adverse effects (Cridge and Rosengren 2013). These untoward side effects have made orthosteric CB_1 ligands challenging to develop into therapeutic agents. To overcome the on-target side effects of CB_1 orthosteric ligands, novel ligands interacting with CB_1 receptors via a new mechanism of action have been vigorously pursued. To this end, several classes of

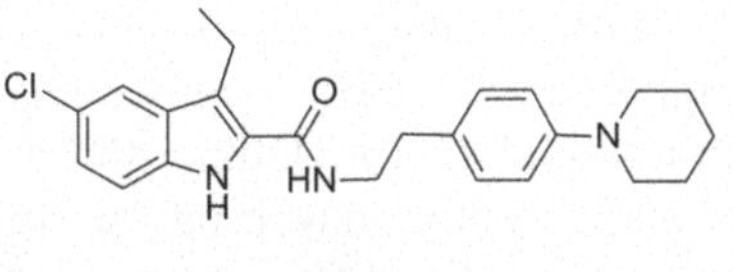

1
Org27569

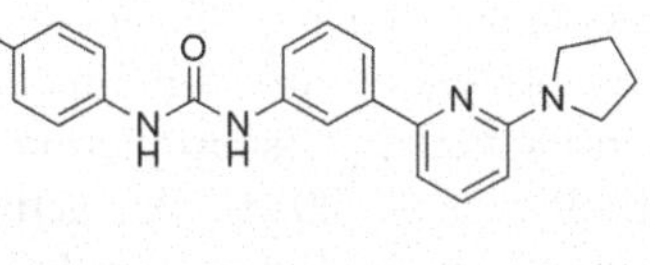

2
PSNCBAM-1

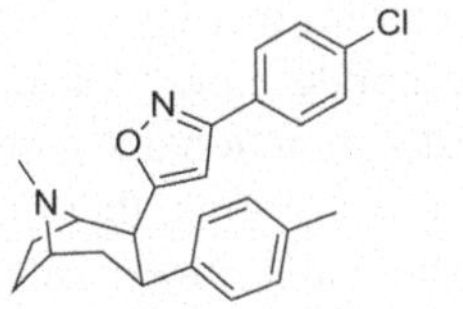

3
RTI-371

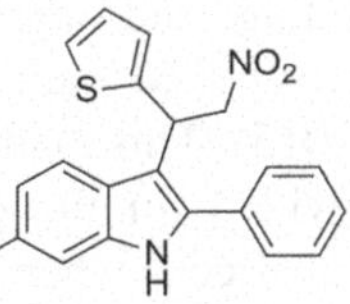

4
ZCZ011

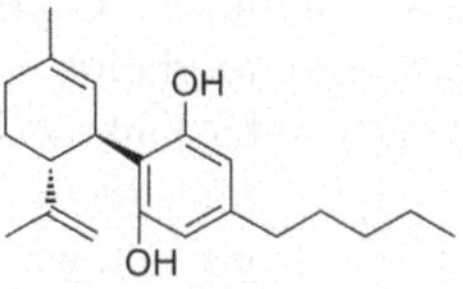

5
Cannabidiol

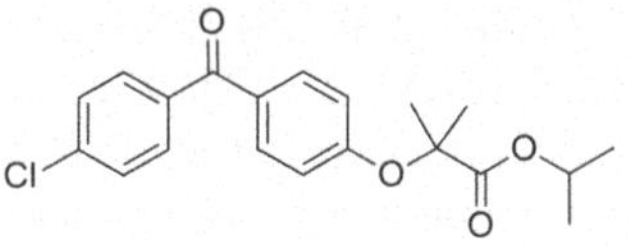

6
Fenofibrate

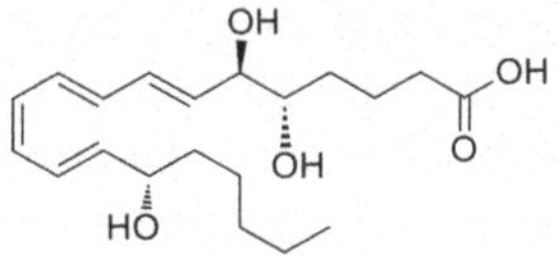

7
Lipoxin A_4

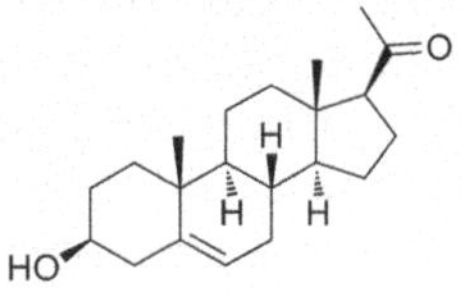

8
Pregnenolone

Arg-Val-Asp-Pro-Val-Asn-Phe-Lys-Leu-Leu-Ser-His

9
Pepcan-12

Fig. 1 Structures of proposed CB_1 receptor allosteric agonists

allosteric modulators, which bind to CB_1 receptor sites different from the orthosteric sites, have been discovered (Fig. 1). These new CB_1 ligands including Org27569 (**1**) (Price et al. 2005), PSNCBAM-1 (**2**) (Horswill et al. 2007), RTI-371 (**3**) (Navarro et al. 2009), ZCZ011 (**4**) (Ignatowska-Jankowska et al. 2015), and others have been suggested (Laprairie et al. 2015; Priestly et al. 2015) including endogenous (Bauer et al. 2012; Pamplona et al. 2012; Vallee et al. 2014) molecules. Theoretically, a receptor can form a multitude of active and inactive conformations through selective stabilization by various ligands. Allosteric modulators can induce receptor conformations distinct from those stabilized by orthosteric agonists and antagonists but are generally substrates of active or inactive receptor conformations. Thus, novel mechanisms of action from ligand binding to cytosolic signal transduction can be achieved. Preliminary studies of these allosteric modulators have revealed new mechanisms of action in regulating CB_1 receptor function. For instance, Org27569 enhances binding of CB_1 orthosteric agonists and promotes β-arrestin-1-mediated phosphorylation of ERK1/2 and is a positive allosteric modulator (PAM). This allosteric modulator also inhibits G-protein binding and CB_1 agonist-induced G-protein-mediated phosphorylation of c-Jun N-terminal kinase (JNK) (Ahn et al. 2013; Baillie et al. 2013). An active form of the receptor may produce signal transduction (e.g., and phosphorylation of some kinases) that differs depending on the nature of the coupling partner (e.g., isoform of G protein and/or β-arrestin). Unlike Org27569, the CB_1 allosteric modulator ZCZ011 enhanced the CB_1-stimulated G-protein binding and augmented G-protein-mediated ERK1/2 phosphorylation induced by CB_1 agonists anandamide and CP55,940 (Ignatowska-Jankowska et al. 2015). This evidence suggested functional selectivity in signal transduction and provided for the possibility of separating therapeutic effects from untoward adverse effects when the physiologically important CB_1 receptors are manipulated with allosteric modulators.

Translational research using preclinical models of several disorders have shown that the CB_1 PAM ZCZ011 and its analogs exhibit exciting promise for potentiating CB_1 receptor activity without eliciting adverse effects typically found in the CB_1 orthosteric agonists (Ignatowska-Jankowska et al. 2015; Cairns et al. 2017; Slivicki et al. 2018b). On the other hand, the well-characterized CB_1 PAM Org27569 failed to show CB_1-dependent anorectic activity in a mouse model (Gamage et al. 2014), whereas it attenuated both cue- and drug-induced reinstatement of cocaine- and methamphetamine-seeking behavior in experimental rats (Jing et al. 2014).

To date, growing evidence from in vitro and in vivo characterization indicate that allosteric modulators of the CB_1 receptor can regulate the function of the CB_1 receptor with novel mechanisms of action. To translate the exciting in vitro pharmacological activities of this class of CB_1 ligands into clinical relevant therapies demand further investigations.

2.4 CB_1 Receptor Functional Selectivity (Biased Agonism)

GPCR signaling is multifaceted, and different ligands can induce multiple receptor micro-conformations that generate diverse pharmacological responses (Luttrell 2014). Multiple micro-conformations give rise to a variety of activated receptor sub-states that best couple to different G proteins (e.g., $G_{i/o\ subtypes}$, G_s, G_q, etc.) or β-arrestins (1 or 2). Both orthosteric (Lauckner et al. 2005; Mukhopadhyay and Howlett 2005) and allosteric (Khurana et al. 2017) ligands can induce a preference for coupling and downstream signaling. Allosteric modulators that evoke β-arrestin-1 binding to signal include ORG27569 (Ahn et al. 2013) and PSNCBAM-1 (Jagla et al. 2019).

Fay and Farrens (2015) used a fluorescence probe to examine changes in the orientation of helices with ORG27659 binding. They found that ORG27569 binding precludes outward movements of helix 6 that are key to G-protein activation. Further, this and movement of helix 7 (and helix 8 on the carboxy-terminus) may help explain alternative signal transduction by β-arrestin. It is also possible that allosteric modulator binding to the CB_1 receptor is in the same region as G-protein or β-arrestin binding, physically precluding some coupling agents from a receptor interaction. Functional selectivity via an allosteric modulator, with or without probe dependence of orthosteric ligand binding, gives one strategy for providing specificity of a therapeutic response.

2.5 CB_2 Receptors

A major impetus for the development of new synthetic cannabinoids was to create molecules that retained therapeutic actions without the occurrence of cannabimimetic side effects. To this end, the CB_2 receptor (Munro et al. 1993) offers great promise. This receptor shares approximately 44% amino acid homology with the CB_1 receptor. Similar to the CB_1 receptor, it is coupled predominantly to $G_{i/o}$ proteins and linked to signaling cascades that involve adenylyl cyclase and cAMP, mitogen-activated protein kinase (MAPK), and the regulation of intracellular calcium. In addition, an extensive characterization of a panel of ligands binding CB_2 receptors revealed compelling evidence of biased agonism with respect to GTPγS, cAMP, β-arrestin, pMAPKs, and G-protein-gated inwardly rectifying potassium channel (GIRKs) (Soethoudt et al. 2017). Several agonists emerged as highly selective for CB_2 receptors, including HU910, HU308, and JWH133. Unlike the CB_1 receptor, the CB_2 receptor is sparsely expressed in the CNS, but it is highly expressed in cells of the immune system. A great deal of effort dedicated to developing selective CB_2 receptor agonists as research tools and candidate medications has revealed that these drugs produce antinociceptive actions without the occurrence of cannabimimetic side effects (for reviews, see Anand et al. 2009; Donvito et al. 2018). Although a variety of CB_2 receptor agonists lacked efficacy in clinical trials, trials are underway with other compounds for a variety of chronic pain conditions (Aghazadeh Tabrizi et al. 2016).

3 The Endocannabinoids and Their Enzymatic Regulation

The cannabinoid receptors discussed in Sect. 2 mediate most of the psychomimetic effects of *Cannabis*. Yet the evolutionary significance of CB_1 and CB_2 receptors is greater than their activation by *Cannabis* in that they are primarily acted upon by endogenous cannabinoid ligands (endocannabinoids), which together form a neuromodulatory network.

Several unique properties of the endocannabinoid system set it apart from the functional profile of a classical neurotransmitter system. These differences include the direction of endocannabinoid cell-to-cell communication, the unique biosynthesis of endocannabinoid lipids in location and temporal regulation, and the manner of achieving endocannabinoid signaling selectivity. The first property, retrograde neurotransmission, distinguishes endocannabinoids from classical neurotransmitters by their release and action sites and as such their direction of cell-to-cell communication. In contrast to classical neurotransmitters that are released from presynaptic terminals to act at postsynaptic neurons, endocannabinoids are released from the postsynaptic neuron and travel retrogradely across the synaptic cleft to act at presynaptic CB_1 receptors. The activation of presynaptic cannabinoid receptors ultimately dampens presynaptic neurotransmitter release (Mackie 2006b), which is how endocannabinoids modulate synaptic strength. This functional consequence gives the endocannabinoid system its label as a neuromodulatory system.

A second property, biosynthesis of endocannabinoids, is also dramatically different from classical neurotransmitters which are synthesized in the cell body and packaged into secretory vesicles, transported to axon terminals, and stored for release upon propagation of an action potential. Endocannabinoid biosynthesis occurs "on demand" in response to increased intracellular Ca^{2+} (Kondo et al. 1998) or activation of the phospholipase C pathway (Prescott and Majerus 1983; Sugiura et al. 1995) at the level of the plasma membrane from phospholipids present within the cell membrane. The manner by which these highly bioactive yet hydrophobic lipids traverse the aqueous environment of the synaptic space as well as following reuptake in the aqueous intracellular environment remains to be fully understood, though carrier proteins such as fatty acid-binding proteins (FABPs) are likely candidates (Haj-Dahmane et al. 2018). The location of the endocannabinoid biosynthetic machinery at the cellular membrane and their hydrophobic nature all contribute to their localized sites of action (20 μm area (Wilson and Nicoll 2001)) and short half-life (less than 5 min (Willoughby et al. 1997)), all of which makes endocannabinoid signaling directed, short lived, and occurring in response to discrete stimuli.

A third property, signaling specificity, also distinguishes the endocannabinoid system from that of classical neurotransmission. In traditional neurotransmission, differential activation of signaling pathways are achieved through binding of distinct receptor subtypes by one single neurotransmitter (Siegel 1999). However, endogenous cannabinoids produce functional selectivity at CB_1 and CB_2 receptors. The endocannabinoid ligands and their abundance and action at cannabinoid receptors are a key component of the endocannabinoid system. However, the anatomical and cellular distribution of their biosynthetic and degradative enzymes exerts precise regulatory control of the actions of these endogenous cannabinoid ligands.

3.1 *N*-Arachidonylethanolamine (Anandamide)

Anandamide acts as a partial agonist at CB_1 and CB_2 receptors (Hillard 2000), as well as binding to TRPV1 receptors (Melck et al. 1999; Zygmunt et al. 1999) and GPR55 (Baker et al. 2006). The best-characterized biosynthetic pathway for anandamide is the conversion of *N*-acylphosphatidylethanolamines (NAPEs) by NAPE phospholipase D-type (NAPE-PLD) (Okamoto et al. 2004). NAPE-PLD is highly expressed in the brain as well as kidney, spleen, lung, heart, and liver (Degenhardt et al. 2013). However studies using NAPE-PLD knockout mice show no changes in brain anandamide levels suggesting the existence of alternative biosynthetic pathways (Leung et al. 2006). A unique feature of anandamide biosynthesis is the existence of several further redundant pathways: the conversion of *N*-acyl-lysophosphatidylethanolamine by a lysophospholipase-D (lyso-PLD) (Sun et al. 2004); the conversion of NAPE or lyso-NAPE by α/β-hydrolase 4 (Simon and Cravatt 2006); and finally the hydrolysis of NAPE by phospholipase C to phosphoanandamide which is then dephosphorylated to anandamide (Liu et al. 2006). The multiple redundant pathways of anandamide biosynthesis perhaps suggest an evolutionarily conserved mechanism for the importance of preserving endocannabinoid tone. The primary deactivation enzyme of anandamide is fatty acid amide hydrolase (FAAH) (Cravatt et al. 1996, 2001), the degradative product of which is arachidonic acid. FAAH is found in soma and dendrites of the postsynaptic neuron and is associated with membranes of cytoplasmic organelles (Gulyas et al. 2004) in areas such as the neocortex, cerebellar cortex, and hippocampus (Egertova et al. 1998). Other enzymes are also responsible for anandamide degradation, specifically through oxidation. Cyclooxygenase-2 (Kozak et al. 2001), lipoxygenases (Hampson et al. 1995), and cytochrome P450 monooxygenases (Snider et al. 2010), all of which convert anandamide to oxygenated derivatives that have biological activity of their own in eicosanoid inflammatory pathways.

3.2 2-Arachidonoylglycerol (2-AG)

2-AG acts as a high-efficacy agonist at both CB_1 and CB_2 receptors (Hillard 2000), as well as binds $GABA_A$ receptors (Sigel et al. 2011). The biosynthesis of 2-AG occurs through the conversion of diacylglycerols (DAG) by the diacylglycerol lipases (DAGL) (Bisogno et al. 2003), in which DAGL-α is predominantly expressed on neurons and DAGL-β is expressed on immune cells (Yoshida et al. 2006; Hsu et al. 2012). The distribution of DAGLs markedly differs between development and adulthood. In the developing mouse forebrain projection neuron, DAGLs are located on elongating axons (co-expressed with CB_1 receptors) and implicated in growth cone guidance (Bisogno et al. 2003). Post-development, DAGLs accumulate on postsynaptic dendrites and participate in endocannabinoid-mediated modulation of synaptic strength (Keimpema et al. 2011). Additional, but less well-studied, 2-AG biosynthetic pathways include PLA1 activation of lysophospholipase C (lyso-PLC) (Higgs and Glomset 1994) and dephosphorylation of arachidonoyl-lysophosphatidic acid (Nakane et al. 2002).

2-AG inactivation occurs by a variety of enzymes which either hydrolyze 2-AG into its component parts (arachidonic acid and glycerol) or transform it by acylation or phosphorylation. The hydrolysis of 2-AG occurs primarily through monoacylglycerol lipase (MAGL) (Dinh et al. 2002; Blankman et al. 2007), which is highly expressed at presynaptic terminals (Gulyas et al. 2004) in brain areas including the cortex, hippocampus, cerebellum, and thalamus (Dinh et al. 2002) and functions in the bulk clearance of 2-AG. To a lesser extent ($<10\%$), 2-AG is also hydrolyzed by ABHD6 and ABHD12 (Blankman et al. 2007) as well as FAAH (Di Marzo et al. 1998). Both ABHD6 and ABHD12 are postsynaptic integral membrane proteins, but ABHD6 has an intracellular facing active site, and the active site of ABHD12 is extracellular. The location of ABHD6/12 and their modest contributions to 2-AG metabolism contribute to the hypothesis that they might act as a form of regulatory break for 2-AG production. Enzymes that participate in the deactivation of 2-AG through transformation include COX-2 (Kozak et al. 2000), cytochrome P450 (Chen et al. 2008), lipoxygenases (Maccarrone et al. 2000), as well as MAG kinases (Kanoh et al. 1986) and MAG acyltransferases (Coleman and Haynes 1986).

2-AG levels are 1,000 times more abundant in the brain than those of AEA. This high level of production is particularly pertinent given that the metabolism of 2-AG contributes to the availability of free arachidonic acid, the major precursor for the production of pro-inflammatory eicosanoids. Specifically, MAGL is the rate-limiting enzyme for free arachidonic acid production in the brain, liver, and lung (Nomura et al. 2011). As such, MAGL not only serves as the major enzyme terminates 2-AG signaling but also plays an important role in the production of free arachidonic acid production in a tissue-specific manner. Importantly, MAGL does not mediate the production of arachidonic acid in the gastrointestinal tract. Ultimately 2-AG production and metabolism serve to facilitate both neuromodulation and immunoregulation, respectively (an extensive review of 2-AG biosynthesis and degradation can be found in Murataeva et al. 2014).

3.3 Other Endocannabinoids, Hemopressins, and Related Lipids

Endocannabinoids are not restricted to AEA or 2-AG. They are members of an ever-growing family of bioactive lipids (Di Marzo 2018). Other described endocannabinoids with cannabimimetic properties include noladin ether (Hanus et al. 2001), N-Arachidonoyl dopamine (Bisogno et al. 2000), virodhamine (Porter et al. 2002), and lysophosphatidylinositol (Pineiro and Falasca 2012). Fatty acid amides such as palmitoylethanolamine and oleoylethanolamine while lacking affinity for CB_1 or CB_2 receptors (O'Sullivan and Kendall 2010) activate GPR55 and GPR119 receptors (Godlewski et al. 2009), as well as enhance AEA and 2-AG activity by competition for FAAH (Ben-Shabat et al. 1998; Jonsson et al. 2001). Hemopressin is a nonapeptide produced from the cleavage of hemoglobin which acts as an inverse agonist at CB_1 receptors (Heimann et al. 2007). Hemopressin shows several physiological effects such as antinociception, hypophagy, and hypotension (Heimann et al. 2007; Monti et al. 2016). Indeed, docking studies have shown that hemopressin binds to the same CB_1 receptor pocket as SR141716, a CB_1 receptor competitive antagonist/ inverse agonist used for metabolic syndrome, but withdrawn from the European market in 2009 due to psychiatric side effects (Motaghedi et al. 2011).

4 Drug Interactions

The endocannabinoid system can interact with a wide range of other neurotransmitter systems including opioids, GABA, glutamate, dopamine, etc. and modulate the effects of ethanol, NSAIDs, and substrates for various enzymes. Here we will focus on two such interactions: the potential of drugs targeting the endocannabinoid system to increase opioid potency (termed opioid-sparing effects) which minimizes side effects and cannabinoid competition for cytochrome P450 (CYP) enzymes making them a potential contraindication for diseases with CYP dysregulation or patients taking drugs metabolized through these enzymes.

4.1 Opioid-Sparing Effects

One consequence of the opioid epidemic crisis is the need to identify alternative drug classes of analgesics that can replace opioids or can reduce the dose of opioids necessary to ameliorate pain. Modulating the endocannabinoid system represents a promising strategy to reduce the effective analgesic doses of opioids while concomitantly decreasing opioid abuse liability as well as unwanted dose-dependent side effects such as constipation and respiratory depression. Substantial preclinical evidence suggests that cannabinoid agonists might produce opioid-sparing effects (for reviews see Nielsen et al. 2017; Donvito et al. 2018). THC represents the most widely selected cannabinoid evaluated in combination with opioids in rodent models of pain. The Welch group pioneered this area of research by employing an isobolographic approach revealing that THC synergistically enhances the antinociceptive effects of various opioids in rodent models of acute pain (Welch and Stevens 1992; Smith et al. 1998; Cichewicz et al. 1999, 2001, 2005; Cox et al. 2007). Likewise, the synthetic cannabinoids CP55,940 and WIN55,212-2 augmented the antinociceptive effects of morphine, but did not affect the discriminative stimulus effects of morphine or heroin self-administration in rhesus monkeys (Maguire et al. 2013). The periaqueductal gray (Wilson-Poe et al. 2012, 2013) has been implicated as a potential brain site contributing to the augmented antinociceptive effects resulting from combined administration of opioids and cannabinoids. Inhibitors of endocannabinoid catabolic enzymes also augment the antinociceptive effects of opioids. Combination of the brain-penetrant FAAH inhibitor URB597 or peripherally restricted FAAH inhibitor URB937 plus morphine produced synergistic antinociceptive effects in the mouse paclitaxel model of neuropathic pain (Slivicki et al. 2018a). Similarly, combined injections of the MAGL inhibitor MJN110 and morphine produced synergistic antinociceptive effects in the mouse chronic constrictive injury model of neuropathic pain (Wilkerson et al. 2016). Curiously, co-administration of the dual FAAH-MAGL inhibitor and morphine produced an additive antinociceptive effect in this assay (Wilkerson et al. 2017).

In contrast to the well-established findings from preclinical studies showing that cannabinoids augment the antinociceptive effects of opioids, translation to clinical settings remains to be established, as discussed in a recent meta-analysis (Nielsen et al. 2017). Based on preclinical studies, clinical case reports, and a highly cited population study (Bachhuber et al. 2014), the idea of opioid-sparing effects of cannabinoid agonists has been touted as rationale for the legalization of "medical" *Cannabis*. While large controlled clinical studies provide some evidence of analgesic benefits of THC, opioid dose changes have rarely been reported (Seeling et al.

2006; Johnson et al. 2010). However, three recent phase 3 clinical trials failed to achieve statistical significance of the primary endpoint (average pain Numerical Rating Scale) of nabiximols (an oral-mucosal spray consisting of approximately equal parts of THC and CBD) in advanced cancer patients with chronic pain not alleviated by optimized opioid treatment (Fallon et al. 2017; Lichtman et al. 2018). However, nabiximols showed efficacy on secondary endpoints including sleep disruption as well as patient (Subject Global Impression of Change and Patient Satisfaction Questionnaire) and physician (Physician Global Impression of Change) questionnaires. Substantial differences (e.g., endpoints, species differences, type of pain, etc.) exist between preclinical studies of pain and treatment of clinical pain (Negus 2018, 2019). Moreover, preclinical studies typically use opioid-naïve or non-tolerant laboratory animal subjects, whereas patients in clinical trials have generally been on large-dose regimens for prolonged periods of time. Thus, it would be advantageous in future clinical investigations to initiate cannabinoid treatment in cancer pain patients prior to establishing an aggressive opioid treatment regimen. In addition, it is possible that cannabinoid drugs produce opioid-sparing effects for only specific types of cancer pain or in certain patients.

4.2 Cytochrome P450 Enzymes

Cytochrome P450 enzymes are highly expressed in the liver and intestine among other tissues and are necessary for the metabolism of steroid hormones, cholesterol, vitamin D, bile acids, and eicosanoids (Hasler et al. 1999). Diseases of CYP dysregulation include hypertension, hepatotoxicity, infection, and chronic inflammation among many others (Setchell et al. 1998; Hiratsuka et al. 2006; Capdevila et al. 2007) (for a full review of CYP roles in disease, see Pikuleva and Waterman 2013). CYP activity is also a major factor in the pharmacokinetics of drugs and thus drug responses (Zanger and Schwab 2013). Endocannabinoids, phytocannabinoids (specifically THC and CBD), as well as synthetic cannabinoids are all substrates of various CYP enzymes (for a full review of cannabinoid interactions with CYP enzymes, see Zendulka et al. 2016). As such, binding of phytocannabinoids to CYP enzymes could potentially produce treatment failure if taken with clinically co-administered drugs. Competitive inhibition of CYP enzymes raises concerns of drug toxicity from clinical medications. Medications metabolized by CYP enzymes taken in combination with phytocannabinoids or synthetic cannabinoids may interfere with metabolism, thereby increasing drug blood levels and/or extending duration of action. Thus, consideration is needed for the potential risk of clinically significant drug interactions between cannabinoid-based drugs and medications metabolized by CYP. Given the increased use of "medical" and recreational cannabis, a great need exists to understand the metabolic and pharmacodynamic interactions between cannabinoid-based drugs and other pharmaceuticals.

5 Conclusions

Since antiquity, *Cannabis* has been recognized for its wide range of therapeutic actions as well as for its intoxicating effects. Studies identifying the active constituents of *Cannabis* provoked an enormous body of research that led to the creation of new research probes revealing mechanisms underlying its pharmacological effects, the discovery of the endocannabinoid system, and cannabinoid-based medications approved by the FDA. However, further research is needed to understand the pharmacological effects and the mechanisms of action underlying the minor phytocannabinoids and terpenes, both alone and in combination. Further work geared toward exploiting promising therapeutic targets within the endocannabinoid system (e.g., allosteric sites on the CB_1 receptor, CB_2 receptors, FAAH, MAGL, FABPs) may yield new medicines. In particular, preclinical research demonstrates that phytocannabinoids, synthetic cannabinoids, and inhibitors of endocannabinoid-regulating enzymes produce antinociception and augment the antinociceptive effects of opioids in a great variety of acute and chronic models of pain. An enormous amount of preclinical studies demonstrate potential efficacy of drugs acting upon the endocannabinoid system in various laboratory animal models of disease and injury. Thus, it remains to examine whether this basic knowledge translates into the clinic. Moreover, given the wide availability of *Cannabis*, *Cannabis* extracts, and phytocannabinoids in dispensaries throughout the US and availability of CBD derived from hemp, a tremendous need exists for evidenced-based practice for therapeutic needs (e.g., mental illness and *Cannabis* Use Disorder), which includes understanding potential harms and minimizing abuse of synthetic cannabinoids. A great need also exists for further research to understand the long-term consequences of *Cannabis* on the developing brain, not only in developing fetuses but also in adolescent and young adults. In sum, great strides have been achieved in the understanding of cannabinoid pharmacology, including the tremendous complexity existing between the endogenous cannabinoid system and the numerous physiological systems it regulates.

Acknowledgments This work was supported by R01 DA039942 (DAK, LD, AHL), R01 DA042157 (ACH), P50 DA006634 (ACH), and VCU School of Pharmacy start-up funds (AHL).

References

Abood ME, Ditto KA, Noel MA et al (1997) Isolation and expression of mouse CB1 cannabinoid receptor gene: comparison of binding properties with those of native CB1 receptors in mouse brain and N18TG2 neuroblastoma cells. Biochem Pharmacol 53:207–214

Adams R, Aycock BF, Loewe S (1948a) Tetrahydrocannabinol homologs. J Am Chem Soc 70:662–664. https://doi.org/10.1021/ja01182a067

Adams R, Mackenzie S, Loewe S (1948b) Tetrahydrocannabinol homologs with doubly branched alkyl groups in the 3-position. J Am Chem Soc 70:664–668. https://doi.org/10.1021/ja01182a068

Aghazadeh Tabrizi M, Baraldi PG, Borea PA, Varani K (2016) Medicinal chemistry, pharmacology, and potential therapeutic benefits of cannabinoid CB2 receptor agonists. Chem Rev 116:519–560. https://doi.org/10.1021/acs.chemrev.5b00411

Ahn H, Mahmoud MM, Shim JY, Kendall DA (2013) Distinct roles of beta-arrestin 1 and beta-arrestin 2 in ORG27569-induced biased signaling and internalization of the cannabinoid receptor 1 (CB1). J Biol Chem 288:9790–9800

Anand P, Whiteside G, Fowler CJ, Hohmann AG (2009) Targeting CB2 receptors and the endocannabinoid system for the treatment of pain. Brain Res Rev 60:255–266. https://doi.org/10.1016/j.brainresrev.2008.12.003

Araque A, Castillo PE, Manzoni OJ, Tonini R (2017) Synaptic functions of endocannabinoid signaling in health and disease. Neuropharmacology 124:13–24

Bachhuber MA, Saloner B, Cunningham CO, Barry CL (2014) Medical cannabis laws and opioid analgesic overdose mortality in the United States, 1999-2010. JAMA Intern Med 174:1668–1673. https://doi.org/10.1001/jamainternmed.2014.4005

Bagher AM, Laprairie RB, Kelly ME, Denovan-Wright EM (2013) Co-expression of the human cannabinoid receptor coding region splice variants (hCB(1)) affects the function of hCB (1) receptor complexes. Eur J Pharmacol 721:341–354

Baillie GL, Horswill JG, Anavi-Goffer S et al (2013) CB(1) receptor allosteric modulators display both agonist and signaling pathway specificity. Mol Pharmacol 83:322–338

Baker D, Pryce G, Davies WL, Hiley CR (2006) In silico patent searching reveals a new cannabinoid receptor. Trends Pharmacol Sci 27(1):1–4

Bari M, Battista N, Fezza F et al (2005) Lipid rafts control signaling of type-1 cannabinoid receptors in neuronal cells. J Biol Chem 280:12212–12220

Barnett-Norris J, Lynch D, Reggio PH (2005) Lipids, lipid rafts and caveolae: their importance for GPCR signaling and their centrality to the endocannabinoid system. Life Sci 77:1625–1639

Barrus DG, Lefever TW, Wiley JL (2018) Evaluation of reinforcing and aversive effects of voluntary Δ9-tetrahydrocannabinol ingestion in rats. Neuropharmacology 137:133–140

Bauer M, Chicca A, Tamborrini M et al (2012) Identification and quantification of a new family of peptide endocannabinoids (Pepcans) showing negative allosteric modulation at CB1 receptors. J Biol Chem 287:36944–36967

Beardsley PM, Scimeca JA, Martin BR (1987) Studies on the agonistic activity of delta 9-11-tetrahydrocannabinol in mice, dogs and rhesus monkeys and its interactions with delta 9-tetrahydrocannabinol. J Pharmacol Exp Ther 241:521–526

Benard G, Massa F, Puente N et al (2012) Mitochondrial CB(1) receptors regulate neuronal energy metabolism. Nat Neurosci 15:558–564

Ben-Shabat S, Fride E, Sheskin T et al (1998) An entourage effect: inactive endogenous fatty acid glycerol esters enhance 2-arachidonoyl-glycerol cannabinoid activity. Eur J Pharmacol 353:23–31

Bisogno T, Melck D, Gretskaya NM et al (2000) N-acyl-dopamines: novel synthetic CB(1) cannabinoid-receptor ligands and inhibitors of anandamide inactivation with cannabimimetic activity in vitro and in vivo. Biochem J 351:817–824

Bisogno T, Howell F, Williams G et al (2003) Cloning of the first sn1-DAG lipases points to the spatial and temporal regulation of endocannabinoid signaling in the brain. J Cell Biol 163:463–468

Blankman JL, Cravatt BF (2013) Chemical probes of endocannabinoid metabolism. Pharmacol Rev 65:849–871. https://doi.org/10.1124/pr.112.006387

Blankman JL, Simon GM, Cravatt BF (2007) A comprehensive profile of brain enzymes that hydrolyze the endocannabinoid 2-arachidonoylglycerol. Chem Biol 14:1347–1356

Bonner TI (1996) Molecular biology of cannabinoid receptors. J Neuroimmunol 69:15–17

Braida D, Pozzi M, Parolaro D, Sala M (2001) Intracerebral self-administration of the cannabinoid receptor agonist CP 55,940 in the rat: interaction with the opioid system. Eur J Pharmacol 413:227–234

Braida D, Losue S, Pegorini S, Sala M (2004) Delta9-tetrahydrocannabinol-induced conditioned place preference and intracerebroventricular self-administration in rats. Eur J Pharmacol 506:63–69

Breivogel CS, Puri V, Lambert JM et al (2013) The influence of beta-arrestin2 on cannabinoid CB1 receptor coupling to G-proteins and subcellular localization and relative levels of beta-arrestin1 and 2 in mouse brain. J Recept Signal Transduct Res 33:367–379

Buckley NE, McCoy KL, Mezey É et al (2000) Immunomodulation by cannabinoids is absent in mice deficient for the cannabinoid CB2 receptor. Eur J Pharmacol 396:141–149. https://doi.org/10.1016/S0014-2999(00)00211-9

Cairns EA, Szczesniak AM, Straiker AJ et al (2017) The in vivo effects of the CB1-positive allosteric modulator GAT229 on intraocular pressure in ocular normotensive and hypertensive mice. J Ocul Pharmacol Ther 33:582–590

Capdevila JH, Falck JR, Imig JD (2007) Roles of the cytochrome P450 arachidonic acid monooxygenases in the control of systemic blood pressure and experimental hypertension. Kidney Int 72:683–689

Celofiga A, Koprivsek J, Klavz J (2014) Use of synthetic cannabinoids in patients with psychotic disorders: case series. J Dual Diagn 10:168–173

Chakrabarti A, Onaivi ES, Chaudhuri G (1995) Cloning and sequencing of a cDNA encoding the mouse brain-type cannabinoid receptor protein. DNA Seq 5:385–388

Chen JK, Chen J, Imig JD et al (2008) Identification of novel endogenous cytochrome p450 arachidonate metabolites with high affinity for cannabinoid receptors. J Biol Chem 283:24514–24524

Chen X, Zheng C, Qian J et al (2014) Involvement of beta-arrestin-2 and clathrin in agonist-mediated internalization of the human cannabinoid CB2 receptor. Curr Mol Pharmacol 7:67–80

Cichewicz DL, Martin ZL, Smith FL, Welch SP (1999) Enhancement mu opioid antinociception by oral delta9-tetrahydrocannabinol: dose-response analysis and receptor identification. J Pharmacol Exp Ther 289:859–867

Cichewicz DL, Haller VL, Welch SP (2001) Changes in opioid and cannabinoid receptor protein following short-term combination treatment with delta(9)-tetrahydrocannabinol and morphine. J Pharmacol Exp Ther 297:121–127

Cichewicz DL, Welch SP, Smith FL (2005) Enhancement of transdermal fentanyl and buprenorphine antinociception by transdermal Δ9-tetrahydrocannabinol. Eur J Pharmacol 525:74–82. https://doi.org/10.1016/j.ejphar.2005.09.039

Clarke R, Merlin M (2013) Cannabis: evolution and ethnobotany. University of California Press, Berkeley

Coleman RA, Haynes EB (1986) Monoacylglycerol acyltransferase. Evidence that the activities from rat intestine and suckling liver are tissue-specific isoenzymes. J Biol Chem 261:224–228

Compton DR, Martin BR (1990) Pharmacological evaluation of water soluble cannabinoids and related analogs. Life Sci 46:1575–1585. https://doi.org/10.1016/0024-3205(90)90391-4

Compton DR, Gold LH, Ward SJ et al (1992a) Aminoalkylindole analogs: cannabimimetic activity of a class of compounds structurally distinct from delta 9-tetrahydrocannabinol. J Pharmacol Exp Ther 263:1118–1126

Compton DR, Johnson MR, Melvin LS, Martin BR (1992b) Pharmacological profile of a series of bicyclic cannabinoid analogs: classification as cannabimimetic agents. J Pharmacol Exp Ther 260:201–209

Compton DR, Rice KC, De Costa BR et al (1993) Cannabinoid structure-activity relationships: correlation of receptor binding and in vivo activities. J Pharmacol Exp Ther 265:218–226

Console-Bram L, Marcu J, Abood ME (2012) Cannabinoid receptors: nomenclature and pharmacological principles. Prog Neuropsychopharmacol Biol Psychiatry 38:4–15

Cox ML, Haller VL, Welch SP (2007) Synergy between delta9-tetrahydrocannabinol and morphine in the arthritic rat. Eur J Pharmacol 567:125–130

Cravatt BF, Giang DK, Mayfield SP et al (1996) Molecular characterization of an enzyme that degrades neuromodulatory fatty-acid amides. Nature 384:83–87

Cravatt BF, Demarest K, Patricelli MP et al (2001) Supersensitivity to anandamide and enhanced endogenous cannabinoid signaling in mice lacking fatty acid amide hydrolase. Proc Natl Acad Sci U S A 98:9371–9376

Cridge BJ, Rosengren RJ (2013) Critical appraisal of the potential use of cannabinoids in cancer management. Cancer Manag Res 5:301–313

Daigle TL, Kearn CS, Mackie K (2008) Rapid CB1 cannabinoid receptor desensitization defines the time course of ERK1/2 MAP kinase signaling. Neuropharmacology 54:36–44

Dalton GD, Howlett AC (2012) Cannabinoid CB1 receptors transactivate multiple receptor tyrosine kinases and regulate serine/threonine kinases to activate ERK in neuronal cells. Br J Pharmacol 165:2497–2511

Degenhardt L, Ferrari AJ, Calabria B et al (2013) The global epidemiology and contribution of Cannabis use and dependence to the global burden of disease: results from the GBD 2010 study. PLoS One 8:e76635

Devane WA, Dysarz FA III, Johnson MR et al (1988) Determination and characterization of a cannabinoid receptor in rat brain. Mol Pharmacol 34:605–613

Devane WA, Hanus L, Breuer A et al (1992) Isolation and structure of a brain constituent that binds to the cannabinoid receptor. Science 258:1946–1949

Di Marzo V (2018) New approaches and challenges to targeting the endocannabinoid system. Nat Rev Drug Discov 17(9):623–639

Di Marzo V, Bisogno T, Sugiura T et al (1998) The novel endogenous cannabinoid 2-arachidonoylglycerol is inactivated by neuronal- and basophil-like cells: connections with anandamide. Biochem J 331:15–19

Diaz-Alonso J, Guzman M, Galve-Roperh I (2012) Endocannabinoids via CB_1 receptors act as neurogenic niche cues during cortical development. Philos Trans R Soc Lond B Biol Sci 367:32293241

Dinh TP, Carpenter D, Leslie FM et al (2002) Brain monoglyceride lipase participating in endocannabinoid inactivation. Proc Natl Acad Sci U S A 99:10819–10824

Donvito G, Nass SR, Wilkerson JL et al (2018) The endogenous cannabinoid system: a budding source of targets for treating inflammatory and neuropathic pain. Neuropsychopharmacology 43:52–79. https://doi.org/10.1038/npp.2017.204

Egertova M, Giang DK, Cravatt BF, Elphick MR (1998) A new perspective on cannabinoid signalling: complementary localization of fatty acid amide hydrolase and the CB1 receptor in rat brain. Proc Natl Acad Sci U S A 265:2081–2085

Eldeeb K, Leone-Kabler S, Howlett AC (2016) CB1 cannabinoid receptor-mediated increases in cyclic AMP accumulation are correlated with reduced Gi/o function. J Basic Clin Physiol Pharmacol 27(3):311–322

Eldeeb K, Leone-Kabler S, Howlett AC (2017) Mouse neuroblastoma CB1 cannabinoid receptor-stimulated [(35)S]GTPS binding: total and antibody-targeted G alpha protein-specific scintillation proximity assays. Methods Enzymol 593:1–21

ElSohly MA, Radwan MM, Gul W et al (2017) Phytochemistry of Cannabis sativa L. Prog Chem Org Nat Prod 103:1–36

Fallon MT, Albert Lux E, McQuade R et al (2017) Sativex oromucosal spray as adjunctive therapy in advanced cancer patients with chronic pain unalleviated by optimized opioid therapy: two double-blind, randomized, placebo-controlled phase 3 studies. Br J Pain 11:119–133. https://doi.org/10.1177/2049463717710042

Fattore L, Cossu G, Martellotta CM, Fratta W (2001) Intravenous self-administration of the cannabinoid CB1 receptor agonist WIN 55,212-2 in rats. Psychopharmacology 156:410–416

Fay X, Farrens Y (2015) Structural dynamics and energetics underlying allosteric inactivation of the cannabinoid receptor CB1. Proc Natl Acad Sci U S A 112:8469–8474

Flores-Sanchez IJ, Verpoorte R (2008) Secondary metabolism in Cannabis. Phytochem Rev 7:615–639

Ford BM, Tai S, Fantegrossi WE, Prather PL (2017) Synthetic pot: not your grandfather's marijuana. Trends Pharmacol Sci 38:257–276. https://doi.org/10.1016/j.tips.2016.12.003

Franklin JM, Vasiljevik T, Prisinzano TE, Carrasco GA (2013) Cannabinoid agonists increase the interaction between beta-arrestin 2 and ERK1/2 and upregulate beta-arrestin 2 and 5-HT(2A) receptors. Pharmacol Res 68:46–58

Freeman MJ, Rose DZ, Myers MA et al (2013) Ischemic stroke after use of the synthetic marijuana "spice". Neurology 81:2090–2093

Gaffuri AL, Ladarre D, Lenkei Z (2012) Type-1 cannabinoid receptor signaling in neuronal development. Pharmacology 90:19–39

Galiegue S, Mary S, Marchand J et al (1995) Expression of central and peripheral cannabinoid receptors in human immune tissues and leukocyte subpopulations. Eur J Biochem 232:54–61

Gamage TF, Ignatowska-jankowska BM, Wiley JL et al (2014) In-vivo pharmacological evaluation of the CB1-receptor allosteric modulator Org-27569. Behav Pharmacol 25:182–185

Gaoni Y, Mechoulam R (1964) Isolation, structure, and partial synthesis of an active constituent of hashish. J Am Chem Soc 86:1646–1647. https://doi.org/10.1021/ja01062a046

Garcia AB, Soria-Gomez E, Bellocchio L, Marsicano G (2016) Cannabinoid receptor type-1: breaking the dogmas. F1000Res 5:990

Gerard CM, Mollereau C, Vassart G, Parmentier M (1991) Molecular-cloning of a human cannabinoid receptor which is also expressed in testis. Biochem J 279:129–134

Gerostamoulos D, Drummer OH, Woodford NW (2015) Deaths linked to synthetic cannabinoids. Forensic Sci Med Pathol 11:478

Glass M, Northup JK (1999) Agonist selective regulation of G proteins by cannabinoid CB(1) and CB(2) receptors. Mol Pharmacol 56:1362–1369

Glass M, Dragunow M, Faull RL (1997) Cannabinoid receptors in the human brain: a detailed anatomical and quantitative autoradiographic study in the fetal, neonatal and adult human brain. Neuroscience 77:299–318

Godlewski G, Offertaler L, Wagner JA, Kunos G (2009) Receptors for acylethanolamides-GPR55 and GPR119. Prostaglandins Other Lipid Mediat 89:3–4

Grim TW, Morales AJ, Gonek MM et al (2016) Stratification of cannabinoid 1 receptor (CB1R) agonist efficacy: manipulation of CB1R density through use of transgenic mice reveals congruence between in vivo and in vitro assays. J Pharmacol Exp Ther 359:329–339

Grim TW, Morales AJ, Thomas BF et al (2017) Apparent CB1 receptor rimonabant affinity estimates: combination with THC and synthetic cannabinoids in the mouse in vivo triad model. J Pharmacol Exp Ther 362:210–218. https://doi.org/10.1124/jpet.117.240192

Grotenhermen F, Muller-Vahl K (2012) The therapeutic potential of cannabis and cannabinoids. Dtsch Arztebl Int 109:495–501

Gulyas AI, Cravatt BF, Bracey MH et al (2004) Segregation of two endocannabinoid-hydrolyzing enzymes into pre- and postsynaptic compartments in the rat hippocampus, cerebellum and amygdala. Eur J Neurosci 20:441–458

Haj-Dahmane S, Shen RY, Elemes MW et al (2018) Fatty-acid-binding protein 5 controls retrograde endocannabinoid signaling at central glutamate synapses. Proc Natl Acad Sci U S A 115:3482–3487

Hampson AJ, Hill WA, Zan-Phillips M et al (1995) Anandamide hydroxylation by brain lipoxygenase: metabolite structures and potencies at the cannabinoid receptor. Biochim Biophys Acta 1259:173–179

Han J, Kesner P, Metna-Laurent M et al (2012) Acute cannabinoids impair working memory through astroglial CB1 receptor modulation of hippocampal LTD. Cell 148:1039–1050

Hanus L, Abu-Lafi S, Fride E et al (2001) 2-arachidonyl glycerol ether, an endogenous agonist of the cannabinoid CB1 receptor. Proc Natl Acad Sci U S A 98:3662–3665

Hasin DS, Kerridge BT, Saha TD et al (2016) Prevalence and correlates of DSM-5 Cannabis use disorder, 2012-2013: findings from the national epidemiologic survey on alcohol and related conditions–III. Am J Psychiatry 173:588–599

Hasler JA, Estabrook RMM, Pikuleva IA et al (1999) Human cytochromes P450. Mol Asp Med 20:1–137

Heimann AS, Gomes I, Dale CS et al (2007) Hemopressin is an inverse agonist of CB1 cannabinoid receptors. Proc Natl Acad Sci U S A 104:20588–20593

Hempel BJ, Wakeford AG, Clasen MM et al (2016) Delta-9-tetrahydrocannabinol (THC) history fails to affect THC's ability to induce place preferences in rats. Pharmacol Biochem Behav 144:1–6

Henriksson BG, Johansson JO, Järbe TUC (1975) Δ9-tetrahydrocannabinol produced discrimination in pigeons. Pharmacol Biochem Behav 5:771–774. https://doi.org/10.1016/0091-3057(75)90105-7

Herkenham M, Lynn AB, Little MD et al (1990) Cannabinoid receptor localization in brain. Proc Natl Acad Sci U S A 87:1932–1936

Higgs HN, Glomset JA (1994) Identification of a phosphatidic acid-preferring phospholipase A1 from bovine brain and testis. Proc Natl Acad Sci U S A 91:9574–9578

Hillard CJ (2000) Biochemistry and pharmacology of the endocannabinoids arachidonylethanolamide and 2-arachidonylglycerol. Prostaglandins Other Lipid Mediat 61:3–18

Hillard CJ, Harris RA, Bloom AS (1985) Effects of the cannabinoids on physical properties of brain membranes and phospholipid vesicles: fluorescence studies. J Pharmacol Exp Ther 232:579–588

Hillard CJ, Pounds JJ, Boyer DR, Bloom AS (1990) Studies of the role of membrane lipid order in the effects of delta 9-tetrahydrocannabinol on adenylate cyclase activation in heart. J Pharmacol Exp Ther 252:1075–1082

Hiratsuka M, Nozawa H, Katsumoto Y et al (2006) Genetic polymorphisms and haplotype structures of the CYP4A22 gene in a Japanese population. Mutat Res 599:98–104

Ho BY, Zhao J (1996) Determination of the cannabinoid receptors in mouse x rat hybridoma NG108-15 cells and rat GH4C1 cells. Neurosci Lett 212:123–126

Horswill JG, Bali U, Shaaban S et al (2007) PSNCBAM-1, a novel allosteric antagonist at cannabinoid CB1 receptors with hypophagic effects in rats. Br J Pharmacol 2:805–814

Houston DB, Howlett AC (1993) Solubilization of the cannabinoid receptor from rat brain and its functional interaction with guanine nucleotide-binding proteins. Mol Pharmacol 43:17–22

Howlett AC, Abood ME (2017) CB1 and CB2 receptor pharmacology. Adv Pharmacol 80:169–206

Howlett AC, Qualy JM, Khachatrian LL (1986) Involvement of Gi in the inhibition of adenylate cyclase by cannabimimetic drugs. Mol Pharmacol 29:307–313

Howlett AC, Johnson MR, Melvin LS, Milne GM (1988) Nonclassical cannabinoid analgetics inhibit adenylate cyclase: development of a cannabinoid receptor model. Mol Pharmacol 33:297–302

Howlett AC, Barth F, Bonner TI et al (2002) International Union of Pharmacology. XXVII. Classification of cannabinoid receptors. Pharmacol Rev 54:161–202

Hsu KL, Tsuboi K, Adibekian A et al (2012) DAGLβ inhibition perturbs a lipid network involved in macrophage inflammatory responses. Nat Chem Biol 8:999–1007

Huffman JW, Zengin G, Wu MJ et al (2005) Structure–activity relationships for 1-alkyl-3-(1-naphthoyl)indoles at the cannabinoid CB1 and CB2 receptors: steric and electronic effects of naphthoyl substituents. New highly selective CB2 receptor agonists. Bioorg Med Chem 13:89–112

Ignatowska-Jankowska BM, Baillie GL, Kinsey S et al (2015) A cannabinoid CB1 receptor-positive allosteric modulator reduces neuropathic pain in the mouse with no psychoactive effects. Neuropsychopharmacology 40:2948–2959

Ilyasov AA, Milligan CE, Pharr EP, Howlett AC (2018) The endocannabinoid system and oligodendrocytes in health and disease. Front Neurosci 12:733

Jagla CAD, Scott CE, Tang Y et al (2019) Primidinyl bipheylureas act as allosteric modulators to activate cannabinoid receptor 1 and initiate B-arrestin-dependent responses. Mol Pharmacol 95:1–10

Järbe TUC, Gifford RS (2014) "Herbal incense": designer drug blends as cannabimimetics and their assessment by drug discrimination and other in vivo bioassays. Life Sci 97:64–71. https://doi.org/10.1016/j.lfs.2013.07.011

JÄrbe TUC, Henriksson BG (1973) Acute effects of two tetrahydrocannabinols (Δ9-THC and Δ8-THC) on water intake in water deprived rats: implications for behavioral studies on marijuana compounds. Psychopharmacologia 30:315–322. https://doi.org/10.1007/BF00429190

JÄrbe TUC, Henriksson BG (1974) Discriminative response control produced with hashish, tetrahydrocannabinols (δ8-THC and δ9-THC), and other drugs. Psychopharmacologia 40(1):1–16. https://doi.org/10.1007/BF00429443

Jarbe TU, Henriksson BG, Ohlin GC (1977) Delta9-THC as a discriminative cue in pigeons: effects of delta8-THC, CBD, and CBN. Arch Int Pharmacodyn Ther 228:68–72

Järbe TUC, Lemay BJ, Halikhedkar A et al (2014) Differentiation between low- and high-efficacy CB 1 receptor agonists using a drug discrimination protocol for rats. Psychopharmacology 231:489–500. https://doi.org/10.1007/s00213-013-3257-8

Järbe TUC, Gifford RS, Zvonok A, Makriyannis A (2016a) Δ9-Tetrahydrocannabinol discriminative stimulus effects of AM2201 and related aminoalkylindole analogs in rats. Behav Pharmacol 27:211–214. https://doi.org/10.1097/FBP.0000000000000196

Järbe TUC, Lemay BJ, Thakur GA, Makriyannis A (2016b) A high efficacy cannabinergic ligand (AM4054) used as a discriminative stimulus: generalization to other adamantyl analogs and Δ9-THC in rats. Pharmacol Biochem Behav 148:46–52. https://doi.org/10.1016/j.pbb.2016.06.001

Jiang HE, Zhao YX, Ferguson DK et al (2006) A new insight into Cannabis sativa (Cannabaceae) utilization from 2500-year-old Yanghai Tombs, Xinjiang, China. J Ethnopharmacol 108:414–422

Jing L, Qiu Y, Zhang Y, Li JX (2014) Effects of the cannabinoid CB1 receptor allosteric modulator ORG 27569 on reinstatement of cocaine-and methamphetamine-seeking behavior in rats. Drug Alcohol Depend 143:251–256

John WS, Martin TJ, Nader MA (2017) Behavioral determinants of cannabinoid self-administration in old world monkeys. Neuropsychopharmacology 42:1522–1530

Johnson JR, Burnell-Nugent M, Lossignol D et al (2010) Multicenter, double-blind, randomized, placebo-controlled, parallel-group study of the efficacy, safety, and tolerability of THC:CBD extract and THC extract in patients with intractable cancer-related pain. J Pain Symptom Manag 39:167–179

Jonsson KO, Vandevoorde SV, Lambert DM et al (2001) Effects of homologues and analogues of palmitoylethanolamide upon the inactivation of the endocannabinoid anandamide. Br J Pharmacol 133:1263–1275

Justinova Z, Tanda G, Redhi GH, Goldberg SR (2003) Self-administration of delta9-tetrahydrocannabinol (THC) by drug naive squirrel monkeys. Psychopharmacology 169:135–140

Kano M (2014) Control of synaptic function by endocannabinoid-mediated retrograde signaling. Proc Jpn Acad Ser B Phys Biol Sci 90:235–250

Kanoh H, Iwata T, Ono T, Suzuki T (1986) Immunological characterization of sn-1,2-diacylglycerol and sn-2-monoacylglycerol kinase from pig brain. J Biol Chem 261:5597–5602

Katona I, Sperlagh B, Sik A et al (1999) Presynaptically located CB1 cannabinoid receptors regulate GABA release from axon terminals of specific hippocampal interneurons. J Neurosci 19:4544–4558

Keimpema E, Mackie K, Harkany T (2011) Molecular model of cannabis sensitivity in developing neuronal circuits. Trends Pharmacol Sci 32:551–561

Khurana L, Mackie K, Piomelli D, Kendall DA (2017) Modulation of CB1 cannabinoid receptor by allosteric ligands: pharmacological and therapeutic opportunities. Neuropharmacology 124:3–12

Kondo S, Kondo H, Nakane S et al (1998) 2-Arachidonoylglycerol, an endogenous cannabinoid receptor agonist: identification as one of the major species of monoacylglycerols in various rat tissues, and evidence for its generation through CA2+-dependent and -independent mechanisms. FEBS Lett 429:152–156

Kozak KR, Rowlinson SW, Marnett LJ (2000) Oxygenation of the endocannabinoid, 2-arachidonylglycerol, to glyceryl prostaglandins by cyclooxygenase-2. J Biol Chem 275:33744–33749

Kozak KR, Crews BC, Ray JL et al (2001) Metabolism of prostaglandin glycerol esters and prostaglandin ethanolamides in vitro and in vivo. J Biol Chem 276:36993–36998

Laprairie R, Bagher A, Kelly M, Denovan-Wright EM (2015) Cannabidiol is a negative allosteric modulator of the cannabinoid CB1 receptor. Br J Pharmacol 172:4790–4805

Lauckner JE, Hille B, Mackie K (2005) The cannabinoid agonist WIN55,212-2 increases intracellular calcium via CB1 receptor coupling to G(q/11) G proteins. Proc Natl Acad Sci U S A 102:19144–19149

Lawrence DK, Gill EW (1975) The effects of delta1-tetrahydrocannabinol and other cannabinoids on spin-labeled liposomes and their relationship to mechanisms of general anesthesia. Mol Pharmacol 11:595–602

Ledent C, Valverde O, Cossu G et al (1999) Unresponsiveness to cannabinoids and reduced addictive effects of opiates in CB1 receptor knockout mice. Science 283:401–404. https://doi.org/10.1126/science.283.5400.401

Lee MA (2013) Smoke signals: a social history of marijuana – medical, recreational and scientific. Scribner, New York

Lefever TW, Marusich JA, Antonazzo KR, Wiley JL (2014) Evaluation of WIN 55,212-2 self-administration in rats as a potential cannabinoid abuse liability model. Pharmacol Biochem Behav 118:30–35

Leung D, Saghatelian A, Simon GM, Cravatt BF (2006) Inactivation of N-acyl phosphatidylethanolamine phospholipase D reveals multiple mechanisms for the biosynthesis of endocannabinoids. Biochemistry 45:4720–4726. https://doi.org/10.1021/bi0601631

Lichtman AH, Wiley JL, Lavecchia KL et al (1998) Effects of SR 141716A after acute or chronic cannabinoid administration in dogs. Eur J Pharmacol 357:139–148. https://doi.org/10.1016/S0014-2999(98)00558-5

Lichtman AH, Lux EA, McQuade R et al (2018) Results of a double-blind, randomized, placebo-controlled study of nabiximols oromucosal spray as an adjunctive therapy in advanced cancer patients with chronic uncontrolled pain. J Pain Symptom Manag 55:179–188. https://doi.org/10.1016/j.jpainsymman.2017.09.001

Ligresti A, De PL, Di MV (2016) From phytocannabinoids to cannabinoid receptors and endocannabinoids: pleiotropic physiological and pathological roles through complex pharmacology. Physiol Rev 96:1593–1659

Little PJ, Compton DR, Johnson MR et al (1988) Pharmacology and stereoselectivity of structurally novel cannabinoids in mice. J Pharmacol Exp Ther 247:1046–1051

Little PJ, Compton DR, Mechoulam R, Martin BR (1989) Stereochemical effects of 11-OH-Δ8-THC-dimethylheptyl in mice and dogs. Pharmacol Biochem Behav 32:661–666. https://doi.org/10.1016/0091-3057(89)90014-2

Liu J, Wang L, Harvey-White J et al (2006) A biosynthetic pathway for anandamide. Proc Natl Acad Sci U S A 103:13345–13350

Lu HC, Mackie K (2016) An introduction to the endogenous cannabinoid system. Biol Psychiatry 79:516–525

Luttrell LM (2014) More than just a hammer: ligand "Bias" and pharmaceutical discovery. Mol Endocrinol 28:281–294

Lyon RC, McComb JA, Schreurs J, Goldstein DB (1981) A relationship between alcohol intoxication and the disordering of brain membranes by a series of short-chain alcohols. J Pharmacol Exp Ther 218:669–675

Maccarrone M, Salvati S, Bari M, Finazzi A (2000) Anandamide and 2-arachidonoylglycerol inhibit fatty acid amide hydrolase by activating the lipoxygenase pathway of the arachidonate cascade. Biochem Biophys Res Commun 278:576–583

Maccarrone M, Guzman M, Mackie K et al (2014) Programming of neural cells by (endo) cannabinoids: from physiological rules to emerging therapies. Nat Rev Neurosci 15:786–801

Mackie K (2006a) Cannabinoid receptors as therapeutic targets. Annu Rev Pharmacol Toxicol 46:101–122

Mackie K (2006b) Mechanisms of CB1 receptor signaling: endocannabinoid modulation of synaptic strength. Int J Obes 30:S19–S23

Maguire DR, Yang W, France CP (2013) Interactions between mu-opioid receptor agonists and cannabinoid receptor agonists in rhesus monkeys: antinociception, drug discrimination, and drug self-administration. J Pharmacol Exp Ther 345:354–362. https://doi.org/10.1124/jpet.113.204099

Mahavadi S, Sriwai W, Huang J et al (2014) Inhibitory signaling by CB1 receptors in smooth muscle mediated by GRK5/beta-arrestin activation of ERK1/2 and Src kinase. Am J Physiol Gastrointest Liver Physiol 306:G535–G545

Martin BR (1986) Cellular effects of cannabinoids. Pharmacol Rev 38:45–74

Martin BR, Dewey WL, Harris LS et al (1975) Marihuana like activity of new synthetic tetrahydrocannabinols. Pharmacol Biochem Behav 5:849–853. https://doi.org/10.1016/S0090-3752(76)80023-3

Martin BR, Jeanne Kallman M, Kaempf GF et al (1984) Pharmacological potency of R- and S-3′-hydroxy-Δ9-tetrahydrocannabinol: additional structural requirement for cannabinoid activity. Pharmacol Biochem Behav 21:61–65. https://doi.org/10.1016/0091-3057(84)90131-X

Matsuda LA, Lolait SJ, Brownstein MJ et al (1990) Structure of a cannabinoid receptor and functional expression of the cloned cDNA. Nature 346:561–564

McAllister SD, Glass M (2002) CB(1) and CB(2) receptor-mediated signalling: a focus on endocannabinoids. Prostaglandins Leukot Essent Fatty Acids 66:161–171

McPartland JM, Glass M, Pertwee RG (2007) Meta-analysis of cannabinoid ligand binding affinity and receptor distribution: interspecies differences. Br J Pharmacol 152:583–593

Mechoulam R, Shvo Y (1963) Hashish I. The structure of cannabidiol. Tetrahedron 19:2073–2078. https://doi.org/10.1016/0040-4020(63)85022-X

Mechoulam R, McCallum N, Burstein S (1976) Recent advances in the chemistry and biochemistry of cannabis. Chem Rev 76:75–112

Mechoulam R, Ben-Shabat S, Hanus L et al (1995) Identification of an endogenous 2-monoglyceride, present in canine gut, that binds to cannabinoid receptors. Biochem Pharmacol 50:83–90

Mechoulam R, Hanus LO, Pertwee R, Howlett AC (2014) Early phytocannabinoid chemistry to endocannabinoids and beyond. Nat Rev Neurosci 15:757–764

Melck D, Bisogno T, De Petrocellis L et al (1999) Unsaturated long-chain N-acyl-vanillyl-amides (N-AVAMs): vanilloid receptor ligands that inhibit anandamide-facilitated transport and bind to CB1 cannabinoid receptors. Biochem Biophys Res Commun 262:275–284

Mendizabal V, Zimmer A, Maldonado R (2006) Involvement of kappa/dynorphin system in WIN 55, 212-2 self-administration in mice. Neuropsychopharmacology 31:1957–1966

Monti L, Steanucci A, Pieretti S et al (2016) Evaluation of the analgesic effect of 4-anilidopiperidine scaffold containing ureas and carbamates. J Enzyme Inhib Med Chem 31:1638–1647

Motaghedi R, Lipman EG, Hogg JE et al (2011) Psychiatric adverse effects of Rimonobant in adults with Prader-Willi syndrome. Eur J Med 54:14–18

Mukhopadhyay S, Howlett AC (2001) CB1 receptor-G protein association. Subtype selectivity is determined by distinct intracellular domains. Eur J Biochem 268:499–505

Mukhopadhyay S, Howlett AC (2005) Chemically distinct ligands promote differential CB1 cannabinoid receptor-Gi protein interactions. Mol Pharmacol 67:2016–2024

Mukhopadhyay S, McIntosh HH, Houston DB, Howlett AC (2000) The CB(1) cannabinoid receptor juxtamembrane C-terminal peptide confers activation to specific G proteins in brain. Mol Pharmacol 57:162–170

Munro S, Thomas KL, Abu-Shaar M (1993) Molecular characterization of a peripheral receptor for cannabinoids. Nature 365:61–65

Murataeva N, Straiker A, Mackie K (2014) Parsing the players: 2-arachidonoylglycerol synthesis and degradation in the CNS. Br J Pharmacol 171:1379–1391

Nakane S, Oka S, Arai S et al (2002) 2-Arachidonoyl-sn-glycero-3-phosphate, an arachidonic acid-containing lysophosphatidic acid: occurrence and rapid enzymatic conversion to 2-arachidonoyl-sn-glycerol, a cannabinoid receptor ligand, in rat brain. Arch Biochem Biophys 402:51–58

Navarro HA, Howard JL, Pollard GT, Carroll F (2009) Positive allosteric modulation of the human cannabinoid (CB1) receptor by RTI-371, a selective inhibitor of the dopamine transporter. Br J Pharmacol 156:1178–1184

Negus SS (2018) Addressing the opioid crisis: the importance of choosing translational endpoints in analgesic drug discovery. Trends Pharmacol Sci 39:327–330. https://doi.org/10.1016/j.tips.2018.02.002

Negus SS (2019) Core outcome measures in preclinical assessment of candidate analgesics. Pharmacol Rev 71:225–266. https://doi.org/10.1124/pr.118.017210

Nielsen S, Sabioni P, Trigo JM et al (2017) Opioid-sparing effect of cannabinoids: a systematic review and meta-analysis. Neuropsychopharmacology 42:1752–1765

Nogueras-Ortiz C, Yudowski GA (2016) The multiple waves of cannabinoid 1 receptor signaling. Mol Pharmacol 90:620–626

Nomura DK, Morrison BE, Blankman JL et al (2011) Endocannabinoid hydrolysis generates brain prostaglandins that promote neuroinflammation. Science 334:809–813

O'Sullivan SE, Kendall DA (2010) Cannabinoid activation of peroxisome proliferator-activated receptors: potential for modulation of inflammatory disease. Immunobiology 215:611–616

Okamoto Y, Morishita J, Tsuboi K et al (2004) Molecular characterization of a phospholipase D generating anandamide and its congeners. J Biol Chem 279:5298–5305

Okazaki H, Kobayashi M, Momohara A et al (2011) Early Holocene coastal environment change inferred from deposits at Okinoshima archeological site, Boso Peninsula, Central Japan. Quat Int 230:87–94

Oliveira da Cruz JF, Robin LM, Drago F et al (2016) Astroglial type-1 cannabinoid receptor (CB1): a new player in the tripartite synapse. Neuroscience 323:35–42

Owens RA, Mustafa MA, Ignatowska-Jankowska BM et al (2017) Inhibition of the endocannabinoid-regulating enzyme monoacylglycerol lipase elicits a CB1 receptor-mediated discriminative stimulus in mice. Neuropharmacology 125:80–86. https://doi.org/10.1016/j.neuropharm.2017.06.032

Pacher P, Batkai S, Kunos G (2006) The endocannabinoid system as an emerging target of pharmacotherapy. Pharmacol Rev 58:389–462

Pamplona FA, Ferreira J, Menezes de Lima O et al (2012) Anti-inflammatory lipoxin A4 is an endogenous allosteric enhancer of CB1 cannabinoid receptor. Proc Natl Acad Sci U S A 109:21134–21139

Pars HG, Granchelli FE, Razdan RK et al (1976) Drugs derived from cannabinoids. 1. nitrogen analogs, benzopyranopyridines and benzopyranopyrroles. J Med Chem 19(4):445–454. https://doi.org/10.1021/jm00226a001

Pertwee RG (2015) Endocannabinoids and their pharmacological actions. Handb Exp Pharmacol 231:1–37. https://doi.org/10.1007/978-3-319-20825-1_1

Pertwee RG, Howlett AC, Abood ME et al (2010) International Union of Basic and Clinical Pharmacology. LXXIX. Cannabinoid receptors and their ligands: beyond CB and CB. Pharmacol Rev 62:588–631

Pikuleva IA, Waterman MR (2013) Cytochromes p450: roles in diseases. J Biol Chem 288:17091–17098

Pineiro R, Falasca M (2012) Lysophosphatidylinositol signalling: new wine from an old bottle. Biochim Biophys Acta 1821:694–705

Pisanti S, Bifulco M (2019) Medical Cannabis: a plurimillennial history of an evergreen. J Cell Physiol 234:8342–8351

Porter AC, Sauer JM, Knierman MD et al (2002) Characterization of a novel endocannabinoid, virodhamine, with antagonist activity at the CB1 receptor. J Pharmacol Exp Ther 301:1020–1024

Prather PL, Martin NA, Breivogel CS, Childers SR (2000) Activation of cannabinoid receptors in rat brain by WIN 55212-2 produces coupling to multiple G protein alpha-subunits with different potencies. Mol Pharmacol 57:1000–1010

Prescott SM, Majerus PW (1983) Characterization of 1,2-diacylglycerol hydrolysis in human platelets. Demonstration of an arachidonoyl monoacylglycerol intermediate. J Biol Chem 258:764–769

Price MR, Baillie GL, Thomas A et al (2005) Allosteric modulation of the cannabinoid CB1 receptor. Mol Pharmacol 68:1484–1495

Priestly RS, Nickolls SA, Alexander SP, Kendall DA (2015) A potential role for cannabinoid receptors in the therapeutic action of fenofibrate. FASEB J 29:1446–1455

Puighermanal E, Marsicano G, Busquets-Garcia A et al (2009) Cannabinoid modulation of hippocampal long-term memory is mediated by mTOR signaling. Nat Neurosci 12:1152–1158

Rinaldi-Carmona M, Barth F, Héaulme M et al (1994) SR141716A, a potent and selective antagonist of the brain cannabinoid receptor. FEBS Lett 350:240–244. https://doi.org/10.1016/0014-5793(94)00773-X

Rinaldi-Carmona M, Calandra B, Shire D et al (1996) Characterization of two cloned human CB1 cannabinoid receptor isoforms. J Pharmacol Exp Ther 278:871–878

Rinaldi-Carmona M, Barth F, Millan J et al (1998) SR 144528, the first potent and selective antagonist of the CB2 cannabinoid receptor. J Pharmacol Exp Ther 284:644–650

Rubino T, Vigano D, Premoli F et al (2006) Changes in the expression of G protein-coupled receptor kinases and beta-arrestins in mouse brain during cannabinoid tolerance: a role for RAS-ERK cascade. Mol Neurobiol 33:199–213

Ryberg E, Vu HK, Larsson N et al (2005) Identification and characterisation of a novel splice variant of the human CB1 receptor. FEBS Lett 579:259–264

SAMHSA (2017) Results from the 2016 national survey on drug use and health: detailed tables. In: Prevalence estimates, standard errors, P values, and sample sizes. Substance Abuse and Mental Health Services Administration, Center for Behavioral Health Statistics and Quality, Rockville

Seeling W, Kneer L, Buchele B et al (2006) DELTA9-tetrahydrocannabinol and the opioid receptor agonist piritramide do not act synergistically in postoperative pain. Anaesthesist 55:391–400

Seeman P (1972) The membrane actions of anesthetics and tranquilizers. Pharmacol Rev 24(4):583–655

Setchell KD, Schwarz M, O'Connell NC et al (1998) Identification of a new inborn error in bile acid synthesis: mutation of the oxysterol 7α-hydroxylase gene causes severe neonatal liver disease. J Clin Invest 102:1690–1703

Shire D, Carillon C, Kaghad M et al (1995) An amino-terminal variant of the central cannabinoid receptor resulting from alternative splicing. J Biol Chem 270:3726–3731

Siegel GJ (1999) Synaptic transmission and cellular signaling: an overview. In: Agranoff MD, Albers BW, Fisher RW, Uhler SK (eds) Basic neurochemistry. Lippincott-R, Philadelphia

Sigel E, Baur R, Racz I et al (2011) The major central endocannabinoid directly acts at GABA (A) receptors. Proc Natl Acad Sci U S A 108:18150–18155

Simon GM, Cravatt BF (2006) Endocannabinoid biosynthesis proceeding through glycerophospho-N-acyl ethanolamine and a role for alpha/beta-hydrolase 4 in this pathway. J Biol Chem 281:26465–26472

Slivicki RA, Saberi SA, Iyer V et al (2018a) Brain-permeant and -impermeant inhibitors of fatty acid amide hydrolase synergize with the opioid analgesic morphine to suppress chemotherapy-induced neuropathic nociception without enhancing effects of morphine on gastrointestinal transit. J Pharmacol Exp Ther 367:551–563. https://doi.org/10.1124/jpet.118.252288

Slivicki RA, Xu Z, Kulkarni PM et al (2018b) Positive allosteric modulation of cannabinoid receptor type 1 suppresses pathological pain without producing tolerance or dependence. Biol Psychiatry 84:722–733

Smith FL, Cichewicz D, Martin ZL, Welch SP (1998) The enhancement of morphine antinociception in mice by Δ9-tetrahydrocannabinol. Pharmacol Biochem Behav 60:559. https://doi.org/10.1016/S0091-3057(98)00012-4

Snider NT, Walker VJ, Hollenberg PF (2010) Oxidation of the endogenous cannabinoid arachidonoyl ethanolamide by the cytochrome P450 monooxygenases: physiological and pharmacological implications. Pharmacol Rev 62:136–154

Soethoudt M, Grether U, Fingerle J et al (2017) Cannabinoid CB 2 receptor ligand profiling reveals biased signalling and off-target activity. Nat Commun 8:13958. https://doi.org/10.1038/ncomms13958

Solinas M, Panlilio LV, Justinova Z et al (2006) Using drug-discrimination techniques to study the abuse-related effects of psychoactive drugs in rats. Nat Protoc 1:1194–1206. https://doi.org/10.1038/nprot.2006.167

Stella N (2010) Cannabinoid and cannabinoid-like receptors in microglia, astrocytes, and astrocytomas. Glia 58:1017–1030

Straiker A, Wager-Miller J, Hutchens J, Mackie K (2012) Differential signalling in human cannabinoid CB1 receptors and their splice variants in autaptic hippocampal neurons. Br J Pharmacol 165:2660–2671

Sugiura T, Kondo S, Sukagawa A et al (1995) 2-Arachidonoylglycerol: a possible endogenous cannabinoid receptor ligand in brain. Biochem Biophys Res Commun 215:89–97

Sun YX, Tsuboi K, Okamoto Y et al (2004) Biosynthesis of anandamide and N-palmitoylethanolamine by sequential actions of phospholipase A2 and lysophospholipase D. Biochem J 380:749–756

Szabo B, Schlicker E (2005) Effects of cannabinoids on neurotransmission. Handb Exp Pharmacol 168:327–365

Tanda G (2016) Preclinical studies on the reinforcing effects of cannabinoids. A tribute to the scientific research of Dr. Steve Goldberg. Psychopharmacology 233:1845–1866. https://doi.org/10.1007/s00213-016-4244-7

Tarasov P, Bezrukova E, Karabanov E et al (2007) Vegetation and climate dynamics during the Holocene and Eemian interglacials derived from Lake Baikal pollen records. Palaeogeogr Palaeoclimatol Palaeoecol 252:440–457

Thomas BF, Compton DR, Martin BR (1990) Characterization of the lipophilicity of natural and synthetic analogs of delta 9-tetrahydrocannabinol and its relationship to pharmacological potency. J Pharmacol Exp Ther 255:624–630

Thomas BF, Adams IB, Mascarella SW et al (1996) Structure-activity analysis of anandamide analogs: relationship to a cannabinoid pharmacophore. J Med Chem 39:471–479. https://doi.org/10.1021/jm9505167

Tsou K, Brown S, Sanudo-Pena MC et al (1998) Immunohistochemical distribution of cannabinoid CB1 receptors in the rat central nervous system. Neuroscience 83:393–411

Turu G, Hunyady L (2010) Signal transduction of the CB1 cannabinoid receptor. J Mol Endocrinol 44:75–85

Vallee M, Vitiello S, Bellocchio L et al (2014) Pregnenolone can protect the brain from cannabis intoxication. Science 343:94–98

Wakeford AGP, Wetzell BB, Pomfrey RL et al (2017) The effects of cannabidiol (CBD) on Delta (9)-tetrahydrocannabinol (THC) self-administration in male and female Long-Evans rats. Exp Clin Psychopharmacol 25:242–248

Walton RP, Martin LF, Keller JH (1938) The relative activity of various purified products obtained from American hashish. J Pharmacol Exp Ther 62:239–251

Welch SP, Stevens DL (1992) Antinociceptive activity of intrathecally administered cannabinoids alone, and in combination with morphine, in mice. J Pharmacol Exp Ther 262:10–18

Whiting PF, Wolff RF, Deshpande S et al (2015) Cannabinoids for medical use: a systematic review and meta-analysis. J Am Med Assoc 313:2456–2473

Wiley JL, Martin BR (2003) Cannabinoid pharmacological properties common to other centrally acting drugs. Eur J Pharmacol 471:185–193. https://doi.org/10.1016/S0014-2999(03)01856-9

Wiley JL, Lowe JA, Balster RL, Martin B (1995) Antagonism of the discriminative stimulus effects of in rats and rhesus monkeys. J Pharmacol Exp Ther 275:1–6

Wiley JL, Compton DR, Dai D et al (1998) Structure-activity relationships of indole- and pyrrole-derived cannabinoids. J Pharmacol Exp Ther 285:995–1004

Wiley JL, Marusich JA, Thomas BF (2017) Combination chemistry: structure-activity relationships of novel psychoactive cannabinoids. Curr Top Behav Neurosci 32:231–248. https://doi.org/10.1007/7854_2016_17

Wiley JL, Owens RA, Lichtman AH (2018) Discriminative stimulus properties of phytocannabinoids, endocannabinoids, and synthetic cannabinoids. Curr Top Behav Neurosci 39:153–173. https://doi.org/10.1007/7854_2016_24

Wilkerson JL, Niphakis MJ, Grim TW et al (2016) The selective monoacylglycerol lipase inhibitor MJN110 produces opioid-sparing effects in a mouse neuropathic pain model. J Pharmacol Exp Ther 357:145–156

Wilkerson JL, Ghosh S, Mustafa M et al (2017) The endocannabinoid hydrolysis inhibitor SA-57: intrinsic antinociceptive effects, augmented morphine-induced antinociception, and attenuated heroin seeking behavior in mice. Neuropharmacology 114:156–167. https://doi.org/10.1016/j.neuropharm.2016.11.015

Willoughby KA, Moore SF, Martin BR, Ellis EF (1997) The biodisposition and metabolism of anandamide in mice. J Pharmacol Exp Ther 282:243–247

Wilson RI, Nicoll RA (2001) Endogenous cannabinoids mediate retrograde signaling at hippocampal synapses. Nature 410:588–592

Wilson-Poe AR, Morgan MM, Aicher SA, Hegarty DM (2012) Distribution of CB1 cannabinoid receptors and their relationship with mu-opioid receptors in the rat periaqueductal gray. Neuroscience 103:449–449. https://doi.org/10.1016/j.neuroscience.2012.03.038

Wilson-Poe AR, Pocius E, Herschbach M, Morgan MM (2013) The periaqueductal gray contributes to bidirectional enhancement of antinociception between morphine and cannabinoids. Pharmacol Biochem Behav 103:449–449. https://doi.org/10.1016/j.pbb.2012.10.002

Xiao JC, Jewell JP, Lin LS et al (2008) Similar in vitro pharmacology of human cannabinoid CB1 receptor variants expressed in CHO cells. Brain Res 1238:36–43

Yoshida T, Fukaya M, Uchigashima M et al (2006) Localization of diacylglycerol lipase-alpha around postsynaptic spine suggests close proximity between production site of an endocannabinoid, 2-arachidonoyl-glycerol, and presynaptic cannabinoid CB1 receptor. J Neurosci 26:4740–4751

Zangen A, Solinas M, Ikemoto S et al (2006) Two brain sites for cannabinoid reward. J Neurosci 26:4901–4907

Zanger UM, Schwab M (2013) Cytochrome P450 enzymes in drug metabolism: regulation of gene expression, enzyme activities, and impact of genetic variation. Pharmacol Ther 138:103–141

Zendulka O, Dovrtelova G, Noskova K et al (2016) Cannabinoids and cytochrome P450 interactions. Curr Drug Metab 17:206–226

Zimmer A, Zimmer AM, Hohmann AG et al (1999) Increased mortality, hypoactivity, and hypoalgesia in cannabinoid CB1 receptor knockout mice. Proc Natl Acad Sci U S A 96:5780–5785

Zygmunt PM, Petersson J, Andersson DA et al (1999) Vanilloid receptors on sensory nerves mediate the vasodilator action of anandamide. Nature 400:452–457

Pharmacotherapies for Cannabis Use Disorders: Clinical Challenges and Promising Therapeutic Agents

Suzanne Nielsen, Pamela Sabioni, Linda Gowing, and Bernard Le Foll

Contents

1 Background ... 356
1.1 Acute Effects of Cannabis ... 357
1.2 Long-Term Effects of Cannabis and Cannabis Use Disorders ... 357
1.3 Neurobiology of Cannabis Use ... 359
2 Pharmacotherapies Tested for CUD ... 360
2.1 Medications of Limited or No Value ... 360
2.2 Medications of Uncertain Value ... 363
2.3 Medications Warranting Further Research ... 364
3 CUD in Special Populations ... 366
3.1 Pharmacotherapy for CUD in People with Concurrent Mental Health Conditions ... 366
3.2 Pregnancy ... 367
4 Future Directions ... 367
4.1 CUD in the Context of Therapeutic Use ... 367

S. Nielsen
Monash Addiction Research Centre, Monash University, Peninsula Campus, Frankston, VIC, Australia

P. Sabioni
Translational Addiction Research Laboratory, Campbell Family Mental Health Research Institute, Centre for Addiction and Mental Health, Toronto, ON, Canada

L. Gowing
Discipline of Pharmacology, University of Adelaide, Adelaide, SA, Australia

B. Le Foll (✉)
Translational Addiction Research Laboratory, Campbell Family Mental Health Research Institute, Centre for Addiction and Mental Health, Toronto, ON, Canada

Acute Care Program, Centre for Addiction and Mental Health, Toronto, ON, Canada

Departments of Family and Community Medicine, Pharmacology and Toxicology, Psychiatry, Institute of Medical Science, University of Toronto, Toronto, ON, Canada

Campbell Family Mental Health Research Institute, Centre for Addiction and Mental Health, Toronto, ON, Canada
e-mail: bernard.lefoll@camh.ca

M. A. Nader, Y. L. Hurd (eds.), *Substance Use Disorders*,
Handbook of Experimental Pharmacology 258, https://doi.org/10.1007/164_2019_258

4.2 Future Research 368
References 368

Abstract
This chapter reviews pharmacotherapies that have been trialled for cannabis dependence, identifying those that warrant further research and those of little or uncertain value. A diverse range of medicines have been tested, representing a broad range of pharmacological strategies. These include tetrahydrocannabinol preparations, various types of antidepressant, anxiolytics, a glutamatergic modulator and the neuropeptide oxytocin. Cannabinoid agonists warrant further research. For the FAAH inhibitor PF-04457845, oxytocin, varenicline and gabapentin, although there is a signal to indicate further research is warranted, these medications do not yet have sufficient evidence to support clinical use, and larger, longer-term trials are needed in representative treatment-seeking populations. Special populations that warrant consideration are those with cannabis dependence and concurrent mental health conditions and those that develop dependence through therapeutic use.

Keywords
Cannabis · Cannabis dependence · Cannabis use disorder · Pharmacotherapy · Treatment

1 Background

Cannabis refers to a genus of plant originally from Asia, now grown around the world, of which the most common species is *Cannabis sativa*. Cannabis contains hundreds of chemical substances, though its two main constituents are the phytocannabinoids, delta 9-tetrahydrocannabinol (THC) and cannabidiol (CBD). CBD has been researched due to its potential therapeutic use (as a neuroprotective, antipsychotic, anxiolytic, anti-seizure and anti-inflammatory) (Rong et al. 2017; Fasinu et al. 2016); THC is more well known for its psychoactive effects, though it has also been proposed to have a wide range of potential therapeutic uses.

Cannabis is currently the most widely used drug (excluding alcohol and tobacco) around the world. According to the 2018 United Nations Office of Drug Control (UNODC) report, it is estimated that around 4% of the global population aged 15–64 years consumed the drug at least once in 2016, which represents approximately 192 million people (United Nations Publilcation SNEX 2018). Past-month cannabis use in the United States, as assessed in the National Survey on Drug Use and Health (NSDUH), among those aged 18–25 years increased from 17% in 2002 to 20% in 2014, with the rise happening mostly after 2007. Although the increase occurred across gender, region, educational level and employment status, higher rates were found among males and unemployed participants (Azofeifa et al. 2016). The National Epidemiologic Survey on Alcohol and Related Conditions-III

(NESARC-III) conducted in 2012–2013 demonstrated past-year prevalence in adult cannabis use at approximately 10%, a significant increase from 4% in 2001–2002 NESARC (Hasin et al. 2015).

1.1 Acute Effects of Cannabis

The typical preferred route of administration is inhalation of cannabis smoke (from cigarettes, cigars, pipes, and water pipes) due to the rapid onset of its effects; such effects are commonly described as relaxing and pleasant sensations that last for about 2–3 h. With oral ingestion (e.g. with edible products), the onset of action is slower, peaking after 2–3 h and lasting longer (4–12 h) (Grotenhermen 2003). The intensity of the effects varies according to the dose of THC, consumption habits (e.g. occasional vs. regular use) and predisposition to mental illness and personality traits (Karila et al. 2014). Cannabis effects are characterised by a combination of euphoria, laugher, sedation, alteration of time perception, increased sensitivity to external stimuli and memory gaps (Panlilio et al. 2015). Increased appetite and dry mouth are also commonly experienced by people who use cannabis. Some of the adverse events experienced include panic attacks, dysphoria, psychotic episodes, anxiety and paranoia (Karila et al. 2014). Cannabis use also adversely impacts short-term memory, attention, coordination and reaction time (Karila et al. 2014; Hall 2015).

High doses of THC might result in more frequent and more serious adverse events from acute intoxication, leading to emergency room visits and hospitalisations. Those are more commonly experienced with the use of synthetic cannabinoids, which are more potent than THC, with most severe and unpredictable negative effects impacting especially younger, naïve users. Acute intoxication with synthetic cannabinoids can include symptoms like extreme agitation, dysphoria, delusions, hallucinations, seizures and suicidal ideation (Spaderna et al. 2013; van Amsterdam et al. 2015).

1.2 Long-Term Effects of Cannabis and Cannabis Use Disorders

Long-term use of cannabis is associated with negative neurological, psychological and general health outcomes (Volkow et al. 2014a). When started in adolescence, the regular use of cannabis is associated with altered brain development, poor educational outcomes and cognitive impairment with lower IQ. The lasting effects of regular use of cannabis during adolescence include decreased performance in brain regions associated with learning, memory and executive functioning, which might be responsible for the lowered IQ (Volkow et al. 2014a; Cadet et al. 2014). Although multiple epidemiological studies support this negative impact on brain function (Meier et al. 2012), it should be noted that recent twin cohort studies suggest that those changes may be related to pre-existing vulnerability and not necessarily to cannabis exposure per se (Jackson et al. 2016).

The chronic or heavy use of cannabis is associated with an increased risk of developing cannabis use disorders (CUD), described in the 5th edition of the *Diagnostic and Statistical Manual of Mental Disorders* (DSM-5) of the American Psychiatric Association. The diagnostic criteria for CUD is similar to those of other substance disorders (i.e. the continued use of the substance despite clinically significant impairment and impact of substance use on daily activities). The main features of the DSM-5 criteria for CUD include:

1. Continuing to use cannabis in larger amounts or for longer than initially intended
2. Being unable to reduce or control the amount of cannabis used, despite repeated attempts to do so
3. Spending a lot of time acquiring cannabis or recovering from its use
4. Strong urges or cravings to use cannabis
5. Repeatedly failing to fulfil obligations at work, in education or in the home
6. Continuing to use cannabis despite repeatedly experiencing negative effects on relationships
7. Giving up a range of important activities (e.g. social, work or recreational activities) as a result of cannabis use
8. Using cannabis in ways that place a person at risk of harm
9. Continuing to use cannabis despite knowing that it is making physical or mental health problems worse
10. Needing to use more cannabis to get the same effect or experiencing less effects from the same amount
11. Experiencing withdrawal symptoms after ceasing use

Experiencing at least two of the above symptoms in a 12-month period is required to meet the criteria for CUD, with meeting 4–5 symptoms representing a moderate use disorder and meeting 6 or more symptoms fulfilling the criteria for a severe use disorder.

Cannabis withdrawal was not included in the DSM-IV due to the lack of data identifying symptoms; however, research has identified withdrawal symptoms that result in significant clinical impairment, such that the revised DSM-5 recognises these symptoms (Hasin et al. 2008). Cannabis withdrawal symptoms are reported by about 30% of people who use cannabis regularly in the general population (Hasin et al. 2008) and by up to 95% of people who report heavy cannabis use (Copersino et al. 2006).

Typical symptoms of cannabis withdrawal include irritability, anger or aggression, nervousness or anxiety, sleep difficulty (e.g. insomnia, disturbing dreams), decreased appetite or weight loss, restlessness, depressed mood, abdominal pain, shakiness/tremors, sweating, fever, chills or headache.

The trajectory and likelihood of developing CUD in the general population are not fully understood. Research suggests that the lifetime risk of developing CUD among regular cannabis users is approximately 9%, increasing to about 17% if the use is started during adolescence, and up to 50% of those who are people who use cannabis daily (Volkow et al. 2014a). The 2012–2013 NESARC-III estimated the prevalence of lifetime CUD around 6.5% among people aged 18 years or older (Grant et al. 2014, 2015).

1.3 Neurobiology of Cannabis Use

All psychoactive drugs stimulate brain reward systems. Dopamine (DA) is the main neurotransmitter associated with the drug's rewarding or 'high' effects, produced by a fast and abrupt release of DA into the ventral striatum (Koob and Volkow 2016).

The two main cannabinoid receptors are cannabinoid receptor type-1 (CB1) and cannabinoid receptor type-2 (CB2), both largely expressed in brain structures such as the neocortex, basal ganglia and hippocampus (Micale et al. 2013). THC is a CB1 and CB2 partial agonist (Felder et al. 1992), though its psychoactive effects are mediated through CB1 receptors. Dopaminergic neurons are also modulated by the endocannabinoid ligands, anandamide and 2-arachidonoyglycerol (2-AG) (Solinas et al. 2008). Both ligands are rich in dopaminergic pathways and elicit DA release in the nucleus accumbens (NAc) (Solinas et al. 2006; de Luca et al. 2014). This effect is blocked by the CB1 antagonist rimonabant, suggesting that the dopaminergic modulation of endocannabinoids involve CB1 receptors similarly to THC (Bloomfield et al. 2016).

The effects of THC on the dopaminergic system differ according to the length of exposure. Evidence from clinical and preclinical research demonstrates acute changes in the dopaminergic system in response to THC administration. Acute THC administration stimulates striatal DA release in rodents (Ng Cheong Ton et al. 1988) and humans (Bloomfield et al. 2016; Bossong et al. 2015), indicating that THC elicits DA release similarly to other drugs of abuse.

Human imaging studies offer insights on dopaminergic changes associated with cannabis use through the evaluation of brain activity in areas with dopaminergic projections. A positron emission tomography (PET) study found that acute THC is associated with increased metabolic activities of the orbitofrontal cortex, prefrontal cortex and basal ganglia in people who use cannabis (Volkow et al. 1996).

Molecular imaging studies have assessed the effects of acute THC administration on DA changes and have shown that THC in fact elicits DA release in the ventral striatum in the human brain (Bossong et al. 2015). The magnitude of this effect appears limited, but we are still in the early days of exploration of this response in humans, as few studies have been conducted (Thiruchselvam et al. 2017).

Contrarily, there is more evidence for reduced dopaminergic function in regular, chronic cannabis users. PET studies have demonstrated reduced capacity of DA synthesis in chronic cannabis users, which may explain reduced response to rewarding effects of cannabis and reduced motivation (Bloomfield et al. 2014a, b). The striatal DA release in people who use cannabis regularly was reduced in response to stimulant challenges and inversely correlated with addiction severity and craving (Volkow et al. 2014b; van de Giessen et al. 2017). There is also indication of decreased DA transporter density in people who use cannabis chronically (Leroy et al. 2012).

Chronic THC use has been shown to downregulate CB1 receptors though this downregulation of CB1 receptors has been shown to quickly reverse following withdrawal in cannabis-dependent subjects (D'Souza et al. 2016). Downregulation of fatty acid amide hydrolase (FAAH) has also been reported in heavy cannabis users (Boileau et al. 2016) indicating important changes in the cannabinoid system associated with CUD (see Sloan et al. 2019 for a recent review on studies evaluating endocannabinoid signaling in psychiatric disorders).

2 Pharmacotherapies Tested for CUD

To date, there are no approved medications for the treatment of CUD. A range of different pharmacological approaches have been tested with the aim of assisting people with CUD to reduce their cannabis use through reducing withdrawal symptoms, craving and addressing other cognitive factors. The results of these studies vary, and are summarised in Table 1, and described in more detail below. We previously carried out a systematic (Cochrane) review on this topic (Nielsen et al. 2019), and here we extend these findings and consider specific needs of different populations and future directions for the field.

2.1 Medications of Limited or No Value

Many tested medicines have shown no evidence of efficacy, evidence of poor tolerability and/or poorer clinical outcomes compared to placebo. These medicines appear to offer little or no value for further research or clinical treatment in CUD. They are described below.

2.1.1 Antidepressants

Numerous clinical trials have been conducted with antidepressants for CUD with limited evidence of any value in reducing cannabis use or withdrawal symptoms. Antidepressants trialled include selective serotonin reuptake inhibitors (SSRI)

Table 1 Summary of medications that have been tested for CUD

Further research	Uncertain	Little value
Nabiximols, dronabinol, nabilone	Dronabinol + lofexidine	Fluoxetine, vilazodone, escitalopram, nefazodone, mirtazapine, venlafaxine
Gabapentin	Topiramate	Lithium, divalproex sodium, baclofen
Oxytocin	Buproprion	Buspirone
FAAH inhibitor (PF-04457845)	*N*-acetylcysteine, varenicline, injectable naltrexone	Atomoxetine, quetiapine

(fluoxetine, vilazodone and escitalopram) and mixed action antidepressants (bupropion, nefazodone, mirtazapine and venlafaxine). Below is a summary of the studies and outcomes.

Fluoxetine Fluoxetine is the first agent of the SSRI class of antidepressants. SSRIs are potent inhibitors of serotonin (5-HT) transporter protein, enhancing the actions of serotonin on $5HT_{1A}$ receptors. Fluoxetine has been approved for the treatment of major depression disorder, panic disorder, obsessive compulsive disorder (OCD), bulimia nervosa, post-traumatic stress and premenstrual dysphoric disorder.

Fluoxetine was tested in two randomised trials ($n = 104$ across the two studies) in adolescents ($n = 34$) and young adults ($n = 70$) with major depression and CUD (Cornelius et al. 2010; Findling et al. 2009). In these studies, fluoxetine was well tolerated but was not more effective than placebo for depressive or cannabis-related symptoms.

Vilazodone A randomised trial ($n = 76$) that compared vilazodone (an SSRI and partial 5-HT_{1A} agonist) to placebo found no benefit in vilazodone on cannabis use outcomes (McRae-Clark et al. 2016). This study also identified important gender differences where women had worse cannabis use outcomes with vilazodone compared to placebo (McRae-Clark et al. 2016).

Escitalopram A randomised trial ($n = 52$) of the SSRI escitalopram combined with cognitive behavioural therapy found a high (50%) rate of dropout and low rate of abstinence with escitalopram compared to placebo suggested limited value in this medication, though the very high dropout rate complicates interpretation of these study findings (Weinstein et al. 2014).

Buproprion and Nefazodone Buproprion, an atypical antidepressant, selectively inhibits the neuronal reuptake of DA, norepinephrine (NE) and 5-HT. Bupropion was examined in one lab study and two randomised trials. In an early laboratory study ($n = 10$), some cannabis withdrawal symptoms were increased with bupropion administration (ratings of irritability, restlessness, depression and trouble sleeping) compared to placebo (Haney et al. 2001). A similar laboratory study ($n = 7$) found nefazodone (5-HT_2 and α1-adrenergic receptors antagonist) decreased some symptoms (such as anxiety) but did not improve overall mood, and participants still reported discomfort during withdrawal (Haney et al. 2003).

These atypical antidepressants (bupropion and nefazodone) were later tested in treatment-seeking individuals. A small ($n = 22$) two-arm pilot study found that withdrawal symptoms and craving were improved in the bupropion group, compared to placebo (Penetar et al. 2012). A three-arm trial ($n = 106$) comparing bupropion, nefazodone and placebo found no effect of either drug (compared to placebo) on cannabis use or cannabis withdrawal symptoms (Carpenter et al. 2009). Taken together, there is limited evidence to suggest that bupropion or nefazodone merit further study.

Mirtazapine Mirtazapine is an antagonist of α2-adrenergic receptors, inhibiting negative feedback to the presynaptic nerve and causing an increase of 5-HT and NE release. Mirtazapine is a potent antagonist to 5-HT_2, 5-HT_3 and histamine 1 (H1) receptors, with a weak antagonism action on 5-HT_1 receptors. Mirtazapine was tested in a randomised study of 81 adults which found that mirtazapine offered no benefit over placebo on cannabis use or withdrawal outcomes, though sleep efficiency and quality improved (but not daily sleep disturbances) (Frewen 2009). These results were consistent with a laboratory study ($n = 11$) which tested a model of cannabis withdrawal and relapse (Haney et al. 2010). This study found that compared to placebo, mirtazapine resulted in improved sleep during abstinence and increased food intake but had no effect on cannabis withdrawal symptoms (Haney et al. 2010).

Venlafaxine Venlafaxine is a 5-HT-NE reuptake inhibitor (SNRI) antidepressant. Venlafaxine may assist with mood but shows little promise for treating CUD. In a study of 103 adults with CUD and depression, those randomised to receive venlafaxine had improvements in mood yet significantly lower rates of abstinence (11.8%) compared to placebo (36.5%) (Levin et al. 2013). A secondary analysis of this same study ($n = 103$) compared withdrawal symptoms between patients receiving venlafaxine and placebo and found that those in the venlafaxine group had more severe withdrawal symptoms (Kelly et al. 2014). The authors concluded that noradrenergic agents, such as venlafaxine, may negatively affect outcomes of patients attempting to cease cannabis use.

2.1.2 Anticonvulsants and Mood Stabilisers

Lithium and Divalproex Sodium Two randomised trials examined medications classed as anticonvulsants and mood stabilisers, lithium and divalproex sodium. An inpatient study of 38 cannabis-dependent adults compared lithium carbonate to placebo (Johnston et al. 2014). No differences in cannabis use outcomes were found between the two groups, though some improvements in sleep outcomes were noted in the lithium group (Johnston et al. 2014; Allsop et al. 2015). The precise mechanism of action of lithium is unknown. It is possible that its effects are due to its interaction with the transport of monovalent or divalent cations in neurons. Similarly, the mechanism of divalproex sodium's therapeutic actions is not well understood; it may act by increasing gamma-aminobutyric acid (GABA) levels in the brain or by altering the properties of voltage-dependent sodium channels.

An outpatient study of 52 cannabis-dependent adults randomised to divalproex sodium or placebo also found that there was no group difference on either the frequency or amount of cannabis used (Levin et al. 2004). The study also found that irritability decreased in divalproex and placebo groups, with no group difference (Levin et al. 2004).

2.1.3 Other Medications

Baclofen Baclofen, a GABA-B receptor agonist, was tested in a laboratory study and showed little effect on mood during abstinence from cannabis and worsened cognitive performance in both abstinence and active use phases of the study (Haney et al. 2010). An open-label study reported common side effects of sedation and lethargy (Nanjayya et al. 2010).

Buspirone Two trials examined the anxiolytic, buspirone. Buspirone is a 5-HT_{1A} partial agonist and DA D2 receptor antagonist. There were promising results in an initial smaller trial ($n = 50$) (McRae-Clark et al. 2009), but in a larger study ($n = 175$), buspirone was no more effective than placebo at reducing cannabis use or cannabis withdrawal symptoms (McRae-Clark et al. 2015). Women had worse cannabis use outcomes compared with men with buspirone (McRae-Clark et al. 2015).

Atomoxetine Atomoxetine, a NE reuptake inhibitor that is approved for treating attention deficit hyperactivity disorder (ADHD), was tested in a smaller trial of 38 cannabis-dependent adults with ADHD (McRae-Clark et al. 2010). No effects were seen on cannabis use or craving measures, with the authors concluding that atomoxetine may improve ADHD symptoms but does not reduce cannabis use.

Quetiapine Quetiapine is an atypical or second-generation antipsychotic that is often used off-label for its sedative effects. Quetiapine is a selective antagonist with high affinity for 5-HT_2 and DA D2 receptors. It also acts as antagonist on 5-HT_{1A}, 5-HT2, DA D1, histamine H1 and adrenergic $\alpha 1$ and $\alpha 2$ receptors. Quetiapine was tested in a laboratory study ($n = 14$) with people who regularly used cannabis but were not seeking treatment (Cooper et al. 2013). In this study, quetiapine improved sleep quality, increased caloric intake and decreased weight loss but increased cannabis craving and self-administration during relapse phase, indicating that quetiapine would be an unlikely candidate as a treatment for CUD.

2.2 Medications of Uncertain Value

Naltrexone There is some evidence of cross-modulating effects of the opioid and cannabinoid systems (Notzon et al. 2018). An open-label pilot study tested injectable naltrexone (an opioid antagonist that is used as 'relapse prevention' medication in alcohol use disorder). This small ($n = 12$) study of cannabis-dependent people found that injectable naltrexone decreased the frequency but not the quantity of cannabis use (Notzon et al. 2018). Adjunct medication was required for cannabis withdrawal symptoms up to 2 weeks after an injection, potentially complicating the use of this medication. Further studies are required to determine if naltrexone may play any role in the treatment of CUD.

Topiramate Topiramate, an anticonvulsant that enhances GABA-activated chloride channels, was tested in a randomised trial with 66 adolescents who were regularly using cannabis (Gray et al. 2018; Miranda et al. 2017). Compared with placebo, topiramate was associated with reduced amount of cannabis smoked, without increasing abstinence. Side effects were common, notably poorer cognitive function, which was the major reason for dropout (Gray et al. 2018). A secondary analysis of the study data established that greater cannabis use was associated with lower likelihood of dropping out (Gray et al. 2018), and among those that remained in the study, none reported cognitive side effects. Further research may establish if this is a valuable medication for specific subpopulations.

***N*-Acetylcysteine** Two trials have examined *n*-acetylcysteine (NAC). The mechanism of action of NAC is complex, but it seems that it produces neuropsychoactive effects through the modulation of NMDA receptors and increasing glutamate release. An early trial with NAC showed promising results in adolescents ($n = 116$) (Gray et al. 2012). However, these findings were not replicated in a later larger study of adults ($n = 302$) (Gray et al. 2017). The authors concluded that an attempt should be made to replicate the earlier promising findings in adolescents.

Lofexidine + Dronabinol A number of trials have tested different cannabinoid agonists (see following section). A single study examined adding lofexidine (a potent α2-adrenergic receptor agonist with moderate agonist effects towards α1-adrenergic, 5-HT_{1A}, 5-HT_7, 5-HT_{2C} and 5-HT_{1D} receptors) in combination with dronabinol (synthetic form of THC) (Levin et al. 2016). The study found no difference in rates of abstinence from cannabis between dronabinol-lofexidine and placebo groups, concluding that the addition of lofexidine does not add benefit to that provided with cannabinoid agonists alone.

2.3 Medications Warranting Further Research

Five pharmacological approaches hold promise for further study. Those medications considered to hold promise have either been tested in multiple studies and shown promising results (in the case of cannabinoid agonists) or are considered promising because only single studies have been conducted which suggest further studies are warranted (FAAH inhibitor PF-04457845, oxytocin, varenicline and gabapentin).

2.3.1 Cannabinoid Agonists

The clinical approach that has been most studied is that of using cannabinoid agonists as either a withdrawal treatment or a maintenance treatment (with a similar pharmacological approach to nicotine replacement therapy or methadone or buprenorphine in opioid agonist treatment). Three cannabinoid preparations have been tested: two pharmaceutical cannabinoids (nabilone and dronabinol) and a cannabinoid extract (containing a 1:1 ratio of THC and cannabidiol), known as nabiximols.

In a laboratory study ($n = 11$), nabilone was able to attenuate cannabis withdrawal symptoms with once per day dosing, and prevented a 'relapse' in the laboratory model, while showing low abuse liability (Haney et al. 2013). Another laboratory study ($n = 11$) suggested the combination of nabilone and zolpidem may improve cannabis use outcomes (Herrmann et al. 2016). These studies suggest nabilone may hold promise for testing in clinical settings as a cannabinoid agonist pharmacotherapy, though to date studies have been limited to laboratory settings.

In a larger randomised controlled trial ($n = 156$), dronabinol improved treatment retention and withdrawal symptoms but did not improve abstinence relative to placebo (Levin et al. 2011).

Two published trials have examined nabiximols. An inpatient withdrawal study ($n = 51$) found that nabiximols reduced cannabis withdrawal symptoms and craving, but not cannabis use, at follow-up, compared to placebo (Allsop et al. 2014). A later outpatient study ($n = 40$) examined 12 weeks of nabiximols in combination with motivational enhancement treatment and found no difference in abstinence from cannabis between nabiximols and placebo, though rates of cannabis use in the nabiximols group appeared lower at the end of treatment (Trigo et al. 2018), notably in the groups using a high quantity of nabiximols.

This body of evidence suggests that the approach of 'cannabis agonist treatment' is promising, though larger, longer-term treatment studies are required before this can be recommended.

2.3.2 Other Pharmacological Approaches to Explore

The *FAAH inhibitor*, PF-04457845, was tested in cannabis-dependent males ($n = 70$) (D'Souza et al. 2018). Participants were randomised with a 2:1 ratio (active to placebo). The study design involved 5 days of initial inpatient treatment and the remainder of the 4 weeks with medication supplied in an outpatient setting. The short-term (4-week) study found that those randomised to PF-04457845 reported fewer cannabis withdrawal symptoms and reported less cannabis use at 4 weeks.

A pilot randomised trial of *oxytocin* ($n = 16$) examined the hypothesis that oxytocin would enhance efficacy of motivational enhancement therapy (Sherman et al. 2017). The study was not powered to provide conclusive results; however, participants receiving oxytocin showed reductions in amount of cannabis used daily and number of sessions of cannabis use per day that were not seen in the placebo group. Further research may determine if this is a potential pharmacological strategy to improve the effectiveness of psychological treatments.

Varenicline, a nicotine partial agonist, was tested in people who were using cannabis and tobacco and were in opioid treatment. This small-scale ($n = 7$) cross-over study suggests varenicline is well tolerated and may reduce cannabis craving (Adams et al. 2018), though larger studies on more representative populations are required.

Gabapentin is a GABA analog anticonvulsant. It increases GABA's synaptic concentration and GABA effects in neuronal tissues and reduces the release of monoaminergic neurotransmitters. A proof of concept study examining the effect of gabapentin on cannabis use, withdrawal symptoms and executive functioning in people who were cannabis-dependent ($n = 50$) found that, compared to placebo, both cannabis use and withdrawal symptoms were reduced in the gabapentin group (Mason et al. 2012). Improvements in executive functioning were seen in the gabapentin group, suggesting that gabapentin may help with the neural dysregulation associated with long-term cannabis use.

For the FAAH inhibitor PF-04457845, oxytocin, varenicline and gabapentin, although there is a signal to indicate further research is warranted, these medications do not yet have sufficient evidence to support clinical use, and larger, longer-term trials are needed in representative treatment-seeking populations.

3 CUD in Special Populations

3.1 Pharmacotherapy for CUD in People with Concurrent Mental Health Conditions

The association between cannabis use and psychosis and the prevalence of cannabis use worldwide have led to identification of concurrent cannabis use and mental health disorders as an area of concern (Alharbi and El-Guebaly 2016). Lifetime substance use among people with schizophrenia has been reported to be as high as 50% (Akerele and Levin 2007). As with the general population, the most prevalent substances used are alcohol, tobacco and cannabis.

Use of cannabis and other psychoactive substances by people with serious mental health disorders has been associated with exacerbation of mental health, poor treatment compliance, disruption of role functioning and increased rates of relapse and rehospitalisation (Akerele and Levin 2007; Brunette et al. 2011). The rationale for treating cannabis use in people with schizophrenia spectrum disorders is that it may allow for more appropriate treatment and better prognosis of the psychotic illness (Hjorthoj et al. 2009).

Antipsychotics are DA blockers and hence should act to reduce positive reinforcement of drug use (Akerele and Levin 2007). Typical antipsychotic medications do not appear to limit cannabis or other substance use in people with schizophrenia, but the different antipsychotics vary in their affinity for the DA D2 receptor (Machielsen et al. 2014). Preliminary results with small numbers suggest that the atypical antipsychotic, clozapine, might reduce cannabis use. Use of clozapine is restricted due to side effects, but an area of research is the investigation of other atypical antipsychotics that might reduce cannabis use with less side effects (Brunette et al. 2011).

In a systematic (Cochrane) review, Temmingh et al. (2018) compared risperidone with other antipsychotics in people with serious mental illness and co-occurring substance misuse. The only outcome related to cannabis that was reported was craving, and the evidence was assessed as being very low quality. Other outcomes reported in the systematic review were specific to serious mental illness. Temmingh et al. found that clozapine was associated with lower levels of craving for cannabis compared to risperidone (1 RCT, $n = 28$, MD 7.00, 95% CI 2.37 to 11.63) while there was no clear difference in craving for risperidone compared to olanzapine (1 RCT, $n = 41$, MD 5.00 95% CI −4.86 to 14.86). The authors concluded that there is not sufficient good quality evidence available to determine the effects of risperidone compared to other antipsychotics in people with a dual diagnosis.

A second Cochrane review focused on cannabis and schizophrenia (McLoughlin et al. 2014), considering specific psychological therapies for cannabis use, the effects of cannabidiol on the symptoms of schizophrenia and the effects of different antipsychotics on cannabis use. Temmingh et al. (2018) found that no one treatment showed superiority for reduction in cannabis use.

3.2 Pregnancy

Possible harmful effects of using cannabis during pregnancy include premature birth, longer labours, respiratory problems for mothers and mood and other psychological problems for the mother. Some of these effects are likely to be due to smoking as the means of cannabis use, and some may be due to the specific effects of psychoactive components of cannabis. Currently there is insufficient evidence to determine whether low-risk use of cannabis during pregnancy is possible, so it is generally recommended that women who are pregnant or intending to become pregnant should cease cannabis use. WHO guidelines (WHO 2014) recommend the use of psychological therapies to support cessation of cannabis use in pregnancy due to a lack of evidence on the efficacy of pharmacological therapies.

4 Future Directions

The availability of cannabis and cannabinoid therapeutics is changing in many countries. Increasing legal access for therapeutic and recreational use will result in a change in the way cannabis is used and a change in populations who may use it. This may bring new challenges and result in new populations seeking treatment for use disorders.

4.1 CUD in the Context of Therapeutic Use

CUD is one of the most prevalent substance use disorders in the general population (Goldstein et al. 2015; Mewton et al. 2013), though these have typically been associated with nonmedical use. Given that CUD is commonly associated with regular use, it would be expected that a small but important number of people using cannabinoids for therapeutic purposes might also develop use disorders. Most clinical trials of cannabinoids have not followed patients up for long enough or specifically assessed prevalence of developing use disorders to enable an estimate of how common this might be. Nevertheless, it is likely that there will be patients who receive clinical benefits from cannabis-based medicines but also display features of use disorders including loss of control of the amount used and adverse effects of the use of cannabinoids on their life. This is a similar paradigm to the development of opioid dependence among patients prescribed opioids for pain. There are recommended frameworks for monitoring these outcomes with opioids using a 'universal precautions' framework to assess risk (Gourlay et al. 2005), implementing appropriate risk-mitigation strategies and monitoring clinical outcomes to ensure that benefits for patients outweigh any adverse effects that the patient may be experiencing. Adapting and validating these frameworks for therapeutic use with cannabinoids would be a worthy endeavour as therapeutic use of cannabinoids expands.

4.2 Future Research

Future work may also look to better understand the roles of CB1 antagonists and FAAH inhibitors as potential molecules for treating CUD and may elucidate if there are optimal THC/CBD ratios for the management of CUD and also for a range of other proposed therapeutic uses. Continuing to conduct detailed population-level and cohort studies will also provide new information on how exposure to cannabis and regulation of cannabis may be related to developing use disorders, including identifying protective factors and vulnerabilities.

In conclusion, we are currently in a dynamic time of rapidly changing cannabis use and changing roles of cannabinoids as therapeutics. Although many potential therapeutic approaches have not yielded strong results, it is likely that the evidence base and use will rapidly develop in the coming years. This increased use means that interest in pharmacotherapies for CUD is likely to remain, therefore developing our understanding of effective treatments will continue to be a priority.

Conflict of Interest Dr. Le Foll has/will received some in-kind donation of cannabis product from Canopy and Aurora and medication donation from Pfizer and Bioprojet and was provided a coil for TMS study from Brainsway. Dr. Le Foll has/will perform research with industry funding obtained from Canopy, Bioprojet, ACS and Alkermes. Dr. Le Foll has received in-kind donations of nabiximols from GW Pharma for past studies funded by CIHR and NIH.

References

Adams TA, Arnsten JH, Ning Y, Nahvi S (2018) Feasibility and preliminary effectiveness of varenicline for treating co-occurring cannabis and tobacco use. J Psychoactive Drugs 50 (1):12–18

Akerele E, Levin FR (2007) Comparison of olanzapine to risperidone in substance-abusing individuals with schizophrenia. Am J Addict 16:260–268

Alharbi FF, El-Guebaly N (2016) Cannabis and amphetamine-type stimulant-induced psychoses: a systematic overview. Addict Disord Treat 15(4):190–200

Allsop DJ, Copeland J, Lintzeris N, Dunlop AJ, Montebello M, Sadler C et al (2014) Nabiximols as an agonist replacement therapy during cannabis withdrawal: a randomized clinical trial. JAMA Psychiat 71(3):281–291

Allsop DJ, Bartlett DJ, Johnston J, Helliwell D, Winstock A, McGregor IS et al (2015) The effects of lithium carbonate supplemented with nitrazepam on sleep disturbance during cannabis abstinence. J Clin Sleep Med 11(10):1153–1162

Azofeifa A, Mattson ME, Schauer G, McAfee T, Grant A, Lyerla R (2016) National estimates of marijuana use and related indicators - national survey on drug use and health, United States, 2002–2014. MMWR Surveill Summ 65(11):1–28

Bloomfield MA, Morgan CJ, Egerton A, Kapur S, Curran HV, Howes OD (2014a) Dopaminergic function in cannabis users and its relationship to cannabis-induced psychotic symptoms. Biol Psychiatry 75(6):470–478

Bloomfield MA, Morgan CJ, Kapur S, Curran HV, Howes OD (2014b) The link between dopamine function and apathy in cannabis users: an [18F]-DOPA PET imaging study. Psychopharmacology 231(11):2251–2259

Bloomfield MA, Ashok AH, Volkow ND, Howes OD (2016) The effects of delta(9)-tetrahydrocannabinol on the dopamine system. Nature 539(7629):369–377

Boileau I, Mansouri E, Williams B, Le Foll B, Rusjan P, Mizrahi R et al (2016) Fatty acid amide hydrolase binding in brain of cannabis users: imaging with the novel radiotracer [(11)C]CURB. Biol Psychiatry 80(9):691–701

Bossong MG, Mehta MA, van Berckel BN, Howes OD, Kahn RS, Stokes PR (2015) Further human evidence for striatal dopamine release induced by administration of 9-tetrahydrocannabinol (THC): selectivity to limbic striatum. Psychopharmacology 232(15):2723–2729

Brunette MF, Dawson R, O'Keefe CD, Narasimhan M, Noordsy DL, Wojcik J et al (2011) A randomized trial of clozapine vs. other antipsychotics for cannabis use disorder in patients with schizophrenia. J Dual Diagn 7(1–2):50–63

Cadet JL, Bisagno V, Milroy CM (2014) Neuropathology of substance use disorders. Acta Neuropathol 127(1):91–107

Carpenter KM, McDowell D, Brooks DJ, Cheng WY, Levin FR (2009) A preliminary trial: double-blind comparison of nefazodone, bupropion-sr, and placebo in the treatment of cannabis dependence. Am J Addict 18(1):53–64

Cooper ZD, Foltin RW, Hart CL, Vosburg SK, Comer SD, Haney M (2013) A human laboratory study investigating the effects of quetiapine on marijuana withdrawal and relapse in daily marijuana smokers. Addict Biol 18(6):993–1002

Copersino ML, Boyd SJ, Tashkin DP, Huestis MA, Heishman SJ, Dermand JC et al (2006) Cannabis withdrawal among non-treatment-seeking adult cannabis users. Am J Addict 15 (1):8–14

Cornelius JR, Bukstein OG, Douaihy AB, Clark DB, Chung TA, Daley DC et al (2010) Double-blind fluoxetine trial in comorbid MDD-CUD youth and young adults. Drug Alcohol Depend 112(1–2):39–45

D'Souza DC, Cortes-Briones JA, Ranganathan M, Thurnauer H, Creatura G, Surti T et al (2016) Rapid changes in cannabinoid 1 receptor availability in cannabis-dependent male subjects after abstinence from cannabis. Biol Psychiatry Cogn Neurosci Neuroimaging 1(1):60–67

D'Souza DC, Cortes-Briones J, Creatura G, Bluez G, Thurnauer H, Deaso E et al (2018) Efficacy and safety of a fatty acid amide hydrolase inhibitor (PF-04457845) in the treatment of cannabis withdrawal and dependence in men: a double-blind, placebo-controlled, parallel group, phase 2a single-site randomised controlled trial. Lancet Psychiatry 6:35–45

de Luca MA, Valentini V, Bimpisidis Z, Cacciapaglia F, Caboni P, di Chiara G (2014) Endocannabinoid 2-arachidonoylglycerol self-administration by Sprague-Dawley rats and stimulation of in vivo dopamine transmission in the nucleus accumbens shell. Front Psych 5:140

Fasinu PS, Phillips S, ElSohly MA, Walker LA (2016) Current status and prospects for cannabidiol preparations as new therapeutic agents. Pharmacotherapy 36(7):781–796

Felder CC, Veluz JS, Williams HL, Briley EM, Matsuda LA (1992) Cannabinoid agonists stimulate both receptor- and non-receptor-mediated signal transduction pathways in cells transfected with and expressing cannabinoid receptor clones. Mol Pharmacol 42(5):838–845

Findling RL, Pagano ME, McNamara NK, Stansbrey RJ, Faber JE, Lingler J et al (2009) The short-term safety and efficacy of fluoxetine in depressed adolescents with alcohol and cannabis use disorders: a pilot randomized placebo-controlled trial. Child Adolesc Psychiatry Ment Health 3:11

Frewen AR (2009) An examination of withdrawal symptoms and their relationship with outcomes in a combined behavioural and pharmacological intervention for dependent cannabis users. Macquarie University, Macquarie Park

Goldstein RB, Chou SP, Smith SM, Jung J, Zhang H, Saha TD et al (2015) Nosologic comparisons of DSM-IV and DSM-5 alcohol and drug use disorders: results from the national epidemiologic survey on alcohol and related conditions–III. J Stud Alcohol Drugs 76(3):378–388

Gourlay DL, Heit HA, Almahrezi A (2005) Universal precautions in pain medicine: a rational approach to the treatment of chronic pain. Pain Med 6(2):107–112

Grant BF, Chu A, Sigman R, Amsbary M, Kali J, Sugawara Y et al (2014) Source and accuracy statement: national epidemiologic survey on alcohol and related conditions-III (NESARC-III). National Institute on Alcohol Abuse and Alcoholism, Rockville

Grant BF, Goldstein RB, Saha TD, Chou SP, Jung J, Zhang H et al (2015) Epidemiology of DSM-5 alcohol use disorder: results from the national epidemiologic survey on alcohol and related conditions III. JAMA Psychiat 72(8):757–766

Gray KM, Carpenter MJ, Baker NL, DeSantis SM, Kryway E, Hartwell KJ et al (2012) A double-blind randomized controlled trial of N-acetylcysteine in cannabis-dependent adolescents. Am J Psychiatry 169(8):805–812

Gray KM, Sonne SC, McClure EA, Ghitza UE, Matthews AG, McRae-Clark AL et al (2017) A randomized placebo-controlled trial of N-acetylcysteine for cannabis use disorder in adults. Drug Alcohol Depend 177:249–257

Gray JC, Treloar Padovano H, Wemm SE, Miranda R (2018) Predictors of topiramate tolerability in heavy cannabis-using adolescents and young adults: a secondary analysis of a randomized, double-blind, placebo-controlled trial. J Clin Psychopharmacol 38(2):134–137

Grotenhermen F (2003) Pharmacokinetics and pharmacodynamics of cannabinoids. Clin Pharmacokinet 42(4):327–360

Hall W (2015) What has research over the past two decades revealed about the adverse health effects of recreational cannabis use? Addiction 110(1):19–35

Haney M, Ward AS, Comer SD, Hart CL, Foltin RW, Fischman MW (2001) Bupropion SR worsens mood during marijuana withdrawal in humans. Psychopharmacology 155(2):171–179

Haney M, Hart CL, Ward AS, Foltin RW (2003) Nefazodone decreases anxiety during marijuana withdrawal in humans. Psychopharmacology 165:157–165

Haney M, Hart CL, Vosburg SK, Comer SD, Reed SC, Cooper ZD et al (2010) Effects of baclofen and mirtazapine on a laboratory model of marijuana withdrawal and relapse. Psychopharmacology 211:233–244

Haney M, Cooper ZD, Bedi G, Vosburg SK, Comer SD, Foltin RW (2013) Nabilone decreases marijuana withdrawal and a laboratory measure of marijuana relapse. Neuropsychopharmacology 38(8):1557–1565

Hasin DS, Keyes KM, Alderson D, Wang S, Aharonovich E, Grant BF (2008) Cannabis withdrawal in the United States: results from NESARC. J Clin Psychiatry 69(9):1354–1363

Hasin DS, Saha TD, Kerridge BT, Goldstein RB, Chou SP, Zhang H et al (2015) Prevalence of marijuana use disorders in the United States between 2001-2002 and 2012-2013. JAMA Psychiat 72(12):1235–1242

Herrmann ES, Cooper ZD, Bedi G, Ramesh D, Reed SC, Comer SD et al (2016) Effects of zolpidem alone and in combination with nabilone on cannabis withdrawal and a laboratory model of relapse in cannabis users. Psychopharmacology 233(13):2469–2478

Hjorthoj C, Fohlmann A, Nordentoft M (2009) Treatment of cannabis use disorders in people with schizophrenia spectrum disorders - a systematic review. Addict Behav 34(6–7):520–525

Jackson NJ, Isen JD, Khoddam R, Irons D, Tuvblad C, Iacono WG et al (2016) Impact of adolescent marijuana use on intelligence: results from two longitudinal twin studies. Proc Natl Acad Sci U S A 113(5):E500–E508

Johnston J, Lintzeris N, Allsop DJ, Suraev A, Booth J, Carson DS et al (2014) Lithium carbonate in the management of cannabis withdrawal: a randomized placebo-controlled trial in an inpatient setting. Psychopharmacology 231(24):4623–4636

Karila L, Roux P, Rolland B, Benyamina A, Reynaud M, Aubin HJ et al (2014) Acute and long-term effects of cannabis use: a review. Curr Pharm Des 20(25):4112–4118

Kelly MA, Pavlicova M, Glass A, Mariani JJ, Bisaga A, Sullivan MA et al (2014) Do withdrawal-like symptoms mediate increased marijuana smoking in individuals treated with venlafaxine-XR? Drug Alcohol Depend 144:42–46

Koob GF, Volkow ND (2016) Neurobiology of addiction: a neurocircuitry analysis. Lancet Psychiatry 3(8):760–773

Leroy C, Karila L, Martinot JL, Lukasiewicz M, Duchesnay E, Comtat C et al (2012) Striatal and extrastriatal dopamine transporter in cannabis and tobacco addiction: a high-resolution PET study. Addict Biol 17(6):981–990

Levin FR, McDowell D, Evans SM, Nunes E, Akerele E, Donovan S et al (2004) Pharmacotherapy for marijuana dependence: a double-blind, placebo-controlled pilot study of divalproex sodium. Am J Addict 13:21–32

Levin FR, Mariani JJ, Brooks DJ, Pavlicova M, Cheng W, Nunes EV (2011) Dronabinol for the treatment of cannabis dependence: a randomized, double-blind, placebo-controlled trial. Drug Alcohol Depend 116(1–3):142–150

Levin FR, Mariani J, Brooks DJ, Pavlicova M, Nunes EV, Agosti V et al (2013) A randomized double-blind, placebo-controlled trial of venlafaxine-extended release for co-occurring cannabis dependence and depressive disorders. Addiction 108:1084–1094

Levin FR, Mariani JJ, Pavlicova M, Brooks D, Glass A, Mahony A et al (2016) Dronabinol and lofexidine for cannabis use disorder: a randomized, double-blind, placebo-controlled trial. Drug Alcohol Depend 159:53–60

Machielsen MWJ, Veltman DJ, van den Brink W, de Haan L (2014) The effect of clozapine and risperidone on attentional bias in patients with schizophrenia and a cannabis use disorder: an fMRI study. J Psychopharmacol 28(7):633–642

Mason BJ, Crean R, Goodell V, Light JM, Quello S, Shadan F et al (2012) A proof-of-concept randomized controlled study of gabapentin: effects on cannabis use, withdrawal and executive function deficits in cannabis-dependent adults. Neuropsychopharmacology 37(7):1689–1698

McLoughlin BC, Pushpa-Rajah JA, Gillies D, Rathbone J, Variend H, Kalakouti E et al (2014) Cannabis and schizophrenia. Cochrane Database Syst Rev 10:CD004837

McRae-Clark AL, Carter RE, Killeen TK, Carpenter MJ, Wahlquist AE, Simpson SA et al (2009) A placebo-controlled trial of buspirone for the treatment of marijuana dependence. Drug Alcohol Depend 105:132–138

McRae-Clark AL, Carter RE, Killeen TK, Carpenter MJ, White KG, Brady KT (2010) A placebo-controlled trial of atomoxetine in marijuana-dependent individuals with attention deficit hyperactivity disorder. Am J Addict 19(6):481–489

McRae-Clark AL, Baker NL, Gray KM, Killeen TK, Wagner AM, Brady KT et al (2015) Buspirone treatment of cannabis dependence: a randomized, placebo-controlled trial. Drug Alcohol Depend 156:29–37

McRae-Clark AL, Baker NL, Gray KM, Killeen T, Hartwell KJ, Simonian SJ (2016) Vilazodone for cannabis dependence: a randomized, controlled pilot trial. Am J Addict 25(1):69–75

Meier MH, Caspi A, Ambler A, Harrington H, Houts R, Keefe RS et al (2012) Persistent cannabis users show neuropsychological decline from childhood to midlife. Proc Natl Acad Sci U S A 109(40):E2657–E2664

Mewton L, Slade T, Teesson M (2013) An evaluation of the proposed DSM-5 cannabis use disorder criteria using Australian national survey data. J Stud Alcohol Drugs 74(4):614–621

Micale V, Di Marzo V, Sulcova A, Wotjak CT, Drago F (2013) Endocannabinoid system and mood disorders: priming a target for new therapies. Pharmacol Ther 138(1):18–37

Miranda R, Treloar H, Blanchard A, Justus A, Monti PM, Chun T et al (2017) Topiramate and motivational enhancement therapy for cannabis use among youth: a randomized placebo-controlled pilot study. Addict Biol 22(3):779–790

Nanjayya SB, Shivappa M, Chand PK, Murthy P, Benegal V (2010) Baclofen in cannabis dependence syndrome. Biol Psychiatry 68(3):e9–e10

Ng Cheong Ton JM, Gerhardt GA, Friedemann M, Etgen AM, Rose GM, Sharpless NS et al (1988) The effects of delta 9-tetrahydrocannabinol on potassium-evoked release of dopamine in the rat caudate nucleus: an in vivo electrochemical and in vivo microdialysis study. Brain Res 451 (1–2):59–68

Nielsen S, Gowing L, Sabioni P, Le Foll B (2019) Pharmacotherapies for cannabis dependence. Cochrane Database Syst Rev 1:Cd008940

Notzon DP, Kelly MA, Choi CJ, Pavlicova M, Mahony AL, Brooks DJ et al (2018) Open-label pilot study of injectable naltrexone for cannabis dependence. Am J Drug Alcohol Abuse 44 (6):619–627

Panlilio LV, Goldberg SR, Justinova Z (2015) Cannabinoid abuse and addiction: clinical and preclinical findings. Clin Pharmacol Ther 97(6):616–627

Penetar DM, Looby AR, Ryan ET, Maywalt MA, Lukas SE (2012) Bupropion reduces some of the symptoms of marihuana withdrawal in chronic marihuana users: a pilot study. Subst Abuse Res Treat 6(1):63–71

Rong C, Lee Y, Carmona NE, Cha DS, Ragguett RM, Rosenblat JD et al (2017) Cannabidiol in medical marijuana: research vistas and potential opportunities. Pharmacol Res 121:213–218

Sherman BJ, Baker NL, McRae-Clark AL (2017) Effect of oxytocin pretreatment on cannabis outcomes in a brief motivational intervention. Psychiatry Res 249:318–320

Sloan ME, Grant CW, Gowin JL, Ramchandani VA, Le Foll B (2019) Endocannabinoid signaling in psychiatric disorders: a review of positron emission tomography studies. Acta Pharmacol Sin 40(3):342–350

Solinas M, Justinova Z, Goldberg SR, Tanda G (2006) Anandamide administration alone and after inhibition of fatty acid amide hydrolase (FAAH) increases dopamine levels in the nucleus accumbens shell in rats. J Neurochem 98(2):408–419

Solinas M, Goldberg SR, Piomelli D (2008) The endocannabinoid system in brain reward processes. Br J Pharmacol 154(2):369–383

Spaderna M, Addy PH, D'Souza DC (2013) Spicing things up: synthetic cannabinoids. Psychopharmacology 228(4):525–540

Temmingh HS, Williams T, Siegfried N, Stein DJ (2018) Risperidone versus other antipsychotics for people with severe mental illness and co-occurring substance misuse. Cochrane Database Syst Rev 1:CD011057

Thiruchselvam T, Malik S, Le Foll B (2017) A review of positron emission tomography studies exploring the dopaminergic system in substance use with a focus on tobacco as a co-variate. Am J Drug Alcohol Abuse 43(2):197–214

Trigo JM, Soliman A, Quilty LC, Fischer B, Rehm J, Selby P et al (2018) Nabiximols combined with motivational enhancement/cognitive behavioral therapy for the treatment of cannabis dependence: a pilot randomized clinical trial. PLoS One 13(1):e0190768

United Nations Publilcation SNEX. World drug report 2018

van Amsterdam J, Brunt T, van den Brink W (2015) The adverse health effects of synthetic cannabinoids with emphasis on psychosis-like effects. J Psychopharmacol 29(3):254–263

van de Giessen E, Weinstein JJ, Cassidy CM, Haney M, Dong Z, Ghazzaoui R et al (2017) Deficits in striatal dopamine release in cannabis dependence. Mol Psychiatry 22(1):68–75

Volkow ND, Gillespie H, Mullani N, Tancredi L, Grant C, Valentine A et al (1996) Brain glucose metabolism in chronic marijuana users at baseline and during marijuana intoxication. Psychiatry Res 67(1):29–38

Volkow ND, Compton WM, Weiss SR (2014a) Adverse health effects of marijuana use. N Engl J Med 371(9):879

Volkow ND, Wang GJ, Telang F, Fowler JS, Alexoff D, Logan J et al (2014b) Decreased dopamine brain reactivity in marijuana abusers is associated with negative emotionality and addiction severity. Proc Natl Acad Sci U S A 111(30):E3149–E3156

Weinstein AM, Miller H, Bluvstein I, Rapoport E, Schreiber S, Bar-Hamburger R et al (2014) Treatment of cannabis dependence using escitalopram in combination with cognitive-behavior therapy: a double-blind placebo-controlled study. Am J Drug Alcohol Abuse 40(1):16–22

World Health Organization (2014) WHO Guidelines Approved by the Guidelines Review Committee. Guidelines for the identification and management of substance use and substance use disorders in pregnancy. World Health Organization, Geneva

Molecular Mechanisms Associated with Nicotine Pharmacology and Dependence

Christie D. Fowler, Jill R. Turner, and M. Imad Damaj

Contents

1 Introduction 374
2 Basic Neurocircuitry of Nicotine Addiction 375
3 Role of Nicotinic Receptors in Nicotine Dependence and Brain Function 376
4 Modulatory Factors That Influence nAChR Expression and Signaling 378
5 Genomics and Genetics of Nicotine Dependence 379
  5.1 Overview 379
  5.2 Human and Animal Genetic Studies 379
  5.3 Transcriptionally Adaptive Changes 380
6 Other Constituents in Nicotine and Tobacco Products Mediating Dependence 381
7 Therapeutic Approaches for Tobacco and Nicotine Dependence 383
  7.1 Nicotine Replacement Therapies 383
  7.2 Varenicline and Bupropion 383
  7.3 Novel Approaches 384
8 Conclusion 385
References 385

Abstract

Tobacco dependence is a leading cause of preventable disease and death worldwide. Nicotine, the main psychoactive component in tobacco cigarettes, has also

C. D. Fowler
Department of Neurobiology and Behavior, University of California Irvine, Irvine, CA, USA

J. R. Turner
Department of Pharmaceutical Sciences, College of Pharmacy, University of Kentucky, Lexington, KY, USA

M. Imad Damaj (✉)
Department of Pharmacology and Toxicology, Virginia Commonwealth University, Richmond, VA, USA

Translational Research Initiative for Pain and Neuropathy at VCU, Richmond, VA, USA
e-mail: m.damaj@vcuhealth.org

M. A. Nader, Y. L. Hurd (eds.), *Substance Use Disorders*,
Handbook of Experimental Pharmacology 258, https://doi.org/10.1007/164_2019_252

been garnering increased popularity in its vaporized form, as derived from e-cigarette devices. Thus, an understanding of the molecular mechanisms underlying nicotine pharmacology and dependence is required to ascertain novel approaches to treat drug dependence. In this chapter, we review the field's current understanding of nicotine's actions in the brain, the neurocircuitry underlying drug dependence, factors that modulate the function of nicotinic acetylcholine receptors, and the role of specific genes in mitigating the vulnerability to develop nicotine dependence. In addition to nicotine's direct actions in the brain, other constituents in nicotine and tobacco products have also been found to alter drug use, and thus, evidence is provided to highlight this issue. Finally, currently available pharmacotherapeutic strategies are discussed, along with an outlook for future therapeutic directions to achieve to the goal of long-term nicotine cessation.

Keywords
Neurobiology nicotine dependence · Nicotine · Nicotinic receptors · Smoking cessation

1 Introduction

Cigarette smoking is the principal cause of premature death and disability in the United States. In 2014, about 480,000 deaths in the United States were caused by cigarette smoking. Globally, smoking-related illnesses result in over four million deaths annually. However, despite enormous educational efforts about the health hazards of smoking and other tobacco control efforts, many smokers continue to encounter extreme difficulty quitting and staying tobacco-free in the long-term. The 2017 CDC report estimated that 15.1% of the US population was "current smokers," (11.2% (75%) of them are daily smokers).

Addiction to tobacco smoking depends not only on the positive reinforcing and hedonic actions of nicotine but also on escape from the aversive consequences of nicotine withdrawal. Many studies suggest that avoidance of the negative emotional state produced by nicotine withdrawal represents a motivational component that promotes continued tobacco use and relapse after smoking cessation. The difficulty in overcoming nicotine dependence is illustrated by the poor success rates among smokers who try to quit. While the majority of smokers (~70%) report an interest in quitting, and around 55% have attempted to quit in the previous year, ~7% of smokers are abstinent at 1 month after their quit date, and fewer than 2% are abstinent 1 year after quitting when they do not receive assistance in smoking cessation (CDC 2015).

While several smoking cessation therapies are available, the success rate of these therapies after 1 year remains only about 20–25% (Gonzales et al. 2006). Therefore, understanding the various mechanisms and factors involved in the different aspects of nicotine dependence is crucial to develop successful prevention and intervention approaches, including newer and more effective pharmacotherapies.

2 Basic Neurocircuitry of Nicotine Addiction

Tobacco smoke contains about 9,000 chemicals, among which about 70 are known carcinogens. However, nicotine is the major psychoactive ingredient in tobacco smoke and the component most associated with tobacco dependence. The development and persistence of dependence on tobacco is due to the actions of nicotine, acting at neuronal nicotinic acetylcholine receptors (nAChRs). nAChRs belong to the Cys-loop receptor family, which are ligand-gated ion channels that form pentamers arranged around a water-filled pore and allow for the influx of both Na+ and Ca^{2+} (Changeux et al. 1998). The subunits of mammalian neuronal nAChRs range from α2–α7, α9, α10, to β2–β4, which form multiple combinations of homomeric and heteromeric receptor subtypes having varying function (Changeux et al. 1998). These receptors have three broad conformational states: resting closed states, open states, and desensitized states (Changeux et al. 1998). The typical resting closed state is induced when the orthosteric site (traditional ligand binding site) is unoccupied and the cation channel is closed. Upon binding of an orthosteric agonist, the cation channel is opened, allowing for cation influx into the cell. Following the open state, the receptor is then desensitized; despite agonist binding, the cation channel is closed, rendering the receptor inactive (Changeux et al. 1998). Due to their predominant presynaptic location, nAChRs in the CNS primarily function via modulation of neurotransmitter release (Mansvelder and McGehee 2000). This modulation, in turn, results in long-term synaptic plasticity, which is a prominent neuronal signature of exposure to nicotine (Ji et al. 2001). The most abundant nAChRs found in the mammalian brain are the low-affinity homomeric α7 and the high-affinity heteromeric α4β2 containing (α4β2∗), which have diverse characteristics (Hill et al. 1993). The α7 nAChR has high calcium permeability, low probability of opening, and rapid desensitization (in milliseconds) (Williams et al. 2011). In contrast, the α4β2∗ nAChR has a high probability of opening and desensitizes at a slower rate (in seconds) (Li and Steinbach 2010). These differing characteristics, however, do not necessarily drive divergent effects on neuronal plasticity. For example, previous studies have shown that both α4β2∗ and α7 nAChR activation can either elicit (Lagostena et al. 2008; Tang and Dani 2009; Welsby et al. 2009) or prevent (Alkondon and Albuquerque 2001; Alkondon et al. 1997; Ji et al. 2001) long-term potentiation (LTP) in the hippocampus, with these variable effects attributed to activation of differing subtypes on specific interneuron populations. Further, accessory nAChR subunits, such as α5 and β3, can integrate into the α4β2, α3β4, or α3β2 nAChR subtypes to alter receptor function. For instance, insertion of the α5 subunit into the α4β2 or α3β2 nAChR subtypes results in increased ligand-mediated receptor activation, rate of desensitization, and conductance (Gerzanich et al. 1998; Ramirez-Latorre et al. 1996).

Nicotine initiates its rewarding effects by activating nAChRs in the natural reward system of the brain, the mesolimbic pathway. This pathway is comprised of dopaminergic neurons originating in the ventral tegmental area (VTA) that project to regions such as the nucleus accumbens (NAc), prefrontal cortex (PFC), amygdala, and hippocampus (De Biasi and Dani 2011; Lisman and Grace 2005).

Dopamine release, especially in the NAc, is associated with the rewarding and reinforcing effects of all drugs of abuse. nAChRs are localized throughout the mesolimbic circuitry and when activated, increase dopaminergic firing and release (De Biasi and Dani 2011; Di Chiara 2000). Further, infusion of nAChR antagonists directly into the VTA attenuates nicotine self-administration (Corrigall et al. 1994). This pathway has a complex circuitry that also involves other neurotransmitters; for instance, glutamatergic, GABAergic, and cholinergic inputs converge on dopamine neurons to modulate dopamine release (Dani and Bertrand 2007). Cholinergic neurons in the laterodorsal tegmentum and the pedunculopontine tegmentum initiate excitation of dopamine neurons in VTA that project to the NAc (Maskos 2010; Omelchenko and Sesack 2005), and these cells in the pedunculopontine tegmentum have been shown to regulate nicotine self-administration (Lanca et al. 2000). In opposition to reward-related signaling, dense nAChR expression is also found in the projection from the medial habenula (MHb) to the interpeduncular nucleus (IPN), a circuit involved in aversive processing and nicotine withdrawal (Fowler et al. 2011; Salas et al. 2009). The major neurotransmitters of this pathway are acetylcholine, glutamate, and substance P, and it is thought that presynaptic nAChRs on MHb axons facilitate glutamate release from cholinergic and glutamatergic coexpressing axons in the IPN to mediate the aversive signal to high doses of nicotine (Fowler et al. 2011; Girod and Role 2001), which serves to limit drug intake.

3 Role of Nicotinic Receptors in Nicotine Dependence and Brain Function

The utilization of genetically mutant mice, pharmacological interventions, and viral reexpression approaches have implicated particular brain areas and specific nAChR subtypes in nicotine dependence. For instance, in a β2 knockout mouse model, the β2∗ nAChRs have been shown to be required for nicotine reward and reinforcement, as revealed in nicotine conditioned place preference (CPP) and intravenous self-administration studies (Orejarena et al. 2012; Picciotto et al. 1998; Walters et al. 2006). The β2 subunit co-assembles with the α6 and α4 subunits to form several α6β2∗, α4β2∗, and α4α6β2∗ nAChR subtypes, which are notably expressed in the VTA-NAc circuit (Champtiaux et al. 2003; Klink et al. 2001; Salminen et al. 2004). These findings are consistent with the fact that stimulation of α4β2∗ high-affinity nAChRs located on the dopaminergic cells in the VTA shifts firing from tonic to phasic modes, resulting in increased DA release in both the NAc and the PFC (Dani et al. 2011). Nicotine CPP revealed a critical role of the α4, α6, and β2 subunits in the NAc via genetic mutant mice and site-specific infusions (Sanjakdar et al. 2015). In addition, genetic ablation of the β2, α6, and α4 nAChR subunits attenuated nicotine self-administration in mice, an effect which could be rescued by reexpression of these subunits in the VTA via a lentiviral vector (Picciotto et al. 1998; Pons et al. 2008). Furthermore, α4 "knock-in" mice (Leu9' Ala mutation renders animals hypersensitive to nicotine) demonstrated a preference for nicotine at a dose 50-fold lower than the typical nicotine dose that induces a preference in wild-type (WT) mice in the CPP test (Tapper et al. 2004).

Reward systems in the brain undergo neuroadaptations after chronic exposure to nicotine in tobacco products, which likely underlie nicotine dependence. Cessation from cigarette smoking induces a withdrawal syndrome comprised of physical, affective, and cognitive symptoms. The severity of these symptoms is a risk factor for relapse (Le Foll and Goldberg 2005; Markou and Kenny 2002), and nAChRs are important mediators of nicotine withdrawal symptoms. The nonselective nAChR antagonist mecamylamine is known to precipitate nicotine withdrawal signs in nicotine-dependent rodents (Damaj et al. 2003). Pharmacological interventions and mouse knockout studies have revealed that nAChR subunits modulate different aspects of the nicotine withdrawal syndrome. For example, some affective signs of withdrawal such as aversion-, anxiety-, and anhedonia-like measures are mediated by the β2, α6, β4, and α7 nAChR subunits (Jackson et al. 2008, 2009). The physical signs of the nicotine withdrawal syndrome are mediated by α3, α5, α2, and β4 (Jackson et al. 2008, 2013; Salas et al. 2009), and a subset are mediated by α7 subunits (Stoker et al. 2012). One interesting feature of chronic nicotine exposure is the upregulation of nAChRs, most notably α4β2∗ (Flores et al. 1992). This phenomenon has been observed both in vitro and in vivo and in human imaging studies (Kassiou et al. 2001; Marks et al. 1983; Perry et al. 1999). Interestingly, rodent and human studies suggest a positive correlation of nicotine withdrawal signs with upregulation of α4β2∗ nAChRs (Cosgrove et al. 2010; Turner et al. 2011). Furthermore, the MHb-IPN pathway has been selectively implicated in withdrawal-induced somatic signs with α5∗ and β4∗ nAChRs (Salas et al. 2009). In addition, infusion of the α6∗ nAChR-selective antagonist α-conotoxin MII in the MHb attenuated anxiety-like behavior in nicotine-withdrawn mice (Pang et al. 2016). Aberrant synaptic and circuitry function is also thought to underlie abnormal behavioral phenotypes, including nicotine withdrawal phenotypes like cognitive impairments and affective dysfunction (Ashare et al. 2014; Turner et al. 2013). For example, the hippocampus and the orbitofrontal cortex (OFC) are two well-described circuits impinging upon these nicotine withdrawal symptoms (Schoenbaum et al. 2016; Turner et al. 2011; Zhou et al. 2018), including impulsivity, altered affect, and cognition in humans. Supporting data in human (Dani and Harris 2005) and animal (Jackson et al. 2008) models link hippocampal function with nicotine withdrawal-induced symptoms, which are reliable determinants for smoking cessation outcomes. Functional imaging studies in smokers have shown that activation of the hippocampus can be correlated with both cognitive and affective withdrawal symptoms (Froeliger et al. 2010; McClernon and Gilbert 2004). Additionally, human studies report a correlation between hippocampal volume and successful quit attempts (Froeliger et al. 2010). This link may be due to nAChRs present at both excitatory and inhibitory terminals (Alkondon and Albuquerque 2001; Jones and Yakel 1997; Wada et al. 1989), well-positioning nicotinic signaling to influence the balance of excitatory and inhibitory transmission within the hippocampus (John and Berg 2015). The OFC regulates impulsivity, affective value of reinforcers, and emotion-attention interactions (Schoenbaum et al. 2016). Previous studies reported that nicotine self-administration in rodents alters synaptic morphology in the OFC (Vazquez-Sanroman et al. 2016), while tobacco smokers display both morphological and functional connectivity changes within this region (Claus et al. 2013; Li et al. 2015). For example, smoking has been consistently shown to reduce the thickness of gray matter volume in the OFC (Kuhn et al. 2010; Li et al. 2015), and acute nicotine increases blood oxygen level-dependent fMRI signal in the striato-thalamo-orbitofrontal circuit (Ashare et al. 2014). However, the neuronal mechanisms underlying these effects are not easily examined, given that nicotine modulates the release of a number of neurotransmitters, including glutamate, GABA, and dopamine, and can lead to both facilitation and suppression of neuronal firing. For example, electrophysiological experiments have shown that nicotine impacts long-term potentiation (LTP) generation in the orbitofrontal cortex (Couey et al. 2007; Zhou et al. 2018). Classical LTP is based on the observation that a neuron's excitability to a particular synaptic input is increased following high-frequency stimulation, representing the molecular basis for Hebb's postulate, which states that when two connected cells fire simultaneously, the connection between them is strengthened. Previous studies examining nicotine's effect on this phenomenon have reported enhancement of LTP in a number of brain regions, such as the hippocampus (Nakauchi and Sumikawa 2012), amygdala (Huang et al. 2008), and VTA (Mansvelder and McGehee 2000). However, these effects diverge in the OFC. Zhou and colleagues (Zhou et al. 2018) demonstrated that acute nicotine application to the OFC during LTP induction resulted in nicotine-mediated conversion of LTP to LTD, a form of "metaplasticity," due to enhanced GABAergic transmission. These effects were in agreement with studies in nearby frontal cortical regions, where nicotine was observed to raise the threshold for LTP induction via enhancing GABAergic transmission (Couey et al. 2007). As appreciation grows for the importance of frontocortical excitatory/inhibitory balance in nicotine dependence (Pittaras et al. 2016), understanding nicotine's effects in this region may not only lead to better understanding of circuit-level mechanisms of nicotine dependence but also to potential therapeutic interventions.

4 Modulatory Factors That Influence nAChR Expression and Signaling

Several mechanisms that regulate nAChR expression, assembly, and trafficking were reported in the last two decades. Recent studies have shown that nicotine can act as a "chaperone" which expedites the transport of nAChR subunits, including α4 and β2 nAChRs, to the endoplasmic reticulum and facilitates the passage and insertion of assembled nAChRs to the plasma membrane (Henderson et al. 2014; Srinivasan et al. 2011). In this context, this pharmacological chaperone mechanism may represent an important molecular mechanism of the first step in neuroadaptation to chronic nicotine and possibility of the emergence of neuronal adaptations underlying nicotine dependence. Another class of nAChR signaling modulators is represented by the Ly-6/neurotoxin gene superfamily of proteins that exhibit cellular specific expression patterns in the brain and include Lynx1, Lynx2, and Lypd6. These proteins are negative modulators of nAChR signaling and feature a three-looped fold, a structural characteristically shared with the snake venom toxin α-bungarotoxin. Thus, as endogenous prototoxins, these proteins can bind directly to the extracellular face of nAChRs (Arvaniti et al. 2016; Miwa et al. 1999). The presence of Lynx1 and Lynx2 increases the desensitization rate and decreases ligand binding efficiency for multiple nAChR subtypes (George et al. 2017; Ibanez-Tallon et al. 2002; Lyukmanova et al. 2011; Tekinay et al. 2009). In cortex, Lynx1 is expressed in both glutamatergic and γ-aminobutyric acid-ergic (GABAergic) neurons, whereas Lynx2 has been mainly localized in glutamatergic neurons (Demars and Morishita 2014). Results suggest that lynx proteins can modulate nAChR function in the brain with important consequences for cholinergic-dependent synaptic plasticity (reviewed in Miwa et al. 2011; Miwa and Walz 2012; Thomsen and Mikkelsen 2012). Recently, Nissen and colleagues reported that the antinociceptive effect of nicotine and epibatidine in acute thermal pain tests is enhanced in Lynx1 knockout mice (Nissen et al. 2018). Further, computer simulations predict preferential binding affinity of Lynx1 to the α:α interface that exists in the stoichiometry of the low sensitivity $(\alpha4)3(\beta2)2$ nAChRs.

5 Genomics and Genetics of Nicotine Dependence

5.1 Overview

Nicotine addiction is a complex disorder with multiple factors contributing to its dependence. Though a large host of factors contribute to nicotine dependence, reward, withdrawal effects, and relapse, twin studies have shown that genetics play a pivotal role (Li et al. 2003; Sullivan and Kendler 1999). Approximately 70% of the variability in nicotine dependence and smoking persistence has been attributed to genetic influences (Broms et al. 2006; Carmelli et al. 1992; Kendler et al. 2000; Li et al. 2003). Furthermore, twin studies have shown that ~50% of the individual differences that contribute to smoking relapse can be attributed to heritability (Xian et al. 2003). Ongoing studies examining not only genetics, but genomics and epigenetics, are increasing our understanding of how individual differences drive vulnerability or resilience to nicotine dependence.

5.2 Human and Animal Genetic Studies

In recent years, genome-wide association studies in humans revealed that a variant in the CHRNA5/A3/B4 gene cluster (encodes α3, α5, β4 nAChR subunits), located in chromosome region 15q25, serves as a risk factor for lung cancer and nicotine dependence (Berrettini et al. 2008; Liu et al. 2010; Saccone et al. 2009). More specifically, a single nucleotide polymorphism (SNP) in the CHRNA5 gene (rs16969968) (D398N), which encodes the α5 nAChR subunit, has been repeatedly linked to increased risk for tobacco dependence (Bierut et al. 2008; Kuryatov et al. 2011). The mechanisms behind this increased risk have been investigated in in vitro and in vivo functional studies. The α5 SNP was shown to reduce the function of the α3β4 and α4β2 nAChR subtypes that incorporate the mutant subunit (Bierut et al. 2008), a loss of function that subsequently was shown to influence addiction-like behaviors in vivo. Initial studies were conducted in α5 nAChR subunit gene knockout mice (Fowler et al. 2011). The α5 knockout mice were found to exhibit far greater motivation to consume large quantities of nicotine, and reexpression of α5 subunits within this pathway attenuated nicotine intake to wild-type levels (Fowler et al. 2011). Further, decreased expression of α5 subunits in rats similarly increased nicotine intake while decreasing the inhibitory effects of higher nicotine doses on brain reward circuitries (Fowler et al. 2011, 2013). Similar observations occurred in the nicotine CPP paradigm where α5 knockout mice exhibited a maintained nicotine preference at higher doses not maintained by α5 wild-type mice (Jackson et al. 2010). In addition, in mice expressing the α5 human mutation, an increase in nicotine self-administration was reported (Wilking and Stitzel 2015). Furthermore, using rats carrying the α5 human mutation, Forget et al. (2018) found greater nicotine intake in the SNP-expressing mutant rats compared with wild-type rats, as well as an increase in nicotine motivation mutant rats. In addition, the SNP-expressing rats exhibited a higher reinstatement of nicotine-seeking lever-pressing responses than the wild-type rats (Forget et al. 2018). Collectively, these studies suggest that the α5 subunit acts as an inhibitory signal that limits nicotine consumption and rewarding effects in smokers.

5.3 Transcriptionally Adaptive Changes

A potential way smoking and genetics may interact is through transcriptionally driven adaptive changes. It is now clear that continued drug use induces adaptive changes in the central nervous system that lead to drug dependence. Long-term adaptations in cellular signaling mechanisms are likely part of the maintenance of drug dependence, which may be necessary for their development and persistence. One well-characterized protein responsible for regulating gene expression is the transcription factor cAMP response element binding protein (CREB). Both human and animal studies have shown that CREB-dependent transcription is an important molecular mechanism underlying dependence on multiple drugs of abuse, including nicotine (Nestler 2005). In human studies, CREB expression correlates with the number of cigarettes smoked per day (Lenz et al. 2010). In adult mice, CREB activation is necessary for nicotine reward (Walters et al. 2005). These studies and others suggest a role for CREB in mediating the neuroplasticity changes that characterize nicotine dependence (Kenney et al. 2012; Portugal et al. 2012; Turner et al. 2014). For example, Turner and colleagues (Fisher et al. 2017; Turner et al. 2014) showed that hippocampal CREB signaling and the associated changes in synaptic plasticity impacted nicotine withdrawal phenotypes in mice. Further studies (Fisher et al. 2017) then demonstrated that site-specific CREB deletion in the hippocampus impacted both cognitive and affective nicotine withdrawal phenotypes due to reduced CREB-mediated transcription of neuroplasticity-related genes, such as Arc and TrkB. However, while CREB is an important regulator of transcription, its widespread function precludes its use for development of targeted therapeutics. Instead, current studies are examining genomic CREB targets as potential therapeutics. For example, CREB ChIP-Seq data show that CREB's activation by chronic nicotine and withdrawal differentially modulate its binding to the genome and network pathway analyses of these data highlight the importance of different families of neuroplasticity genes, such as neurotrophin, netrin, and neuregulin family members (Turner et al. 2014).

Genes encoding a member of the epidermal growth factor family, neuregulin 3 (NRG3), and its receptor, ErbB4, have been recently linked to smoking cessation outcomes (Loukola et al. 2014; Turner et al. 2014). NRG3 is present on excitatory cells and signals transsynaptically through the ErbB4 receptor, which is found on select inhibitory cell types (Vullhorst et al. 2017). Genetic variation in this pathway has been demonstrated to impact multiple dimensions of smoking behavior, including smoking initiation, amount smoked, and nicotine dependence (Loukola et al. 2008, 2014). In particular, single nucleotide polymorphisms in the gene for NRG3 result in impaired ability to quit smoking in the clinical population (Turner et al. 2014). Conserved and consistent association of variants in this pathway with nicotine dependence measures lends confidence to future mechanistic evaluation of these associations. Furthermore, these data suggest that while therapeutic interventions for molecules such as CREB are unlikely, evaluation of those gene families regulated by CREB has great potential for future therapeutic development. For example, compounds targeting downstream effectors of ErbB4, the receptor for the CREB target gene NRG3, are already being developed for clinical use in psychiatric conditions such as schizophrenia (Law et al. 2012), a condition highly comorbid with nicotine dependence.

6 Other Constituents in Nicotine and Tobacco Products Mediating Dependence

While the field has focused on nicotine as the main psychoactive constituent in cigarettes and e-cigarettes, it is important to consider other compounds in the products that may alter the pharmacokinetics of nicotine and/or exert independent reinforcing effects on the substance user. Accumulating research has provided evidence that some non-nicotine constituents have innate reinforcing properties, which may thereby increase product use. For instance, anatabine, anabasine, cotinine, and myosmine have all been shown to increase the reinforcing properties of nicotine (Clemens et al. 2009; Hall et al. 2014). Mesolimbic dopamine levels are also increased in the presence of cotinine, acetaldehyde, and nornicotine at a level similar to that found for other substances of abuse (Bardo et al. 1999; Dwoskin et al. 1993, 1999; Foddai et al. 2004). Acetaldehyde and several minor alkaloids have also been shown to act as reinforcers (Myers et al. 1982; Peana et al. 2010; Smith et al. 2015), although it is debatable as to whether this potentiative effect occurs at the concentrations of product consumed by humans. Another potential candidate mediating the enhanced reinforcing effect of nicotine in tobacco cigarettes is MAO inhibition with chronic exposure (Fowler et al. 1996, 2000). Consistent with the findings in humans, pharmacological inhibition of MAO in rodents has been shown to increase low-dose nicotine self-administration (Smith et al. 2015). Furthermore, the β-carbolines, harman and norharman, appear to inhibit MAO and may partially explain the effects found with tobacco consumption (Truman et al. 2017). With specific regard to e-cigarettes, several factors may interact to affect nicotine absorption and bioavailability, including pH, concentration of propylene glycol to glycerine vehicle, alcohol, nicotyrine, temperature, concentration of nicotine, and user characteristics (e.g., puff topography, level of experience) (DeVito and Krishnan-Sarin 2018). In addition, propylene glycol has been shown to decrease the aversive effects of high-dose nicotine, which may subsequently promote higher levels of nicotine consumption (Harris et al. 2018).

Various flavorant additives are also found in tobacco and e-cigarette products, and this topic has garnered recent attention since product flavor has been reported to be a main reason for the initiation of e-cigarette use among adolescents (Kong et al. 2015). Interestingly, a fMRI study found that e-cigarette advertisements showing sweet- and fruit-flavored products elicited a greater increase in nucleus accumbens activity compared to tobacco e-cigarette advertisements or control images of sweets and fruits (Garrison et al. 2018), thus demonstrating the strong cue-associated effects of these flavorants on brain reward circuity. In addition to enhancing the attractiveness and palatability of the cigarette, the additives may additionally interact with nicotine or other constituents at a biological level. For instance, menthol, a common flavoring additive to cigarettes and e-cigarettes, has garnered much attention recently given the preferential use of mentholated products among youth, adult women, and racial/ethnic minorities (FDA 2013; Villanti et al. 2017). In addition to focused marketing in targeted communities, the disproportional use by these populations has been proposed to be due to underlying genetic or biological factors, such as differences in nAChR expression or nicotine metabolism. Indeed, the presence of menthol in cigarettes has been demonstrated to alter nicotine's effects in smokers (Benowitz et al. 2004; Williams et al. 2007), which may be due to menthol-mediated inhibition of nicotine metabolism (Caraballo et al. 2011; Fagan et al. 2016) and potentiative effects on nicotine-mediated dopamine release in brain reward pathways (Zhang et al. 2018). Furthermore, menthol has also been shown to allosterically modulate α7 nAChRs (Ashoor et al. 2013) and can further upregulate nAChR expression (Alsharari et al. 2015). Thus, the pharmacological and addictive properties of nicotine may be enhanced and prolonged in the presence of menthol. This is further evidenced by the finding that mentholated cigarette smokers are less successful in maintaining abstinence following cessation (Caraballo et al. 2011; Fagan et al. 2016; Okuyemi et al. 2007).

7 Therapeutic Approaches for Tobacco and Nicotine Dependence

7.1 Nicotine Replacement Therapies

Nicotine replacement therapies (NRT) represent one of the first effective strategies to promote smoking cessation. In most formulations, nicotine is slowly administered over a prolonged period of time; this approach is thought to attenuate the negative somatic and cognitive effects found during drug withdrawal, while minimizing the reinforcing properties of the drug. A variety of available products include nicotine containing gums, lozenges, and patches. In controlled studies, NRT has been shown to be moderately efficacious in the short-term (days to weeks) (Hartmann-Boyce et al. 2018). However, over longer periods, relapse is often found in most individuals (Hartmann-Boyce et al. 2018), thus necessitating the development of alternate approaches. Along these lines, e-cigarette devices were developed as an NRT and harm reduction product. Compared to the traditional tobacco cigarette, e-cigarettes have been promoted as reducing exposure to carcinogens while providing reinforcing properties of nicotine via inhalation and quick delivery of the drug to the brain. Although e-cigarettes have been reported to assist some individuals in tobacco cessation, the emerging incidence of e-cigarette use among never smokers has represented a concerning trend for the promotion of nicotine dependence, especially among adolescents (Miech et al. 2019). Indeed, while e-cigarettes may be less harmful than tobacco cigarettes, they are by no means harmless, as evidenced by the multitude of chemicals and carcinogens emitted (Goniewicz et al. 2018). It is currently debatable as to whether electronic nicotine delivery devices should be employed by physicians for tobacco cessation since inconsistent findings have been reported with effectiveness and the potential harmful effects with short- and long-term use remain to be resolved (Livingston et al. 2019).

7.2 Varenicline and Bupropion

Given the direct action of nicotine on $\alpha4\beta2*$ nAChRs to mediate the reinforcing properties of the drug, it is perhaps not surprising that the most efficacious pharmacotherapeutics available is varenicline, a partial agonist of $\alpha4\beta2*$ nAChRs. Varenicline also has full agonist, but less potent, effects at $\alpha7$ and $\alpha3\beta4*$ nAChRs and serotonin 5-HT_3 receptors. Approved by the FDA in 2006, varenicline has been shown to have similar or greater effectiveness in promoting smoking cessation compared to NRT and other approved therapeutics, such as bupropion (Gonzales et al. 2006). Bupropion was first characterized as a dopamine and norepinephrine reuptake inhibitor with antidepressant actions but more recently became approved as a first-line treatment for tobacco cessation. In addition to its actions as a catecholamine reuptake inhibitor, bupropion has also been shown to result in noncompetitive antagonism of $\alpha4\beta2*$ and $\alpha3\beta4*$ nAChRs (Carroll et al. 2014) and negative allosteric modulation of serotonin $5HT_{3A}$ receptors (Pandhare et al. 2017), either of which may underlie the beneficial effects found for smoking cessation. In addition to NRT, varenicline, and bupropion, the tricyclic antidepressant nortriptyline and the α-adrenergic agonist clonidine have also been prescribed for smoking cessation, although studies have generally found them to be less effective than the aforementioned therapeutics (Dodd et al. 2018).

7.3 Novel Approaches

With advances in our understanding of the biological mechanisms underlying nicotine's physiological, reinforcing, and aversive effects, novel approaches for therapeutic development hold the promise of achieving substantial long-term clinical outcomes. Since α5∗ nAChRs in the MHb-IPN pathway have been demonstrated to mediate the aversive properties of nicotine that limit intake (Fowler et al. 2011), drug development efforts are focused on generating positive allosteric modulators of these receptors, with the idea of enhancing aversive processing in the presence of nicotine to decrease further drug intake (Jin et al. 2014). Another compound, AT-1001, which is an α3β4 partial agonist, has been shown to reduce nicotine relapse-related behaviors in rodents (Yuan et al. 2017), likely through action on the α3β4∗ nAChRs expressed in the MHb. GLP-1 receptor signaling has also been implicated in MHb-IPN modulation of nicotine intake (Tuesta et al. 2017), and a GLP-1 receptor agonist, liraglutide, is currently being tested for smoking cessation in a clinical trial (Ashare 2019). Another potentially beneficial strategy is to inhibit the main enzyme responsible for metabolizing nicotine, CYP2A6. The foundation of this approach is based on the observation that individuals with allelic variation in the CYP2A6 enzyme exhibit lower levels of nicotine consumption and greater abstinence rates when attempting to quit (Strasser et al. 2007). With CYP2A6 inhibition, lower levels of drug consumption would result in higher levels of nicotine intake, which may thereby lead either to an aversive effect with moderate levels of nicotine consumption or a reinforcing effect at lower levels of nicotine. Methoxsalen, a CYP2A5/CYP2A6 inhibitor, was a promising candidate as it was shown to decrease nicotine dependence-associated behaviors in rodents (Alsharari et al. 2014; Bagdas et al. 2014), but this drug was not further advanced for smoking cessation due to carcinogenic side effects that were unrelated to the CYP2A6 inhibitor actions. As such, current drug development efforts are ongoing to derive alternative CYP2A6 inhibitors. In addition to pharmacotherapeutics, nicotine vaccines have been under development. Conceptually, vaccination results in the generation of antibodies that bind to nicotine in the blood, thereby reducing the amount of nicotine capable of entering the brain. However, double-blind randomized trials have failed to demonstrate sustained benefit in long-term cessation (Hartmann-Boyce et al. 2012; Tonstad et al. 2013), likely due to insufficiently sustained antibody levels. In another approach to minimize nicotine entry into the brain, NicA2-J1 has been developed as a reengineered nicotine-degrading enzyme (Kallupi et al. 2018). Interestingly, while NicA2-J1 did not induce significant differences from the control in nicotine intake, an attenuation of withdrawal and relapse-related behaviors was found in rats (Kallupi et al. 2018).

8 Conclusion

Tobacco use disorder is the leading cause of preventable disease and death in the United States and worldwide. The health consequences of nicotine addiction resulting from prolonged drug use are tremendous and devastating. After more than three decades of research on the neurobiology of nicotine dependence, health professionals can now turn to several efficacious pharmacotherapies to treat smoking. These agents often double the odds for quitting over placebo and in some cases (i.e., varenicline) almost triple the odds of quitting over those of placebo. However, despite these advances, many smokers relapse, and unfortunately the long-term abstinence rates among smokers attempting to quit remain low. Therefore, a better understanding of the various genetic, behavioral, and biological mechanisms mediating the various aspects of nicotine dependence is paramount.

References

Alkondon M, Albuquerque EX (2001) Nicotinic acetylcholine receptor alpha7 and alpha4beta2 subtypes differentially control GABAergic input to CA1 neurons in rat hippocampus. J Neurophysiol 86:3043–3055

Alkondon M, Pereira EF, Barbosa CT, Albuquerque EX (1997) Neuronal nicotinic acetylcholine receptor activation modulates gamma-aminobutyric acid release from CA1 neurons of rat hippocampal slices. J Pharmacol Exp Ther 283:1396–1411

Alsharari SD, Siu EC, Tyndale RF, Damaj MI (2014) Pharmacokinetic and pharmacodynamics studies of nicotine after oral administration in mice: effects of methoxsalen, a CYP2A5/6 inhibitor. Nicotine Tob Res 16:18–25

Alsharari SD, King JR, Nordman JC, Muldoon PP, Jackson A, Zhu AZ, Tyndale RF, Kabbani N, Damaj MI (2015) Effects of menthol on nicotine pharmacokinetic, pharmacology and dependence in mice. PLoS One 10:e0137070

Arvaniti M, Jensen MM, Soni N, Wang H, Klein AB, Thiriet N, Pinborg LH, Muldoon PP, Wienecke J, Imad Damaj M, Kohlmeier KA, Gondre-Lewis MC, Mikkelsen JD, Thomsen MS (2016) Functional interaction between Lypd6 and nicotinic acetylcholine receptors. J Neurochem 138:806–820

Ashare R (2019) Daily liraglutide for nicotine dependence. USNLB, ClinicalTrials.gov. NCT03712098

Ashare RL, Falcone M, Lerman C (2014) Cognitive function during nicotine withdrawal: implications for nicotine dependence treatment. Neuropharmacology 76(Pt B):581–591

Ashoor A, Nordman JC, Veltri D, Yang KH, Al Kury L, Shuba Y, Mahgoub M, Howarth FC, Sadek B, Shehu A, Kabbani N, Oz M (2013) Menthol binding and inhibition of alpha7-nicotinic acetylcholine receptors. PLoS One 8:e67674

Bagdas D, Muldoon PP, Zhu AZ, Tyndale RF, Damaj MI (2014) Effects of methoxsalen, a CYP2A5/6 inhibitor, on nicotine dependence behaviors in mice. Neuropharmacology 85:67–72

Bardo MT, Green TA, Crooks PA, Dwoskin LP (1999) Nornicotine is self-administered intravenously by rats. Psychopharmacology 146:290–296

Benowitz NL, Herrera B, Jacob P (2004) Mentholated cigarette smoking inhibits nicotine metabolism. J Pharmacol Exp Ther 310:1208–1215

Berrettini W, Yuan X, Tozzi F, Song K, Francks C, Chilcoat H, Waterworth D, Muglia P, Mooser V (2008) Alpha-5/alpha-3 nicotinic receptor subunit alleles increase risk for heavy smoking. Mol Psychiatry 13:368–373

Bierut LJ, Stitzel JA, Wang JC, Hinrichs AL, Grucza RA, Xuei X, Saccone NL, Saccone SF, Bertelsen S, Fox L, Horton WJ, Breslau N, Budde J, Cloninger CR, Dick DM, Foroud T, Hatsukami D, Hesselbrock V, Johnson EO, Kramer J, Kuperman S, Madden PA, Mayo K, Nurnberger J Jr, Pomerleau O, Porjesz B, Reyes O, Schuckit M, Swan G, Tischfield JA, Edenberg HJ, Rice JP, Goate AM (2008) Variants in nicotinic receptors and risk for nicotine dependence. Am J Psychiatry 165:1163–1171

Broms U, Silventoinen K, Madden PAF, Heath AC, Kaprio J (2006) Genetic architecture of smoking behavior: a study of Finnish adult twins. Twin Res Hum Genet 9:64–72

Caraballo RS, Holiday DB, Stellman SD, Mowery PD, Giovino GA, Muscat JE, Eriksen MP, Bernert JT, Richter PA, Kozlowski LT (2011) Comparison of serum cotinine concentration within and across smokers of menthol and nonmenthol cigarette brands among non-Hispanic black and non-Hispanic white U.S. adult smokers, 2001–2006. Cancer Epidemiol Biomarkers Prev 20:1329–1340

Carmelli D, Swan GE, Robinette D, Fabsitz R (1992) Genetic influence on smoking – a study of male twins. New Engl J Med 327:829–833

Carroll FI, Blough BE, Mascarella SW, Navarro HA, Lukas RJ, Damaj MI (2014) Bupropion and bupropion analogs as treatments for CNS disorders. Adv Pharmacol 69:177–216

CDC (2015) Smoking-attributable mortality, years of potential life lost, and productivity losses – United States, 2000–2004. MMWR Morb Mortal Wkly Rep 57(45):1226–1228. Updated 4 Mar 2015

Champtiaux N, Gotti C, Cordero-Erausquin M, David DJ, Przybylski C, Lena C, Clementi F, Moretti M, Rossi FM, Le Novere N, McIntosh JM, Gardier AM, Changeux JP (2003) Subunit composition of functional nicotinic receptors in dopaminergic neurons investigated with knock-out mice. J Neurosci 23:7820–7829

Changeux JP, Bertrand D, Corringer PJ, Dehaene S, Edelstein S, Lena C, Le Novere N, Marubio L, Picciotto M, Zoli M (1998) Brain nicotinic receptors: structure and regulation, role in learning and reinforcement. Brain Res Brain Res Rev 26:198–216

Claus ED, Blaine SK, Filbey FM, Mayer AR, Hutchison KE (2013) Association between nicotine dependence severity, BOLD response to smoking cues, and functional connectivity. Neuropsychopharmacology 38:2363–2372

Clemens KJ, Caille S, Stinus L, Cador M (2009) The addition of five minor tobacco alkaloids increases nicotine-induced hyperactivity, sensitization and intravenous self-administration in rats. Int J Neuropsychopharmacol 12:1355–1366

Corrigall WA, Coen KM, Adamson KL (1994) Self-administered nicotine activates the mesolimbic dopamine system through the ventral tegmental area. Brain Res 653:278–284

Cosgrove KP, Esterlis I, McKee S, Bois F, Alagille D, Tamagnan GD, Seibyl JP, Krishnan-Sarin S, Staley JK (2010) Beta2∗ nicotinic acetylcholine receptors modulate pain sensitivity in acutely abstinent tobacco smokers. Nicotine Tob Res 12:535–539

Couey JJ, Meredith RM, Spijker S, Poorthuis RB, Smit AB, Brussaard AB, Mansvelder HD (2007) Distributed network actions by nicotine increase the threshold for spike-timing-dependent plasticity in prefrontal cortex. Neuron 54:73–87

Damaj MI, Kao W, Martin BR (2003) Characterization of spontaneous and precipitated nicotine withdrawal in the mouse. J Pharmacol Exp Ther 307:526–534

Dani JA, Bertrand D (2007) Nicotinic acetylcholine receptors and nicotinic cholinergic mechanisms of the central nervous system. Annu Rev Pharmacol Toxicol 47:699–729

Dani JA, Harris RA (2005) Nicotine addiction and comorbidity with alcohol abuse and mental illness. Nat Neurosci 8:1465–1470

Dani JA, Jenson D, Broussard JI, De Biasi M (2011) Neurophysiology of nicotine addiction. J Addict Res Ther S1. pii: 001

De Biasi M, Dani JA (2011) Reward, addiction, withdrawal to nicotine. Annu Rev Neurosci 34:105–130

Demars MP, Morishita H (2014) Cortical parvalbumin and somatostatin GABA neurons express distinct endogenous modulators of nicotinic acetylcholine receptors. Mol Brain 7:75

DeVito EE, Krishnan-Sarin S (2018) E-cigarettes: impact of e-liquid components and device characteristics on nicotine exposure. Curr Neuropharmacol 16:438–459

Di Chiara G (2000) Role of dopamine in the behavioural actions of nicotine related to addiction. Eur J Pharmacol 393:295–314

Dodd S, Arancini L, Gomez-Coronado N, Gasser R, Lubman DI, Dean OM, Berk M (2018) Considerations when selecting pharmacotherapy for nicotine dependence. Expert Opin Pharmacother 20:1–6

Dwoskin LP, Buxton ST, Jewell AL, Crooks PA (1993) S(−)-Nornicotine increases dopamine release in a calcium-dependent manner from superfused rat striatal slices. J Neurochem 60:2167–2174

Dwoskin LP, Teng L, Buxton ST, Crooks PA (1999) (S)-(−)-Cotinine, the major brain metabolite of nicotine, stimulates nicotinic receptors to evoke [3H]dopamine release from rat striatal slices in a calcium-dependent manner. J Pharmacol Exp Ther 288:905–911

Fagan P, Pokhrel P, Herzog TA, Pagano IS, Franke AA, Clanton MS, Alexander LA, Trinidad DR, Sakuma KL, Johnson CA, Moolchan ET (2016) Nicotine metabolism in young adult daily menthol and nonmenthol smokers. Nicotine Tob Res 18:437–446

FDA (2013) Preliminary scientific evaluation of the possible public health effects of menthol versus nonmenthol cigarettes. http://www.fda.gov/downloads/UCM361598.pdf. Accessed Apr 2017

Fisher ML, LeMalefant RM, Zhou L, Huang G, Turner JR (2017) Distinct roles of CREB within the ventral and dorsal Hippocampus in mediating nicotine withdrawal phenotypes. Neuropsychopharmacology 42:1599–1609

Flores CM, Rogers SW, Pabreza LA, Wolfe BB, Kellar KJ (1992) A subtype of nicotinic cholinergic receptor in rat brain is composed of alpha 4 and beta 2 subunits and is up-regulated by chronic nicotine treatment. Mol Pharmacol 41:31–37

Foddai M, Dosia G, Spiga S, Diana M (2004) Acetaldehyde increases dopaminergic neuronal activity in the VTA. Neuropsychopharmacology 29:530–536

Forget B, Scholze P, Langa F, Morel C, Pons S, Mondoloni S, Besson M, Durand-de Cuttoli R, Hay A, Tricoire L, Lambolez B, Mourot A, Faure P, Maskos U (2018) A human polymorphism in CHRNA5 is linked to relapse to nicotine seeking in transgenic rats. Curr Biol 28:3244–3253. e7

Fowler JS, Volkow ND, Wang GJ, Pappas N, Logan J, Shea C, Alexoff D, MacGregor RR, Schlyer DJ, Zezulkova I, Wolf AP (1996) Brain monoamine oxidase A inhibition in cigarette smokers. Proc Natl Acad Sci U S A 93:14065–14069

Fowler JS, Wang GJ, Volkow ND, Franceschi D, Logan J, Pappas N, Shea C, MacGregor RR, Garza V (2000) Maintenance of brain monoamine oxidase B inhibition in smokers after overnight cigarette abstinence. Am J Psychiatry 157:1864–1866

Fowler CD, Lu Q, Johnson PM, Marks MJ, Kenny PJ (2011) Habenular alpha5 nicotinic receptor subunit signalling controls nicotine intake. Nature 471:597–601

Fowler CD, Tuesta L, Kenny PJ (2013) Role of alpha5* nicotinic acetylcholine receptors in the effects of acute and chronic nicotine treatment on brain reward function in mice. Psychopharmacology 229(3):503–513

Froeliger B, Kozink RV, Rose JE, Behm FM, Salley AN, McClernon FJ (2010) Hippocampal and striatal gray matter volume are associated with a smoking cessation treatment outcome: results of an exploratory voxel-based morphometric analysis. Psychopharmacology 210:577–583

Garrison KA, O'Malley SS, Gueorguieva R, Krishnan-Sarin S (2018) A fMRI study on the impact of advertising for flavored e-cigarettes on susceptible young adults. Drug Alcohol Depend 186:233–241

George AA, Bloy A, Miwa JM, Lindstrom JM, Lukas RJ, Whiteaker P (2017) Isoform-specific mechanisms of alpha3beta4*-nicotinic acetylcholine receptor modulation by the prototoxin lynx1. FASEB J 31:1398–1420

Gerzanich V, Wang F, Kuryatov A, Lindstrom J (1998) Alpha 5 subunit alters desensitization, pharmacology, Ca++ permeability and Ca++ modulation of human neuronal alpha 3 nicotinic receptors. J Pharmacol Exp Ther 286:311–320

Girod R, Role LW (2001) Long-lasting enhancement of glutamatergic synaptic transmission by acetylcholine contrasts with response adaptation after exposure to low-level nicotine. J Neurosci 21:5182–5190

Goniewicz ML, Smith DM, Edwards KC, Blount BC, Caldwell KL, Feng J, Wang L, Christensen C, Ambrose B, Borek N, van Bemmel D, Konkel K, Erives G, Stanton CA, Lambert E, Kimmel HL, Hatsukami D, Hecht SS, Niaura RS, Travers M, Lawrence C, Hyland AJ (2018) Comparison of nicotine and toxicant exposure in users of electronic cigarettes and combustible cigarettes. JAMA Netw Open 1:e185937

Gonzales D, Rennard SI, Nides M, Oncken C, Azoulay S, Billing CB, Watsky EJ, Gong J, Williams KE, Reeves KR, Varenicline Phase 3 Study Group (2006) Varenicline, an alpha4beta2 nicotinic acetylcholine receptor partial agonist, vs sustained-release bupropion and placebo for smoking cessation: a randomized controlled trial. JAMA 296:47–55

Hall BJ, Wells C, Allenby C, Lin MY, Hao I, Marshall L, Rose JE, Levin ED (2014) Differential effects of non-nicotine tobacco constituent compounds on nicotine self-administration in rats. Pharmacol Biochem Behav 120:103–108

Harris AC, Muelken P, Haave Z, Swain Y, Smethells JR, LeSage MG (2018) Propylene glycol, a major electronic cigarette constituent, attenuates the adverse effects of high-dose nicotine as measured by intracranial self-stimulation in rats. Drug Alcohol Depend 193:162–168

Hartmann-Boyce J, Cahill K, Hatsukami D, Cornuz J (2012) Nicotine vaccines for smoking cessation. Cochrane Database Syst Rev 8:CD007072

Hartmann-Boyce J, Chepkin SC, Ye W, Bullen C, Lancaster T (2018) Nicotine replacement therapy versus control for smoking cessation. Cochrane Database Syst Rev 5:CD000146

Henderson BJ, Srinivasan R, Nichols WA, Dilworth CN, Gutierrez DF, Mackey ED, McKinney S, Drenan RM, Richards CI, Lester HA (2014) Nicotine exploits a COPI-mediated process for chaperone-mediated up-regulation of its receptors. J Gen Physiol 143:51–66

Hill JA Jr, Zoli M, Bourgeois JP, Changeux JP (1993) Immunocytochemical localization of a neuronal nicotinic receptor: the beta 2-subunit. J Neurosci 13:1551–1568

Huang YY, Kandel ER, Levine A (2008) Chronic nicotine exposure induces a long-lasting and pathway-specific facilitation of LTP in the amygdala. Learn Mem 15:603–610

Ibanez-Tallon I, Miwa JM, Wang HL, Adams NC, Crabtree GW, Sine SM, Heintz N (2002) Novel modulation of neuronal nicotinic acetylcholine receptors by association with the endogenous prototoxin lynx1. Neuron 33:893–903

Jackson KJ, Martin BR, Changeux JP, Damaj MI (2008) Differential role of nicotinic acetylcholine receptor subunits in physical and affective nicotine withdrawal signs. J Pharmacol Exp Ther 325:302–312

Jackson KJ, Kota DH, Martin BR, Damaj MI (2009) The role of various nicotinic receptor subunits and factors influencing nicotine conditioned place aversion. Neuropharmacology 56:970–974

Jackson KJ, Marks MJ, Vann RE, Chen X, Gamage TF, Warner JA, Damaj MI (2010) Role of alpha5 nicotinic acetylcholine receptors in pharmacological and behavioral effects of nicotine in mice. J Pharmacol Exp Ther 334:137–146

Jackson KJ, Sanjakdar SS, Muldoon PP, McIntosh JM, Damaj MI (2013) The alpha3beta4* nicotinic acetylcholine receptor subtype mediates nicotine reward and physical nicotine withdrawal signs independently of the alpha5 subunit in the mouse. Neuropharmacology 70:228–235

Ji D, Lape R, Dani JA (2001) Timing and location of nicotinic activity enhances or depresses hippocampal synaptic plasticity. Neuron 31:131–141

Jin Z, Khan P, Shin Y, Wang J, Lin L, Cameron MD, Lindstrom JM, Kenny PJ, Kamenecka TM (2014) Synthesis and activity of substituted heteroaromatics as positive allosteric modulators for alpha4beta2alpha5 nicotinic acetylcholine receptors. Bioorg Med Chem Lett 24:674–678

John D, Berg DK (2015) Long-lasting changes in neural networks to compensate for altered nicotinic input. Biochem Pharmacol 97:418–424

Jones S, Yakel JL (1997) Functional nicotinic ACh receptors on interneurons in the rat hippocampus. J Physiol 504(Pt 3):603–610

Kallupi M, Xue S, Zhou B, Janda KD, George O (2018) An enzymatic approach reverses nicotine dependence, decreases compulsive-like intake, and prevents relapse. Sci Adv 4:eaat4751

Kassiou M, Eberl S, Meikle SR, Birrell A, Constable C, Fulham MJ, Wong DF, Musachio JL (2001) In vivo imaging of nicotinic receptor upregulation following chronic (−)-nicotine treatment in baboon using SPECT. Nucl Med Biol 28:165–175

Kendler KS, Thornton LM, Pedersen NL (2000) Tobacco consumption in Swedish twins reared apart and reared together. Arch Gen Psychiatry 57:886–892

Kenney JW, Poole RL, Adoff MD, Logue SF, Gould TJ (2012) Learning and nicotine interact to increase CREB phosphorylation at the jnk1 promoter in the hippocampus. PLoS One 7:e39939

Klink R, de Kerchove d'Exaerde A, Zoli M, Changeux JP (2001) Molecular and physiological diversity of nicotinic acetylcholine receptors in the midbrain dopaminergic nuclei. J Neurosci 21:1452–1463

Kong G, Morean ME, Cavallo DA, Camenga DR, Krishnan-Sarin S (2015) Reasons for electronic cigarette experimentation and discontinuation among adolescents and young adults. Nicotine Tob Res 17:847–854

Kuhn S, Schubert F, Gallinat J (2010) Reduced thickness of medial orbitofrontal cortex in smokers. Biol Psychiatry 68:1061–1065

Kuryatov A, Berrettini W, Lindstrom J (2011) Acetylcholine receptor (AChR) alpha5 subunit variant associated with risk for nicotine dependence and lung cancer reduces (alpha4beta2) alpha5 AChR function. Mol Pharmacol 79:119–125

Lagostena L, Trocme-Thibierge C, Morain P, Cherubini E (2008) The partial alpha7 nicotine acetylcholine receptor agonist S 24795 enhances long-term potentiation at CA3-CA1 synapses in the adult mouse hippocampus. Neuropharmacology 54:676–685

Lanca AJ, Adamson KL, Coen KM, Chow BL, Corrigall WA (2000) The pedunculopontine tegmental nucleus and the role of cholinergic neurons in nicotine self-administration in the rat: a correlative neuroanatomical and behavioral study. Neuroscience 96:735–742

Law AJ, Wang Y, Sei Y, O'Donnell P, Piantadosi P, Papaleo F, Straub RE, Huang W, Thomas CJ, Vakkalanka R, Besterman AD, Lipska BK, Hyde TM, Harrison PJ, Kleinman JE, Weinberger DR (2012) Neuregulin 1-ErbB4-PI3K signaling in schizophrenia and phosphoinositide 3-kinase-p110delta inhibition as a potential therapeutic strategy. Proc Natl Acad Sci U S A 109:12165–12170

Le Foll B, Goldberg SR (2005) Control of the reinforcing effects of nicotine by associated environmental stimuli in animals and humans. Trends Pharmacol Sci 26:287–293

Lenz B, Klafki HW, Hillemacher T, Killisch N, Schaller G, Frieling H, Clepce M, Gossler A, Thuerauf N, Winterer G, Kornhuber J, Bleich S (2010) Smoking behaviour is associated with expression and phosphorylation of CREB in human buffy coat. Int J Neuropsychopharmacol 13:207–215

Li P, Steinbach JH (2010) The neuronal nicotinic alpha4beta2 receptor has a high maximal probability of being open. Br J Pharmacol 160:1906–1915

Li MD, Cheng R, Ma JZ, Swan GE (2003) A meta-analysis of estimated genetic and environmental effects on smoking behavior in male and female adult twins. Addiction 98:23–31

Li Y, Yuan K, Cai C, Feng D, Yin J, Bi Y, Shi S, Yu D, Jin C, von Deneen KM, Qin W, Tian J (2015) Reduced frontal cortical thickness and increased caudate volume within fronto-striatal circuits in young adult smokers. Drug Alcohol Depend 151:211–219

Lisman JE, Grace AA (2005) The hippocampal-VTA loop: controlling the entry of information into long-term memory. Neuron 46:703–713

Liu JZ, Tozzi F, Waterworth DM, Pillai SG, Muglia P, Middleton L, Berrettini W, Knouff CW, Yuan X, Waeber G, Vollenweider P, Preisig M, Wareham NJ, Zhao JH, Loos RJ, Barroso I, Khaw KT, Grundy S, Barter P, Mahley R, Kesaniemi A, McPherson R, Vincent JB, Strauss J, Kennedy JL, Farmer A, McGuffin P, Day R, Matthews K, Bakke P, Gulsvik A, Lucae S, Ising M, Brueckl T, Horstmann S, Wichmann HE, Rawal R, Dahmen N, Lamina C, Polasek O, Zgaga L, Huffman J, Campbell S, Kooner J, Chambers JC, Burnett MS, Devaney JM, Pichard AD, Kent KM, Satler L, Lindsay JM, Waksman R, Epstein S, Wilson JF, Wild SH, Campbell H, Vitart V, Reilly MP, Li M, Qu L, Wilensky R, Matthai W, Hakonarson HH, Rader DJ, Franke A, Wittig M, Schafer A, Uda M, Terracciano A, Xiao X, Busonero F, Scheet P, Schlessinger D, St Clair D, Rujescu D, Abecasis GR, Grabe HJ, Teumer A, Volzke H, Petersmann A, John U, Rudan I, Hayward C, Wright AF, Kolcic I, Wright BJ, Thompson JR, Balmforth AJ, Hall AS, Samani NJ, Anderson CA, Ahmad T, Mathew CG, Parkes M, Satsangi J, Caulfield M, Munroe PB, Farrall M, Dominiczak A, Worthington J, Thomson W, Eyre S, Barton A, Mooser V, Francks C, Marchini J (2010) Meta-analysis and imputation refines the association of 15q25 with smoking quantity. Nat Genet 42:436–440

Livingston CJ, Freeman RJ, Costales VC, Westhoff JL, Caplan LS, Sherin KM, Niebuhr DW (2019) Electronic nicotine delivery systems or e-cigarettes: American College of Preventive Medicine's practice statement. Am J Prev Med 56:167–178

Loukola A, Broms U, Maunu H, Widen E, Heikkila K, Siivola M, Salo A, Pergadia ML, Nyman E, Sammalisto S, Perola M, Agrawal A, Heath AC, Martin NG, Madden PA, Peltonen L, Kaprio J (2008) Linkage of nicotine dependence and smoking behavior on 10q, 7q and 11p in twins with homogeneous genetic background. Pharmacogenomics J 8:209–219

Loukola A, Wedenoja J, Keskitalo-Vuokko K, Broms U, Korhonen T, Ripatti S, Sarin AP, Pitkaniemi J, He L, Happola A, Heikkila K, Chou YL, Pergadia ML, Heath AC, Montgomery GW, Martin NG, Madden PA, Kaprio J (2014) Genome-wide association study on detailed profiles of smoking behavior and nicotine dependence in a twin sample. Mol Psychiatry 19:615–624

Lyukmanova EN, Shenkarev ZO, Shulepko MA, Mineev KS, D'Hoedt D, Kasheverov IE, Filkin SY, Krivolapova AP, Janickova H, Dolezal V, Dolgikh DA, Arseniev AS, Bertrand D, Tsetlin VI, Kirpichnikov MP (2011) NMR structure and action on nicotinic acetylcholine receptors of water-soluble domain of human LYNX1. J Biol Chem 286:10618–10627

Mansvelder HD, McGehee DS (2000) Long-term potentiation of excitatory inputs to brain reward areas by nicotine. Neuron 27:349–357

Markou A, Kenny PJ (2002) Neuroadaptations to chronic exposure to drugs of abuse: relevance to depressive symptomatology seen across psychiatric diagnostic categories. Neurotox Res 4:297–313

Marks MJ, Burch JB, Collins AC (1983) Effects of chronic nicotine infusion on tolerance development and nicotinic receptors. J Pharmacol Exp Ther 226:817–825

Maskos U (2010) Role of endogenous acetylcholine in the control of the dopaminergic system via nicotinic receptors. J Neurochem 114:641–646

McClernon FJ, Gilbert DG (2004) Human functional neuroimaging in nicotine and tobacco research: basics, background, and beyond. Nicotine Tob Res 6:941–959

Miech R, Johnston L, O'Malley PM, Bachman JG, Patrick ME (2019) Adolescent vaping and nicotine use in 2017–2018 – U.S. National Estimates. N Engl J Med 380:192–193

Miwa JM, Walz A (2012) Enhancement in motor learning through genetic manipulation of the Lynx1 gene. PLoS One 7:e43302

Miwa JM, Ibanez-Tallon I, Crabtree GW, Sanchez R, Sali A, Role LW, Heintz N (1999) Lynx1, an endogenous toxin-like modulator of nicotinic acetylcholine receptors in the mammalian CNS. Neuron 23:105–114

Miwa JM, Freedman R, Lester HA (2011) Neural systems governed by nicotinic acetylcholine receptors: emerging hypotheses. Neuron 70:20–33

Myers WD, Ng KT, Singer G (1982) Intravenous self-administration of acetaldehyde in the rat as a function of schedule, food deprivation and photoperiod. Pharmacol Biochem Behav 17:807–811

Nakauchi S, Sumikawa K (2012) Endogenously released ACh and exogenous nicotine differentially facilitate long-term potentiation induction in the hippocampal CA1 region of mice. Eur J Neurosci 35:1381–1395

Nestler EJ (2005) Is there a common molecular pathway for addiction? Nat Neurosci 8:1445–1449

Nissen NI, Anderson KR, Wang H, Lee HS, Garrison C, Eichelberger SA, Ackerman K, Im W, Miwa JM (2018) Augmenting the antinociceptive effects of nicotinic acetylcholine receptor activity through lynx1 modulation. PLoS One 13:e0199643

Okuyemi KS, Faseru B, Sanderson Cox L, Bronars CA, Ahluwalia JS (2007) Relationship between menthol cigarettes and smoking cessation among African American light smokers. Addiction 102:1979–1986

Omelchenko N, Sesack SR (2005) Laterodorsal tegmental projections to identified cell populations in the rat ventral tegmental area. J Comp Neurol 483:217–235

Orejarena MJ, Herrera-Solis A, Pons S, Maskos U, Maldonado R, Robledo P (2012) Selective re-expression of beta2 nicotinic acetylcholine receptor subunits in the ventral tegmental area of the mouse restores intravenous nicotine self-administration. Neuropharmacology 63:235–241

Pandhare A, Pappu AS, Wilms H, Blanton MP, Jansen M (2017) The antidepressant bupropion is a negative allosteric modulator of serotonin type 3A receptors. Neuropharmacology 113:89–99

Pang X, Liu L, Ngolab J, Zhao-Shea R, McIntosh JM, Gardner PD, Tapper AR (2016) Habenula cholinergic neurons regulate anxiety during nicotine withdrawal via nicotinic acetylcholine receptors. Neuropharmacology 107:294–304

Peana AT, Muggironi G, Diana M (2010) Acetaldehyde-reinforcing effects: a study on oral self-administration behavior. Front Psych 1:23

Perry DC, Davila-Garcia MI, Stockmeier CA, Kellar KJ (1999) Increased nicotinic receptors in brains from smokers: membrane binding and autoradiography studies. J Pharmacol Exp Ther 289:1545–1552

Picciotto MR, Zoli M, Rimondini R, Lena C, Marubio LM, Pich EM, Fuxe K, Changeux JP (1998) Acetylcholine receptors containing the beta2 subunit are involved in the reinforcing properties of nicotine. Nature 391:173–177

Pittaras EC, Faure A, Leray X, Moraitopoulou E, Cressant A, Rabat AA, Meunier C, Fossier P, Granon S (2016) Neuronal nicotinic receptors are crucial for tuning of E/I balance in prelimbic cortex and for decision-making processes. Front Psych 7:171

Pons S, Fattore L, Cossu G, Tolu S, Porcu E, McIntosh JM, Changeux JP, Maskos U, Fratta W (2008) Crucial role of alpha4 and alpha6 nicotinic acetylcholine receptor subunits from ventral tegmental area in systemic nicotine self-administration. J Neurosci 28:12318–12327

Portugal GS, Wilkinson DS, Turner JR, Blendy JA, Gould TJ (2012) Developmental effects of acute, chronic, and withdrawal from chronic nicotine on fear conditioning. Neurobiol Learn Mem 97:482–494

Ramirez-Latorre J, Yu CR, Qu X, Perin F, Karlin A, Role L (1996) Functional contributions of alpha5 subunit to neuronal acetylcholine receptor channels. Nature 380:347–351

Saccone NL, Wang JC, Breslau N, Johnson EO, Hatsukami D, Saccone SF, Grucza RA, Sun L, Duan W, Budde J, Culverhouse RC, Fox L, Hinrichs AL, Steinbach JH, Wu M, Rice JP, Goate AM, Bierut LJ (2009) The CHRNA5-CHRNA3-CHRNB4 nicotinic receptor subunit gene cluster affects risk for nicotine dependence in African-Americans and in European-Americans. Cancer Res 69:6848–6856

Salas R, Sturm R, Boulter J, De Biasi M (2009) Nicotinic receptors in the habenulo-interpeduncular system are necessary for nicotine withdrawal in mice. J Neurosci 29:3014–3018

Salminen O, Murphy KL, McIntosh JM, Drago J, Marks MJ, Collins AC, Grady SR (2004) Subunit composition and pharmacology of two classes of striatal presynaptic nicotinic acetylcholine receptors mediating dopamine release in mice. Mol Pharmacol 65:1526–1535

Sanjakdar SS, Maldoon PP, Marks MJ, Brunzell DH, Maskos U, McIntosh JM, Bowers MS, Damaj MI (2015) Differential roles of alpha6beta2* and alpha4beta2* neuronal nicotinic receptors in nicotine- and cocaine-conditioned reward in mice. Neuropsychopharmacology 40:350–360

Schoenbaum G, Chang CY, Lucantonio F, Takahashi YK (2016) Thinking outside the box: orbitofrontal cortex, imagination, and how we can treat addiction. Neuropsychopharmacology 41:2966–2976

Smith TT, Schaff MB, Rupprecht LE, Schassburger RL, Buffalari DM, Murphy SE, Sved AF, Donny EC (2015) Effects of MAO inhibition and a combination of minor alkaloids, beta-carbolines, and acetaldehyde on nicotine self-administration in adult male rats. Drug Alcohol Depend 155:243–252

Srinivasan R, Pantoja R, Moss FJ, Mackey ED, Son CD, Miwa J, Lester HA (2011) Nicotine up-regulates alpha4beta2 nicotinic receptors and ER exit sites via stoichiometry-dependent chaperoning. J Gen Physiol 137:59–79

Stoker AK, Olivier B, Markou A (2012) Role of alpha7- and beta4-containing nicotinic acetylcholine receptors in the affective and somatic aspects of nicotine withdrawal: studies in knockout mice. Behav Genet 42:423–436

Strasser AA, Malaiyandi V, Hoffmann E, Tyndale RF, Lerman C (2007) An association of CYP2A6 genotype and smoking topography. Nicotine Tob Res 9:511–518

Sullivan PF, Kendler KS (1999) The genetic epidemiology of smoking. Nicotine Tob Res 1(Suppl 2):S51–S57; discussion S69–70

Tang J, Dani JA (2009) Dopamine enables in vivo synaptic plasticity associated with the addictive drug nicotine. Neuron 63:673–682

Tapper AR, McKinney SL, Nashmi R, Schwarz J, Deshpande P, Labarca C, Whiteaker P, Marks MJ, Collins AC, Lester HA (2004) Nicotine activation of alpha4* receptors: sufficient for reward, tolerance, and sensitization. Science 306:1029–1032

Tekinay AB, Nong Y, Miwa JM, Lieberam I, Ibanez-Tallon I, Greengard P, Heintz N (2009) A role for LYNX2 in anxiety-related behavior. Proc Natl Acad Sci U S A 106:4477–4482

Thomsen MS, Mikkelsen JD (2012) Type I and II positive allosteric modulators differentially modulate agonist-induced up-regulation of alpha7 nicotinic acetylcholine receptors. J Neurochem 123:73–83

Tonstad S, Heggen E, Giljam H, Lagerback PA, Tonnesen P, Wikingsson LD, Lindblom N, de Villiers S, Svensson TH, Fagerstrom KO (2013) Niccine(R), a nicotine vaccine, for relapse prevention: a phase II, randomized, placebo-controlled, multicenter clinical trial. Nicotine Tob Res 15:1492–1501

Truman P, Grounds P, Brennan KA (2017) Monoamine oxidase inhibitory activity in tobacco particulate matter: are harman and norharman the only physiologically relevant inhibitors? Neurotoxicology 59:22–26

Tuesta LM, Chen Z, Duncan A, Fowler CD, Ishikawa M, Lee BR, Liu XA, Lu Q, Cameron M, Hayes MR, Kamenecka TM, Pletcher M, Kenny PJ (2017) GLP-1 acts on habenular avoidance circuits to control nicotine intake. Nat Neurosci 20:708–716

Turner JR, Castellano LM, Blendy JA (2011) Parallel anxiolytic-like effects and upregulation of neuronal nicotinic acetylcholine receptors following chronic nicotine and varenicline. Nicotine Tob Res 13:41–46

Turner JR, Wilkinson DS, Poole RL, Gould TJ, Carlson GC, Blendy JA (2013) Divergent functional effects of sazetidine-a and varenicline during nicotine withdrawal. Neuropsychopharmacology 38:2035–2047

Turner JR, Ray R, Lee B, Everett L, Xiang J, Jepson C, Kaestner KH, Lerman C, Blendy JA (2014) Evidence from mouse and man for a role of neuregulin 3 in nicotine dependence. Mol Psychiatry 19:801–810

Vazquez-Sanroman DB, Monje RD, Bardo MT (2016) Nicotine self-administration remodels perineuronal nets in ventral tegmental area and orbitofrontal cortex in adult male rats. Addict Biol 22(6):1743–1755

Villanti AC, Johnson AL, Ambrose BK, Cummings KM, Stanton CA, Rose SW, Feirman SP, Tworek C, Glasser AM, Pearson JL, Cohn AM, Conway KP, Niaura RS, Bansal-Travers M, Hyland A (2017) Flavored tobacco product use in youth and adults: findings from the first wave of the PATH study (2013–2014). Am J Prev Med 53(2):139–151

Vullhorst D, Ahmad T, Karavanova I, Keating C, Buonanno A (2017) Structural similarities between Neuregulin 1-3 isoforms determine their subcellular distribution and signaling mode in central neurons. J Neurosci 37:5232–5249

Wada E, Wada K, Boulter J, Deneris E, Heinemann S, Patrick J, Swanson LW (1989) Distribution of alpha 2, alpha 3, alpha 4, and beta 2 neuronal nicotinic receptor subunit mRNAs in the central nervous system: a hybridization histochemical study in the rat. J Comp Neurol 284:314–335

Walters CL, Cleck JN, Kuo YC, Blendy JA (2005) Mu-opioid receptor and CREB activation are required for nicotine reward. Neuron 46:933–943

Walters CL, Brown S, Changeux JP, Martin B, Damaj MI (2006) The beta2 but not alpha7 subunit of the nicotinic acetylcholine receptor is required for nicotine-conditioned place preference in mice. Psychopharmacology 184:339–344

Welsby PJ, Rowan MJ, Anwyl R (2009) Intracellular mechanisms underlying the nicotinic enhancement of LTP in the rat dentate gyrus. Eur J Neurosci 29:65–75

Wilking JA, Stitzel JA (2015) Natural genetic variability of the neuronal nicotinic acetylcholine receptor subunit genes in mice: consequences and confounds. Neuropharmacology 96:205–212

Williams JM, Gandhi KK, Steinberg ML, Foulds J, Ziedonis DM, Benowitz NL (2007) Higher nicotine and carbon monoxide levels in menthol cigarette smokers with and without schizophrenia. Nicotine Tob Res 9:873–881

Williams DK, Stokes C, Horenstein NA, Papke RL (2011) The effective opening of nicotinic acetylcholine receptors with single agonist binding sites. J Gen Physiol 137:369–384

Xian H, Scherrer JF, Madden PAF, Lyons MJ, Tsuang M, True WR, Eisen SA (2003) The heritability of failed smoking cessation and nicotine withdrawal in twins who smoked and attempted to quit. Nicotine Tob Res 5:245–254

Yuan M, Malagon AM, Yasuda D, Belluzzi JD, Leslie FM, Zaveri NT (2017) The alpha3beta4 nAChR partial agonist AT-1001 attenuates stress-induced reinstatement of nicotine seeking in a rat model of relapse and induces minimal withdrawal in dependent rats. Behav Brain Res 333:251–257

Zhang M, Harrison E, Biswas L, Tran T, Liu X (2018) Menthol facilitates dopamine-releasing effect of nicotine in rat nucleus accumbens. Pharmacol Biochem Behav 175:47–52

Zhou L, Fisher ML, Cole RD, Gould TJ, Parikh V, Ortinski PI, Turner JR (2018) Neuregulin 3 signaling mediates nicotine-dependent synaptic plasticity in the orbitofrontal cortex and cognition. Neuropsychopharmacology 43:1343–1354

Randomized Clinical Trials Investigating Innovative Interventions for Smoking Cessation in the Last Decade

Marie N. S. Gendy, Christine Ibrahim, Matthew E. Sloan, and Bernard Le Foll

Contents

1 Introduction 2
2 Cholinergic System 3
  2.1 Agonists 3
  2.2 Antagonists 4
  2.3 Positive Allosteric Modulators and Acetylcholinesterase Inhibitors 4
3 Endocannabinoid System 5

Marie N. S. Gendy and Christine Ibrahim contributed equally to this work.

M. N. S. Gendy · C. Ibrahim
Translational Addiction Research Laboratory, Centre for Addiction and Mental Health, Toronto, ON, Canada

Department of Pharmacology, University of Toronto, Toronto, ON, Canada

M. E. Sloan
Department of Psychiatry, Yale University School of Medicine, New Haven, CT, USA

B. Le Foll (✉)
Translational Addiction Research Laboratory, Centre for Addiction and Mental Health, Toronto, ON, Canada

Department of Pharmacology, University of Toronto, Toronto, ON, Canada

Addictions Division, Campbell Family Mental Health Research Institute, Centre for Addiction and Mental Health, Toronto, ON, Canada

Division of Brain and Therapeutics, Department of Psychiatry, University of Toronto, Toronto, ON, Canada

Institute of Medical Sciences, University of Toronto, Toronto, ON, Canada

Alcohol Research and Treatment Clinic, Centre for Addiction and Mental Health, Toronto, ON, Canada

Department of Family and Community Medicine, University of Toronto, Toronto, ON, Canada
e-mail: Bernard.LeFoll@camh.ca

M. A. Nader, Y. L. Hurd (eds.), *Substance Use Disorders*,
Handbook of Experimental Pharmacology 258, https://doi.org/10.1007/164_2019_253

3.1 CB1 Receptor Inverse Agonists 6
3.2 Cannabidiol 6
4 Naltrexone 6
5 Lorcaserin 7
6 Antidepressants 8
6.1 Selective Serotonin Reuptake Inhibitors 8
6.2 Monoamine Oxidase Inhibitors 9
6.3 Tricyclic Antidepressants 9
6.4 Nontraditional Antidepressants 10
7 The Noradrenergic System 10
8 Anti-epileptic Drugs 11
8.1 Gabapentin and Pregabalin 11
8.2 Topiramate and Zonisamide 11
9 Gamma-Aminobutyric Acid (GABA) Receptors 12
10 Glucagon-Like Peptide-1 (GLP-1) Receptor Agonists 12
11 Statins 13
12 Stimulants and Atomoxetine 13
12.1 Attention Deficit Hyperactivity Disorder (ADHD) Medications 13
12.2 Atomoxetine 14
12.3 Modafinil 14
13 N-Acetylcysteine 14
14 N-Methyl-D-Aspartate (NMDA) Receptors 15
15 Progesterone 15
16 Conclusion 16
References 17

Abstract

Every year, billions of dollars are spent treating smoking and related conditions, yet smoking-related morbidity and mortality continue to rise. There are currently only three FDA-approved medications for smoking cessation: nicotine replacement therapy, bupropion, and varenicline. Although these medications increase abstinence rates, most individuals relapse following treatment. This chapter reviews clinical trials published within the past 10 years investigating novel smoking cessation pharmacotherapies. Among these pharmacotherapies, some showed promising results, such as cytisine and endocannabinoid modulators, whereas others failed to produce significant effects. More research is needed to develop drugs that produce higher rates of long-term abstinence and to determine which subgroups of patients benefit from a given treatment.

Keywords

Anticonvulsants · Antidepressive agents · Cannabinoid receptor modulators · Cholinergic agents · Randomized controlled trial · Smoking cessation · Smoking cessation agents · Tobacco use disorder

1 Introduction

Smoking addiction, now referred to by the DSM-5 as tobacco use disorder (TUD), is a complex condition that is thought to be caused by a combination of psychosocial and pharmacological factors (Mitchell and Potenza 2014). It is estimated that there are over one billion smokers worldwide. Tobacco-related morbidity is thought to lead to seven million deaths per year, and this number is expected to increase to eight to ten million deaths per year by 2030 (Burki 2015; Forouzanfar et al. 2015; Gowing et al. 2015). Unfortunately, quitting smoking is extremely difficult; less than 5% of quit attempts per year are considered successful despite the fact that 70% of smokers wish to quit (Schauer et al. 2015).

Nicotine is the most addictive ingredient in cigarettes (Le Foll and Goldberg 2006). Nicotine binds to nicotinic cholinergic receptors (nAChRs), which are ligand-gated ion channels. The reinforcing effects of nicotine are mediated through the release of various neurotransmitters including dopamine, which plays a fundamental role in reward, as well as acetylcholine, vasopressin, serotonin, norepinephrine, glutamate, gamma-aminobutyric acid (GABA), and beta-endorphins (David et al. 2014; Le Foll 2013). Researchers are continuously searching for medications that target one or more of these neurotransmitter systems in the hopes of finding new effective smoking cessation aids (Bozinoff and Le Foll 2018).

There are currently three pharmacotherapies for smoking cessation that are approved by the Food and Drug Administration (FDA): nicotine replacement therapy (NRT), bupropion hydrochloride, and varenicline tartrate (Le Foll and George 2007; Prochaska and Benowitz 2016). NRT products include gum, patches, inhalers, nasal and oral sprays, and lozenges, and their main benefits are the reduction of craving and withdrawal symptoms induced by tobacco cessation (Stead et al. 2012). Bupropion hydrochloride acts by blocking nAChRs, as well as norepinephrine and dopamine reuptake, which reduces smoking cessation-induced craving, withdrawal symptoms, and negative mood (Kotlyar et al. 2011; McCarthy et al. 2008). Varenicline tartrate, a selective $\alpha 4\beta 2*$ nicotinic receptor partial agonist (the asterisk indicates the potential presence of other subunits) (Cahill et al. 2013), is thought to be the most effective medication for smoking cessation. Although FDA-approved medications increase abstinence rates, relapse remains the most likely outcome, with abstinence rates of only 20–30% at 1 year posttreatment (Cahill et al. 2007). New pharmacotherapies are needed for TUD in order to achieve higher rates of long-term abstinence.

2 Cholinergic System

The addictive effects of tobacco are thought to arise from activation of nicotinic acetylcholine receptors (nAChRs) in the ventral tegmental area and the nucleus accumbens (Weinberger and Sofuoglu 2009). Hence, a great deal of smoking cessation research has focused on drugs that target nAChRs. However, not all drugs targeting nAChRs act in the same way. For instance, varenicline acts as a partial agonist at $\alpha4\beta2*$ (Coe et al. 2005), whereas bupropion is a noncompetitive antagonist at $\alpha3\beta2$, $\alpha4\beta2*$, and less effectively at $\alpha7$ (Slemmer et al. 2000). The different nAChR subtypes have been extensively characterized in preclinical studies (Benowitz 2010; Mineur and Picciotto 2008).

2.1 Agonists

In the past decade, three nAChR agonists without FDA approval have been tested for use as smoking cessation aids: dianicline, encenicline, and cytisine. Dianicline is a partial agonist of the $\alpha4\beta2*$ nicotinic acetylcholine receptor subtype. It showed promising effects in Phase I and II studies. However, in a Phase III trial, researchers found no benefit of dianicline treatment on abstinence rates compared to placebo (Tonstad et al. 2011), and the drug was withdrawn from future development. Around the same time, it was shown that binding affinity to $\alpha4\beta2*$ nAChRs is two orders of magnitude lower for dianicline compared to varenicline (Rollema et al. 2010). Similarly, encenicline, an $\alpha7$ nAChR partial agonist, did not show any benefit for smoking cessation when compared to placebo or when co-administered with nicotine replacement therapy (Schuster et al. 2018).

Cytisine is a partial agonist of $\alpha4\beta2*$ derived from plants of the Leguminosae (Fabaceae) family (Izaddoost et al. 1976). In 1964, cytisine (Tabex®) was marketed as a smoking cessation aid in Central and Eastern Europe (Tutka and Zatonski 2006). However, it still has not been approved in Western countries, except in Canada where it was approved as a natural health product in 2016 (Government of Canada 2018). Cytisine has been shown to be both a beneficial smoking cessation aid and a cost-effective treatment. A typical course of treatment with cytisine lasts 25 days and costs as little as $20, whereas varenicline treatment typically lasts 12 weeks and costs around $500 (Prochaska et al. 2013). Many clinical trials have demonstrated beneficial effects of cytisine, such as one study that found that 10.6% of participants given cytisine were continuously abstinent after 26 weeks, as compared to 1.2% of participants given placebo (Vinnikov et al. 2008). A similar trial was conducted investigating abstinence rates at 12 months (West et al. 2011). Rates of abstinence in the cytisine group were 8.4%, compared to 2.4% in the placebo group. When compared to nicotine replacement therapy, cytisine was found to be superior at 1 week, 1 month, 2 months, and 6 months of follow-up (Walker et al. 2014). It should be noted that over the 6 months, those given cytisine reported more adverse effects, mainly nausea, vomiting, and sleep disorders. The next step will be to determine whether cytisine is as effective as varenicline. Currently, there is an ongoing clinical trial investigating this in Maori smokers (Clinicaltrial.gov identifier NCT02957786) (Walker et al. 2018).

2.2 Antagonists

Mecamylamine is a nonselective and noncompetitive nAChR antagonist (Philip et al. 2012). Earlier smoking cessation trials with mecamylamine have demonstrated mixed results (Glover et al. 2007; Rose et al. 1994, 1996). More recently, researchers reanalyzed the results of a randomized placebo-controlled clinical trial evaluating the use of mecamylamine to treat alcohol use disorder in smokers and non-smokers (Roberts et al. 2018). They found no effect on smoking outcomes. However, it should be noted that motivation to quit smoking was not measured as this study was focused on the treatment of alcohol use disorder; hence participants may not have been interested in quitting smoking.

2.3 Positive Allosteric Modulators and Acetylcholinesterase Inhibitors

Positive allosteric modulators (PAM) of nicotinic acetylcholine receptors have been developed for smoking cessation. JNJ-39393406 is a PAM of the α7 subtype of nAChRs recently developed by Janssen Research and Development LLC. A group of researchers ran two studies, one with healthy smokers ($n = 31$) and another with smokers with schizophrenia ($n = 56$), but both studies were negative (Perkins et al. 2018). JNJ-39393406 did not improve abstinence rates, craving, or withdrawal when compared to placebo. Although this was not a large clinical trial, the researchers concluded that further research is not warranted at this particular dose (100 mg BID).

Two acetylcholinesterase inhibitors have recently been tested for smoking cessation. Galantamine, in addition to being an acetylcholinesterase inhibitor, is also a PAM of the α4β2* receptor. A recent 7-week trial randomized participants ($n = 60$) to 8 or 16 mg of galantamine per day or placebo (MacLean et al. 2018). During the pre-quit period, both doses of galantamine reduced urine cotinine levels and smoking in a laboratory choice task compared to placebo, but did not decrease self-reported cigarette smoking. Results following the quit attempt have not yet been published. Another acetylcholinesterase inhibitor, rivastigmine, has also been tested in alcohol-dependent smokers and methamphetamine-dependent smokers. In the alcohol dependence study, participants ($n = 26$) were randomized to either 6 mg/day of rivastigmine or placebo for 4 weeks. Rivastigmine was found to decrease the number of daily cigarettes consumed (−30%), tobacco craving (−18%), and carbon monoxide (CO) levels (−32%) (Diehl et al. 2009). In the methamphetamine dependence study, participants were randomized to 3 or 6 mg of rivastigmine or placebo for 9 days. They found that rivastigmine did not have any effects on smoking measures, but a trend was observed for reduction in urges to smoke (De la Garza and Yoon 2011). However, it should be noted that the sample size was small ($n = 13$), the participants were nontreatment seeking, and the duration of treatment was short. Further studies are necessary to determine whether rivastigmine is effective in smokers without comorbid addiction.

3 Endocannabinoid System

Weight gain is a serious concern for smokers who wish to quit, especially females. It is thought that nicotine increases basal metabolic rate and smoking cessation can lead to increased appetite and decreased energy consumption (Filozof et al. 2004). The current FDA-approved medications are not effective at preventing the weight gain associated with smoking cessation. For example, bupropion and NRT delay weight gain to some extent, but their effects do not last after treatment cessation (Parsons et al. 2009). It would be an asset if one agent could reduce both smoking rates and abstinence-related weight gain.

The endocannabinoid system is one of the central nervous system's neuromodulator systems. It is formed of cannabinoid receptors, endogenous cannabinoids (endocannabinoids), and various enzymes responsible for the synthesis or the degradation of the endocannabinoids. The cannabinoid receptors 1 and 2 (CB1 and CB2) are the main cannabinoid receptors which mediate the actions of endocannabinoids as well as the exogenous cannabinoids (Lu and Anderson 2017). Endocannabinoid system modulators facilitate weight loss in obesity (Drewnowski et al. 1995; King et al. 2013) and have also been shown to decrease nicotine self-administration in animal models (Cohen et al. 2002). These medications might be helpful in individuals who have difficulty quitting due to fear of weight gain or in individuals who relapse following smoking cessation-induced weigh gain.

3.1 CB1 Receptor Inverse Agonists

Rimonabant is a CB1 inverse agonist and has been previously used as a treatment for obesity (Curioni and Andre 2006; Sloan et al. 2017). Recently, the results of several large clinical trials for smoking cessation were published (Robinson et al. 2018). An analysis of the pooled data from these three trials ($n = 2097$) found that individuals treated with 20 mg of rimonabant had significantly higher rates of abstinence even at 48 weeks post-quit date compared to placebo (OR = 1.50, 95% CI: 1.03, 2.17) (Robinson et al. 2018). Nevertheless, the rimonabant group showed higher rates of side effects such as nausea, vomiting, diarrhea, and anxiety. The high rate of psychiatric side effects led to the voluntary withdrawal of rimonabant from the European market in 2008.

Other CB1 inverse agonists were also examined for smoking cessation. For example, surinabant was assessed at three different doses, 2.5 mg/day ($n = 199$), 5 mg/day ($n = 204$), or 10 mg/day ($n = 205$) vs. placebo ($n = 202$), during an 8-week treatment phase and 6-week follow-up and was not found to be effective (Tonstad and Aubin 2012). Another CB1 inverse agonist, taranabant, was also ineffective (Morrison et al. 2010). The poor efficacy of CB1 inverse agonists in these studies may have been at least partially due to the unfavorable side effect profile of these medications.

3.2 Cannabidiol

Cannabidiol (CBD), a non-psychoactive exogenous cannabinoid, acts on multiple non-cannabinoid receptors including serotonin 1A (5HT1A), peroxisome proliferator-activated receptor gamma (PPAR γ), and transient receptor potential vanilloid 1 (TRPV1) cation channels (Laprairie et al. 2015). Although CBD was previously thought to antagonize CB1 (Pertwee 2008), recent evidence suggests that it may actually function as a negative allosteric modulator (Tham et al. 2018). In a recent small trial ($n = 24$), smokers were randomized to treatment with cannabidiol (400 μg) or placebo inhalers. Those treated with cannabidiol showed a 40% decrease in the number of cigarettes smoked during the treatment period (1 week) and at follow-up (2 weeks after treatment) compared to those treated with placebo (Morgan et al. 2013). However, this trial was limited by the small sample size, short duration of follow-up, and the use of smoking reduction rather than cessation as an outcome. Nevertheless, given that CBD seems to have a better safety profile than rimonabant (Bergamaschi et al. 2011), further investigation remains worthwhile.

4 Naltrexone

Mu-opioid receptor antagonists may facilitate smoking cessation and weight reduction (Epstein and King 2004; Hutchison et al. 1999; King and Meyer 2000; Lee et al. 2005; Wewers et al. 1998). Naltrexone is a mu-opioid receptor antagonist that is FDA approved to treat alcohol and opioid use disorders. Researchers have considered its use as an adjunctive agent to augment the effect of nicotine replacement and to prevent weight gain following smoking cessation (King et al. 2006; O'Malley et al. 2006).

A recent randomized trial found that naltrexone in combination with NRT ($n = 162$) decreased weight gain and increased quit rates versus NRT with placebo ($n = 154$). The weight gain reduction was observed more in females (King et al. 2012). However, in 2013, a Cochrane review pooled data from 8 trials and concluded that naltrexone (25–100 mg/day) was not effective as a long-term smoking cessation aid either alone or in combination with NRT (RR 0.97; 95% CI 0.76–1.24, 1,213 participants) (David et al. 2013). It should be noted that many trials used nontreatment-seeking smokers and different groups tested different dosages, monitoring processes, and quitting plans, all of which could have affected the end results.

Naltrexone has also been examined in combination with bupropion, as this combination has been approved for weight loss in individuals with obesity. It is thought that weight loss is achieved through dual action: naltrexone decreases food reward by blocking endorphins and bupropion inhibits appetite (Tek 2016). Obese smokers were treated with naltrexone and bupropion in an open-label trial for 24 weeks. The results showed a decrease in tobacco use but no change in weight (Wilcox et al. 2010). A 24-week clinical trial using the combination of naltrexone and bupropion was also conducted in individuals with schizophrenia, who have high rates of both smoking and obesity (Marder et al. 2004; Morisano et al. 2009). This trial did not show a significant effect of treatment with naltrexone plus bupropion ($n = 11$) over placebo ($n = 10$) for either smoking cessation or weight reduction (Lyu et al. 2018).

5 Lorcaserin

Lorcaserin (Belviq®) is a drug approved by the FDA for weight loss (US Food and Drug Administration 2018a). It is a selective serotonin 5-HT_{2C} receptor agonist. In humans, 5-HT_{2C} receptors are mainly located in the central nervous system, primarily in the choroid plexus, prefrontal cortex, basal ganglia, and hippocampus (Roth et al. 1998). Given that obesity and drug addiction are thought to share similar neurobiological mechanisms (Volkow and Wise 2005), pharmacotherapies that are effective for obesity could potentially be used to treat substance use disorders as well.

In rats, lorcaserin has been found to reduce nicotine self-administration and nicotine-seeking behavior (Higgins et al. 2012; Levin et al. 2011). These favorable results led to the first clinical trial investigating lorcaserin for smoking cessation. A 12-week randomized controlled trial was conducted in which 603 participants were randomized to 10 mg of lorcaserin once a day (QD), 10 mg twice a day (BID), or placebo (Shanahan et al. 2017). At the end of 3 months of treatment, the BID group had a significantly higher abstinence rate compared to QD and placebo groups (15.3% for BID, 8.7% for QD, and 5.6% for placebo). Participants assigned to 10 mg BID of lorcaserin had the highest CO-confirmed abstinence rate, although these results did not reach significance. A single-arm trial investigating a combination of varenicline and lorcaserin for smoking cessation and post-cessation weight gain has also been published (Hurt et al. 2017). Among the 20 participants, 10 achieved prolonged smoking abstinence at the end of 12 weeks of treatment. Waist circumference increased by 0.2 ± 6.0 cm and weight increased by 1.1 ± 3.9 kg. There is also a completed clinical trial evaluating a combination of lorcaserin and the nicotine patch for smoking cessation, but to our knowledge, no data have been published as of yet (Clinicaltrial.gov identifier NCT02906644).

6 Antidepressants

Antidepressants constitute several classes of medication including selective serotonin reuptake inhibitors (SSRIs), serotonin and norepinephrine reuptake inhibitors (SNRIs), monoamine oxidase inhibitors (MAOIs), and tricyclic antidepressants (TCAs). The idea of treating TUD with antidepressants stemmed from observations that smokers were more likely to have a history of depression than non-smokers and that quitting smoking may lead to depression (Anda et al. 1990; Benowitz and Wilson Peng 2000). There have been even higher levels of interest in antidepressants as smoking cessation aids ever since bupropion (Zyban®), an antidepressant which inhibits norepinephrine and dopamine reuptake, was approved as a smoking cessation treatment (Richmond and Zwar 2003).

6.1 Selective Serotonin Reuptake Inhibitors

Selective serotonin reuptake inhibitors (SSRIs) are a class of antidepressants that function by blocking the reuptake of serotonin in presynaptic nerve terminals (Stahl 1998), thereby increasing synaptic levels of serotonin. There are various SSRIs on the market including fluoxetine, fluvoxamine, paroxetine, sertraline, citalopram, and escitalopram. Fluoxetine is the most studied SSRI for smoking cessation. There is evidence that its efficacy may be dependent on the population studied. For example, smokers with symptoms of depression or past history of major depressive disorder have been shown to benefit most from fluoxetine (Blondal et al. 1999; Dalack et al. 1995), although not all studies have found long-term efficacy (Spring et al. 2007). Nonetheless, these studies led researchers to focus on fluoxetine as a treatment for smokers with depressive symptoms.

Within the past decade, two clinical trials have been completed using fluoxetine for smoking cessation, both directed at smokers with depressive symptoms. Researchers evaluated whether administration of fluoxetine for longer periods prior to the target quit date would improve abstinence rates (Brown et al. 2014). They found that administering fluoxetine for 8 weeks instead of 2 weeks prior to the target quit date was more beneficial. However, the decrease in point prevalence abstinence was more evident at 6-month follow-up than 12-month follow-up, indicating a potential lack of long-term effectiveness. Another study found that treatment with fluoxetine 8 weeks prior to the target quit date did not affect abstinence rates compared to placebo (Minami et al. 2014). However, this study found that fluoxetine treatment reduced pre-quit depressive symptoms and craving in women and withdrawal-related negative affect in men, suggesting potential sex-specific effects.

6.2 Monoamine Oxidase Inhibitors

Monoamine oxidases (MAO) are enzymes that metabolize monoamine and indolamine neurotransmitters (e.g., dopamine, serotonin, norepinephrine) leading to their inactivation (Fiedorowicz and Swartz 2004). MAOs are divided into two subtypes, MAO-A and MAO-B. MAO-A selectivity metabolizes norepinephrine, serotonin, epinephrine, and dopamine, whereas MAO-B selective metabolizes dopamine and β-phenylethylamine (Krishnan 2007). Studies have shown smokers to have reduced MAO activity compared to non-smokers (Lewis et al. 2007; Rose et al. 2001). The rationale for using MAO inhibitors in smoking cessation is to mimic the reduced enzymatic activity found in smokers, which was hypothesized to facilitate quitting.

Selegiline, a selective inhibitor of monoamine oxidase B that is currently used to treat treatment-resistant depression (US Food and Drug Administration 2018b) and Parkinson's disease (US Food and Drug Administration 2018c), has been tested as a smoking cessation aid. Oral selegiline was initially shown to improve abstinence rates when compared to placebo or when used in conjunction with nicotine replacement therapy (NRT) (Biberman et al. 2003; George et al. 2003). However, these results are inconsistent with more recent trials. One trial testing oral selegiline for 8 weeks found that subjects given placebo had numerically higher rates of abstinence at the end of treatment (16% for selegiline and 20% for placebo) (Weinberger et al. 2010). Transdermal selegiline was also found to have no benefit in two other trials (Kahn et al. 2012; Killen et al. 2010). Most recently, EVT302, a new monoamine oxidase B inhibitor, was tested in a Phase II trial. EVT302 showed no superiority over placebo. Administering a nicotine patch along with EVT302 also did not show any additional benefit (Berlin et al. 2012).

6.3 Tricyclic Antidepressants

Tricyclic antidepressants are another class of antidepressant that affects serotonin and norepinephrine signaling (Feighner 1999). One particular tricyclic antidepressant, nortriptyline, has been studied extensively and is approved as a smoking cessation aid in New Zealand (Hughes et al. 2014). A meta-analysis of six clinical trials demonstrated a significant benefit of nortriptyline monotherapy on long-term smoking cessation rates compared to placebo (Hughes et al. 2014). More recently, two clinical trials were completed testing nortriptyline in conjunction with NRT. One study ($n = 901$) found that although both individual therapies were effective, combining the two treatments did not provide further benefits (Aveyard et al. 2008). Another study in a prison population ($n = 425$) also found no increased benefit of combining nortriptyline with NRT (Richmond et al. 2013). When these recent trials were analyzed together with two older but similar trials, there was insufficient evidence to suggest that the combination of nortriptyline and NRT was superior to NRT monotherapy (Hughes et al. 2014).

6.4 Nontraditional Antidepressants

Two nontraditional antidepressants, available primarily as supplements, have been tested for smoking cessation in healthy smokers. St. John's wort is an herbal supplement that is thought to inhibit the reuptake and metabolism of norepinephrine, dopamine, and serotonin (Butterweck 2003). In mice, St. John's wort decreased signs of nicotine withdrawal (Catania et al. 2003). However, when tested in a randomized clinical trial, various doses of St. John's wort did not increase smoking abstinence rates or decrease nicotine withdrawal when compared to placebo (Sood et al. 2010a). The dietary supplement, S-adenosyl-L-methionine (SAMe), is also thought to increase dopamine, norepinephrine, and serotonin levels (Sood et al.

2012) and is used as an antidepressant. When tested for smoking cessation, it was found that SAMe, like St. John's wort, did not increase abstinence rates or decrease tobacco withdrawal (Sood et al. 2012).

7 The Noradrenergic System

Preclinical studies indicate that the noradrenergic system may play a critical role in mediating nicotine reinforcement and nicotine seeking (Forget et al. 2010). Noradrenergic modulators such as labetalol, clonidine, and guanfacine have shown some success at decreasing nicotine craving in human laboratory paradigms (McKee et al. 2015; Sofuoglu et al. 2003) and some clinical trials (Gourlay et al. 2004). Clonidine is a centrally acting α2-adrenergic receptor agonist which lowers heart rate and peripheral resistance. A placebo-controlled trial testing clonidine showed weak evidence for its use as a smoking cessation aid based on abstinence results at 12 weeks of treatment (Gourlay et al. 2004). Side effects such as dizziness, dry mouth, and postural hypotension might limit its use. Doxazocin is an α1-adrenergic receptor antagonist. Its ability to reduce alcohol and cocaine use has been shown in prior studies (Kenna et al. 2016; O'Neil et al. 2013; Shorter et al. 2013). In a pilot study, titrated doses of doxazocin from 4–8 mg/day over 21 days showed a significant reduction in stress-precipitated smoking lapse and tobacco craving compared to placebo (Verplaetse et al. 2017). Large randomized controlled trials (RCTs) with longer follow-up duration are needed to investigate noradrenergic modulators as smoking cessation aids.

8 Anti-epileptic Drugs

8.1 Gabapentin and Pregabalin

Gabapentin is a drug that binds to the α_2-δ subunit of voltage-gated calcium channels and reduces the release of neuronal glutamate. It is also thought to increase the concentration of GABA in the brain (Sood et al. 2007). The clinical evidence for gabapentin's use as a smoking cessation aid is limited. One study found bupropion to be associated with higher abstinence rates compared to gabapentin (White et al. 2005). An open-label study investigated the effects of 8 weeks of gabapentin 600 mg 3 times/day and found an abstinence rate of 24% at 6 months and a significant decrease in the number of cigarettes smoked compared with baseline (Sood et al. 2007). However, a follow-up study that compared two doses of gabapentin, 600 mg 3 times/day or 900 mg 3 times/day, to placebo found no significant difference in abstinence rates between groups at 12 weeks posttreatment (Sood et al. 2010b). Pregabalin, like gabapentin, also binds to voltage-gated calcium channels and has been tested as a smoking cessation aid. A double-blind study compared 300 mg/day of pregabalin to placebo for a 4-day duration and found no benefit on smoking behavior but some reduction in withdrawal symptoms (Herman et al. 2012).

Unfortunately, this trial was of insufficient duration to determine whether pregabalin has any clinical utility.

8.2 Topiramate and Zonisamide

Topiramate is an FDA-approved anticonvulsant and prophylactic treatment for migraine. It has multiple mechanisms of action. It antagonizes glutamatergic receptors, inhibits sodium and L-type calcium channels, and increases GABAergic neurotransmission via GABA-A receptors (Johnson 2004). These actions have been postulated to counterbalance the effects of nicotine, although subjective effects of nicotine are not affected by topiramate (Le Foll et al. 2008a). In 2008, the first randomized, double-blind, placebo-controlled trial investigating topiramate for smoking cessation found sex-specific effects, such that men taking topiramate were almost 16 times more likely to quit smoking compared to women receiving treatment (Anthenelli et al. 2008). A subsequent three-arm pilot study comparing the effects of topiramate and NRT, topiramate monotherapy, and placebo found that topiramate in conjunction with NRT increased continuous abstinence rates compared to placebo (37% vs. 5%, respectively) (Oncken et al. 2014). Topiramate monotherapy also produced higher abstinence rates compared to placebo, but this did not reach significance. However, since there was no NRT monotherapy group, it is unclear if topiramate plus NRT is superior to NRT alone. Several studies testing topiramate in men concurrently diagnosed with alcohol use disorder and TUD have also been conducted. A 12-week trial comparing topiramate (300 mg/day) to naltrexone (50 mg/day) and placebo found reductions in cigarettes smoked per day in the topiramate versus placebo groups and a trend for greater effect in the topiramate versus naltrexone group (Baltieri et al. 2009). On the other hand, a trial with 129 alcohol-dependent smokers who were given topiramate (200 mg/day) or placebo for 12 weeks found no effects on smoking cessation or alcohol relapse (Anthenelli et al. 2017). Zonisamide is an anti-epileptic drug that functions similarly to topiramate but has less adverse side effects (Verrotti et al. 2013). One trial tested a 300 mg dose in combination with varenicline for 10 weeks (Dunn et al. 2016). The combination of zonisamide and varenicline decreased self-reported smoking, nicotine withdrawal, and craving compared to varenicline and placebo, but did not produce any significant differences in cotinine measurements.

9 Gamma-Aminobutyric Acid (GABA) Receptors

Baclofen is a GABA-B receptor agonist that is FDA approved for the treatment of spasticity and has also been extensively studied as a treatment for alcohol use disorder. It has been suggested that this medication may be effective as a smoking cessation aid (Le Foll et al. 2008b; Malcolm 2003; Markou et al. 2004). A 9-week, double-blind, placebo-controlled trial in treatment-seeking smokers showed that 80 mg/day of baclofen reduced the number of cigarettes smoked per day compared to placebo (Franklin et al. 2009). However, there was a high rate of non-completion in this trial. Currently, the same group is running a Phase II trial investigating the effects of baclofen on brain and behavior in cigarette smokers (ClinicalTrials.gov identifier NCT01821560). The study has been completed, but to our knowledge, results have not yet been published. Another single-arm trial tested baclofen (60 mg/d) in combination with bupropion (300 mg/day) for 7-week duration (White et al. (2011). Eleven out of the 20 participants maintained continuous abstinence over the last 4 weeks of treatment. These preliminary results show early promise for baclofen as a smoking cessation aid, but further studies are warranted.

10 Glucagon-Like Peptide-1 (GLP-1) Receptor Agonists

GLP-1 is involved in glucose homeostasis. It functions by increasing insulin secretion and decreasing glucagon release in the periphery (Holst and Seino 2009). GLP-1 also acts centrally on receptors in the hypothalamus and brain stem to produce hypoglycemic effects (Gutniak et al. 1992; Matsuyama et al. 1988). GLP-1 agonists are therefore used as weight control agents for obese diabetic and nondiabetic patients. Preclinical studies indicate that GLP-1 receptor agonists attenuate the substance-induced reward effects of nicotine (Egecioglu et al. 2013a) and other drugs of abuse (Egecioglu et al. 2013a, b, c; Erreger et al. 2012; Graham et al. 2013). This may be due to the fact that GLP-1 receptors are also expressed in the mesolimbic dopamine reward system (Merchenthaler et al. 1999) and may be involved in reward signaling induced by various substances of abuse. Studies showed that the administration of a GLP-1 receptor agonist blunted the rewarding and reinforcing effects of drugs of abuse (Alhadeff et al. 2012). Exenatide, a GLP-1 agonist and a treatment for type 2 diabetes mellitus, is currently being tested as a smoking cessation aid in prediabetic individuals who are overweight ($n = 90$). All smokers received transdermal NRT and behavioral counseling during the 6-week study period (2 weeks of treatment before quit day and 4 weeks after). No results have been published as of yet (ClinicalTrials.gov identifier NCT02975297). There is also an ongoing clinical trial investigating the effects of Dulaglutide, a GLP-1 receptor agonist, on smoking cessation (Clinicaltrial.gov identifier NCT03204396).

11 Statins

Statins are 3-hydroxy-3-methyl-glutaryl-coaenzyme A (HMG CoA) reductase inhibitors that are used to treat hypercholesterolemia (Law and Rudnicka 2006). Statins reduce nicotine-induced reinstatement in animals, although the mechanism for this remains unclear (Chauvet et al. 2016). Only one study has tested a statin for smoking cessation in humans. A 3-month placebo-controlled RCT ($n = 118$) found no effect of 40 mg of simvastatin on craving, number of cigarettes smoked per day, or sustained abstinence. However, the authors suggest that this may have been due to differences in simvastatin brain penetration between animals and humans (Ingrand et al. 2018); therefore studying statins with greater brain penetrance may prove worthwhile.

12 Stimulants and Atomoxetine

12.1 Attention Deficit Hyperactivity Disorder (ADHD) Medications

Individuals with ADHD are at higher risk of developing nicotine dependence and have lower rates of smoking cessation (Pomerleau et al. 1995). The main treatments for ADHD in all age groups are stimulants such as methylphenidate-based and amphetamine-based products (Faraone and Buitelaar 2010; Faraone and Glatt 2010). Two trials have tested stimulants in smokers with ADHD. The first study randomized smokers with ADHD to 72 mg/day of methylphenidate ($n = 127$) or placebo ($n = 128$) for 11 weeks. During the study, brief weekly individual smoking cessation counseling and 21 mg/day nicotine patches were provided. Unfortunately, methylphenidate treatment did not increase smoking cessation rates in this trial (Winhusen et al. 2010). Another trial randomized smokers with ADHD to 70 mg/day of lisdexamfetamine, an amphetamine prodrug, plus NRT, or placebo plus NRT. Lisdexamfetamine significantly reduced ADHD symptoms but did not reduce smoking abstinence rates compared to placebo (Kollins et al. 2014). Therefore, stimulant treatment in combination with NRT has not been found to be effective in smokers with ADHD to date, and it is not known if they provide any efficacy in smokers without ADHD.

12.2 Atomoxetine

Atomoxetine is another medication used to treat ADHD that functions as a noradrenaline reuptake inhibitor (Garnock-Jones and Keating 2009). A small trial investigated atomoxetine in nontreatment-seeking smokers with ADHD ($n = 15$) in experimental laboratory sessions. Atomoxetine reduced nicotine withdrawal symptoms after overnight abstinence (Gehricke et al. 2011). Another human laboratory study in nontreatment-seeking smokers ($n = 50$), which employed a placebo-controlled crossover design, found reduced withdrawal symptoms under the atomoxetine condition (Ray et al. 2009). Finally, a 14-day double-blind trial that treated smokers diagnosed with schizophrenia ($n = 12$) with atomoxetine (0, 40, or 80 mg/day) found that treatment with atomoxetine led to a 22% decrease in the number of cigarettes smoked per day (Sacco et al. 2009). However, it is not clear whether atomoxetine could be used to reduce smoking rates for a sustained period of time.

12.3 Modafinil

Modafinil is a medication that is used to promote wakefulness in individuals with daytime sleepiness (Ballon and Feifel 2006). It was thought that modafinil's putative cognitive enhancing effects could reduce nicotine withdrawal symptoms and improve quit rates (Lerman et al. 2002). A group of researchers tested modafinil (200 mg/day) versus placebo for smoking cessation in treatment-seeking smokers ($n = 157$) for 8 weeks. Interim analyses were negative. Moreover, the group treated with modafinil showed more abstinence-induced negative mood and withdrawal symptoms. Therefore, the trial was discontinued, and it was concluded that modafinil is not a promising smoking cessation aid (Schnoll et al. 2008).

13 N-Acetylcysteine

N-Acetylcysteine (NAC) is a cysteine prodrug used to treat acetaminophen overdose. In the central nervous system, NAC is converted to cystine (Olive et al. 2012), extracellular cystine is then exchanged for intracellular glutamate, thereby leading to higher levels of extracellular glutamate (Baker et al. 2002). NAC was initially studied as a smoking cessation aid due to emerging evidence that glutamate signaling contributed to addiction (Kalivas et al. 2009). For example, preclinical work found that glutamate reduced the rewarding effects of nicotine and decreased withdrawal (Kenny et al. 2003; Liechti et al. 2007).

In 2009, the first placebo-controlled human study investigating NAC for smoking cessation found decreased cigarette smoking in the NAC versus the placebo group, but no differences in CO levels (Knackstedt et al. 2009). Shortly afterward, a small human laboratory study found that participants in the NAC arm rated cigarettes as less rewarding than in the placebo arm (Schmaal et al. 2011). A 12-week double-blind randomized control trial in participants with TUD found that treatment with NAC significantly reduced the number of cigarettes smoked and CO levels. Also, 47.1% of participants treated with NAC quit smoking compared to 21.4% of participants given placebo (Prado et al. 2015). A single-arm pilot trial ($n = 19$) using a combination of NAC (2.4 g/day) and varenicline (2 mg/day) for 4 weeks showed a significant decrease in the number of cigarettes smoked at the screening visit (16 ± 2) compared to the follow-up visit (5 ± 1). However, point prevalence abstinence rates at the end of the treatment remained low. Despite these preliminary results, studies testing NAC to date have employed small samples, short follow-up duration, and variable doses of NAC. Large clinical trials of longer duration need to be conducted before NAC can be used for treatment of TUD.

14 N-Methyl-D-Aspartate (NMDA) Receptors

N-methyl-D-aspartate (NMDA) receptors are thought to modulate drug self-administration and relapse (Kenny et al. 2009; Trujillo 1995) and could represent a potential target for smoking cessation. Preclinical work has shown that GW468816, a selective antagonist at the glycine site on NMDA receptors, prevents nicotine relapse in short- and long-term models of smoking cessation. Despite these promising preclinical findings, a double-blind, placebo-controlled trial in humans demonstrated that GW468816 had no effect on abstinence rates at the end of 5 weeks of treatment (Evins et al. 2011). D-cycloserine, a partial NMDA agonist, is an FDA-approved antibiotic used for the treatment of tuberculosis (US Food and Drug Administration 2018d). It has been studied for its possible role in enhancing cue exposure therapy in the treatment of addictions (Elrashidi and Ebbert 2014). However, three trials found no benefit to adding D-cycloserine to psychotherapy for smoking cessation (Kamboj et al. 2012; Santa Ana et al. 2009; Yoon et al. 2013). Currently, there is an ongoing clinical trial evaluating the effect of D-cycloserine on smoking cessation in motivated smokers with panic attacks (Clinicaltrial.gov identifier NCT01944423).

15 Progesterone

Progesterone is a steroid hormone that is synthesized in the ovaries and adrenal glands (Lynch and Sofuoglu 2010). Progesterone has been shown to interact with multiple receptors such as GABA-A and nicotinic cholinergic receptors (Lynch and Sofuoglu 2010; Pereira et al. 2002). In preclinical studies, female rats were more motivated for nicotine when progesterone levels were low, and nicotine self-administration decreased when females were pregnant with high levels of progesterone (Lesage et al. 2007; Lynch 2009). Clinical work has been limited, but there is some evidence for progesterone as a smoking cessation aid for both men and women. In one study, researchers gave participants a single 200 mg dose of progesterone or placebo followed by intravenous (IV) nicotine (Sofuoglu et al. 2009). They found that those given progesterone rated the nicotine as having worse effects, had lower levels of "drug liking," and a decreased urge to smoke. Another study examined the effects of 200 or 400 mg/day of progesterone compared to placebo on smoking urges and behaviors (Sofuoglu et al. 2011). They found that 400 mg of progesterone reduced smoking urges, but did not affect ad libitum smoking behavior. A 12-week randomized, double-blind, placebo-controlled, trial was conducted in which 46 abstinent postpartum females were given either 400 mg/day of progesterone or placebo. This study found that participants given progesterone had a higher prevalence of abstinence at 4 weeks (Allen et al. 2016). Researchers also looked at the effect of 400 mg/day of progesterone on women who had achieved abstinence during pregnancy (Forray et al. 2017). They were given progesterone treatment or placebo immediately after delivery for 8 weeks. Women in the active treatment arm were 1.8 times more likely to be abstinent at week 8, and the time to relapse was longer (10 vs. 4 weeks), although this finding did not reach statistical significance. There is an ongoing clinical trial assessing the combination of progesterone and nicotine replacement therapy for smoking cessation (Clinicaltrial.gov identifier NCT02685072). This trial is also fairly small; studies that are more adequately powered will be needed to determine if progesterone treatment can be used on a larger scale.

16 Conclusion

Every year, billions of dollars are spent treating smoking and related comorbidities (Goodchild et al. 2018). In spite of this, abstinence rates following pharmacotherapy remain low. A deeper understanding of the complex relationship between the cholinergic system and other neurotransmitter systems will be necessary in order to discover novel treatment targets for TUD. Among the pharmacotherapies investigated in the past 10 years, some candidates show promising results such as cytisine and endocannabinoid modulators, whereas others failed to produce significant effects. However, many trials have been limited by small sample sizes and short duration of follow-up. Larger trials that monitor long-term abstinence rates are necessary.

It is unlikely that one medication will benefit all smokers due to individual variability in neurochemistry and behavior. More research will be needed to determine how to tailor specific pharmacotherapies to subpopulations of smokers such as smokers with obesity, mental illnesses, and other comorbidities with a consideration of possible sex differences. It could also be of interest to investigate if treatment using a combination of drugs yields any benefit. Hopefully such research will provide clinicians with an improved pharmacological arsenal which can be used to curb the growing burden of nicotine addiction.

References

Alhadeff AL, Rupprecht LE, Hayes MR (2012) GLP-1 neurons in the nucleus of the solitary tract project directly to the ventral tegmental area and nucleus accumbens to control for food intake. Endocrinology 153:647–658

Allen SS, Allen AM, Lunos S, Tosun N (2016) Progesterone and postpartum smoking relapse: a pilot double-blind placebo-controlled randomized trial. Nicotine Tob Res 18:2145–2153

Anda RF, Williamson DF, Escobedo LG, Mast EE, Giovino GA, Remington PL (1990) Depression and the dynamics of smoking. A national perspective. JAMA 264:1541–1545

Anthenelli RM, Blom TJ, McElroy SL, Keck PE Jr (2008) Preliminary evidence for gender-specific effects of topiramate as a potential aid to smoking cessation. Addiction 103:687–694

Anthenelli RM, Heffner JL, Wong E, Tibbs J, Russell K, Isgro M, Dinh E, Wehrle C, Worley MJ, Doran N (2017) A randomized trial evaluating whether topiramate aids smoking cessation and prevents alcohol relapse in recovering alcohol-dependent men. Alcohol Clin Exp Res 41:197–206

Aveyard P, Johnson C, Fillingham S, Parsons A, Murphy M (2008) Nortriptyline plus nicotine replacement versus placebo plus nicotine replacement for smoking cessation: pragmatic randomised controlled trial. BMJ 336:1223–1227

Baker DA, Xi ZX, Shen H, Swanson CJ, Kalivas PW (2002) The origin and neuronal function of in vivo nonsynaptic glutamate. J Neurosci 22:9134–9141

Ballon JS, Feifel D (2006) A systematic review of modafinil: potential clinical uses and mechanisms of action. J Clin Psychiatry 67:554–566

Baltieri DA, Daro FR, Ribeiro PL, Andrade AG (2009) Effects of topiramate or naltrexone on tobacco use among male alcohol-dependent outpatients. Drug Alcohol Depend 105:33–41

Benowitz NL (2010) Nicotine addiction. N Engl J Med 362:2295–2303

Benowitz NL, Wilson Peng M (2000) Non-nicotine pharmacotherapy for smoking cessation: mechanisms and prospects. CNS Drugs 13:265–285

Bergamaschi MM, Queiroz RH, Zuardi AW, Crippa JA (2011) Safety and side effects of cannabidiol, a *Cannabis sativa* constituent. Curr Drug Saf 6:237–249

Berlin I, Hunneyball IM, Greiling D, Jones SP, Fuder H, Stahl HD (2012) A selective reversible monoamine oxidase B inhibitor in smoking cessation: effects on its own and in association with transdermal nicotine patch. Psychopharmacology 223:89–98

Biberman R, Neumann R, Katzir I, Gerber Y (2003) A randomized controlled trial of oral selegiline plus nicotine skin patch compared with placebo plus nicotine skin patch for smoking cessation. Addiction 98:1403–1407

Blondal T, Gudmundsson LJ, Tomasson K, Jonsdottir D, Hilmarsdottir H, Kristjansson F, Nilsson F, Bjornsdottir US (1999) The effects of fluoxetine combined with nicotine inhalers in smoking cessation--a randomized trial. Addiction 94:1007–1015

Bozinoff N, Le Foll B (2018) Understanding the implications of the biobehavioral basis of nicotine addiction and its impact on the efficacy of treatment. Expert Rev Respir Med 12:793–804

Brown RA, Abrantes AM, Strong DR, Niaura R, Kahler CW, Miller IW, Price LH (2014) Efficacy of sequential use of fluoxetine for smoking cessation in elevated depressive symptom smokers. Nicotine Tob Res 16:197–207

Burki TK (2015) WHO tobacco report focuses on increased taxation. Lancet Respir Med 3:604

Butterweck V (2003) Mechanism of action of St John's wort in depression: what is known? CNS Drugs 17:539–562

Cahill K, Stead LF, Lancaster T (2007) Nicotine receptor partial agonists for smoking cessation. Cochrane Database Syst Rev 4:CD006103

Cahill K, Stevens S, Perera R, Lancaster T (2013) Pharmacological interventions for smoking cessation: an overview and network meta-analysis. Cochrane Database Syst Rev 5:CD009329

Catania MA, Firenzuoli F, Crupi A, Mannucci C, Caputi AP, Calapai G (2003) *Hypericum perforatum* attenuates nicotine withdrawal signs in mice. Psychopharmacology 169:186–189

Chauvet C, Nicolas C, Lafay-Chebassier C, Jaber M, Thiriet N, Solinas M (2016) Statins reduce the risks of relapse to addiction in rats. Neuropsychopharmacology 41:1588–1597

Coe JW, Brooks PR, Vetelino MG, Wirtz MC, Arnold EP, Huang J, Sands SB, Davis TI, Lebel LA, Fox CB, Shrikhande A, Heym JH, Schaeffer E, Rollema H, Lu Y, Mansbach RS, Chambers LK, Rovetti CC, Schulz DW, Tingley FD, O'Neill BT (2005) Varenicline: an α4β2 nicotinic receptor partial agonist for smoking cessation. J Med Chem 48:3474–3477

Cohen C, Perrault G, Voltz C, Steinberg R, Soubrie P (2002) SR141716, a central cannabinoid (CB (1)) receptor antagonist, blocks the motivational and dopamine-releasing effects of nicotine in rats. Behav Pharmacol 13:451–463

Curioni C, Andre C (2006) Rimonabant for overweight or obesity. Cochrane Database Syst Rev 4: Cd006162

Dalack GW, Glassman AH, Rivelli S, Covey L, Stetner F (1995) Mood, major depression, and fluoxetine response in cigarette smokers. Am J Psychiatry 152:398–403

David SP, Lancaster T, Stead LF, Evins AE, Prochaska JJ (2013) Opioid antagonists for smoking cessation. Cochrane Database Syst Rev 6:CD003086

David SP, Chu IM, Lancaster T, Stead LF, Evins AE, Prochaska JJ (2014) Systematic review and meta-analysis of opioid antagonists for smoking cessation. BMJ Open 4:e004393

De la Garza R 2nd, Yoon JH (2011) Evaluation of the effects of rivastigmine on cigarette smoking by methamphetamine-dependent volunteers. Prog Neuro-Psychopharmacol Biol Psychiatry 35:1827–1830

Diehl A, Nakovics H, Mutschler J, Hermann D, Kiefer F (2009) Rivastigmine reduces tobacco craving in alcohol-dependent smokers. Pharmacopsychiatry 42:89–94

Drewnowski A, Krahn DD, Demitrack MA, Nairn K, Gosnell BA (1995) Naloxone, an opiate blocker, reduces the consumption of sweet high-fat foods in obese and lean female binge eaters. Am J Clin Nutr 61:1206–1212

Dunn KE, Marcus TF, Kim C, Schroeder JR, Vandrey R, Umbricht A (2016) Zonisamide reduces withdrawal symptoms but does not enhance varenicline-induced smoking cessation. Nicotine Tob Res 18:1171–1179

Egecioglu E, Engel JA, Jerlhag E (2013a) The glucagon-like peptide 1 analogue Exendin-4 attenuates the nicotine-induced locomotor stimulation, accumbal dopamine release, conditioned place preference as well as the expression of locomotor sensitization in mice. PLoS One 8: e77284

Egecioglu E, Engel JA, Jerlhag E (2013b) The glucagon-like peptide 1 analogue, exendin-4, attenuates the rewarding properties of psychostimulant drugs in mice. PLoS One 8:e69010

Egecioglu E, Steensland P, Fredriksson I, Feltmann K, Engel JA, Jerlhag E (2013c) The glucagon-like peptide 1 analogue Exendin-4 attenuates alcohol mediated behaviors in rodents. Psychoneuroendocrinology 38:1259–1270

Elrashidi MY, Ebbert JO (2014) Emerging drugs for the treatment of tobacco dependence: 2014 update. Expert Opin Emerg Drugs 19:243–260

Epstein AM, King AC (2004) Naltrexone attenuates acute cigarette smoking behavior. Pharmacol Biochem Behav 77:29–37

Erreger K, Davis AR, Poe AM, Greig NH, Stanwood GD, Galli A (2012) Exendin-4 decreases amphetamine-induced locomotor activity. Physiol Behav 106:574–578

Evins AE, Pachas G, Mischoulon D, Urbanoski K, Carlini S, Sousa J, Bentley K, Rigotti NA, Nino-Gomez J, Loebl T, Janes AC, Kaufman MJ, Fava M (2011) A double-blind, placebo-controlled trial of the NMDA glycine site antagonist, GW468816, for prevention of relapse to smoking in females. J Clin Psychopharmacol 31:597–602

Faraone SV, Buitelaar J (2010) Comparing the efficacy of stimulants for ADHD in children and adolescents using meta-analysis. Eur Child Adolesc Psychiatry 19:353–364

Faraone SV, Glatt SJ (2010) A comparison of the efficacy of medications for adult attention-deficit/ hyperactivity disorder using meta-analysis of effect sizes. J Clin Psychiatry 71:754–763

Feighner JP (1999) Mechanism of action of antidepressant medications. J Clin Psychiatry 60 (Suppl 4):4–11; discussion 12-3

Fiedorowicz JG, Swartz KL (2004) The role of monoamine oxidase inhibitors in current psychiatric practice. J Psychiatr Pract 10:239–248

Filozof C, Fernandez Pinilla MC, Fernandez-Cruz A (2004) Smoking cessation and weight gain. Obes Rev 5:95–103

Forget B, Wertheim C, Mascia P, Pushparaj A, Goldberg SR, Le Foll B (2010) Noradrenergic alpha1 receptors as a novel target for the treatment of nicotine addiction. Neuropsychopharmacology 35:1751–1760

Forouzanfar MH, Alexander L, Anderson HR, Bachman VF, Biryukov S, Brauer M, Burnett R et al (2015) Global, regional, and national comparative risk assessment of 79 behavioural, environmental and occupational, and metabolic risks or clusters of risks in 188 countries, 1990–2013: a systematic analysis for the Global Burden of Disease Study 2013. Lancet 386:2287–2323

Forray A, Gilstad-Hayden K, Suppies C, Bogen D, Sofuoglu M, Yonkers KA (2017) Progesterone for smoking relapse prevention following delivery: a pilot, randomized, double-blind study. Psychoneuroendocrinology 86:96–103

Franklin TR, Harper D, Kampman K, Kildea-McCrea S, Jens W, Lynch KG, O'Brien CP, Childress AR (2009) The GABA B agonist baclofen reduces cigarette consumption in a preliminary double-blind placebo-controlled smoking reduction study. Drug Alcohol Depend 103:30–36

Garnock-Jones KP, Keating GM (2009) Atomoxetine: a review of its use in attention-deficit hyperactivity disorder in children and adolescents. Paediatr Drugs 11:203–226

Gehricke JG, Hong N, Wigal TL, Chan V, Doan A (2011) ADHD medication reduces cotinine levels and withdrawal in smokers with ADHD. Pharmacol Biochem Behav 98:485–491

George TP, Vessicchio JC, Termine A, Jatlow PI, Kosten TR, O'Malley SS (2003) A preliminary placebo-controlled trial of selegiline hydrochloride for smoking cessation. Biol Psychiatry 53:136–143

Glover ED, Laflin MT, Schuh KJ, Schuh LM, Nides M, Christen AG, Glover PN, Strnad JV (2007) A randomized, controlled trial to assess the efficacy and safety of a transdermal delivery system of nicotine/mecamylamine in cigarette smokers. Addiction 102:795–802

Goodchild M, Nargis N, Tursan d'Espaignet E (2018) Global economic cost of smoking-attributable diseases. Tob Control 27:58–64

Gourlay SG, Stead LF, Benowitz NL (2004) Clonidine for smoking cessation. Cochrane Database Syst Rev 3:CD000058

Government of Canada (2018) Licensed natural health products database (LNHPD): product information. Retrieved from https://health-products.canada.ca/lnhpd-bdpsnh/info.do?licence=80072429

Gowing LR, Ali RL, Allsop S, Marsden J, Turf EE, West R, Witton J (2015) Global statistics on addictive behaviours: 2014 status report. Addiction 110:904–919

Graham DL, Erreger K, Galli A, Stanwood GD (2013) GLP-1 analog attenuates cocaine reward. Mol Psychiatry 18:961–962

Gutniak M, Orskov C, Holst JJ, Ahren B, Efendic S (1992) Antidiabetogenic effect of glucagon-like peptide-1 (7-36)amide in normal subjects and patients with diabetes mellitus. N Engl J Med 326:1316–1322

Herman AI, Waters AJ, McKee SA, Sofuoglu M (2012) Effects of pregabalin on smoking behavior, withdrawal symptoms, and cognitive performance in smokers. Psychopharmacology 220:611–617

Higgins GA, Silenieks LB, Rossmann A, Rizos Z, Noble K, Soko AD, Fletcher PJ (2012) The 5-HT2C receptor agonist lorcaserin reduces nicotine self-administration, discrimination, and reinstatement: relationship to feeding behavior and impulse control. Neuropsychopharmacology 37:1177–1191

Holst JJ, Seino Y (2009) GLP-1 receptor agonists: targeting both hyperglycaemia and disease processes in diabetes. Diabetes Res Clin Pract 85:1–3

Hughes JR, Stead LF, Hartmann-Boyce J, Cahill K, Lancaster T (2014) Antidepressants for smoking cessation. Cochrane Database Syst Rev 1:CD000031

Hurt RT, Croghan IT, Schroeder DR, Hays JT, Choi DS, Ebbert JO (2017) Combination varenicline and lorcaserin for tobacco dependence treatment and weight gain prevention in overweight and obese smokers: a pilot study. Nicotine Tob Res 19:994–998

Hutchison KE, Monti PM, Rohsenow DJ, Swift RM, Colby SM, Gnys M, Niaura RS, Sirota AD (1999) Effects of naltrexone with nicotine replacement on smoking cue reactivity: preliminary results. Psychopharmacology 142:139–143

Ingrand I, Solinas M, Ingrand P, Dugast E, Saulnier PJ, Perault-Pochat MC, Lafay-Chebassier C (2018) Lack of effects of simvastatin on smoking cessation in humans: a double-blind, randomized, placebo-controlled clinical study. Sci Rep 8:3836

Izaddoost M, Harris BG, Gracy RW (1976) Structure and toxicity of alkaloids and amino acids of *Sophora secundiflora*. J Pharm Sci 65:352–354

Johnson BA (2004) Topiramate-induced neuromodulation of cortico-mesolimbic dopamine function: a new vista for the treatment of comorbid alcohol and nicotine dependence? Addict Behav 29:1465–1479

Kahn R, Gorgon L, Jones K, McSherry F, Glover ED, Anthenelli RM, Jackson T, Williams J, Murtaugh C, Montoya I, Yu E, Elkashef A (2012) Selegiline transdermal system (STS) as an aid for smoking cessation. Nicotine Tob Res 14:377–382

Kalivas PW, LaLumiere RT, Knackstedt L, Shen H (2009) Glutamate transmission in addiction. Neuropharmacology 56:169–173

Kamboj SK, Joye A, Das RK, Gibson AJ, Morgan CJ, Curran HV (2012) Cue exposure and response prevention with heavy smokers: a laboratory-based randomised placebo-controlled trial examining the effects of D-cycloserine on cue reactivity and attentional bias. Psychopharmacology 221:273–284

Kenna GA, Haass-Koffler CL, Zywiak WH, Edwards SM, Brickley MB, Swift RM, Leggio L (2016) Role of the alpha1 blocker doxazosin in alcoholism: a proof-of-concept randomized controlled trial. Addict Biol 21:904–914

Kenny PJ, Gasparini F, Markou A (2003) Group II metabotropic and α-amino-3-hydroxy-5-methyl-4-isoxazole propionate (AMPA)/kainate glutamate receptors regulate the deficit in brain reward function associated with nicotine withdrawal in rats. J Pharmacol Exp Ther 306:1068–1076

Kenny PJ, Chartoff E, Roberto M, Carlezon WA Jr, Markou A (2009) NMDA receptors regulate nicotine-enhanced brain reward function and intravenous nicotine self-administration: role of the ventral tegmental area and central nucleus of the amygdala. Neuropsychopharmacology 34:266–281

Killen JD, Fortmann SP, Murphy GM Jr, Hayward C, Fong D, Lowenthal K, Bryson SW, Killen DT, Schatzberg AF (2010) Failure to improve cigarette smoking abstinence with transdermal selegiline + cognitive behavior therapy. Addiction 105:1660–1668

King AC, Meyer PJ (2000) Naltrexone alteration of acute smoking response in nicotine-dependent subjects. Pharmacol Biochem Behav 66:563–572

King A, de Wit H, Riley RC, Cao D, Niaura R, Hatsukami D (2006) Efficacy of naltrexone in smoking cessation: a preliminary study and an examination of sex differences. Nicotine Tob Res 8:671–682

King AC, Cao D, O'Malley SS, Kranzler HR, Cai X, deWit H, Matthews AK, Stachoviak RJ (2012) Effects of naltrexone on smoking cessation outcomes and weight gain in nicotine-dependent men and women. J Clin Psychopharmacol 32:630–636

King A, Cao D, Zhang L, Rueger SY (2013) Effects of the opioid receptor antagonist naltrexone on smoking and related behaviors in smokers preparing to quit: a randomized controlled trial. Addiction 108:1836–1844

Knackstedt LA, LaRowe S, Mardikian P, Malcolm R, Upadhyaya H, Hedden S, Markou A, Kalivas PW (2009) The role of cystine-glutamate exchange in nicotine dependence in rats and humans. Biol Psychiatry 65:841–845

Kollins SH, English JS, Itchon-Ramos N, Chrisman AK, Dew R, O'Brien B, McClernon FJ (2014) A pilot study of lis-dexamfetamine dimesylate (LDX/SPD489) to facilitate smoking cessation in nicotine-dependent adults with ADHD. J Atten Disord 18:158–168

Kotlyar M, Drone D, Thuras P, Hatsukami DK, Brauer L, Adson DE, al'Absi M (2011) Effect of stress and bupropion on craving, withdrawal symptoms, and mood in smokers. Nicotine Tob Res 13:492–497

Krishnan KR (2007) Revisiting monoamine oxidase inhibitors. J Clin Psychiatry 68(Suppl 8):35–41

Laprairie RB, Bagher AM, Kelly ME, Denovan-Wright EM (2015) Cannabidiol is a negative allosteric modulator of the cannabinoid CB1 receptor. Br J Pharmacol 172:4790–4805

Law M, Rudnicka AR (2006) Statin safety: a systematic review. Am J Cardiol 97:52C–60C

Le Foll B (2013) Chapter 55 – neuropharmacology of nicotine. In: Miller PM (ed) Biological research on addiction. Academic Press, San Diego, pp 561–571

Le Foll B, George TP (2007) Treatment of tobacco dependence: integrating recent progress into practice. CMAJ 177:1373–1380

Le Foll B, Goldberg SR (2006) Nicotine as a typical drug of abuse in experimental animals and humans. Psychopharmacology 184:367–381

Le Foll B, Justinova Z, Wertheim CE, Barnes C, Goldberg SR (2008a) Topiramate does not alter nicotine or cocaine discrimination in rats. Behav Pharmacol 19:13–20

Le Foll B, Wertheim CE, Goldberg SR (2008b) Effects of baclofen on conditioned rewarding and discriminative stimulus effects of nicotine in rats. Neurosci Lett 443:236–240

Lee YS, Joe KH, Sohn IK, Na C, Kee BS, Chae SL (2005) Changes of smoking behavior and serum adrenocorticotropic hormone, cortisol, prolactin, and endogenous opioids levels in nicotine dependence after naltrexone treatment. Prog Neuro-Psychopharmacol Biol Psychiatry 29:639–647

Lerman C, Roth D, Kaufmann V, Audrain J, Hawk L, Liu A, Niaura R, Epstein L (2002) Mediating mechanisms for the impact of bupropion in smoking cessation treatment. Drug Alcohol Depend 67:219–223

Lesage MG, Keyler DE, Burroughs D, Pentel PR (2007) Effects of pregnancy on nicotine self-administration and nicotine pharmacokinetics in rats. Psychopharmacology 194:413–421

Levin ED, Johnson JE, Slade S, Wells C, Cauley M, Petro A, Rose JE (2011) Lorcaserin, a 5-HT2C agonist, decreases nicotine self-administration in female rats. J Pharmacol Exp Ther 338:890–896

Lewis A, Miller JH, Lea RA (2007) Monoamine oxidase and tobacco dependence. Neurotoxicology 28:182–195

Liechti ME, Lhuillier L, Kaupmann K, Markou A (2007) Metabotropic glutamate 2/3 receptors in the ventral tegmental area and the nucleus accumbens shell are involved in behaviors relating to nicotine dependence. J Neurosci 27:9077–9085

Lu Y, Anderson HD (2017) Cannabinoid signaling in health and disease. Can J Physiol Pharmacol 95:311–327

Lynch WJ (2009) Sex and ovarian hormones influence vulnerability and motivation for nicotine during adolescence in rats. Pharmacol Biochem Behav 94:43–50

Lynch WJ, Sofuoglu M (2010) Role of progesterone in nicotine addiction: evidence from initiation to relapse. Exp Clin Psychopharmacol 18:451–461

Lyu X, Du J, Zhan G, Wu Y, Su H, Zhu Y, Jarskog F, Zhao M, Fan X (2018) Naltrexone and bupropion combination treatment for smoking cessation and weight loss in patients with schizophrenia. Front Pharmacol 9:181

MacLean RR, Waters AJ, Brede E, Sofuoglu M (2018) Effects of galantamine on smoking behavior and cognitive performance in treatment-seeking smokers prior to a quit attempt. Hum Psychopharmacol 33:e2665

Malcolm RJ (2003) GABA systems, benzodiazepines, and substance dependence. J Clin Psychiatry 64(Suppl 3):36–40

Marder SR, Essock SM, Miller AL, Buchanan RW, Casey DE, Davis JM, Kane JM, Lieberman JA, Schooler NR, Covell N, Stroup S, Weissman EM, Wirshing DA, Hall CS, Pogach L, Pi-Sunyer X, Bigger JT Jr, Friedman A, Kleinberg D, Yevich SJ, Davis B, Shon S (2004) Physical health monitoring of patients with schizophrenia. Am J Psychiatry 161:1334–1349

Markou A, Paterson NE, Semenova S (2004) Role of gamma-aminobutyric acid (GABA) and metabotropic glutamate receptors in nicotine reinforcement: potential pharmacotherapies for smoking cessation. Ann N Y Acad Sci 1025:491–503

Matsuyama T, Komatsu R, Namba M, Watanabe N, Itoh H, Tarui S (1988) Glucagon-like peptide-1 (7-36 amide): a potent glucagonostatic and insulinotropic hormone. Diabetes Res Clin Pract 5:281–284

McCarthy DE, Piasecki TM, Lawrence DL, Jorenby DE, Shiffman S, Baker TB (2008) Psychological mediators of bupropion sustained-release treatment for smoking cessation. Addiction 103:1521–1533

McKee SA, Potenza MN, Kober H, Sofuoglu M, Arnsten AF, Picciotto MR, Weinberger AH, Ashare R, Sinha R (2015) A translational investigation targeting stress-reactivity and prefrontal cognitive control with guanfacine for smoking cessation. J Psychopharmacol 29:300–311

Merchenthaler I, Lane M, Shughrue P (1999) Distribution of pre-pro-glucagon and glucagon-like peptide-1 receptor messenger RNAs in the rat central nervous system. J Comp Neurol 403:261–280

Minami H, Kahler CW, Bloom EL, Prince MA, Abrantes AM, Strong DR, Niaura R, Miller IW, Palm Reed KM, Price LH, Brown RA (2014) Effects of sequential fluoxetine and gender on prequit depressive symptoms, affect, craving, and quit day abstinence in smokers with elevated depressive symptoms: a growth curve modeling approach. Exp Clin Psychopharmacol 22:392–406

Mineur YS, Picciotto MR (2008) Genetics of nicotinic acetylcholine receptors: relevance to nicotine addiction. Biochem Pharmacol 75:323–333

Mitchell MR, Potenza MN (2014) Addictions and personality traits: impulsivity and related constructs. Curr Behav Neurosci Rep 1:1–12

Morgan CJA, Das RK, Joye A, Curran HV, Kamboj SK (2013) Cannabidiol reduces cigarette consumption in tobacco smokers: preliminary findings. Addict Behav 38:2433–2436

Morisano D, Bacher I, Audrain-McGovern J, George TP (2009) Mechanisms underlying the comorbidity of tobacco use in mental health and addictive disorders. Can J Psychiatr 54:356–367

Morrison MF, Ceesay P, Gantz I, Kaufman KD, Lines CR (2010) Randomized, controlled, double-blind trial of taranabant for smoking cessation. Psychopharmacology 209:245–253

O'Neil ML, Beckwith LE, Kincaid CL, Rasmussen DD (2013) The alpha1-adrenergic receptor antagonist, doxazosin, reduces alcohol drinking in alcohol-preferring (P) rats. Alcohol Clin Exp Res 37:202–212

Olive MF, Cleva RM, Kalivas PW, Malcolm RJ (2012) Glutamatergic medications for the treatment of drug and behavioral addictions. Pharmacol Biochem Behav 100:801–810

O'Malley SS, Cooney JL, Krishnan-Sarin S, Dubin JA, McKee SA, Cooney NL, Blakeslee A, Meandzija B, Romano-Dahlgard D, Wu R, Makuch R, Jatlow P (2006) A controlled trial of naltrexone augmentation of nicotine replacement therapy for smoking cessation. Arch Intern Med 166:667–674

Oncken C, Arias AJ, Feinn R, Litt M, Covault J, Sofuoglu M, Kranzler HR (2014) Topiramate for smoking cessation: a randomized, placebo-controlled pilot study. Nicotine Tob Res 16:288–296

Parsons AC, Shraim M, Inglis J, Aveyard P, Hajek P (2009) Interventions for preventing weight gain after smoking cessation. Cochrane Database Syst Rev 1:CD006219

Pereira EFR, Hilmas C, Santos MD, Alkondon M, Maelicke A, Albuquerque EX (2002) Unconventional ligands and modulators of nicotinic receptors. J Neurobiol 53:479–500

Perkins KA, Roy Chengappa KN, Karelitz JL, Boldry MC, Michael V, Herb T, Gannon J, Brar J, Ford L, Rassnick S, Brunzell DH (2018) Initial cross-over test of a positive allosteric modulator of alpha-7 nicotinic receptors to aid cessation in smokers with or without schizophrenia. Neuropsychopharmacology 43:1334–1342

Pertwee RG (2008) The diverse CB1 and CB2 receptor pharmacology of three plant cannabinoids: delta9-tetrahydrocannabinol, cannabidiol and delta9-tetrahydrocannabivarin. Br J Pharmacol 153:199–215

Philip NS, Carpenter LL, Tyrka AR, Price LH (2012) The nicotinic acetylcholine receptor as a target for antidepressant drug development. Sci World J 2012:104105

Pomerleau OF, Downey KK, Stelson FW, Pomerleau CS (1995) Cigarette smoking in adult patients diagnosed with attention deficit hyperactivity disorder. J Subst Abus 7:373–378

Prado E, Maes M, Piccoli LG, Baracat M, Barbosa DS, Franco O, Dodd S, Berk M, Vargas Nunes SO (2015) N-acetylcysteine for therapy-resistant tobacco use disorder: a pilot study. Redox Rep 20:215–222

Prochaska JJ, Benowitz NL (2016) The past, present, and future of nicotine addiction therapy. Annu Rev Med 67:467–486

Prochaska JJ, Das S, Benowitz NL (2013) Cytisine, the world's oldest smoking cessation aid. BMJ 347:f5198

Ray R, Rukstalis M, Jepson C, Strasser A, Patterson F, Lynch K, Lerman C (2009) Effects of atomoxetine on subjective and neurocognitive symptoms of nicotine abstinence. J Psychopharmacol 23:168–176

Richmond R, Zwar N (2003) Review of bupropion for smoking cessation. Drug Alcohol Rev 22:203–220

Richmond R, Indig D, Butler T, Wilhelm K, Archer V, Wodak A (2013) A randomized controlled trial of a smoking cessation intervention conducted among prisoners. Addiction 108:966–974

Roberts W, Ralevski E, Verplaetse TL, McKee SA, Petrakis IL (2018) Tobacco use during a clinical trial of mecamylamine for alcohol dependence: medication effects on smoking and associations with reductions in drinking. J Subst Abus Treat 94:91–96

Robinson JD, Cinciripini PM, Karam-Hage M, Aubin HJ, Dale LC, Niaura R, Anthenelli RM (2018) Pooled analysis of three randomized, double-blind, placebo controlled trials with rimonabant for smoking cessation. Addict Biol 23:291–303

Rollema H, Shrikhande A, Ward KM, Tingley FD 3rd, Coe JW, O'Neill BT, Tseng E, Wang EQ, Mather RJ, Hurst RS, Williams KE, de Vries M, Cremers T, Bertrand S, Bertrand D (2010) Pre-clinical properties of the alpha4beta2 nicotinic acetylcholine receptor partial agonists varenicline, cytisine and dianicline translate to clinical efficacy for nicotine dependence. Br J Pharmacol 160:334–345

Rose JE, Behm FM, Westman EC, Levin ED, Stein RM, Ripka GV (1994) Mecamylamine combined with nicotine skin patch facilitates smoking cessation beyond nicotine patch treatment alone. Clin Pharmacol Ther 56:86–99

Rose JE, Westman EC, Behm FM (1996) Nicotine/mecamylamine combination treatment for smoking cessation. Drug Dev Res 38:243–256

Rose JE, Behm FM, Ramsey C, Ritchie JC Jr (2001) Platelet monoamine oxidase, smoking cessation, and tobacco withdrawal symptoms. Nicotine Tob Res 3:383–390

Roth BL, Willins DL, Kristiansen K, Kroeze WK (1998) 5-Hydroxytryptamine2-family receptors (5-hydroxytryptamine2A, 5-hydroxytryptamine2B, 5-hydroxytryptamine2C): where structure meets function. Pharmacol Ther 79:231–257

Sacco KA, Creeden C, Reutenauer EL, Vessicchio JC, Weinberger AH, George TP (2009) Effects of atomoxetine on cognitive function and cigarette smoking in schizophrenia. Schizophr Res 107:332–333

Santa Ana EJ, Rounsaville BJ, Frankforter TL, Nich C, Babuscio T, Poling J, Gonsai K, Hill KP, Carroll KM (2009) D-Cycloserine attenuates reactivity to smoking cues in nicotine dependent smokers: a pilot investigation. Drug Alcohol Depend 104:220–227

Schauer GL, Malarcher AM, Babb SD (2015) Gradual reduction of cigarette consumption as a cessation strategy: prevalence, correlates, and relationship with quitting. Nicotine Tob Res 17:530–538

Schmaal L, Berk L, Hulstijn KP, Cousijn J, Wiers RW, van den Brink W (2011) Efficacy of N-acetylcysteine in the treatment of nicotine dependence: a double-blind placebo-controlled pilot study. Eur Addict Res 17:211–216

Schnoll RA, Wileyto EP, Pinto A, Leone F, Gariti P, Siegel S, Perkins KA, Dackis C, Heitjan DF, Berrettini W, Lerman C (2008) A placebo-controlled trial of modafinil for nicotine dependence. Drug Alcohol Depend 98:86–93

Schuster RM, Pachas GN, Stoeckel L, Cather C, Nadal M, Mischoulon D, Schoenfeld DA, Zhang H, Ulysse C, Dodds EB, Sobolewski S, Hudziak V, Hanly A, Fava M, Evins AE (2018) Phase IIb trial of an alpha7 nicotinic receptor partial agonist with and without nicotine patch for withdrawal-associated cognitive deficits and tobacco abstinence. J Clin Psychopharmacol 38:307–316

Shanahan WR, Rose JE, Glicklich A, Stubbe S, Sanchez-Kam M (2017) Lorcaserin for smoking cessation and associated weight gain: a randomized 12-week clinical trial. Nicotine Tob Res 19:944–951

Shorter D, Lindsay JA, Kosten TR (2013) The alpha-1 adrenergic antagonist doxazosin for treatment of cocaine dependence: a pilot study. Drug Alcohol Depend 131:66–70

Slemmer JE, Martin BR, Damaj MI (2000) Bupropion is a nicotinic antagonist. J Pharmacol Exp Ther 295:321–327
Sloan ME, Gowin JL, Ramchandani VA, Hurd YL, Le Foll B (2017) The endocannabinoid system as a target for addiction treatment: trials and tribulations. Neuropharmacology 124:73–83
Sofuoglu M, Babb D, Hatsukami DK (2003) Labetalol treatment enhances the attenuation of tobacco withdrawal symptoms by nicotine in abstinent smokers. Nicotine Tob Res 5:947–953
Sofuoglu M, Mitchell E, Mooney M (2009) Progesterone effects on subjective and physiological responses to intravenous nicotine in male and female smokers. Hum Psychopharmacol Clin Exp 24:559–564
Sofuoglu M, Mouratidis M, Mooney M (2011) Progesterone improves cognitive performance and attenuates smoking urges in abstinent smokers. Psychoneuroendocrinology 36:123–132
Sood A, Ebbert JO, Schroeder DR, Croghan IT, Sood R, Vander Weg MW, Wong GY, Hays JT (2007) Gabapentin for smoking cessation: a preliminary investigation of efficacy. Nicotine Tob Res 9:291–298
Sood A, Ebbert JO, Prasad K, Croghan IT, Bauer B, Schroeder DR (2010a) A randomized clinical trial of St. John's wort for smoking cessation. J Altern Complement Med 16:761–767
Sood A, Ebbert JO, Wyatt KD, Croghan IT, Schroeder DR, Sood R, Hays JT (2010b) Gabapentin for smoking cessation. Nicotine Tob Res 12:300–304
Sood A, Prasad K, Croghan IT, Schroeder DR, Ehlers SL, Ebbert JO (2012) S-adenosyl-L-methionine (SAMe) for smoking abstinence: a randomized clinical trial. J Altern Complement Med 18:854–859
Spring B, Doran N, Pagoto S, McChargue D, Cook JW, Bailey K, Crayton J, Hedeker D (2007) Fluoxetine, smoking, and history of major depression: a randomized controlled trial. J Consult Clin Psychol 75:85–94
Stahl SM (1998) Mechanism of action of serotonin selective reuptake inhibitors. Serotonin receptors and pathways mediate therapeutic effects and side effects. J Affect Disord 51:215–235
Stead LF, Perera R, Bullen C, Mant D, Hartmann-Boyce J, Cahill K, Lancaster T (2012) Nicotine replacement therapy for smoking cessation. Cochrane Database Syst Rev 11:CD000146
Tek C (2016) Naltrexone HCl/bupropion HCl for chronic weight management in obese adults: patient selection and perspectives. Patient Prefer Adherence 10:751–759
Tham M, Yilmaz O, Alaverdashvili M, Kelly MEM, Denovan-Wright EM, Laprairie RB (2018) Allosteric and orthosteric pharmacology of cannabidiol and cannabidiol-dimethylheptyl at the type 1 and type 2 cannabinoid receptors. Br J Pharmacol 176(10):1455–1469
Tonstad S, Aubin HJ (2012) Efficacy of a dose range of surinabant, a cannabinoid receptor blocker, for smoking cessation: a randomized controlled clinical trial. J Psychopharmacol 26:1003–1009
Tonstad S, Holme I, Tonnesen P (2011) Dianicline, a novel alpha4beta2 nicotinic acetylcholine receptor partial agonist, for smoking cessation: a randomized placebo-controlled clinical trial. Nicotine Tob Res 13:1–6
Trujillo KA (1995) Effects of noncompetitive N-methyl-D-aspartate receptor antagonists on opiate tolerance and physical dependence. Neuropsychopharmacology 13:301–307
Tutka P, Zatonski W (2006) Cytisine for the treatment of nicotine addiction: from a molecule to therapeutic efficacy. Pharmacol Rep 58:777–798
U.S. Food and Drug Administration (2018a) Drugs@FDA: FDA approved drug products. Retrieved from https://www.accessdata.fda.gov/scripts/cder/daf/index.cfm?event=overview.process&ApplNo=022529
U.S. Food and Drug Administration (2018b) Drugs@FDA: FDA approved drug products. Retrieved from https://www.accessdata.fda.gov/scripts/cder/daf/index.cfm?event=overview.process&ApplNo=021336
U.S. Food and Drug Administration (2018c) Drugs@FDA: FDA approved drug products. Retrieved from https://www.accessdata.fda.gov/scripts/cder/daf/index.cfm?event=overview.process&ApplNo=021479

U.S. Food and Drug Administration (2018d) Drugs@FDA: FDA approved drug products. Retrieved from https://www.accessdata.fda.gov/scripts/cder/daf/index.cfm?event=BasicSearch.process

Verplaetse TL, Weinberger AH, Oberleitner LM, Smith KMZ, Pittman BP, Shi JM, Tetrault JM, Lavery ME, Picciotto MR, McKee SA (2017) Effect of doxazosin on stress reactivity and the ability to resist smoking. J Psychopharmacol 31:830–840

Verrotti A, Loiacono G, Di Sabatino F, Zaccara G (2013) The adverse event profile of zonisamide: a meta-analysis. Acta Neurol Scand 128:297–304

Vinnikov D, Brimkulov N, Burjubaeva A (2008) A double-blind, randomised, placebo-controlled trial of cytisine for smoking cessation in medium-dependent workers. J Smok Cessat 3:57–62

Volkow ND, Wise RA (2005) How can drug addiction help us understand obesity? Nat Neurosci 8:555–560

Walker N, Howe C, Glover M, McRobbie H, Barnes J, Nosa V, Parag V, Bassett B, Bullen C (2014) Cytisine versus nicotine for smoking cessation. N Engl J Med 371:2353–2362

Walker N, Smith B, Barnes J, Verbiest M, Kurdziel T, Parag V, Pokhrel S, Bullen C (2018) Cytisine versus varenicline for smoking cessation for Maori (the indigenous people of New Zealand) and their extended family: protocol for a randomised non-inferiority trial. Addiction 114 (2):344–352

Weinberger AH, Sofuoglu M (2009) The impact of cigarette smoking on stimulant addiction. Am J Drug Alcohol Abuse 35:12–17

Weinberger AH, Reutenauer EL, Jatlow PI, O'Malley SS, Potenza MN, George TP (2010) A double-blind, placebo-controlled, randomized clinical trial of oral selegiline hydrochloride for smoking cessation in nicotine-dependent cigarette smokers. Drug Alcohol Depend 107:188–195

West R, Zatonski W, Cedzynska M, Lewandowska D, Pazik J, Aveyard P, Stapleton J (2011) Placebo-controlled trial of cytisine for smoking cessation. N Engl J Med 365:1193–1200

Wewers ME, Dhatt R, Tejwani GA (1998) Naltrexone administration affects ad libitum smoking behavior. Psychopharmacology 140:185–190

White WD, Crockford D, Patten S, El-Guebaly N (2005) A randomized, open-label pilot comparison of gabapentin and bupropion SR for smoking cessation. Nicotine Tob Res 7:809–813

White WD, Crockford DN, Currie SR, Patten S, el-Guebaly N (2011) A prospective single-arm open-label study of baclofen and bupropion SR combination therapy for smoking cessation. Addict Disord Treat 10:101–104

Wilcox CS, Oskooilar N, Erickson JS, Billes SK, Katz BB, Tollefson G, Dunayevich E (2010) An open-label study of naltrexone and bupropion combination therapy for smoking cessation in overweight and obese subjects. Addict Behav 35:229–234

Winhusen TM, Somoza EC, Brigham GS, Liu DS, Green CA, Covey LS, Croghan IT, Adler LA, Weiss RD, Leimberger JD, Lewis DF, Dorer EM (2010) Impact of attention-deficit/hyperactivity disorder (ADHD) treatment on smoking cessation intervention in ADHD smokers: a randomized, double-blind, placebo-controlled trial. J Clin Psychiatry 71:1680–1688

Yoon JH, Newton TF, Haile CN, Bordnick PS, Fintzy RE, Culbertson C, Mahoney JJ, Hawkins RY, LaBounty KR, Ross EL, Aziziyeh AI, La Garza RD (2013) Effects of D-cycloserine on cue-induced craving and cigarette smoking among concurrent cocaine- and nicotine-dependent volunteers. Addict Behav 38:1518–1526

Adolescent Vulnerability to Alcohol Use Disorder: Neurophysiological Mechanisms from Preclinical Studies

Brian A. McCool and Molly M. McGinnis

Contents

1 Background and Overview 422
2 Adolescence and Glutamate/GABA Neurotransmitter Systems 423
3 Adolescent Ethanol Exposure 426
3.1 Adolescent Ethanol Exposure and Glutamate Neurotransmission 426
3.2 Adolescent Ethanol Exposure and GABA Neurotransmission 431
4 Concluding Remarks 433
References 436

Abstract

Adolescent alcohol use in human populations dramatically increases the likelihood of adult alcohol use disorder. This adolescent vulnerability is recapitulated in preclinical models which provide important opportunities to understand basic neurobiological mechanisms. We provide here an overview of GABAergic and glutamatergic neurotransmission and our current understanding of the sensitivity of these systems to adolescent ethanol exposure. As a whole, the preclinical literature suggests that adolescent vulnerability may be directly related to region-specific neurobiological processes that continue to develop during adolescence. These processes include the activity of intrinsic circuits within diverse brain regions (primarily represented by GABAergic neurotransmission) and activity-dependent regulation of synaptic strength at glutamatergic synapses. Furthermore, GABAergic and glutamatergic neurotransmission within regions/circuits that regulate cognitive function, emotion, and their integration appears to be the most vulnerable to adolescent ethanol exposure. Finally, using documented

B. A. McCool (✉) · M. M. McGinnis
Department of Physiology and Pharmacology, Wake Forest School of Medicine, Winston-Salem, NC, USA
e-mail: bmccool@wakehealth.edu

M. A. Nader, Y. L. Hurd (eds.), *Substance Use Disorders*,
Handbook of Experimental Pharmacology 258, https://doi.org/10.1007/164_2019_296

behavioral differences between adolescents and adults with respect to acute ethanol, we highlight additional circuits and regions for future study.

Keywords
AMPAR · $GABA_A$ · NMDAR

1 Background and Overview

There is a robust literature in humans on the vulnerability of adolescents for the development of alcohol use disorders (AUDs) following early drinking experiences. Over seven million individuals ages 12–20 (~19% of all adolescents) report alcohol use in the past month with approximately 77% of these exhibiting "risky" drinking, like heavy or binge-like use (five or more drinks/occasion, SAMHSA 2017). The lifetime prevalence for alcohol dependence drops tenfold as the age of first use increases from early adolescence (~14 years old) into young adulthood (>20 years old; Grant and Dawson 1997). Consistent with these findings, individuals reporting first use of alcohol between the ages of 11 and 14 are five times more likely to repeatedly use alcohol despite persistent negative consequences (abuse) over a subsequent 20-year period and eight times more likely to develop alcohol dependence (inability to quit drinking, withdrawal symptoms, increased tolerance to the acute intoxicating effects) over the next 10 years compared to individuals initiating alcohol use when they were >19 years old (DeWit et al. 2000). Longitudinal studies confirm that adolescents who drink to intoxication during this period are at greatest risk for developing AUD as adults (Warner et al. 2007). These findings all suggest that adolescents are uniquely sensitive to the long-term consequences of ethanol exposure. This age-group is characterized by dramatic development of brain structures involved with fine motor skills, habit formation, executive function, memory, and emotional regulation (Bundy et al. 2017). As a result, understanding both the developmental changes in the neural systems regulating drinking behavior and the neurophysiological consequences of adolescent ethanol exposure is particularly important for defining the neurophysiological mechanisms governing vulnerability to AUD in this population.

Identification of neurobiological mechanisms responsible for adolescent vulnerability to AUD has required the development of preclinical models. These models, primarily rodents but also including some studies in nonhuman primates, have strong face validity. In rats, for example, adolescence is generally defined as the period from postweaning (post-natal day 21–28 or P21–28) to young adulthood (~P60) (Sengupta 2013). Adolescent rats are less sensitive to the locomotor impairing and sedative effects of acute ethanol compared to adults (Pian et al. 2008; Schramm-Sapyta et al. 2010; White et al. 2002). Notably, subjective feelings of intoxication in humans are diminished in the sons of alcoholics (Schuckit 1984) who have greater risk for the development of AUD. Adolescent rats also self-administer greater amounts of ethanol compared to adults in many paradigms (Bell et al. 2011; Vetter et al. 2007; Walker et al. 2008) and are less sensitive to aversive properties of ethanol during noncontingent administration (Morales et al. 2014; Schramm-Sapyta et al. 2010, 2014), although this latter finding may be sex-specific (Morales et al. 2014).

Preclinical studies thus parallel many aspects of human adolescent ethanol abuse and have produced a number of important insights into the adult behavioral consequences resulting from adolescent ethanol dependence-like exposures that produce both heighten negative affective behaviors and acute withdrawal symptoms. There have been a number of exceptional reviews highlighting these advances (Crews and Boettiger 2009; Crews et al. 2016; Doremus-Fitzwater and Spear 2016; Maldonado-Devincci et al. 2010; Spear 2016; Spear and Swartzwelder 2014; White and Swartzwelder 2005). Most relevant for this chapter, adolescent dependence-like exposure in rodents dramatically increases adult ethanol consumption/preference (Alaux-Cantin et al. 2013; Amodeo et al. 2017; Criado and Ehlers 2013; Gass et al. 2014; Pascual et al. 2009), ethanol-seeking behavior (Amodeo et al. 2017), motivation to consume ethanol (Serlin and Torregrossa 2015), and decreases sensitivity to ethanol impairment/aversion (Graham and Diaz-Granados 2006; Jury et al. 2017; Mejia-Toiber et al. 2014). Preclinical models therefore provide opportunities both to understand basic neurophysiological mechanisms conferring adolescent vulnerability and may help identify potential therapeutic targets. This chapter will summarize our understanding of these neurophysiological mechanisms with a specific focus on glutamate and GABA neurotransmission and their alteration by adolescent ethanol exposures.

2 Adolescence and Glutamate/GABA Neurotransmitter Systems

After the perinatal period, glutamate and GABA act as the major excitatory and inhibitory neurotransmitter systems in the central nervous system, respectively. Both systems regulate neuronal activity through ion-conducting (ionotropic) and G protein-coupled (metabotropic) neurotransmitter receptors. Glutamate ionotropic receptors, all cation-conducting channels, consist of at least three pharmacologically and biophysically identifiable subtypes – α-amino-3-hydroxy-5-methyl-4-isoxazolepropionic acid (AMPA), kainate, and *N*-methyl-D-aspartate (NMDA) receptors. AMPA receptors are homomeric or heteromeric assemblies of four subunits arising from four different gene produces (GluA1–GluA4). GluA1–GluA3 are widely expressed throughout the central nervous system at all developmental stages, with GluA4 showing more restricted expression during early development and restricted localization to thalamic subnuclei postweaning period. Kainate receptors, pharmacologically, structurally, and functionally similar to AMPA receptors, are composed of multi-subunit assemblies of tetramers arising from five distinct genes (GluK1–GluK5). Although the neurophysiology of kainate receptors is generally less well-characterized than AMPA receptors, they are highly permeable to calcium and, in many instances, appear to be localized to presynaptic glutamate terminals where they act as feedback facilitators of glutamate release (Huettner 2003; Zhuo 2017). NMDA receptors are also tetrameric assemblies but are believed to consist of two obligatory GluN1 subunits (eight alternatively spliced isoforms) and, at most synapses, two subunits encoded by at least one of four different GluN2 subunits (GluN2A-D). Like kainate receptors, NMDA receptors are also highly permeable to extracellular calcium but are more commonly localized at postsynaptic sites (but see Bouvier et al. 2015; Dore et al. 2017). Postsynaptic NMDA receptors are typically blocked by intracellular magnesium bound to the channel pore which is displaced by membrane depolarizations, usually mediated by AMPA receptors. This type of "coincidence" detection by NMDA receptors, requiring both synaptic glutamate and membrane depolarization, likely underlies their role in the activity-dependent changes in synaptic efficacy (plasticity) that is believed to represent the synaptic correlate of learning and memory. $GABA_A$ receptors, members of the Cys-loop family of ligand-gated ion channels, are all anion-selective channels that mediated much of the "fast" inhibitory neurotransmission in the adult central nervous system. Like other members of the Cys-loop family, these receptors are pentameric assemblies that, for $GABA_A$, contain at least alpha and beta subunits. Synaptic $GABA_A$ receptors are believed to require gamma subunits as part of the pore-forming complex since these subunits contain binding sites for gephyrin which localizes $GABA_A$ receptors to postsynaptic sites. Delta subunits, which can replace gamma subunits in the assembly, dramatically alter complex pharmacology, function, and localization. Delta-containing $GABA_A$ receptors are frequently found in extrasynaptic $GABA_A$ receptors providing "tonic" inhibition mediated by GABA spillover from synaptic site. In addition to ionotropic receptors, glutamate and GABA also bind to heterotrimeric G protein-coupled receptors (mGluR and $GABA_B$, respectively). These receptors couple to a variety of signaling cascades and can regulate the production of second messengers like intracellular calcium, cyclic AMP, and inositol phosphates and can directly regulate the activity of ion channels like voltage-gated calcium channels and inwardly rectifying potassium channels. Compared to the ionotropic receptors, these metabotropic signaling events occur somewhat slowly owing to their localization (generally peripheral to the active zone) and their reliance on multistep signaling processes.

The late prenatal/early postnatal period is defined by rapid development of brain structures and neurotransmitter systems. For example, the expression and synaptic function of $GABA_A$ and ionotropic glutamate receptors generally mature during this period, prior to adolescence. These receptors, as well as their associated postsynaptic anchoring proteins which are involved with receptor trafficking and localization, reach adult levels/distributions prior to weaning in rodents (Dong et al. 1999; Korpi et al. 1993; Martin et al. 1998; Pandey et al. 2015; Virtanen et al. 2018; Yu et al. 2006; Zhong et al. 1995). Similar observations have been reported for mGluRs (Defagot et al. 2002) and $GABA_B$ receptors (Fritschy et al. 1999; Gaiarsa et al. 1995). The developmental trajectories of these various neurotransmitter receptor systems in nonhuman primates appear to be very similar (Gonzalez-Burgos et al. 2008; Shaw et al. 1991). These findings suggest that the functional aspects related to "fast" neurotransmitter systems like glutamate and GABA are largely in place prior to adolescence. However, activity-related "plastic" changes in synaptic function of these neurotransmitter systems appear to develop throughout the adolescent period in many brain regions. For example, long-term potentiation (LTP) at glutamate synapses, most typically characterized as activity-dependent upregulation of synaptic efficacy, is more robust in adults in brain regions like the prefrontal cortex (Konstantoudaki et al. 2018), hippocampal dentate gyrus (Zitman and Richter-Levin 2013), and interpeduncular nucleus (Koppensteiner et al. 2017). In contrast, LTP in the barrel cortex (Konstantoudaki et al. 2018) and nucleus accumbens (Schramm et al. 2002) either develops prior to adolescence (cortex) or is greater in adolescents compared to adults (n. accumbens). These findings suggest that LTP related to sensory processing and reward circuitry develop relatively early while plasticity related to executive control, spatial memory/emotion regulation, and negative control of reward circuitry (interpeduncular nucleus, Nishikawa et al. 1986) occurs postadolescence. On the other hand, long-term depression (LTD) at glutamate synapses is typical in many adolescent brain regions (Bergerot et al. 2013; Zhang et al. 2015) and may reflect processes related to the robust pruning of synapses during this developmental period (Selemon 2013). Recent work also suggests that circuits integrating emotional control and executive function are also established during adolescence. In adults for example, ventral hippocampal (vHC) and basolateral amygdala (BLA) inputs to the prefrontal cortex (PFC) converge to dynamically regulate synaptic plasticity in the latter region. High-frequency stimulation of BLA inputs in vivo produces LTP of PFC synaptic responses, while coincidental stimulation of vHC inputs either de-potentiates (normalizes) or prevents, depending on the temporal sequence of BLA and vHC input activation, BLA-mediated PFC plasticity. vHC de-potentiation/block of BLA-mediated plasticity is notably absent in adolescent rats (Thomases et al. 2014). Similarly, high-frequency stimulation of vHC inputs to the PFC alone produces LTD of local field potentials in the PFC; picrotoxin, a $GABA_A$ receptor noncompetitive antagonist, converts this depression to potentiation. Both this picrotoxin-sensitive LTD and the resulting LTP are expressed in adult animals but not adolescents (Caballero et al. 2014). This suggests a robust developmental regulation of PFC GABAergic control of plasticity in this region. Further, the development of GABAergic control of glutamatergic plasticity in the PFC appears directly related to the maturation of local GABA circuits (Kang et al. 2018; Konstantoudaki et al. 2018; Morishita et al. 2015).

Compared to glutamate synapses, less is known about the adolescent development of GABAergic synaptic plasticity. However, the distribution and localization of synaptic specializations associated with GABA neurotransmission may continue to develop during adolescence as well. For example, gephyrin, the $GABA_A$ receptor anchoring protein which stabilizes these receptors in postsynaptic compartments, declines markedly in axonal initial segments of nonhuman primate medial prefrontal cortical pyramidal neurons during adolescence (Cruz et al. 2009), while gephyrin clusters on the dendritic shafts of these neurons appears to be stable prior to weaning in rodents (Virtanen et al. 2018). These observations suggest a subtle shift in GABAergic control over neuronal excitability during the adolescent period that may be reflected by GABAergic adaptations to adolescent ethanol exposure (below). Thus, while the basal function of many glutamate and GABA synapses may be "adult-like" prior to adolescence, the processes involved with their dynamic, activity-dependent regulation as well as the circuits themselves may continue to develop throughout this period. In particular, adolescent development of glutamatergic and GABAergic synaptic function appears in regions like the prefrontal cortex, hippocampus, and basolateral amygdala. This suggests that integration of emotional information, memory, and executive control continues developing during adolescence and may suggest why these processes are particularly vulnerable to disruption by external influences including ethanol exposure.

3 Adolescent Ethanol Exposure

Longitudinal studies in humans show that adolescents who drink to intoxication are at greatest risk of developing AUD as adults (Warner et al. 2007). Preclinical rodent models have therefore relied primarily upon noncontingent ethanol exposure given the limited self-administration in this species. Although there is limited data currently, adolescent self-administration in nonhuman primates appears to cause disruptions in neurotransmitter function which parallel those using noncontingent exposure in rodents suggesting that the exposure itself is a major factor in adolescent vulnerability. Most rodent preclinical studies utilize repeating cycles of brief, robust intoxication (ethanol delivered intraperitoneally, intragastrically, or through vapor inhalation) followed by short-term withdrawal to mimic the binge-like drinking patterns that are common in human adolescents. These adolescent exposures dysregulate adult behaviors and suggest an overall increase in an "addiction-prone" phenotype. For example, adult rats with a history of adolescent ethanol exposure exhibit greater ethanol-seeking behavior (Amodeo et al. 2017; Gass et al. 2014), consumption (Amodeo et al. 2017; Criado and Ehlers 2013; Pascual et al. 2009), and preference (Pascual et al. 2009). Exceptional reviews highlighting an array of adult behavioral consequences related to adolescent ethanol exposure are in the literature (Crews and Boettiger 2009; Doremus-Fitzwater and Spear 2016; Spear and Swartzwelder 2014; Varlinskaya et al. 2016; White and Swartzwelder 2005). In general, these reviews suggest that adult outcomes can be characterized as a persistent, adolescent-like behavioral phenotype in adults exposed to adolescent intermittent ethanol. These phenotypes include reduced executive function, increased reward sensitivity, and reduced sensitivity to ethanol sedation and motor impairment. While there has been a few reviews integrating these rodent behavioral outcomes in the context of dopamine neurochemistry/neurotransmission (Doremus-Fitzwater and Spear 2016; Maldonado-Devincci et al. 2010; Spear 2016) and neuro-immune function (Crews et al. 2016; Pascual et al. 2014; Ward et al. 2014), the current review will focus on the central role of GABA and glutamate in the central nervous system and their vulnerability to adolescent ethanol exposure.

3.1 Adolescent Ethanol Exposure and Glutamate Neurotransmission

Dendritic Spine Morphology The morphological correlates of glutamatergic neurotransmission are dendritic spines. These postsynaptic specializations oppose presynaptic release sites and contain glutamate receptors and signaling pathways responsible for moment-by-moment synaptic activity as well as activity-dependent changes in synaptic efficacy. During spine morphogenesis, immature spines appear as thin filopodial-like projections that mature into mushroom-shaped specializations. In general, adolescent ethanol exposure appears to influence adult spine density and morphology (hence maturation) in a brain region-dependent manner. There is a dramatic increase in both hippocampal principal neuron dendritic branching and the number of mature spines during adolescence (Aoki et al. 2017); in the dentate gyrus (Mulholland et al. 2018), adolescent ethanol exposure modestly reduces the number of "immature" spines. In contrast, in the CA1 (Risher et al. 2015), adolescent exposure increases the density of immature spines while decreasing the relative number of mature spines. These ethanol-related alterations in adult spine morphology may be an anatomical correlate of memory dysfunction in adults exposed to adolescent ethanol (Swartzwelder et al. 2015).

Adolescent ethanol exposure produces similar outcomes in rat prelimbic cortex. There ethanol exposure increases the density of immature spines (Trantham-Davidson et al. 2017). In contrast, studies with Thy-1 transgenic mice (Jury et al. 2017) found that adolescent exposure had no effect on spine density in prelimbic cortex but instead increased the width of mature spines. Both of these studies utilized intermittent ethanol vapor exposure; it is therefore not clear if the differences between the rat and mouse studies represent distinct, model-dependent outcomes or other procedural differences like the use of pyrazole in mice to stabilize blood-ethanol concentrations or higher blood-ethanol concentrations and longer exposures in the rat study. Regardless, in the same study, Jury et al. also reported adolescent ethanol exposure produced (1) similar effects in the basolateral amygdala (no effect on spine density, increase in the width of mature spines) and (2) a completely novel reduction in spine density and increase in mature spine width in the infralimbic cortex. While changes in spine density and shape are difficult to interpret in the context of synaptic function, these data nicely illustrate that adolescent ethanol exposure alters the synaptic architecture associated with glutamate neurotransmission in a brain region-dependent manner.

Adolescent Ethanol and Glutamate Receptors Similar to the regionally-dependent alterations in dendritic spine density and morphology, adolescent ethanol exposure appears to regulate the expression/function of glutamate receptors in a region- and age-specific manner. In a study comparing the short-term consequences of ethanol exposure during adolescence (P23) and adulthood in rats (P60), Pian et al. (2010) showed that adolescent exposure decreased cortical NR1 subunit protein levels during the exposure which normalized within 24 h post-ethanol. There was no effect on NR2A or NR2B subunit protein expression. In adults, cortical NR1, 2A, and 2B subunit proteins were also decreased immediately after the exposure. While NR1 levels normalized 2 weeks after the exposure (more slowly than adolescents), NR2A and NR2B subunit levels were dramatically elevated at this later time point albeit with distinct time courses. While adolescent exposure likewise decreases hippocampal NR1 and NR2A subunit protein levels, the expression of both proteins is elevated following a 2 week withdrawal. There was no effect on adolescent hippocampal NR2B subunits; exposure-dependent effects on these subunits in adults rapidly normalize within 24 h. A more recent proteomic analysis of adult hippocampal proteins following adolescent ethanol exposure focused on synaptic and extrasynaptic proteins directly associated with the NMDA NR2B subunit (Swartzwelder et al. 2016). This study again did not find significant effects of the adolescent exposure on adult levels of NR2B in either the synaptic or non-synaptic/extrasynaptic subcellular compartments. However, among the dozens of proteins associated with NR2B that were altered by the adolescent ethanol exposure, the treatment up-regulated pathways associated with the actin cytoskeleton in the synaptic compartment providing some indication of the molecular mechanisms controlling changes in spine density/morphology discussed in a previous paragraph.

In the non-synaptic fraction, adult NR1 subunit proteins associated with NR2B were also upregulated by the adolescent ethanol exposure suggesting increased function of NMDA receptors at these extra-synaptic sites. Importantly, extra-synaptic, NR2B-containing NMDA receptors in the hippocampus appear to help mediate long-term, activity-dependent regulation of glutamate neurotransmission (Lu et al. 2001; Yang et al. 2017), excitotoxic insult (Lai et al. 2011; Liu et al. 2007), and neuron excitability/network synchrony (Papouin and Oliet 2014). In contrast to these dynamic effects of ethanol exposure on adolescent NMDA subunit proteins in the cortex and hippocampus, neither adolescent nor adult ethanol exposure alter expression of NMDA receptor NR2 subunit mRNAs in lateral/basolateral amygdala (BLA) tissue (Falco et al. 2009; Floyd et al. 2003) or in individual BLA principal-like neurons (Floyd et al. 2003). However, NR1 subunit mRNA levels in this region are increased by adolescent ethanol; this is associated with increased NMDA receptor-mediated whole-cell currents (Floyd et al. 2003). Notably, the Floyd et al. study also showed that adolescent ethanol exposure increases NMDA current inhibition by the NR2B-selective antagonist, ifenprodil. These data, along with changes in the biophysical properties and calcium permeability of NMDA-mediated currents (Floyd et al. 2003), suggest increased functional contributions by NR2B subunits in BLA principal neurons following adolescent ethanol despite minimal impact of the exposure on subunit mRNAs or protein levels. These data together suggest that adolescent ethanol exposure regulates NMDA receptor expression/function in a regionally-specific manner and can involve transcription, translation, receptor function, and potentially localization.

The sensitivity of adolescent AMPA-type glutamate receptors in general, and particularly in the context of adult outcomes, is less well documented. In a study examining differences between adolescent and adult mouse AMPA receptors in the amygdala immediately following intermittent-access ethanol drinking, Agoglia et al. (2015) found no effects on total protein levels of GluA1 subunit in either the amygdala or striatum. In the amygdala however, adolescent drinking decreased phosphorylation of Serine 831 (Ser831) on the GluA1 subunit, in contrast to adult drinking which increased phosphorylation of this same site. The decreased phosphorylation in adolescents was associated with decreased phosphorylation of the auto-regulatory Threonine 286 site on CamKII suggesting a mechanistic link between decreased CamKII activity and GluA1 phosphorylation at Ser831. In contrast to these findings in mice, a dependence-like ethanol exposure in adolescent rats increased phosphorylation of lateral/basolateral amygdala AMPA subunits GluA1 at Ser831 as well as GluA2 at Ser880. This exposure also increased phosphorylation of the autoregulatory sites, Thr286 and Thr305, on CamKII and the phosphorylation of the PKC substrate, neurogranin (Christian et al. 2012). Like the mouse study, this rat study also found that an adolescent ethanol exposure had little impact on total protein levels of AMPA receptor subunits. Notably, GluA1 phosphorylation at S831 and GluA2 at Ser880 are both associated with increased receptor trafficking to the plasma membrane that is typically observed during activity-dependent synaptic plasticity; increased trafficking of AMPA receptors to the plasma membrane was directly demonstrated in the rat study (Christian et al. 2012). There are numerous procedural differences between the Agoglia and Christian study including exposure paradigm (hence level of intoxication), model system (mouse versus rat), and a specific focus on the cortical-like lateral and basolateral subdivisions in the rat study.

Adolescent Ethanol and Glutamate Synaptic Function In light of the regionally-dependent effects of adolescent ethanol exposure on glutamate receptor expression, it is perhaps no surprise that studies focused on glutamatergic neurotransmission likewise appear to highlight alterations in synaptic function that are again dependent upon the brain region. In the CA1 hippocampus for example, adolescent ethanol exposure increases NMDA-mediated synaptic currents (Swartzwelder et al. 2017) and increases the expression of long-term potentiation measured (LTP) with field recordings (Risher et al. 2015; Sabeti and Gruol 2008). Similar ethanol exposures during late adolescence/young adulthood actually decrease LTP expression (Sabeti and Gruol 2008) suggesting the effects of ethanol on NMDA-mediated synaptic currents and synaptic plasticity are age-dependent.

In the lateral/basolateral amygdala, chronic ethanol and withdrawal differentially modulate pre- and post-synaptic properties of glutamatergic synapses in adolescent rats. The BLA receives qualitatively distinct information from excitatory inputs arising from both cortical and subcortical/thalamic brain regions, which project to the BLA via the lateral external capsule or medial stria terminalis, respectively (Sah et al. 2003). In line with these afferents arising from different brain regions and entering the BLA through different anatomical pathways, the effects of adolescent ethanol exposure on these glutamatergic synapses also differ. For example, the subcortical/thalamic afferents entering the BLA through the medial stria terminalis arise from regions like the medial prefrontal cortex, anterior cingulate cortex, hippocampus, thalamus, and somatosensory cortex. In contrast, afferents entering the BLA through the lateral external capsule originate from lateral cortical areas such as the temporal, occipital, piriform, entorhinal, and insular cortices. Adolescent ethanol exposure increases in 'basal' glutamate synaptic transmission in the BLA, evidenced by increased frequency of spontaneous excitatory postsynaptic currents (sEPSC) as well as an increase in the frequency and amplitude of action potential-independent miniature EPSCs recorded in the presence of the sodium channel blocker, tetrodotoxin (Lack et al. 2007). Notably, this pre- and postsynaptic facilitation of BLA glutamate neurotransmission occurs in an input-specific fashion. Several studies have found increased presynaptic glutamate release following adolescent ethanol exposure when stimulating the medial stria terminalis inputs, with no presynaptic alterations at the lateral external capsule inputs (Christian et al. 2012, 2013; Lack et al. 2009; Morales et al. 2018). Christian et al. (2013) further revealed that this increased presynaptic function was characterized by increased synaptic glutamate concentrations, decreased 'failure-rates' ('no response' following minimal electrical stimulation), and enhanced contributions by the readily releasable pool of synaptic vesicles. These presynaptic physiological responses to adolescent ethanol were also associated with increased levels of vesicle-associated proteins like VAMP2 (part of the SNARE complex) and the vesicular glutamate proteins, VGLUT1, and VGLUT2. Additionally, BLA CB1 cannabinoid receptors located on medial stria terminalis terminals normally inhibit excitatory transmission. Robinson et al. (2016) found that adolescent ethanol exposure impairs CB1 function at these inputs and decreases CB1 protein expression.

Adolescent ethanol increases postsynaptic function, but not presynaptic function, at external capsule afferents onto BLA principal neurons (Christian et al. 2012, 2013; Floyd et al. 2003; Lack et al. 2007, 2009; Morales et al. 2018). Using a strontium (Sr^{2+}) substitution method to specifically separate pre- and postsynaptic function (Dodge et al. 1969) at these external capsule inputs, we found a significant increase in the Sr^{2+}-dependent EPSC (asynchronous EPSCs or aEPSCs) amplitude but not effect on frequency (Christian et al. 2012; Morales et al. 2018). In addition to postsynaptic AMPA receptor function, adolescent ethanol exposure also increases synaptic function of postsynaptic NMDA (Floyd et al. 2003; Lack et al. 2007) and kainate-type glutamate receptors (Lack et al. 2009). Notably, the input-specific alterations in BLA glutamatergic synaptic transmission induced by adolescent ethanol described above are also exposure duration- and sex-dependent. Morales et al. (2018) recently found that increased presynaptic function at medial stria terminalis inputs required shorter exposure durations relative to postsynaptic alterations at lateral external capsule inputs; and this was true for both sexes. However, synaptic alterations in females required longer ethanol exposures than males. These data all suggest that adolescent ethanol up-regulates the synaptic function of all three major subtypes of ionotropic glutamate receptors expressed by BLA principal neurons and increases presynaptic function stria terminalis inputs onto BLA principal neurons.

In contrast to the dynamic regulation of glutamate synapses in hippocampus and lateral/basolateral amygdala, recent work (Cuzon-Carlson et al. 2018) compared striatal miniature EPSC frequency (presynaptic), amplitude (postsynaptic), and biophysical properties in ethanol drinking monkeys across age-at-first-access that included adolescents (4–5 years old, equivalent to 15–18 years old humans), young adults (5–6 years old, 20–24 years old humans), and mature adults (7–11 years old, equivalent to 25–40 years old humans). After 14 months of drinking, the study found no significant age-by-exposure interactions for mEPSC frequency or amplitude in either the caudate or putamen. Similar studies in rodents showed no effect of adolescent exposure on extracellular glutamate concentrations in the caudate (Boutros et al. 2014). These studies together show that the region-specific effects of adolescent exposure on glutamate receptor expression function are likewise reflected at the level of the synapse. Importantly, glutamatergic transmission in reward- and habit-related regions appear to achieve adult-like resilience to ethanol exposure during adolescence while synaptic function in regions involved with executive function and emotional control remain vulnerable.

3.2 Adolescent Ethanol Exposure and GABA Neurotransmission

Adolescent Ethanol and GABA Receptors Like glutamatergic receptors, adolescent ethanol exposure appears to produce region-dependent changes in the expression and localization of $GABA_A$ receptors. In the prelimbic cortex for example, adolescent ethanol exposure does not appear to modulate total protein levels of the $\alpha1$, $\alpha4$, $\alpha5$, δ, or $\gamma2$ subunits and does not appear to alter the plasma membrane levels of delta-containing receptors in adults (Centanni et al. 2017). But this contrasts with substantive changes in $GABA_A$-mediated extrasynaptic currents mediated by delta-containing $GABA_A$ receptors that is produced by a similar exposure (below). In contrast to the prelimbic cortex, $GABA_A$ protein expression in adult hippocampus is dramatically altered by adolescent ethanol exposure. In a separate study, Centanni et al. (2014) used total hippocampus and separated lysates into synaptic and non-synaptic fractions. Adolescent exposure decreased $\alpha4$ subunit protein in the detergent-resistant, synaptic fraction and decreased δ subunit levels in the detergent-soluble, extrasynaptic fraction. Thus, adolescent ethanol appears to shift the subunit composition of adult hippocampal $GABA_A$ receptors. Surprisingly, $\alpha4$ subunit mRNA was increased by the adolescent exposure – a potential compensation to changes in subunit protein levels. Adult ethanol exposure had no effect on either subunit in hippocampus. Similarly, long-term adolescent ethanol drinking did not alter levels of the $GABA_A$ $\alpha1$ subunit mRNA in the lateral/basolateral amygdala; although adult drinking experience increased levels of the subunit mRNA (Falco et al. 2009). This contrasts with studies of $GABA_A$ subunit proteins in this brain region which found that an adolescent dependence-like exposure decreased both $\alpha1$ subunit proteins levels and diminished $\alpha1$-containing receptors found on the plasma membrane (Diaz et al. 2011). Although adult outcomes were not measured in the Diaz et al. study, this work also found that adolescent ethanol increased the levels of $\alpha4$-containing receptors at the cell surface without altering total levels of $\alpha4$ subunit protein. $GABA_A$ gamma2 subunit and gephyrin protein levels were also increased by the adolescent ethanol exposure; these proteins localize $GABA_A$ receptors to postsynaptic specializations (Schweizer et al. 2003). While these findings highlight the region-specific effects of the exposure, they indicate that adolescent ethanol appears to also alter the proteins involved with receptor trafficking/localization. Importantly, trafficking/localization can occur independently from or in conjunction with alterations in protein or mRNA expression.

Adolescent Ethanol and GABAergic Synaptic Function Like the effects on subunit expression, adolescent ethanol exposure exerts region-specific effects on adult GABAergic neurotransmission. Generally, those regions in which GABAergic synaptic function are developing during adolescence remain sensitive to ethanol exposure during this period. In prelimbic cortex for example, adult 'basal' GABAergic synaptic function, reflected by tetrodotoxin-resistant or 'miniature' inhibitory postsynaptic currents (mIPSCs), remains unaltered by adolescent ethanol exposure. However, the amplitude of spontaneous IPSCs – which reflect both basal transmission and the activity of intrinsic cortical GABAergic connections – is decreased by adolescent ethanol (Centanni et al. 2017) highlighting the vulnerability of developing adolescent GABAergic circuits in this brain region. Importantly, adolescent ethanol exposure also decreases electrically-evoked, repetitive firing of prelimbic cortical fast-spiking interneurons (Trantham-Davidson et al. 2017). Together these findings suggest that ethanol-dependent modulation of GABAergic circuitry may reflect direct effects on intrinsic interneurons or their synapses. Importantly, extrasynaptic $GABA_A$ receptors, which mediate the tonic currents expressed by prelimbic principal neurons, are also vulnerable to adolescent ethanol exposure. During the transition from adolescence to adulthood, the number of prelimbic layer 5/6 pyramidal neurons expressing tonic currents increases from roughly 20% of these cells at P45 to 100% of neurons at P90; adolescent ethanol exposure 'freezes' neurons in the adolescent phenotype such that number of adult neurons expressing tonic currents is greatly reduced (Centanni et al. 2017). Thus, both the intrinsic GABAergic circuitry and extrasynaptic GABAergic function in the prelimbic cortex are shaped by adolescent ethanol exposure.

In the hippocampus, acute ethanol potentiates sIPSC frequency to a greater extent in adults compared to adolescents, with minimal effects on mIPSCs (Li et al. 2003, 2006). This again suggests development of intrinsic hippocampal GABAergic circuitry during adolescence. However, in contrast to the cortex, adolescent exposure has no effect on adult sIPSC amplitude or frequency suggesting that hippocampal GABAergic circuitry is more resilient than cortex during this period. In contrast, the amplitude of tonic GABA currents in the dentate decrease from adolescence to adulthood; adolescent exposure accentuates this decline (Fleming et al. 2013). Acute ethanol facilitation of GABA tonic currents is also more pronounced in adolescent-ethanol animals compared (Fleming et al. 2012, 2013). Thus, while adolescent exposure has modest impact on adult GABAergic circuitry in the hippocampus, it produces persistent changes in both the tonic GABAergic currents and the acute effects of ethanol on these extrasynaptic currents.

In the BLA, at least two anatomically and functionally distinct populations of GABAergic interneurons, the lateral pericapsular intercalated cells (LPC) and local interneurons, synapse onto principal neurons. LPCs are GABAergic interneurons found in concentrated clusters along the external capsule while local GABAergic interneurons that are scattered throughout the BLA (Spampanato et al. 2011). Similar to the hippocampus, acute ethanol potentiates $GABA_A$ mediated inhibitory postsynaptic currents (IPSCs) recorded from both distal LPCs and local interneuron synapses in the BLA (Silberman et al. 2008). Chronic adolescent ethanol exposure robustly decreases presynaptic function at LPC GABAergic synapses which provide robust feed-forward inhibition to principal neurons (Diaz et al. 2011). Interestingly, adolescent ethanol does not alter GABAergic release from local interneurons. In addition to these presynaptic changes, Diaz and colleagues reported an increase in the decay kinetics of miniature IPSCs, likely arising from local interneurons which synapse onto principal neuron soma and proximal dendrites, suggesting an ethanol-induced modulation of postsynaptic function in intrinsic BLA GABAergic circuitry. This paralleled changes in the $GABA_A$ receptor subunit composition (described above).

In contrast to the specific vulnerability of adolescent GABAergic synapses/circuits in the cortex, hippocampus, and lateral/basolateral amygdala, adolescent and adult ethanol drinking alter GABAergic neurotransmission in nonhuman primate caudate/putamen to a similar extent. At these synapses, there is a general trend for an age-dependent increase in mIPSC frequency in both brain regions; an ethanol drinking history suppresses mIPSC frequency regardless of age (Cuzon-Carlson et al. 2018). There was no impact of drinking on mIPSC amplitude in these studies. However, sIPSCs were not measured so the impact of ethanol drinking on intrinsic GABAergic circuitry, particularly the excitability of GABA interneurons is not yet certain.

4 Concluding Remarks

A critical observation for GABA and glutamate within this review is that synaptic processes developing during adolescence appear to be the most vulnerable to ethanol exposure. Fundamental aspects of GABAergic and glutamatergic neurotransmission (i.e., presynaptic release, postsynaptic receptor function) are largely intact in many brain region by adolescence with some notable exceptions. But, the literature suggests that substantial components of GABAergic circuitry continue to develop during adolescence. These components can include the localization of GABAergic synapses on principal neurons (reflected by shifts in gephyrin immunoreactivity), GABAergic neuron firing (circuit ‘activity’), and extrasynaptic receptor activity. All these aspects of GABAergic neurotransmission are sensitive to adolescent ethanol exposure. For glutamate synapses, activity-dependent modulation of synaptic efficacy (‘plasticity’) likewise develops during adolescence and appears most vulnerable to ethanol exposure. This may be a product of developing signaling cascades or NMDA receptor function/activity/localization which can be influenced by subunit composition. Although these conclusions are specific for GABA and glutamate, similar outcomes are apparent for other neurotransmitters as well. With dopamine for example, adolescence can be characterized as a ‘reward-focused period’ (Doremus-Fitzwater and Spear 2016). This reward-centric focus is highlighted anatomically by a dramatic peak in dopaminergic projection development, particularly fibers from the ventral tegmental area and substantia nigra to the striatum, nucleus accumbens, and throughout the cortex (Doremus-Fitzwater and Spear 2016). Functionally, there are also peaks in dopamine cell firing rates (Marinelli and McCutcheon 2014) and receptor levels (Doremus-Fitzwater and Spear 2016) during adolescence. Adolescent ethanol exposure modulates the development of these processes. In the prelimbic cortex for example, ethanol exposure reduces dopamine fiber density and decreases D1-mediated regulation of pyramidal cell firing (Boutros et al. 2014; Trantham-Davidson et al. 2017). Similar to dopamine, the cholinergic system continues to develop during the transition from adolescence to adulthood (Carcoba et al. 2014; Nordberg et al. 1992). Also, adolescent ethanol exposure profoundly decreases the number of choline acetyltransferase-positive neurons in the basal forebrain (Boutros et al. 2014; Coleman et al. 2011; Fernandez and Savage 2017; Swartzwelder et al. 2015; Vetreno et al. 2014; Vetreno and Crews 2018). These data all suggest that vulnerability to ethanol exposure is directly related to neural processes which continue to mature during adolescence.

A second, equally important observation from the literature is that adolescent ethanol exposure alters GABA and glutamatergic neurotransmission in a brain region-dependent manner. Exposure-dependent alterations in receptor expression (mRNA or protein), phosphorylation, or localization vary across the regions are highlighted here. However, region-specific disruption in receptor expression is not specific to GABA or glutamate. For example, adolescent ethanol exposure significantly decreasing dopamine D1 and D2 protein levels in the frontal cortex but only D2 protein in the hippocampus and striatum (Pascual et al. 2009). Even subdivisions within the same region can express unique alterations. For example, spine morphology – an anatomical marker for glutamatergic synapses – is differentially impacted by adolescent exposure in hippocampal subregions like dentate gyrus and CA1 (Mulholland et al. 2018; Risher et al. 2015) or in medial prefrontal cortical areas like prelimbic and infralimbic cortex (Jury et al. 2017). It is perhaps no surprise then that synaptic function and circuits are likewise altered by adolescent ethanol in a regionally-specific manner.

A limitation associated with the current preclinical literature is that processes maturing during adolescence remain poorly defined in many instances. The focus of this review has thus been primarily on adolescent ethanol modulation of GABA and glutamate neurotransmission in the context of executive function, memory, and emotion – processes well recognized as exhibiting profound development during adolescence. As highlighted in the Introduction, adolescents and adults also differ in self-administration behavior and are differentially sensitive to ethanol sedation/intoxication and aversion. Circuits and synaptic processes related to these behaviors are therefore important targets for future preclinical studies. For example, outside of the well described dopamine circuits influencing activity of nucleus accumbens neurons (Doremus-Fitzwater and Spear 2016), glutamate and/or GABA signaling in the lateral hypothalamus, dorsal striatum, central amygdala all regulate ethanol self-administration (Hwa et al. 2017). The circuits/processes controlling ethanol sedation/intoxication are less well-defined, but acute ethanol inhibits nicotinic receptors in brainstem nuclei involved with motor performance, attention, and sleep (McDaid et al. 2016). In a recent study with fMRI in humans, ethanol impairment of simulated driving behavior had its greatest effect on hemodynamics in cingulate/orbitofrontal circuits involved with attention and cerebellar/motor cortical circuits involved with gross and fine motor control (Meda et al. 2009). Finally, recent work focused on aversion-like behavior suggests that projections from the lateral habenula (LHb) to the ventral tegmental area (VTA) are promising targets for study as well. The lateral habenula provides glutamatergic input to GABAergic neurons in the rostromedial tegmental nucleus (RMTg) which negatively regulate VTA dopamine neurons projecting to the nucleus accumbens (Lammel et al. 2012). Optogenetic and lesion studies suggest this pathway is intimately involved with conditioned taste aversion (Haack et al. 2014; Lammel et al. 2012). Importantly, electrical stimulation of LHb reduces voluntary ethanol drinking (Li et al. 2016); neuron activity within the LHb-RMTg pathway is highly correlated with ethanol conditioned taste aversion (Glover et al. 2016). While additional circuit mapping studies are needed to understand the brain regions controlling ethanol sedation/intoxication and aversion, a focus on the adolescent development of the systems/circuits will help define synaptic mechanisms impacted by ethanol exposure during this vulnerable period.

Finally, it is worth noting that a detailed neurophysiological understanding of how sex regulates adolescent vulnerability to ethanol is largely missing in preclinical studies. Clinical data suggest the effects of sex are likely to be subtle. For example, sex does not predict lifetime drinking trajectory (i.e., those that go on to develop drinking problems as adults) in adolescent drinkers (Warner et al. 2007). However, lifetime prevalence for alcohol abuse and dependence following adolescent drinking tends to be lower for females compared to males across the entire adolescent period (Grant and Dawson 1997). Factors that influence sex-dependent drinking trajectories are likely to be subtle and potentially species-specific. For example, parental relationships appear to differentially regulate adolescent drinking in males and females, with more 'protective' or 'controlling' relationships reducing alcohol consumption in adolescent females and increasing it in males (Leung et al. 2014). Female humans tend to consume more alcohol during early adolescence with these relationships reversing to more 'adult-like' drinking (males>females) by late adolescence/early adulthood (Patrick and Schulenberg 2013). Importantly, these studies suggest that diagnostic criteria related to clinical interventions may need to be refined to address subtle differences between sexes across the adolescent period. Unfortunately, in a study examining adolescent alcohol and drug use in pediatric care settings, Sterling et al. (2012) found that adolescent males were significantly more likely than females to receive screening for alcohol use. Similar to these human studies, there is a paucity of neurophysiological data in females from preclinical studies. Behavioral studies may give some clue to potential circuits and neurotransmitter systems. For example, there are marginal sex differences with respect to cognitive function (Pavlovian conditioned approach; Madayag et al. 2017) and anxiety-like behavior (Amodeo et al. 2018). Sex differences related to ethanol locomotor impairment are also only evident in adult animals following long-term ethanol drinking that begins during adolescence (Westbrook et al. 2018). Despite this, adolescent male and female rats do differ with respect to the impact of stress (Wille-Bille et al. 2017) and social context (Varlinskaya et al. 2015) on ethanol drinking; sex interacts with social context to influence conditioned aversion to ethanol (Morales et al. 2014; Vetter-O'Hagen et al. 2009), but this may be influenced by both the conditioning paradigm (Pautassi et al. 2011) and rat strain (Schramm-Sapyta et al. 2014). Together, this literature suggests that subtle sex differences, particularly related to affiliative and social relationships, may distinguish the vulnerability within unique adolescent populations.

References

Agoglia AE, Holstein SE, Reid G, Hodge CW (2015) CaMKIIalpha-GluA1 activity underlies vulnerability to adolescent binge alcohol drinking. Alcohol Clin Exp Res 39:1680–1690

Alaux-Cantin S, Warnault V, Legastelois R, Botia B, Pierrefiche O, Vilpoux C, Naassila M (2013) Alcohol intoxications during adolescence increase motivation for alcohol in adult rats and induce neuroadaptations in the nucleus accumbens. Neuropharmacology 67:521–531

Amodeo LR, Kneiber D, Wills DN, Ehlers CL (2017) Alcohol drinking during adolescence increases consumptive responses to alcohol in adulthood in Wistar rats. Alcohol 59:43–51

Amodeo LR, Wills DN, Sanchez-Alavez M, Nguyen W, Conti B, Ehlers CL (2018) Intermittent voluntary ethanol consumption combined with ethanol vapor exposure during adolescence increases drinking and alters other behaviors in adulthood in female and male rats. Alcohol 73:57–66

Aoki C, Chowdhury TG, Wable GS, Chen YW (2017) Synaptic changes in the hippocampus of adolescent female rodents associated with resilience to anxiety and suppression of food restriction-evoked hyperactivity in an animal model for anorexia nervosa. Brain Res 1654:102–115

Bell RL, Rodd ZA, Smith RJ, Toalston JE, Franklin KM, McBride WJ (2011) Modeling binge-like ethanol drinking by peri-adolescent and adult P rats. Pharmacol Biochem Behav 100:90–97

Bergerot A, Rigby M, Bouvier G, Marcaggi P (2013) Persistent posttetanic depression at cerebellar parallel fiber to Purkinje cell synapses. PLoS One 8:e70277

Boutros N, Semenova S, Markou A (2014) Adolescent intermittent ethanol exposure diminishes anhedonia during ethanol withdrawal in adulthood. Eur Neuropsychopharmacol 24:856–864

Bouvier G, Bidoret C, Casado M, Paoletti P (2015) Presynaptic NMDA receptors: roles and rules. Neuroscience 311:322–340

Bundy DAP, de Silva N, Horton S, Patton GC, Schultz L, Jamison DT (2017) Child and adolescent health and development: realizing neglected potential. In: Bundy DAP, de Silva N, Horton S, Jamison DT, Patton GC (eds) Child and adolescent health and development, 3rd edn. The International Bank for Reconstruction and Development/The World Bank, Washington, pp 1–23

Caballero A, Thomases DR, Flores-Barrera E, Cass DK, Tseng KY (2014) Emergence of GABAergic-dependent regulation of input-specific plasticity in the adult rat prefrontal cortex during adolescence. Psychopharmacology 231:1789–1796

Carcoba LM et al (2014) Cholinergic transmission during nicotine withdrawal is influenced by age and pre-exposure to nicotine: implications for teenage smoking. Dev Neurosci 36:347–355

Centanni SW et al (2014) Adolescent alcohol exposure alters GABAA receptor subunit expression in adult hippocampus. Alcohol Clin Exp Res 38:2800–2808

Centanni SW, Burnett EJ, Trantham-Davidson H, Chandler LJ (2017) Loss of delta-GABAA receptor-mediated tonic currents in the adult prelimbic cortex following adolescent alcohol exposure. Addict Biol 22:616–628

Christian DT, Alexander NJ, Diaz MR, Robinson S, McCool BA (2012) Chronic intermittent ethanol and withdrawal differentially modulate basolateral amygdala AMPA-type glutamate receptor function and trafficking. Neuropharmacology 62:2429–2438

Christian DT, Alexander NJ, Diaz MR, McCool BA (2013) Thalamic glutamatergic afferents into the rat basolateral amygdala exhibit increased presynaptic glutamate function following withdrawal from chronic intermittent ethanol. Neuropharmacology 65:134–142

Coleman LG Jr, He J, Lee J, Styner M, Crews FT (2011) Adolescent binge drinking alters adult brain neurotransmitter gene expression, behavior, brain regional volumes, and neurochemistry in mice. Alcohol Clin Exp Res 35:671–688

Crews FT, Boettiger CA (2009) Impulsivity, frontal lobes and risk for addiction. Pharmacol Biochem Behav 93:237–247

Crews FT, Vetreno RP, Broadwater MA, Robinson DL (2016) Adolescent alcohol exposure persistently impacts adult neurobiology and behavior. Pharmacol Rev 68:1074–1109

Criado JR, Ehlers CL (2013) Effects of adolescent onset voluntary drinking followed by ethanol vapor exposure on subsequent ethanol consumption during protracted withdrawal in adult Wistar rats. Pharmacol Biochem Behav 103:622–630

Cruz DA, Lovallo EM, Stockton S, Rasband M, Lewis DA (2009) Postnatal development of synaptic structure proteins in pyramidal neuron axon initial segments in monkey prefrontal cortex. J Comp Neurol 514:353–367

Cuzon-Carlson VC, Grant KA, Lovinger DM (2018) Synaptic adaptations to chronic ethanol intake in male rhesus monkey dorsal striatum depend on age of drinking onset. Neuropharmacology 131:128–142

Defagot MC, Villar MJ, Antonelli MC (2002) Differential localization of metabotropic glutamate receptors during postnatal development. Dev Neurosci 24:272–282

DeWit DJ, Adlaf EM, Offord DR, Ogborne AC (2000) Age at first alcohol use: a risk factor for the development of alcohol disorders. Am J Psychiatry 157:745–750

Diaz MR, Christian DT, Anderson NJ, McCool BA (2011) Chronic ethanol and withdrawal differentially modulate basolateral amygdala paracapsular and local GABAergic synapses. J Pharmacol Exp Ther 337:162–170

Dodge FA Jr, Miledi R, Rahamimoff R (1969) Strontium and quantal release of transmitter at the neuromuscular junction. J Physiol 200:267–283

Dong H, Zhang P, Song I, Petralia RS, Liao D, Huganir RL (1999) Characterization of the glutamate receptor-interacting proteins GRIP1 and GRIP2. J Neurosci 19:6930–6941

Dore K, Stein IS, Brock JA, Castillo PE, Zito K, Sjostrom PJ (2017) Unconventional NMDA receptor signaling. J Neurosci 37:10800–10807

Doremus-Fitzwater TL, Spear LP (2016) Reward-centricity and attenuated aversions: an adolescent phenotype emerging from studies in laboratory animals. Neurosci Biobehav Rev 70:121–134

Falco AM, Bergstrom HC, Bachus SE, Smith RF (2009) Persisting changes in basolateral amygdala mRNAs after chronic ethanol consumption. Physiol Behav 96:169–173

Fernandez GM, Savage LM (2017) Adolescent binge ethanol exposure alters specific forebrain cholinergic cell populations and leads to selective functional deficits in the prefrontal cortex. Neuroscience 361:129–143

Fleming RL, Acheson SK, Moore SD, Wilson WA, Swartzwelder HS (2012) In the rat, chronic intermittent ethanol exposure during adolescence alters the ethanol sensitivity of tonic inhibition in adulthood. Alcohol Clin Exp Res 36:279–285

Fleming RL et al (2013) Binge-pattern ethanol exposure during adolescence, but not adulthood, causes persistent changes in GABAA receptor-mediated tonic inhibition in dentate granule cells. Alcohol Clin Exp Res 37:1154–1160

Floyd DW, Jung KY, McCool BA (2003) Chronic ethanol ingestion facilitates N-methyl-D-aspartate receptor function and expression in rat lateral/basolateral amygdala neurons. J Pharmacol Exp Ther 307:1020–1029

Fritschy JM, Meskenaite V, Weinmann O, Honer M, Benke D, Mohler H (1999) $GABA_B$-receptor splice variants GB1a and GB1b in rat brain: developmental regulation, cellular distribution and extrasynaptic localization. Eur J Neurosci 11:761–768

Gaiarsa JL, Tseeb V, Ben-Ari Y (1995) Postnatal development of pre- and postsynaptic GABAB-mediated inhibitions in the CA3 hippocampal region of the rat. J Neurophysiol 73:246–255

Gass JT et al (2014) Adolescent alcohol exposure reduces behavioral flexibility, promotes disinhibition, and increases resistance to extinction of ethanol self-administration in adulthood. Neuropsychopharmacology 39:2570–2583

Glover EJ, McDougle MJ, Siegel GS, Jhou TC, Chandler LJ (2016) Role for the rostromedial tegmental nucleus in signaling the aversive properties of alcohol. Alcohol Clin Exp Res 40:1651–1661

Gonzalez-Burgos G, Kroener S, Zaitsev AV, Povysheva NV, Krimer LS, Barrionuevo G, Lewis DA (2008) Functional maturation of excitatory synapses in layer 3 pyramidal neurons during postnatal development of the primate prefrontal cortex. Cereb Cortex 18:626–637

Graham DL, Diaz-Granados JL (2006) Periadolescent exposure to ethanol and diazepam alters the aversive properties of ethanol in adult mice. Pharmacol Biochem Behav 84:406–414

Grant BF, Dawson DA (1997) Age at onset of alcohol use and its association with DSM-IV alcohol abuse and dependence: results from the National Longitudinal Alcohol Epidemiologic Survey. J Subst Abus 9:103–110

Haack AK, Sheth C, Schwager AL, Sinclair MS, Tandon S, Taha SA (2014) Lesions of the lateral habenula increase voluntary ethanol consumption and operant self-administration, block yohimbine-induced reinstatement of ethanol seeking, and attenuate ethanol-induced conditioned taste aversion. PLoS One 9:e92701

Huettner JE (2003) Kainate receptors and synaptic transmission. Prog Neurobiol 70:387–407

Hwa L, Besheer J, Kash T (2017) Glutamate plasticity woven through the progression to alcohol use disorder: a multi-circuit perspective. F1000Research 6:298

Jury NJ et al (2017) Chronic ethanol during adolescence impacts corticolimbic dendritic spines and behavior. Alcohol Clin Exp Res 41:1298–1308

Kang S, Cox CL, Gulley JM (2018) High frequency stimulation-induced plasticity in the prelimbic cortex of rats emerges during adolescent development and is associated with an increase in dopamine receptor function. Neuropharmacology 141:158–166

Konstantoudaki X, Chalkiadaki K, Vasileiou E, Kalemaki K, Karagogeos D, Sidiropoulou K (2018) Prefrontal cortical-specific differences in behavior and synaptic plasticity between adolescent and adult mice. J Neurophysiol 119:822–833

Koppensteiner P, Melani R, Ninan I (2017) A cooperative mechanism involving Ca(2+)-permeable AMPA receptors and retrograde activation of GABAB receptors in interpeduncular nucleus plasticity. Cell Rep 20:1111–1122

Korpi ER, Uusi-Oukari M, Kaivola J (1993) Postnatal development of diazepam-insensitive [3H] Ro 15-4513 binding sites. Neuroscience 53:483–488

Lack AK, Diaz MR, Chappell A, DuBois DW, McCool BA (2007) Chronic ethanol and withdrawal differentially modulate pre- and postsynaptic function at glutamatergic synapses in rat basolateral amygdala. J Neurophysiol 98:3185–3196

Lack AK, Christian DT, Diaz MR, McCool BA (2009) Chronic ethanol and withdrawal effects on kainate receptor-mediated excitatory neurotransmission in the rat basolateral amygdala. Alcohol 43:25–33

Lai TW, Shyu WC, Wang YT (2011) Stroke intervention pathways: NMDA receptors and beyond. Trends Mol Med 17:266–275

Lammel S et al (2012) Input-specific control of reward and aversion in the ventral tegmental area. Nature 491:212–217

Leung RK, Toumbourou JW, Hemphill SA (2014) The effect of peer influence and selection processes on adolescent alcohol use: a systematic review of longitudinal studies. Health Psychol Rev 8:426–457

Li Q, Wilson WA, Swartzwelder HS (2003) Developmental differences in the sensitivity of hippocampal $GABA_A$ receptor-mediated IPSCS to ethanol. Alcohol Clin Exp Res 27:2017–2022

Li Q, Wilson WA, Swartzwelder HS (2006) Developmental differences in the sensitivity of spontaneous and miniature IPSCs to ethanol. Alcohol Clin Exp Res 30:119–126

Li J, Zuo W, Fu R, Xie G, Kaur A, Bekker A, Ye JH (2016) High frequency electrical stimulation of lateral habenula reduces voluntary ethanol consumption in rats. Int J Neuropsychopharmacol 27:pyw050

Liu Y et al (2007) NMDA receptor subunits have differential roles in mediating excitotoxic neuronal death both in vitro and in vivo. J Neurosci 27:2846–2857

Lu W, Man H, Ju W, Trimble WS, MacDonald JF, Wang YT (2001) Activation of synaptic NMDA receptors induces membrane insertion of new AMPA receptors and LTP in cultured hippocampal neurons. Neuron 29:243–254

Madayag AC, Stringfield SJ, Reissner KJ, Boettiger CA, Robinson DL (2017) Sex and adolescent ethanol exposure influence Pavlovian conditioned approach. Alcohol Clin Exp Res 41:846–856

Maldonado-Devincci AM, Badanich KA, Kirstein CL (2010) Alcohol during adolescence selectively alters immediate and long-term behavior and neurochemistry. Alcohol 44:57–66

Marinelli M, McCutcheon JE (2014) Heterogeneity of dopamine neuron activity across traits and states. Neuroscience 282:176–197

Martin LJ, Furuta A, Blackstone CD (1998) AMPA receptor protein in developing rat brain: glutamate receptor-1 expression and localization change at regional, cellular, and subcellular levels with maturation. Neuroscience 83:917–928

McDaid J, Abburi C, Wolfman SL, Gallagher K, McGehee DS (2016) Ethanol-induced motor impairment mediated by inhibition of alpha7 nicotinic receptors. J Neurosci 36:7768–7778

Meda SA, Calhoun VD, Astur RS, Turner BM, Ruopp K, Pearlson GD (2009) Alcohol dose effects on brain circuits during simulated driving: an fMRI study. Hum Brain Mapp 30:1257–1270

Mejia-Toiber J, Boutros N, Markou A, Semenova S (2014) Impulsive choice and anxiety-like behavior in adult rats exposed to chronic intermittent ethanol during adolescence and adulthood. Behav Brain Res 266:19–28

Morales M, Schatz KC, Anderson RI, Spear LP, Varlinskaya EI (2014) Conditioned taste aversion to ethanol in a social context: impact of age and sex. Behav Brain Res 261:323–327

Morales M, McGinnis MM, Robinson SL, Chappell AM, McCool BA (2018) Chronic intermittent ethanol exposure modulation of glutamatergic neurotransmission in rat lateral/basolateral amygdala is duration-, input-, and sex-dependent. Neuroscience 371:277–287

Morishita H, Kundakovic M, Bicks L, Mitchell A, Akbarian S (2015) Interneuron epigenomes during the critical period of cortical plasticity: implications for schizophrenia. Neurobiol Learn Mem 124:104–110

Mulholland PJ, Teppen TL, Miller KM, Sexton HG, Pandey SC, Swartzwelder HS (2018) Donepezil reverses dendritic spine morphology adaptations and Fmr1 epigenetic modifications in hippocampus of adult rats after adolescent alcohol exposure. Alcohol Clin Exp Res 42:706–717

Nishikawa T, Fage D, Scatton B (1986) Evidence for, and nature of, the tonic inhibitory influence of habenulointerpeduncular pathways upon cerebral dopaminergic transmission in the rat. Brain Res 373:324–336

Nordberg A, Alafuzoff I, Winblad B (1992) Nicotinic and muscarinic subtypes in the human brain: changes with aging and dementia. J Neurosci Res 31:103–111

Pandey SP, Rai R, Gaur P, Prasad S (2015) Development- and age-related alterations in the expression of AMPA receptor subunit GluR2 and its trafficking proteins in the hippocampus of male mouse brain. Biogerontology 16:317–328

Papouin T, Oliet SH (2014) Organization, control and function of extrasynaptic NMDA receptors. Philos Trans R Soc Lond Ser B Biol Sci 369:20130601

Pascual M, Boix J, Felipo V, Guerri C (2009) Repeated alcohol administration during adolescence causes changes in the mesolimbic dopaminergic and glutamatergic systems and promotes alcohol intake in the adult rat. J Neurochem 108:920–931

Pascual M, Pla A, Minarro J, Guerri C (2014) Neuroimmune activation and myelin changes in adolescent rats exposed to high-dose alcohol and associated cognitive dysfunction: a review with reference to human adolescent drinking. Alcohol Alcohol 49:187–192

Patrick ME, Schulenberg JE (2013) Prevalence and predictors of adolescent alcohol use and binge drinking in the United States. Alcohol Res 35:193–200

Pautassi RM, Myers M, Spear LP, Molina JC, Spear NE (2011) Ethanol induces second-order aversive conditioning in adolescent and adult rats. Alcohol 45:45–55

Pian JP, Criado JR, Walker BM, Ehlers CL (2008) Differential effects of acute alcohol on EEG and sedative responses in adolescent and adult Wistar rats. Brain Res 1194:28–36

Pian JP, Criado JR, Milner R, Ehlers CL (2010) N-methyl-D-aspartate receptor subunit expression in adult and adolescent brain following chronic ethanol exposure. Neuroscience 170:645–654

Risher ML et al (2015) Adolescent intermittent alcohol exposure: persistence of structural and functional hippocampal abnormalities into adulthood. Alcohol Clin Exp Res 39:989–997

Robinson SL, Alexander NJ, Bluett RJ, Patel S, McCool BA (2016) Acute and chronic ethanol exposure differentially regulate CB1 receptor function at glutamatergic synapses in the rat basolateral amygdala. Neuropharmacology 108:474–484

Sabeti J, Gruol DL (2008) Emergence of NMDAR-independent long-term potentiation at hippocampal CA1 synapses following early adolescent exposure to chronic intermittent ethanol: role for sigma-receptors. Hippocampus 18:148–168

Sah P, Faber ES, Lopez De Armentia M, Power J (2003) The amygdaloid complex: anatomy and physiology. Physiol Rev 83:803–834

SAMHSA (2017) Key substance use and mental health indicators in the United States: results from the 2016 National Survey on Drug Use and Health. HHS publication no. SMA 17-5044; NSDUH series H-52. Center for Behavioral Health Statistics and Quality, Substance Abuse and Mental Health Services Administration, Rockville

Schramm NL, Egli RE, Winder DG (2002) LTP in the mouse nucleus accumbens is developmentally regulated. Synapse 45:213–219

Schramm-Sapyta NL et al (2010) Aversive effects of ethanol in adolescent versus adult rats: potential causes and implication for future drinking. Alcohol Clin Exp Res 34:2061–2069

Schramm-Sapyta NL, Francis R, MacDonald A, Keistler C, O'Neill L, Kuhn CM (2014) Effect of sex on ethanol consumption and conditioned taste aversion in adolescent and adult rats. Psychopharmacology 231:1831–1839

Schuckit MA (1984) Subjective responses to alcohol in sons of alcoholics and control subjects. Arch Gen Psychiatry 41:879–884

Schweizer C, Balsiger S, Bluethmann H, Mansuy IM, Fritschy JM, Mohler H, Luscher B (2003) The gamma 2 subunit of GABA(A) receptors is required for maintenance of receptors at mature synapses. Mol Cell Neurosci 24:442–450

Selemon LD (2013) A role for synaptic plasticity in the adolescent development of executive function. Transl Psychiatry 3:e238

Sengupta P (2013) The laboratory rat: relating its age with human's. Int J Prev Med 4:624–630

Serlin H, Torregrossa MM (2015) Adolescent rats are resistant to forming ethanol seeking habits. Dev Cogn Neurosci 16:183–190

Shaw C, Cameron L, March D, Cynader M, Zielinski B, Hendrickson A (1991) Pre- and postnatal development of GABA receptors in Macaca monkey visual cortex. J Neurosci 11:3943–3959

Silberman Y, Shi L, Brunso-Bechtold JK, Weiner JL (2008) Distinct mechanisms of ethanol potentiation of local and paracapsular GABAergic synapses in the rat basolateral amygdala. J Pharmacol Exp Ther 324:251–260

Spampanato J, Polepalli J, Sah P (2011) Interneurons in the basolateral amygdala. Neuropharmacology 60:765–773

Spear LP (2016) Consequences of adolescent use of alcohol and other drugs: studies using rodent models. Neurosci Biobehav Rev 70:228–243

Spear LP, Swartzwelder HS (2014) Adolescent alcohol exposure and persistence of adolescent-typical phenotypes into adulthood: a mini-review. Neurosci Biobehav Rev 45:1–8

Sterling S, Kline-Simon AH, Wibbelsman C, Wong A, Weisner C (2012) Screening for adolescent alcohol and drug use in pediatric health-care settings: predictors and implications for practice and policy. Addict Sci Clin Pract 7:13

Swartzwelder HS, Acheson SK, Miller KM, Sexton HG, Liu W, Crews FT, Risher ML (2015) Adolescent intermittent alcohol exposure: deficits in object recognition memory and forebrain cholinergic markers. PLoS One 10:e0140042

Swartzwelder HS, Risher ML, Miller KM, Colbran RJ, Winder DG, Wills TA (2016) Changes in the adult GluN2B associated proteome following adolescent intermittent ethanol exposure. PLoS One 11:e0155951

Swartzwelder HS, Park MH, Acheson S (2017) Adolescent ethanol exposure enhances NMDA receptor-mediated currents in hippocampal neurons: reversal by gabapentin. Sci Rep 7:13133

Thomases DR, Cass DK, Meyer JD, Caballero A, Tseng KY (2014) Early adolescent MK-801 exposure impairs the maturation of ventral hippocampal control of basolateral amygdala drive in the adult prefrontal cortex. J Neurosci 34:9059–9066

Trantham-Davidson H et al (2017) Binge-like alcohol exposure during adolescence disrupts dopaminergic neurotransmission in the adult prelimbic cortex. Neuropsychopharmacology 42:1024–1036

Varlinskaya EI, Truxell EM, Spear LP (2015) Ethanol intake under social circumstances or alone in Sprague-Dawley rats: impact of age, sex, social activity, and social anxiety-like behavior. Alcohol Clin Exp Res 39:117–125

Varlinskaya EI, Kim EU, Spear LP (2016) Chronic intermittent ethanol exposure during adolescence: effects on stress-induced social alterations and social drinking in adulthood. Brain Res 2:30188–30183

Vetreno RP, Crews FT (2018) Adolescent binge ethanol-induced loss of basal forebrain cholinergic neurons and neuroimmune activation are prevented by exercise and indomethacin. PLoS One 13:e0204500

Vetreno RP, Broadwater M, Liu W, Spear LP, Crews FT (2014) Adolescent, but not adult, binge ethanol exposure leads to persistent global reductions of choline acetyltransferase expressing neurons in brain. PLoS One 9:e113421

Vetter CS, Doremus-Fitzwater TL, Spear LP (2007) Time course of elevated ethanol intake in adolescent relative to adult rats under continuous, voluntary-access conditions. Alcohol Clin Exp Res 31:1159–1168

Vetter-O'Hagen C, Varlinskaya E, Spear L (2009) Sex differences in ethanol intake and sensitivity to aversive effects during adolescence and adulthood. Alcohol Alcohol 44:547–554

Virtanen MA, Lacoh CM, Fiumelli H, Kosel M, Tyagarajan S, de Roo M, Vutskits L (2018) Development of inhibitory synaptic inputs on layer 2/3 pyramidal neurons in the rat medial prefrontal cortex. Brain Struct Funct 223:1999–2012

Walker BM, Walker JL, Ehlers CL (2008) Dissociable effects of ethanol consumption during the light and dark phase in adolescent and adult Wistar rats. Alcohol 42:83–89

Ward RJ, Lallemand F, de Witte P (2014) Influence of adolescent heavy session drinking on the systemic and brain innate immune system. Alcohol Alcohol 49:193–197

Warner LA, White HR, Johnson V (2007) Alcohol initiation experiences and family history of alcoholism as predictors of problem-drinking trajectories. J Stud Alcohol Drugs 68:56–65

Westbrook SR, Kang M, Sherrill LK, O'Hearn D, Krishnamani T, Gulley JM (2018) Sex differences in adolescent ethanol drinking to behavioral intoxication. J Exp Anal Behav 110:54–62

White AM, Swartzwelder HS (2005) Age-related effects of alcohol on memory and memory-related brain function in adolescents and adults. Recent Dev Alcohol 17:161–176

White AM, Truesdale MC, Bae JG, Ahmad S, Wilson WA, Best PJ, Swartzwelder HS (2002) Differential effects of ethanol on motor coordination in adolescent and adult rats. Pharmacol Biochem Behav 73:673–677

Wille-Bille A, Ferreyra A, Sciangula M, Chiner F, Nizhnikov ME, Pautassi RM (2017) Restraint stress enhances alcohol intake in adolescent female rats but reduces alcohol intake in adolescent male and adult female rats. Behav Brain Res 332:269–279

Yang Q et al (2017) Extrasynaptic NMDA receptor dependent long-term potentiation of hippocampal CA1 pyramidal neurons. Sci Rep 7:3045

Yu ZY, Wang W, Fritschy JM, Witte OW, Redecker C (2006) Changes in neocortical and hippocampal GABAA receptor subunit distribution during brain maturation and aging. Brain Res 1099:73–81

Zhang X, Feng ZJ, Chergui K (2015) Induction of cannabinoid- and N-methyl-D-aspartate receptor-mediated long-term depression in the nucleus accumbens and dorsolateral striatum is region and age dependent. Int J Neuropsychopharmacol 18:pyu052

Zhong J, Carrozza DP, Williams K, Pritchett DB, Molinoff PB (1995) Expression of mRNAs encoding subunits of the NMDA receptor in developing rat brain. J Neurochem 64:531–539

Zhuo M (2017) Cortical kainate receptors and behavioral anxiety. Mol Brain 10:16

Zitman FM, Richter-Levin G (2013) Age and sex-dependent differences in activity, plasticity and response to stress in the dentate gyrus. Neuroscience 249:21–30

Medication Development for Alcohol Use Disorder: A Focus on Clinical Studies

Lorenzo Leggio, Daniel E. Falk, Megan L. Ryan, Joanne Fertig, and Raye Z. Litten

Contents

1 Introduction 444
  1.1 Medications That Have Shown Efficacy in Research Clinical Studies for AUD 445
  1.2 Other Promising Medications or Compounds for AUD 454
2 Conclusions 455
References 456

Abstract

Compared to other medical disorders, including other brain diseases, the number of medications approved for alcohol use disorder (AUD) is very small. Disulfiram, naltrexone (oral and long-acting), and acamprosate are approved by the US Food and Drug Administration (FDA) to treat patients with AUD. These medications are also approved in other countries, including in Europe, where the European Medicines Agency (EMA) also approved nalmefene for AUD. Furthermore, baclofen was recently approved for AUD in France. These approved medications have small effect sizes, which are probably the consequence of the fact that they only work for some patients, yet a personalized approach to match the right medication with the right patient is still in its infancy. Therefore,

L. Leggio (✉)
Section on Clinical Psychoneuroendocrinology and Neuropsychopharmacology, National Institute on Alcohol Abuse and Alcoholism, Division of Intramural Clinical and Biological Research and National Institute on Drug Abuse Intramural Research Program, Bethesda, MD, USA

Medication Development Program, National Institute on Drug Abuse Intramural Research Program, Baltimore, MD, USA

Center for Alcohol and Addiction Studies, Brown University, Providence, RI, USA
e-mail: lorenzo.leggio@nih.gov

D. E. Falk · M. L. Ryan · J. Fertig · R. Z. Litten
Division of Medications Development, National Institute on Alcohol Abuse and Alcoholism, Bethesda, MD, USA

M. A. Nader, Y. L. Hurd (eds.), *Substance Use Disorders*,
Handbook of Experimental Pharmacology 258, https://doi.org/10.1007/164_2019_295

research is needed to expand the armamentarium of medications that clinicians can use to treat their patients, as well as to better develop personalized approaches. This book chapter reviews other medications, beyond those approved by the FDA, that have shown efficacy in clinical trials, as well as medications which are still in the early stages of evaluation in human studies.

Keywords
Alcohol use disorder · Clinical studies · Medication development · Pharmacotherapy

1 Introduction

Addictions, including alcohol use disorder (AUD), represent a chronic brain disorder characterized by a compulsive-like seeking behavior and consumption of excessive amounts of alcohol despite the knowledge of its negative consequences. As many other medical disorders, AUD represents a heterogenous disease and is the product of complex gene $\times$ environment interactions. There have been significant advances in the neuroscience field that have shed light on the neurobiological pathways that underline the development and maintenance of AUD. As reviewed in the previous chapter (McCool and McGinnis 2019), we have now a much better understanding of the molecular and neurobiological basis of AUD, and this knowledge has been instrumental in identifying important druggable targets. Studying these targets has resulted, in turn, in the development of medications that, combined with psychosocial and behavioral interventions, may help patients with AUD to reduce or quit drinking and prevent relapse.

In the USA, three medications have been approved by the US Food and Drug Administration (FDA) for the treatment of AUD: disulfiram, naltrexone (oral and extended-release injectable), and acamprosate. These medications are also approved in other countries, including in Europe, where the European Medicines Agency (EMA) also approved nalmefene for AUD. Furthermore, baclofen was recently approved for AUD in France. As it is often the case in medication development, especially in the neuroscience field, clinical trials testing these medications have from time to time generated conflicting results, therefore questioning the efficacy of these medications. Nonetheless, several meta-analyses do support the efficacy of these medications to treat patients with AUD. In particular, one of the most recent and comprehensive meta-analyses indicates that both acamprosate and oral naltrexone are associated with reduction in return to drinking, with no significant differences between these two medications (Jonas et al. 2014).

Compared to other medical disorders, including other brain diseases, the number of medications approved for AUD is very small. Furthermore, their effect sizes (e.g., numbers needed to treat) are small, which is probably the consequence of the fact that these medications only work for some patients; however, a personalized approach to match the right medication with the right patient is still in its infancy (e.g., for a recent systematic review on potential subgroups who may respond better to naltrexone, see Garbutt et al. 2014). Therefore, research is needed to expand the armamentarium of medications that clinicians can use to treat their patients, as well as to better develop personalized approaches. Efforts made to test other medications beyond those approved by the FDA are reviewed in this book chapter. Specifically, here we briefly review medications that have exhibited efficacy in alcohol treatment clinical trials and examples of medications which are still in the early stages of evaluation in human studies.

1.1 Medications That Have Shown Efficacy in Research Clinical Studies for AUD[1]

1.1.1 ABT-436 (Vasopressin V1b Receptor Antagonist)

Preliminary animal studies suggest that blocking the type 1b receptor (V1b) of the antidiuretic hormone vasopressin results in a reduction in alcohol drinking (Edwards et al. 2011; Zhou et al. 2011). Following on these preclinical findings, ABT-436 800 mg/day, a novel selected V1b receptor antagonist, was evaluated in a 12-week multi-site randomized clinical trial (RCT) of 150 alcohol-dependent individuals (Ryan et al. 2017). ABT-436 significantly increased the percent of days abstinent compared with placebo, while there were no significant differences in heavy drinking days nor on other measures of drinking or alcohol craving. Furthermore, in subgroup analyses, individuals reporting higher baseline levels of stress responded better to ABT-436 than to placebo. Tolerability and safety of ABT-436 in this RCT were excellent. Diarrhea was the only side effect to be significantly more frequent in the ABT-436 group than the placebo group, although only four participants stopped ABT-436 as a result of gastrointestinal complaints. The ABT-436 group, compared with the placebo group, had greater rates of anxiety and nausea, although these differences were only at a statistical trend level. Overall, additional future studies with this compound are warranted, but unfortunately, the manufacturer discontinued development of this compound.

1.1.2 Aripiprazole

Aripiprazole is an atypical, antipsychotic drug, approved by the FDA to treat schizophrenia and bipolar disorder and as adjunct treatment for major depression (Litten et al. 2016). Aripiprazole has multiple pharmacological mechanisms, including acting as a partial agonist for the dopamine D_2 and serotonin 5-HT_{1A} receptors and as an antagonist to the 5-HT_2 receptor (Fleischhacker 2005). Common side effects of aripiprazole include fatigue, insomnia, restlessness, somnolence, anxiety, and disturbances in attention.

Human laboratory studies suggest that aripiprazole may affect drinking behavior. Kranzler et al. (2008) reported that aripiprazole (2.5 mg and 10 mg per day) increased alcohol sedating effects and, to a lesser degree, reduced the euphoric effects ($N = 18$). Voronin et al. (2008) showed that, compared to placebo,

[1]Listed in alphabetical order.

aripiprazole (up to 15 mg per day) reduced alcohol drinking but had no effect on self-reported "high," intoxication, or alcohol craving ($N = 30$). Furthermore, Myrick et al. (2010) conducted a neuroimaging study ($N = 30$) which indicated that aripiprazole (15 mg per day) blunted alcohol cue-induced brain activity in the right ventral striatum. A recent human laboratory study of 99 alcohol-dependent individuals found that aripiprazole (15 mg per day) had no main effect on alcohol drinking during the naturalistic outpatient period (Anton et al. 2017). However, aripiprazole significantly decreased alcohol self-administration among individuals with low self-control and delayed the return to drinking in those with high impulsivity compared with placebo (Anton et al. 2017), suggesting the need for precision medicine to elucidate the efficacy of aripiprazole. Further supporting the importance of this future direction, an additional neurogenetic analysis from the same human laboratory study suggested that polymorphisms in the dopamine transporter 1 (DAT1) and other dopamine-related genes may moderate aripiprazole effects on alcohol cue-elicited striatal activation and alcohol self-administration (Schacht et al. 2018).

In a 12-week multi-site RCT ($N = 295$), aripiprazole (titrated up to 30 mg per day) was effective in reducing the number of drinks per drinking day compared with the placebo group and also reduced the blood concentrations of carbohydrate-deficient transferrin (CDT), a biomarker of excessive alcohol use, at weeks 4 and 8 (Anton et al. 2008). However, aripiprazole was not superior to placebo in percent of days abstinent, number of heavy drinking days, and time to first drinking day (Anton et al. 2008). In addition, 15 mg per day may be an optimal dose to test, given the higher dropout rate in the active group, compared to placebo, especially with the 30 mg dose.

At present, a 12-week RCT is under way in outpatients with bipolar I or II disorder (depressed or mixed mood state) and alcohol use disorder, with active alcohol use (NCT02918370).

1.1.3 Baclofen

Several animal studies support that the $GABA_B$ agonist baclofen, currently approved by the FDA for the treatment of muscle spasticity, may play a role in AUD (for a review, see Colombo and Gessa 2018). From a biobehavioral mechanism standpoint, several human laboratory studies suggest that baclofen may affect alcohol drinking by changing the subjective effects of alcohol. These observations have been reported in human laboratory studies with acute baclofen administration (40 mg or 80 mg) in nondependent heavy drinkers ($N = 18$; Evans and Bisaga 2009), as well as in a pilot human laboratory study ($N = 14$; Leggio et al. 2013) and in a relatively larger follow-up human laboratory study ($N = 34$, Farokhnia et al. 2017, 2018) with alcohol-dependent heavy drinkers treated with baclofen 30 mg per day for approximately a week.

In clinical trials, following a positive small 4-week RCT with baclofen 30 mg per day in alcohol-dependent patients ($N = 39$; Addolorato et al. 2002), a relatively larger 12-week RCT ($N = 84$) was conducted in alcohol-dependent patients with liver cirrhosis (Addolorato et al. 2007). This latter RCT indicated that baclofen

30 mg per day was significantly more effective, as compared to placebo, in increasing total alcohol abstinence, increasing the number of days abstinent, and reducing alcohol craving. An additional analysis also showed that, despite the smaller sample analyzed ($N = 24$), baclofen still was significantly effective in promoting total alcohol abstinence in a subgroup of patients with alcohol dependence, liver cirrhosis, and hepatitis C infection (Leggio et al. 2012). In contrast, another 12-week RCT conducted in 80 patients with alcohol dependence (without liver disease) did not find differences between baclofen 30 mg per day and placebo in any of the alcohol-related outcomes (Garbutt et al. 2010).

The mixed results of these studies suggest that baclofen might be an effective medication only in those patients with higher severity of alcohol dependence (Leggio et al. 2010). Consistent with this hypothesis, a 12-week RCT ($N = 30$) with baclofen (80 mg per day) in alcohol-dependent individuals who also were smokers indicated that baclofen, compared with placebo, significantly increased the number of days abstinent from alcohol and tobacco co-use, and this effect was stronger in those patients with higher severity of alcohol dependence (Leggio et al. 2015). Furthermore, it is possible that the fact that baclofen was effective in those alcohol-dependent patients with liver cirrhosis (Addolorato et al. 2007), but not in those without (Garbutt et al. 2010), may indirectly reflect the different severity of alcohol dependence of these patients. Two recent RCTs support this interpretation. Specifically, a 12-week RCT with baclofen 30 mg per day in 180 veteran patients with hepatitis C virus (HCV) coinfection did not find differences between baclofen and placebo on alcohol-related outcomes; notably, the baseline levels of alcohol were quite low in this trial, reflecting an overall low severity of dependence (Hauser et al. 2017). In contrast, another 12-week RCT ($N = 104$) found a significant effect of baclofen (either 30 mg per day or 75 mg per day, without a dose-response effect) on alcohol-related outcomes in patients (with and without alcoholic liver disease), and the effect of baclofen was stronger in those alcohol-dependent patients with alcoholic liver disease than those without (Morley et al. 2018a).

Some anecdotal case reports suggested that significantly higher doses of baclofen, compared to those used in previous RCTs, may be effective in facilitating alcohol abstinence, i.e., up to 140 mg per day (Bucknam 2007) or even up to 300 mg per day (Ameisen 2005). Despite the anecdotal nature of these reports, they prompted significant mass media interest and attention in the scientific community, culminating in a few RCTs that tested high doses of baclofen. Muller et al. (2015) conducted an RCT with baclofen up to 250 mg per day in 56 alcohol-dependent individuals and found that baclofen, compared to placebo, increased the abstinence rate and cumulative abstinence duration. In contrast, Beraha et al. (2016) conducted an RCT of baclofen in 151 alcohol-dependent individuals who were administered a relatively high dose (150 mg per day), a lower dose (30 mg per day), or placebo and found no differences in time to first relapse or abstinence rates among the three groups. In another multi-site 24-week RCT, baclofen (180 mg per day) or placebo was administered to 320 alcohol-dependent individuals (Reynaud et al. 2017). Although the baclofen and placebo group did not differ significantly for abstinence or drinks per day, baclofen was more effective than placebo in reducing drinking in individuals who were drinking heavily at baseline. In conclusion, whether higher doses are more effective remains unclear and controversial, although higher doses may have a greater risk of adverse events, the most common being somnolence, sleep disorders, asthenia, and dizziness. The French drug administration agency recently approved the use of baclofen for AUD, but it limited the approved dose to up to 80 mg per day (Medical Press 2018).

Two RCTs have recently been completed but results have not been published yet. A 16-week RCT conducted in the USA compared placebo to baclofen 30 mg per day and baclofen 90 mg per day in a community sample of alcohol-dependent patients (NCT01980706). Another RCT conducted in France with alcohol-dependent patients managed by primary care physicians compared placebo to baclofen up to 300 mg per day during a 52-week period (NCT01604330).

Notably, a recent international consensus statement highlighted the potential efficacy of baclofen, calling for additional larger studies with baclofen but also emphasizing the importance of tailoring doses based on safety, tolerability, and efficacy (Agabio et al. 2018).

1.1.4 Gabapentin

Gabapentin is approved by the FDA for the treatment of seizures, neuropathic pain, and restless legs syndrome. Its mechanism of action is thought to be related to its inhibition of voltage-gated calcium channels, which indirectly modulate GABA activity (Sills 2006).

An initial human laboratory study with 33 alcohol-dependent individuals indicated that gabapentin (1,200 mg per day) was effective in reducing alcohol craving and improving sleep quality (Mason et al. 2009).

A few short-term small RCTs have indicated the potential efficacy of gabapentin in AUD patients (Furieri and Nakamura-Palacios 2007; Brower et al. 2008). It has been also suggested that gabapentin may work best in patients with significant withdrawal symptoms. Specifically, compared to placebo, gabapentin (up to 1,200 mg per day for about 6 weeks and combined with flumazenil 20 mg per day for first 2 days) led to an increase in the percent of days abstinent and a longer delay to heavy drinking in 60 alcohol-dependent patients; however, this effect was limited to those patients with more alcohol withdrawal symptoms before treatment (Anton et al. 2009).

Two larger single-site RCTs ($N = 150$ in each trial) further support the role of gabapentin in AUD. The first was a 16-week RCT which combined and compared gabapentin to naltrexone and showed that the combined medication group experienced a longer delay to heavy drinking, less heavy drinking days, and fewer drinks per drinking days than the group taking naltrexone alone or receiving placebo (Anton et al. 2011). Additionally, the patients with the combined gabapentin/naltrexone reported significantly better sleep than the other two groups (Anton et al. 2011). The second trial was a 12-week RCT of gabapentin testing two doses: 900 mg per day and 1,800 mg per day. In this second trial, compared to placebo, gabapentin significantly improved the rates of abstinence and no heavy drinking with greater efficacy in the 1,800 mg per day group than the 900 mg per day group

(Mason et al. 2014). Furthermore, gabapentin reduced alcohol craving and improved mood and sleep (Mason et al. 2014).

More recently, results from another RCT conducted in Thailand further supported the efficacy of gabapentin (Chompookham et al. 2018). Specifically, 112 alcohol-dependent patients were treated with either placebo or gabapentin (at least 300 mg per day) for 12 weeks. Gabapentin significantly reduced the percent of heavy drinking days per week and the weekly drinking days (Chompookham et al. 2018). On the other hand, no superiority of gabapentin compared to placebo was found in a large recent RCT in the USA. The latter was a multi-site 6-month RCT in 346 alcohol-dependent patients treated with placebo or gabapentin enacarbil extended-release, a prodrug formulation of gabapentin designed to increase its bioavailability. This trial did not show efficacy of gabapentin enacarbil, compared to placebo, in any of the alcohol-related primary or secondary outcomes (Falk et al. 2019a). A pharmacokinetic analysis, suggested that specific formulation used in this RCT may have resulted in lower than expected absorption of the active medication (Falk et al. 2019a).

Common side effects of gabapentin in these trials included fatigue, insomnia, and headaches. Furthermore, it is important to mention that, while gabapentin is considered to have no abuse potential, a recent report indicates that gabapentin potentially may be misused in individuals with substance use disorder, especially those who abuse opioids (Smith et al. 2016).

Finally, a 16-week RCT is currently ongoing to investigate if gabapentin up to 1,200 mg per day has efficacy in a sample of patients with DSM-5 criteria for AUD and for history of alcohol withdrawal (NCT02349477).

1.1.5 Ondansetron

Ondansetron is a selective serotonin 5-HT_3 receptor antagonist approved by the FDA for the treatment of nausea and vomiting. Initial human laboratory studies indicated that ondansetron reduces the desire to drink and augments the biphasic (i.e., stimulating and sedating) effects of alcohol ($N = 16$ in Johnson et al. 1993; $N = 15$ in Kenna et al. 2009; $N = 12$ in Swift et al. 1996).

In early clinical trials, an RCT by Sellers et al. (1994) tested ondansetron (0.25 mg or 2 mg per day) in 71 alcohol-dependent individuals and found that, compared to placebo, ondansetron significantly decreased alcohol intake in a subgroup of individuals with relatively lower baseline drinking (10 or less drinks per drinking day). Notably, an unexpected reversed dose effect was observed such that the 0.25 mg dose was more efficacious than the 2 mg dose. A subsequent larger 11-week RCT ($N = 271$) tested ondansetron 2 μg/kg, 8 μg/kg, or 32 μg/kg per day in alcohol-dependent individuals divided as early- and late-onset of alcoholism (25-year-old or younger vs. >25-year-old). This trial showed efficacy of ondansetron only in early-onset patients, with 8 μg/kg being the most effective dose (Johnson et al. 2000).

The selective effect of ondansetron in the early-onset subpopulation raised the question of whether pharmacogenetics may further shed light on the potential selective role of ondansetron in AUD. For example, the *SLC6A4* gene encodes the serotonin transporter, 5-HTT, and the *SLC6A4* promoter contains a functional polymorphic region (5′-regulatory region of the 5-HTT; 5′-HTTLPR) with a long form (L) that possesses an additional 44 base pairs that are absent in the short variant (S). Alcohol-dependent individuals with the LL genotype, compared with those with the SS genotype, have significantly less 5-HT uptake and reduced paroxetine binding capacity (Javors et al. 2005; Johnson et al. 2008). Notably, 5′-HTTLPR polymorphisms have been associated with several psychiatric disorders including AUD. Johnson et al. (2011) performed a 11-week RCT of ondansetron (8 μg/kg per day) in 283 alcohol-dependent individuals randomized to 3 different genotypes: LL, LS, and SS genotypes of the main results of this trial showed that LL genotype patients treated with ondansetron had significantly lower drinks per drinking day and higher percentage of days abstinent, as compared to those treated with ondansetron but with the LS/SS genotypes and to those treated with placebo (Johnson et al. 2011). In a subsequent analysis from the same RCT, Johnson et al. (2013) found additional functional genetic polymorphisms in the *HTR3A* and *HTR3B* genes that encode the 5HT3 receptor, including AC polymorphism in the rs17614942 portion in the *HTR3B* gene and AG and GG polymorphisms in the rs1150226 and rs1176713 portions of the *HTR3A* gene, respectively. Ondansetron was more effective than placebo in reducing the number of drinks per drinking day and the number of heavy drinking days and increasing the percent of days abstinent in people carrying one or more of these genetic variants. However, it is important to keep in mind that the potential functionality of rs1150226 and rs1176713 of *HTR3A* and rs17614942 of *HTR3B* is unknown, and therefore their putative molecular mechanisms need to be elucidated. It has been speculated that all three of these polymorphisms may alter mRNA expression levels (Johnson et al. 2013). Finally, consistent with Johnson et al. (2011), Kenna et al. (2014a) conducted a laboratory study of ondansetron and sertraline in 77 nontreatment-seeking alcohol-dependent individuals and found that ondansetron was effective in reducing the amount of drinking per drinking day in LL genotype individuals. The same team also found that female, but not male, participants who had the LL genotype, and equal or greater than seven exon III repeats on the dopamine receptor D4 gene (DRD4), had significantly reduced alcohol intake after taking ondansetron (0.5 mg per day for 3 weeks) (Kenna et al. 2014b). Notably, expression of the 7-repeat allele of DRD4 is associated with a blunted effect of dopamine on cAMP levels in comparison to the 4-repeat allele, with almost a threefold increase in dopamine concentration required to achieve the same level of dopamine-induced cAMP inhibition as the 4-repeat allele (Asghari et al. 1995; Oak et al. 2000). A meta-analysis suggests DRD4 VNTR variation may be a risk factor for problematic alcohol use; however there is a critical need for studies with larger and more inclusive samples that account for sex and genetic ancestry to fully understand this relationship (Daurio et al. 2019).

From a safety standpoint, ondansetron has been typically very well-tolerated in these clinical trials with alcohol-dependent individuals. An FDA safety precaution warns that cardiac QT prolongation is possible at doses typically used for its approved indication (nausea and vomiting; https://www.fda.gov/Drugs/DrugSafety/ucm271913.htm). However, this side effect may not be evident at the lower doses used in the trials with AUD individuals.

The promising pharmacogenetic effect of ondansetron is currently under further investigation in an ongoing multi-site 16-week RCT testing ondansetron (0.33 mg, twice daily) versus placebo in alcohol-dependent patients prospectively randomized based on selected genotypes at the serotonin transporter and receptor genes (NCT02354703).

1.1.6 Prazosin and Doxazosin

Prazosin is a selective α-1 adrenergic receptor antagonist approved by the FDA to treat hypertension and benign prostatic hyperplasia. The off-label use of prazosin in patients with PTSD led to the anecdotal observation that some patients taking prazosin reduced or even stopped drinking alcohol, hence raising the question whether prazosin may be useful in AUD patients. A small treatment 8-week RCT ($N = 24$; Simpson et al. 2009) and a preliminary human laboratory study ($N = 17$; Fox et al. 2012), both conducted in alcohol-dependent individuals, suggested the potential efficacy of prazosin up to 16 mg per day, compared to placebo, in reducing alcohol drinking and craving. Subsequently, Simpson et al. (2015) and Petrakis et al. (2016) conducted two RCTs of prazosin (16 mg per day) in alcohol-dependent patients with comorbid PTSD: one study was a 6-week RCT in 30 patients and found a significant effect of prazosin in reducing alcohol-related outcomes (Simpson et al. 2015). The other was a 13-week RCT in 96 patients and did not find an effect of prazosin versus placebo on the alcohol-related outcomes (Petrakis et al. 2016). Furthermore, neither study found prazosin improving PTSD symptoms.

More recently, Simpson et al. (2018) conducted a relatively larger RCT ($N = 92$) with alcohol-dependent patients (without PTSD) randomized to either prazosin up to 16 mg per day or placebo. Results indicated that the rates of drinking and heavy drinking over time decreased to a larger extent in the prazosin group compared to placebo. Consistent with previous reports, some side effects like drowsiness were more common in the prazosin group.

Similar to prazosin, the α-1 adrenergic receptor antagonist doxazosin is also approved by the FDA to treat hypertension and benign prostatic hyperplasia. However, compared to prazosin, doxazosin has a longer half-life; hence it requires only once-a-day dosing compared with prazosin's two to three dosages per day. Furthermore, frequency of side effects (e.g., drowsiness, dizziness, fatigue) is lower in doxazosin than prazosin; and, unlike prazosin, doxazosin may be taken with or without food (Leggio and Kenna 2013). These properties of doxazosin have made doxazosin a potential intriguing candidate for AUD, given that medication adherence is a critical challenge both in RCTs and in clinical practice. For this reason, Kenna et al. (2015) conducted a 10-week RCT of doxazosin (up to 16 mg per day) in 41 alcohol-dependent individuals. While no significant differences were found in the drinking outcomes between the doxazosin and placebo groups in the whole sample, in a priori subgroup analysis, doxazosin-treated patients with higher density of family history of alcoholism presented with a significant decrease in drinks per week and heavy drinking days per week. Furthermore, in a later analysis from the same RCT, Haass-Koffler et al. (2017) found that doxazosin, compared with placebo, reduced drinks per week and heavy drinking days per week in a subgroup of patients who had higher baseline standing blood pressure. Notably, these latter results have been recently replicated in a 6-week RCT with prazosin ($N = 36$; 16 mg per day) in AUD (Wilcox et al. 2018). Additional work is needed to identify optimal personalized approaches for the use of alpha-1 receptor blockers for AUD (Haass-Koffler et al. 2018b).

1.1.7 Topiramate and Zonisamide

Topiramate is approved by the FDA for treatment of seizures and migraines. Furthermore, the FDA recently approved the combination of topiramate and phentermine for obesity. Topiramate antagonizes α-amino-3-hydroxy-5-methyl-4-isoxazolepropionic acid (AMPA) and kainate receptors, facilitates GABA activity, blocks L-type calcium channels, reduces voltage-dependent sodium channel activity, and inhibits carbonic anhydrase (Arnone 2005).

Human laboratory studies with individuals not seeking treatment for alcohol problems showed that topiramate at doses of 200 mg per day or 300 mg per day reduced alcohol craving, alcohol drinking (heavy drinking or drinking days), and the stimulating effects of alcohol (Miranda et al. 2008, 2016; Haass-Koffler et al. 2018a). Small RCTs with treatment-seeking individuals with AUD also support a role of topiramate in reducing several alcohol drinking outcomes at doses of 300 mg per day (Knapp et al. 2015) and 100 mg per day (Martinotti et al. 2014).

Furthermore, two larger RCTs (a single-site 12-week trial with 150 alcohol-dependent patients and a multi-site 14-week trial with 371 alcohol-dependent individuals) further indicate that topiramate, up to 300 mg per day, resulted in a significant reduction in craving, drinks per day, and heavy drinking days and a significant increase in abstinent days (Johnson et al. 2003, 2007). Side effects included dizziness, paresthesia, psychomotor slowing, memory or concentration impairment, nervousness, taste perversion, pruritus, and weight loss (Johnson et al. 2003, 2007). By contrast, topiramate did not show efficacy in another 12-week RCT testing topiramate 200 mg per day in 129 alcohol-dependent male smokers who were abstinent for 6 months at study entry (Anthenelli et al. 2017). Overall, these RCTs suggest that topiramate may be more effective in initiating and facilitating abstinence in current drinkers rather than in preventing relapse in individuals who are already abstinent (Swift 2003; Litten et al. 2018).

Additional studies suggest a potential pharmacogenetic effect for topiramate in AUD. An initial pilot human laboratory study showed that heavy drinkers with the CC genotype of a single nucleotide polymorphism (SNP), rs2832407, of the GRIK1 gene encoding the glutamate kainate GluK1 receptor had significantly fewer topiramate-related side effects and lower topiramate blood concentrations (Ray et al. 2009). More recently, a 12-week RCT with 138 alcohol-dependent individuals showed that topiramate 200 mg per day led to a significant reduction in heavy drinking days and a significant increase in abstinent days, and these effects were moderated by the rs2832407 SNP, such that topiramate was effective in the CC genotype, but not in the AC and AA genotypes (Kranzler et al. 2014).

Like topiramate, zonisamide is FDA-approved as an adjunct treatment for partial seizures and has similar pharmacological actions, i.e., blocking voltage-sensitive sodium channels and T-type calcium channels, facilitating GABA activity, and serving as a weak inhibitor of carbonic anhydrase (Kothare and Kaleyias 2008). Compared to topiramate, the side effect profile of zonisamide seems more favorable (Kothare and Kaleyias 2008), hence the interest in testing it for AUD. In an initial placebo-controlled human laboratory study of risky drinkers, zonisamide reduced alcohol craving and alcohol self-administration (Sarid-Segal et al. 2009). Similarly, a 12-week RCT with 40 alcohol-dependent patients indicated that, compared to placebo, zonisamide, up to 500 mg per day, significantly reduced the number of heavy drinking days, drinks per week, and alcohol craving (Arias et al. 2010). Finally, Knapp et al. (2015) conducted a multigroup 14-week RCT with 85 alcohol-dependent individuals comparing zonisamide (400 mg per day), topiramate (300 mg per day), levetiracetam (200 mg per day), and placebo. This study indicated comparable results for both zonisamide and topiramate in reducing percent of drinking days per week, drinks per day, and heavy drinking per week (levetiracetam was only effective in decreasing the percent of heavy drinking days per week). Moreover, zonisamide had a more favorable side effect profile than topiramate.

Larger RCTs are currently ongoing to test the efficacy of zonisamide in AUD (NCT02900352; NCT02368431) and to test the pharmacogenetic-based efficacy of topiramate in AUD (NCT02371889).

1.1.8 Varenicline

Varenicline, a partial agonist at $\alpha4\beta2$ and a full agonist at $\alpha7$, nicotinic acetylcholine receptors (Mihalak et al. 2006), is currently approved by the FDA for smoking cessation. Several proof-of-concept human laboratory studies in alcohol-dependent individuals have indicated that varenicline reduced drinking, alcohol craving, alcohol self-administration, and the subjective reinforcing effects of alcohol ($N = 20$ in McKee et al. 2009; $N = 77$ in Roberts et al. 2017a; $N = 60$ in Roberts et al. 2017b; and $N = 35$ in Schacht et al. 2014). Small treatment randomized clinical trials have also tested varenicline (titrated up to 2 mg per day) in heavy drinkers with AUD. These preliminary studies found that, compared to placebo, varenicline reduced alcohol craving ($N = 30$ in Fucito et al. 2011; $N = 40$ in Plebani et al. 2013), heavy drinking days (Fucito et al. 2011), and drinks per week ($N = 64$; Mitchell et al. 2012).

More recently, these studies led to a larger 13-week multi-site RCT of varenicline (2 mg per day) in alcohol-dependent individuals ($N = 200$), approximately 40% of whom were smokers (Litten et al. 2013). Compared to placebo, varenicline significantly reduced alcohol craving and alcohol consumption outcomes, including heavy drinking days, drinks per day, and drinks per drinking day. Furthermore, a subgroup analysis suggested that varenicline was most effective in individuals with less severe AUD and in those who reduced their smoking (Falk et al. 2015). However, another multi-site 12-week RCT ($N = 160$) conducted in Sweden did not show the same efficacy in favor of varenicline. Specifically, there were no differences in self-reported drinking outcomes or reduction in smoking between the varenicline and placebo groups. However, there were significant reductions in alcohol craving, the number of reported AUD symptoms (measured using the Alcohol Use Disorders

Identification Test [AUDIT]), and blood levels of phosphatidyl ethanol (PEth), a specific biomarker of alcohol consumption (de Bejczy et al. 2015).

Given that varenicline is approved for smoking cessation, a recent two-site RCT in the USA tested its efficacy in patients with alcohol use disorder and comorbid smoking seeking alcohol treatment and further evaluated its secondary effects on smoking abstinence. A total of 131 patients were treated with either varenicline 2 mg per day or placebo (O'Malley et al. 2018). There were no differences between the two groups on the percentage of heavy drinking days in the whole group, although a subgroup analysis indicated that varenicline may reduce the percentage of heavy drinking days in men more than in women. Furthermore, varenicline increased smoking abstinence in the overall sample (O'Malley et al. 2018).

Consistent with this latter trial, the potential role of varenicline for tobacco and alcohol use comorbidity has been also investigated in combination with naltrexone. Indeed, based on the promising results of an initial human lab study with heavy drinking, daily smokers (Ray et al. 2014), a larger RCT is ongoing to test concomitant smoking cessation and alcohol use reduction using a three group medication design consisting of varenicline alone (2 mg per day), naltrexone alone (50 mg per day), and the combination of both varenicline and naltrexone at the same doses as in the monotherapy conditions (NCT02698215).

Varenicline is generally well-tolerated with typically mild to moderate side effects which include nausea, constipation, and abnormal dreams. Notably, the FDA recently removed the box warning on varenicline about possible neuropsychiatric side effects but issued a warning that varenicline may change the way patients respond to alcohol, affecting their ability to tolerate its effects. Moreover, in rare accounts, seizures have been reported in patients taking varenicline (https://www.fda.gov/Drugs/DrugSafety/ucm436494.htm).

1.2 Other Promising Medications or Compounds for AUD

In addition to the medications above, preclinical or preliminary proof-of-concept human studies support the potential role of other medications on novel compounds for the treatment of AUD (for details, see also Litten et al. 2018). Examples are the glucocorticoid receptor antagonist mifepristone (Richardson et al. 2008; Simms et al. 2012; Vendruscolo et al. 2012; Vendruscolo et al. 2015), the hormone oxytocin (for reviews, see Kenna et al. 2012; Lee et al. 2016), the nonselective phosphodiesterase inhibitor ibudilast (Bell et al. 2013; Ray et al. 2017), D-cycloserine (a partial agonist at the glycine modulatory site of the glutamate NMDA receptor; Seif et al. 2015; Watson et al. 2011; Hofmann et al. 2012; MacKillop et al. 2015, Kiefer et al. 2015), *N*-acetylcysteine (Morley et al. 2018b), and blockade of the receptor of the hormone ghrelin (Lee et al. 2018; see also reviews: Zallar et al. 2017; Morris et al. 2018; Farokhnia et al. 2019).

2 Conclusions

This is an exciting time for medication development for AUD and addiction in general. As basic neuroscience research starts to unfold the mechanisms that underline the development and maintenance of AUD, new targets are identified. These targets may lead to the development of novel medications to be tested for their safety and efficacy in patients with AUD. As such, the discovery of novel and more effective targets is clearly a high priority. This is of paramount importance, given that at present, we only have three medications approved by the FDA for AUD.

However, the history of these approved medications, as well as of the additional medications tested in the past decades and reviewed in this chapter, also tells us that no medication will work for all patients with AUD. AUD is a complex and heterogenous disorder; hence it is conceivable that different medications may work best in certain subgroups of patients. Indeed, the challenge rests on identifying precision medicine approaches where the right medication is matched with the right patient (Litten et al. 2015, 2016, 2018). The literature reviewed above provides some examples, including pharmacogenetics (e.g., ondansetron and topiramate); family history or physiological markers (prazosin and doxazosin); severity of dependence and/or medical comorbidity, like liver disease (baclofen); and severity of alcohol withdrawal (gabapentin). However, it is very unlikely that a single factor is able to predict a positive outcome for a specific medication. Rather, it is conceivable that multiple factors will need to be taken into account toward the identification of effective precision medicine approaches (Heilig and Leggio 2016; Litten et al. 2018).

Another important aspect to consider is that various RCTs have often used different primary outcomes to define the efficacy of a specific medication. While it may be important to tailor the specific outcome to the medication under investigation (e.g., whether its mechanism of action is more likely to lead to reduction in heavy alcohol drinking, abstinence, or release prevention), on the other hand, standardization may also be critical. This is particularly important from a regulatory standpoint in terms of acceptable outcomes for pivotal RCTs, especially given growing evidence that non-abstinence-oriented outcomes may be quite beneficial, e.g., percentage of subjects with no heavy drinking days (Falk et al. 2010) and reductions in World Health Organization (WHO)-based drinking risk levels (Falk et al. 2019b).

Last, but not least, medications for AUD are dramatically underutilized; therefore, basic science and human research efforts will need to be accompanied with translational practice approaches, where effective novel medications and precision medicine approaches are effectively translated from the research settings to the clinical practice.

Acknowledgments The authors would like to thank the support of the National Institute on Alcohol Abuse and Alcoholism (LL, DEF, MLR, JF, RZL) and of the National Institute on Drug Abuse (LL). The authors would also like to thank Brittney Browning, B.Sc. (Section on Clinical Psychoneuroendocrinology and Neuropsychopharmacology, National Institute on Alcohol Abuse and Alcoholism and National Institute on Drug Abuse), for providing support with the preparation of the manuscript.

References

Addolorato G, Caputo F, Capristo E, Domenicali M, Bernardi M, Janiri L, Agabio R, Colombo G, Gessa GL, Gasbarrini G (2002) Baclofen efficacy in reducing alcohol craving and intake: a preliminary double-blind randomized controlled study. Alcohol Alcohol 37:504–508

Addolorato G, Leggio L, Ferrulli A, Cardone S, Vonghia L, Mirijello A, Abenavoli L, D'Angelo C, Caputo F, Zambon A, Haber PS, Gasbarrini G (2007) Effectiveness and safety of baclofen for maintenance of alcohol abstinence in alcohol-dependent patients with liver cirrhosis: randomised, double-blind controlled study. Lancet 370:1915–1922

Agabio R, Sinclair JMA, Addolorato G, Aubin HJ, Beraha EM, Caputo F, Chick JD, de La Selle P, Franchitto N, Garbutt JC, Haber PS, Heydtman M, Jaury P, Lingford-Hughes AR, Morley KC, Müller CA, Owens L, Pastor A, Paterson L, Pélissier F, Rolland B, Stafford A, Thompson A, van den Brink W, de Beaurepaire R, Leggio L (2018) The use of baclofen to treat patients with alcohol use disorder: the Cagliari statement. Lancet Psychiatry 5:957–960

Ameisen O (2005) Complete and prolonged suppression of symptoms and consequences of alcohol-dependence using high-dose baclofen: a self-case report of a physician. Alcohol Alcohol 40:147–150

Anthenelli RM, Heffner JL, Wong E, Tibbs J, Russell K, Isgro M, Dinh E, Wehrle C, Worley MJ, Doran N (2017) A randomized trial evaluating whether topiramate aids smoking cessation and prevents alcohol relapse in recovering alcohol-dependent men. Alcohol Clin Exp Res 41:197–206

Anton RF, Kranzler H, Breder C, Marcus RN, Carson WH, Han J (2008) A randomized, multicenter, double-blind, placebo-controlled study of the efficacy and safety of aripiprazole for the treatment of alcohol dependence. J Clin Psychopharmacol 28:5–12

Anton RF, Myrick H, Baros AM, Latham PK, Randall PK, Wright TM, Stewart SH, Waid R, Malcolm R (2009) Efficacy of a combination of flumazenil and gabapentin in the treatment of alcohol dependence: relationship to alcohol withdrawal symptoms. J Clin Psychopharmacol 29:334–342

Anton RF, Myrick H, Wright TM, Latham PK, Baros AM, Waid LR, Randall PK (2011) Gabapentin combined with naltrexone for the treatment of alcohol dependence. Am J Psychiatry 168:709–717

Anton RF, Schacht JP, Voronin KE, Randall PK (2017) Aripiprazole suppression of drinking in a clinical laboratory paradigm: influence of impulsivity and self-control. Alcohol Clin Exp Res 41:1370–1380

Arias A, Feinn R, Oncken C, Covault J, Kranzler HR (2010) Placebo-controlled trial of zonisamide for the treatment of alcohol dependence. J Clin Psychopharmacol 30:318–322

Arnone D (2005) Review of the use of topiramate for treatment of psychiatric disorders. Ann Gen Psychiatry 4:5

Asghari V, Sanyal S, Buchwaldt S, Paterson A, Jovanovic V, van Tol HH (1995) Modulation of intracellular cyclic AMP levels by different human dopamine D4 receptor variants. J Neurochem 65:1157–1165

Bell RL, Lopez MF, Cui C, Egli M, Johnson KW, Franklin KM, Becker HC (2013) Ibudilast reduces alcohol drinking in multiple animal models of alcohol dependence. Addict Biol 20:38–42

Beraha EM, Salemink E, Goudriaan AE, Bakker A, de Jong D, Smits N, Zwart JW, van Geest D, Bodewits P, Schiphof T, Defourny H, van Tricht M, van den Brink W, Wiers RW (2016) Efficacy and safety of high-dose baclofen for the treatment of alcohol dependence: a multicenter, randomized, double-blind controlled trial. Eur Neuorpsychopharmacol 26:1950–1959

Brower KJ, Myra Kim H, Strobbe S, Karam-Hage MA, Consens F, Zucker RA (2008) A randomized double-blind pilot trial of gabapentin versus placebo to treat alcohol dependence and comorbid insomnia. Alcohol Clin Exp Res 32(8):1429–1438

Bucknam W (2007) Suppression of symptoms of alcohol dependence and craving using high-dose baclofen. Alcohol Alcohol 42:158–160

Chompookham P, Rukngan W, Nilaban S, Suwanmajo S, Yoosom P, Kalayasiri R (2018) A randomized trial of low-dose gabapentin for post hospitalization relapse prevention in a Thai clinical sample of alcohol dependence. Psychiatry Res 270:34–40

Colombo G, Gessa GL (2018) Suppressing effect of baclofen on multiple alcohol-related behaviors in laboratory animals. Front Psych 9:475

Daurio AM, Deschaine SL, Modabbernia A, Leggio L (2019) Parsing out the role of dopamine D4 receptor gene (DRD4) on alcohol-related phenotypes: a meta-analysis and systematic review. Addict Biol:e12770. https://doi.org/10.1111/adb.12770

de Bejczy A, Lof E, Walther L, Gutertstam J, Hammarbeg A, Asanovska G, Franck J, Isaksson A, Soderpalm B (2015) Varenicline for treatment of alcohol dependence: a randomized, placebo-controlled trial. Alcohol Clin Exp Res 39:2189–2199

Edwards S, Guerrero M, Ghoneim OM, Roberts E, Koob GF (2011) Evidence that vasopressin V1b receptors mediate the transition to excessive drinking in ethanol-dependent rats. Addict Biol 17:76–85

Evans SM, Bisaga A (2009) Acute interaction of baclofen in combination with alcohol in heavy social drinkers. Alcohol Clin Exp Res 33:19–30

Falk D, Wang XQ, Liu L, Fertig J, Mattson M, Ryan M, Johnson B, Stout R, Litten RZ (2010) Percentage of subjects with no heavy drinking days: evaluation as an efficacy endpoint for alcohol clinical trials. Alcohol Clin Exp Res 34:2022–2034

Falk DE, Castle IJP, Ryan M, Fertig J, Litten RZ (2015) Moderators of varenicline treatment effects in a double-blind, placebo-controlled trial for alcohol dependence: an exploratory analysis. J Addict Med 9:296–303

Falk DE, Ryan ML, Fertig JB, Devine EG, Cruz R, Brown ES, Burns H, Salloum IM, Newport DJ, Mendelson J, Galloway G, Grant T, Kampman K, Brooks C, Green AI, Brunette MF, Rosenthal RN, Dunn KE, Strain EC, Ray L, Shoptaw S, Ait-Daoud Tiouririne N, Gunderson EW, Random J, Scott C, Leggio L, Caras S, Mason B, Litten RZ, The National Institute on Alcohol Abuse and Alcoholism Clinical Investigations Group (NCIG) Study Group (2019a) Gabapentin enacarbil extended-release for alcohol use disorder: a randomized, double-blind, placebo-controlled, multisite trial assessing efficacy and safety. Alcohol Clin Exp Res 43:158–169

Falk DE, O'Malley SS, Witkiewitz K, Anton RF, Litten RZ, Slater M, Kranzler HR, Mann KF, Hasin DS, Johnson B, Meulien D, Ryan M, Fertig J, Alcohol Clinical Trials Initiative (ACTIVE) Workgroup (2019b) Evaluation of drinking risk levels as outcomes in alcohol pharmacotherapy trials: a secondary analysis of 3 randomized clinical trials. JAMA Psychiatry 76:374–381

Farokhnia M, Schwandt ML, Lee MR, Bollinger JW, Farinelli LA, Amodio JP, Sewell L, Lionetti TA, Spero DE, Leggio L (2017) Biobehavioral effects of baclofen in anxious alcohol-dependent individuals: a randomized, double-blind, placebo-controlled, laboratory study. Transl Psychiatry 7:e1108

Farokhnia M, Deschaine SL, Sadighi A, Farinelli LA, Lee MR, Akhlaghi F, Leggio L (2018) A deeper insight into how GABA-B receptor agonism via baclofen may affect alcohol seeking and consumption: lessons learned from a human laboratory investigation. Mol Psychiatry. https://doi.org/10.1038/s41380-018-0287-y

Farokhnia M, Faulkner ML, Piacentino D, Lee MR, Leggio L (2019) Ghrelin: from a gut hormone to a potential therapeutic target for alcohol use disorder. Physiol Behav 204:49–57

Fleischhacker WW (2005) Aripiprazole. Expert Opin Pharmacother 6:2091–2101

Fox HC, Anderson GM, Tuit K, Hansen J, Kimmerling A, Siedlarz KM, Morgan PT, Sinha R (2012) Prazosin effects on stress-and cue-induced craving and stress response in alcohol-dependent individuals: preliminary findings. Alcohol Clin Exp Res 36:351–360

Fucito LM, Toll BA, Wu R, Romano DM, Tek E, O'Malley SS (2011) A preliminary investigation of varenicline for heavy drinking smokers. Psychopharmacology 215:655–663

Furieri FA, Nakamura-Palacios EM (2007) Gabapentin reduces alcohol consumption and craving: a randomized, double-blind, placebo-controlled trial. J Clin Psychiatry 68(11):1691–1700

Garbutt JC, Kampov-Polevoy AB, Gallop R, Kalka-Juhl L, Flannery BA (2010) Efficacy and safety of baclofen for alcohol dependence: a randomized, double-blind, placebo-controlled trial. Alcohol Clin Exp Res 34(11):1849–1857

Garbutt JC, Greenblatt AM, West SL, Morgan LC, Kampov-Polevoy A, Jordan HS, Bobashev GV (2014) Clinical and biological moderators of response to naltrexone in alcohol dependence: a systematic review of the evidence. Addiction 109(8):1274–1284

Haass-Koffler CL, Goodyear K, Zywiak WH, Magill M, Eltinge SE, Wallace PM, Long VM, Jayaram-Lindstrom N, Swift RM, Kenna GA, Leggio L (2017) Higher pressure in associated with greater alcohol drinking reduction in alcohol-dependent individuals treated with doxazosin. Drug Alcohol Depend 177:23–28

Haass-Koffler CL, Goodyear K, Zywiak WH, Leggio L, Kenna GA, Swift RM (2018a) Comparing and combining topiramate and aripiprazole on alcohol-related outcomes in a human laboratory study. Alcohol Alcohol 53(3):268–276

Haass-Koffler CL, Swift RM, Leggio L (2018b) Noradrenergic targets for the treatment of alcohol use disorder. Psychopharmacology 235(6):1625–1634

Hauser P, Fuller B, Ho SB, Thuras P, Kern S, Dieperink E (2017) The safety and efficacy of baclofen to reduce alcohol use in veterans with chronic hepatitis C: a randomized controlled trial. Addiction 112(7):1173–1183

Heilig M, Leggio L (2016) What the alcohol doctor ordered from the neuroscientist: theragnostic biomarkers for personalized treatments. Prog Brain Res 224:401–418

Hofmann SG, Huweler R, MacKillop JM, Kantak K (2012) Effects of D-cycloserine on craving to alcohol cues in problem drinkers: preliminary findings. Am J Drug Alcohol Abuse 38:101–107

Javors MA, Seneviratne C, Roache JD, Ait-Daoud N, Bergeson SE, Walss-Bass MC, Akhtar FZ, Johnson BA (2005) Platelet serotonin uptake and paroxetine binding among allelic genotypes of the serotonin transporter in alcoholics. Prog Neuro-Psychopharmacol Biol Psychiatry 29:7–13

Johnson BA, Campling GM, Griffiths P, Cowen PJ (1993) Attention of some alcohol-induced mood changes and the desire to drink by 5-HT3 receptor blockade: a preliminary study I healthy male volunteers. Psychopharmacology 112:142–144

Johnson BA, Roache JD, Javors MA, DiClemente CC, Cloninger CR, Prihoda TJ, Bordnick PS, Ait-Daoud N, Hensler J (2000) Ondansetron for reduction of drinking among biologically predisposed alcoholic patients: a randomized controlled trial. JAMA 284(8):963–971

Johnson BA, Ait-Daoud N, Bowden CL, DiClemente CC, Roache JD, Lawson K, Javors MA, Ma JZ (2003) Oral topiramate for treatment of alcohol dependence: a randomised controlled trial. Lancet 361:1677–1685

Johnson BA, Rosenthal N, Capece JA, Wiegund F, Mao L, Beyers K, McKay A, Ait-Daoud N, Anton RF, Ciraulo DA, Kranzler HR, Mann K, O'Malley SS, Swift RM (2007) Topiramate for treating alcohol dependence: a randomized controlled trial. JAMA 198(14):1641–1651

Johnson BA, Javors MA, Roache JD, Seneviratne C, Bergeson SE, Ait-Daoud N, Dawes MA, Ma JZ (2008) Can serotonin transporter genotype predict serotonergic function, chronicity, and severity of drinking? Prog Neuro-Psychopharmacol Biol Psychiatry 32:209–216

Johnson BA, Ait-Daoud N, Seneviratne C, Roach JD, Javors MA, Wang XQ, Liu L, Penberthy JK, Di Clemente CC, Li MD (2011) Pharmacogenetic approach at the serotonin transporter gene as a method of reducing the severity of alcohol drinking. Am J Psychiatry 168:265–275

Johnson BA, Seneviratne C, Wang XQ, Ait-Daoud N, Li MD (2013) Determination of genotype combinations that can predict the outcome of the treatment of alcohol dependence using the 5-HT$_3$ antagonist ondansetron. Am J Psychiatry 170:1020–1031

Jonas DE, Amick HR, Feltner C, Bobashev G, Thomas K, Wines R, Kim MM, Shanahan E, Gass CE, Rowe CJ, Garbutt JC (2014) Pharmacotherapy for adults with alcohol use disorders in outpatient settings: a systematic review and meta-analysis. JAMA 311(18):889–900

Kenna GA, Zywiak WH, McGeary JE, Leggio L, McGeary C, Wang S, Grenga A, Swift RM (2009) A within-group design of nontreatment seeking 5-HTTLPR genotyped alcohol-dependent subjects receiving ondansetron and sertraline. Alcohol Clin Exp Res 33:315–323

Kenna GA, Swift RM, Hillemacher T, Leggio L (2012) The relationship of appetitive, reproductive and posterior pituitary hormones to alcoholism and craving in humans. Neuropsychol Rev 22 (3):211–228

Kenna GA, Zywiak WH, Swiftt RM, McGeary JE, Cliifford JS, Shoaff JR, Vuittonet C, Fricchione S, Brickley M, Beaucage K, Haass-Koffler CL, Leggio L (2014a) Ondansetron reduces naturalistic drinking in nontreatment-seeking alcohol-dependent individuals with the LL 5′-HTTLPR genotype: a laboratory study. Alcohol Clin Exp Res 38:1567–1574

Kenna GA, Zwiak WH, Swift RM, McGeary JE, Clifford JS, Shoaff JR, Fricchione S, Brickley M, Beaucage K, Haass-Koffler CL, Leggio L (2014b) Ondansetron and sertraline may interact with 5-HTTLPR and DRD4 polymorphisms to reduce drinking in non-treatment seeking alcohol-dependent women: exploratory findings. Alcohol 48:515–522

Kenna GA, Haass-Koffler CL, Zywiak WH, Edwards SM, Brickley MB, Swift RM, Leggio L (2015) Role of the α1 blocker doxazosin in alcoholism: a proof-of-concept randomized controlled trial. Addict Biol 21:904–914

Kiefer F, Kirsch M, Bach P, Hoffmann S, Reinhard I, Jorde A, von der Goltz C, Spanagel R, Mann K, Loeber S, Vollstadt-Klein S (2015) Effects of D-cycloserine on extinction of mesolimbic cue reactivity in alcoholism: a randomized placebo-controlled trial. Psychopharmacology 232(13):2353–2362

Knapp CM, Ciraulo DA, Sarid-Segal O, Richardson MA, Devine E, Streeter CC, Oscar-Berman M, Surprise C, Colaneri L, Putnam M, Waters M, Richambault C (2015) Zonisamide, topiramate, and levetiracetam: efficacy and neuropsychological effects in alcohol use disorders. J Clin Psychopharmacol 35:1–9

Kothare S, Kaleyias J (2008) Zonisamide: review of pharmacology, clinical efficacy, tolerability, and safety. Expert Opin Drug Metab Toxicol 4:493–506

Kranzler HR, Covault J, Pierucci-Lagha A, Chan G, Douglas K, Arias AJ, Oncken C (2008) Effects of aripiprazole on subjective and physiological responses to alcohol. Alcohol Clin Exp Res 32:1–7

Kranzler HR, Covault J, Feinn R, Armeli S, Tennen H, Arias AJ, Gelernter J, Pond T, Oncken C, Kampman KM (2014) Topiramate treatment for heavy drinkers: moderation by a *GRIK1* polymorphism. Am J Psychiatry 171:445–452

Lee MR, Rohn MCH, Tanda G, Leggio L (2016) Targeting the oxytocin system to treat addictive disorders: rationale and progress to date. CNS Drugs 30(2):109–123

Lee MR, Tapocik JD, Ghareeb M, Schwandt ML, Dias AA, Le AN, Cobbina E, Farinelli LA, Bouhlal S, Farokhnia M, Heilig M, Akhlaghi F, Leggio L (2018) The novel ghrelin receptor inverse agonist PF-5190457 administered with alcohol: preclinical safety experiments and a phase 1b human laboratory study. Mol Psychiatry. https://doi.org/10.1038/s41380-018-0064-y

Leggio L, Kenna GA (2013) Commentary: doxazosin for alcoholism. Alcohol Clin Exp Res 37:191–193

Leggio L, Garbutt JC, Addolorato G (2010) Effectiveness and safety of baclofen in the treatment of alcohol dependent patients. CNS Neurol Disord 9:33–44

Leggio L, Ferrulli A, Zambon A, Caputo F, Kenna GA, Swift RM, Addolorato G (2012) Baclofen promotes alcohol abstinence in alcohol dependent cirrhotic patients with hepatitis C virus (HCV) infection. Addict Behav 37(4):561–564

Leggio L, Zywiak WH, McGeary JE, Edwards S, Fricchione SR, Shoaff JR, Addolorato G, Swift RM, Kenna GA (2013) A human laboratory pilot study with baclofen in alcoholic individuals. Pharmacol Biochem Behav 103:784–791

Leggio L, Zywiak WH, Edwards SM, Tidey JW, Swift RM, Kenna G (2015) A preliminary double-blind, placebo-controlled randomized study of baclofen effects in alcoholic smokers. Psychopharmacology 232:233–243

Litten RZ, Ryan ML, Fertig JB, Falk DE, Johnson B, Dunn KE, Green AI, Pettinati HM, Ciraulo DA, Sarid-Segal O, Kampman K, Brunette MF, Strain EC, Tiouririne NA, Ransom J, Scott C, Stout R (2013) A double-blind, placebo-controlled trial assessing the efficacy of varenicline tartrate for alcohol dependence. J Addict Med 7:277–286

Litten RZ, Ryan ML, Falk DE, Reilly M, Fertig JB, Koob GF (2015) Heterogeneity of alcohol use disorder: understanding mechanisms to advance personalized treatment. Alcohol Clin Exp Res 39:579–584

Litten RZ, Falk DE, Ryan ML, Fertig JB (2016) Discovery, development, and adoption of medications to treat alcohol use disorder: goals for the phases of medications development. Alcohol Clin Exp Res 40:1368–1379

Litten RZ, Falk DE, Ryan ML, Fertig J, Leggio L (2018) Advances in pharmacotherapy development: human clinical studies. Handb Exp Pharmacol 248:579–613

MacKillop J, Few LR, Stojek MK, Murphy CM, Malutinok SF, Johnson FT, Hofmann SG, McGeary JE, Swift RM, Monti PM (2015) D-cycloserine to enhance extinction of cue-elicited craving for alcohol: a translational approach. Transl Psychiatry 5(4):e544

Martinotti G, DiNicola M, De Vita O, Hatzigiakoumis DS, Guglielmo R, Santucci B, Aliotta F, Romanelli R, Verrastro V, Petruccelli F, Di Giannantonio M, Janiri L (2014) Low-dose topiramate in alcohol dependence: a single-blind, placebo-controlled study. J Clin Psychopharmacol 34:709–715

Mason BJ, Light JM, Williams LD, Drobes DJ (2009) Proof-of-concept human laboratory study for protracted abstinence in alcohol dependence: effects of gabapentin. Addict Biol 14(1):73–83

Mason BJ, Quello S, Goodell V, Shadan F, Kyle M, Begovic A (2014) Gabapentin treatment for alcohol dependence: a randomized clinical trial. JAMA Intern Med 174:70

McCool BA, McGinnis MM (2019) Adolescent vulnerability to alcohol use disorder: neurophysiological mechanisms from preclinical studies. Handb Exp Pharmacol. https://doi.org/10.1007/164_2019_296

McKee SA, Harrison ELR, O'Malley SS, Krishnan-Sarin S, Shi J, Tetrault JM, Picciotto MR, Petrakis IL, Estevez N, Balchunas E (2009) Varenicline reduces alcohol self-administration in heavy-drinking smokers. Biol Psychiatry 66:185–195

Medical Press (2018) France clears use of anti-spasm drug to treat alcoholism. https://medicalxpress.com/news/2018-10-france-anti-spasm-drug-alcoholism.html. Accessed 31 May 2019

Mihalak KB, Carroll FI, Luetje CW (2006) Varenicline is a partial agonist at $\alpha 4\beta 2$ and a full agonist at $\alpha 7$ neuronal nicotinic receptors. Mol Pharmacol 70:801–805

Miranda R, MacKillop J, Monti PM, Rohsenow DJ, Tidey J, Gwaltney C, Swift R, Ray L, McGeary J (2008) Effects of topiramate on urge to drink and the subjective effects of alcohol: a preliminary laboratory study. Alcohol Clin Exp Res 32:489–497

Miranda R, MacKillop J, Treloar H, Blanchard A, Tidey JW, Swift R, Chun T, Rohsenow DJ, Monti PM (2016) Biobehavioral mechanisms of topiramate's effects on alcohol use: an investigation pairing laboratory and ecological momentary assessments. Addict Biol 21:171–182

Mitchell JM, Teague CH, Kayser AS, Bartlett SE, Fields HL (2012) Varenicline decreases alcohol consumption in heavy-drinking smokers. Psychopharmacology 223:299–306

Morley KC, Baillie A, Fraser I, Furneaux-Bate A, Dore G, Roberts M, Abdalla A, Phung N, Haber PS (2018a) Baclofen in the treatment of alcohol dependence with or without liver disease: multisite, randomised, double-blind, placebo-controlled trial. Br J Psychiatry 212(6):362–369

Morley KC, Baillie A, van den Brink W, Chitty KE, Brady K, Back SE, Seth D, Sutherland G, Leggio L, Haber PS (2018b) N-acetyl cysteine in the treatment of alcohol use disorder in patients with liver disease: rationale for further research. Expert Opin Investig Drugs 27 (8):667–675

Morris LS, Voon V, Leggio L (2018) Stress, motivation, and the gut-brain axis: a focus on the ghrelin system and alcohol use disorder. Alcohol Clin Exp Res 42:1378

Muller CA, Geisel O, Petz P, Higl V, Kruger J, Stickel A, Beck A, Wernecke KD, Hellweg R, Heinz A (2015) High-dose baclofen for the treatment of alcohol dependence (BACLAD study): a randomized, placebo-controlled trial. Eur Neuropsychopharmacol 25:1167–1177

Myrick H, Li X, Randall PK, Henderson S, Voronin K, Anton RF (2010) The effect of aripiprazole in cue-induced brain activation and drinking parameters in alcoholics. J Clin Psychopharmacol 30:365–372

Oak JN, Oldenhof J, van Tol HH (2000) The dopamine D4 receptor: one decade of research. Eur J Pharmacol 405:303–327

O'Malley SS, Zweben A, Fucito LM, Wu R, Piepmeier ME, Ockert DM, Bold KW, Petrakis I, Muvvala S, Jatlow P, Gueorguieva R (2018) Effect of varenicline combined with medical management on alcohol use disorder with comorbid cigarette smoking: a randomized clinical trial. JAMA Psychiat 75:129–138

Petrakis IL, Desai N, Gueorguieva R, Arias A, O'Brien E, Jane JS, Sevarino K, Southwick S, Ralevski E (2016) Prazosin for veterans with posttraumatic stress disorder and comorbid alcohol dependence: a clinical trial. Alcohol Clin Exp Res 40:178–186

Plebani JG, Lynch KG, Rennert L, Pettinati HM, O'Brien CP, Kampman KM (2013) Results from a pilot clinical trial of varenicline for the treatment of alcohol dependence. Drug Alcohol Depend 133(2):754–758

Ray LA, Miranda R, MacKillop J, McGeary J, Tidey JW, Rohsenow DJ, Gwaltney C, Swift RW, Monti PM (2009) A preliminary pharmacogenetic investigation of adverse events from topiramate in heavy drinkers. Exp Clin Psychopharmacol 17:122–129

Ray LA, Courtney KE, Ghahremani DG, Miotto K, Brody A, London ED (2014) Varenicline, low dose naltrexone, and their combination for heavy-drinking smokers: human laboratory findings. Psychopharmacology 231:3843–3853

Ray LA, Bujarski S, Shoptaw S, Roche DJ, Heinzerling K, Miotto K (2017) Development of the neuroimmune modulator ibudilast for the treatment of alcoholism: a randomized, placebo-controlled, human laboratory trial. Neuropsychopharmacology 42(9):1776–1788

Reynaud M, Aubin HJ, Trinquet F, Zakine B, Dano C, Dematteis M, Trojak B, Paille F, Detilleux M (2017) A randomized, placebo-controlled study of high-dose baclofen in alcohol-dependent patients – the ALPADIR study. Alcohol Alcohol 52(4):439–446

Richardson HN, Lee SY, O'Dell LE, Koob GF, Rivier CL (2008) Alcohol self-administration acutely stimulates the hypothalamic-pituitary-adrenal axis, but alcohol dependence leads to a dampened neuroendocrine state. Eur J Neurosci 28:1641–1653

Roberts W, Harrison ELR, McKee SA (2017a) Effects of varenicline on alcohol cue reactivity in heavy drinkers. Psychopharmacology 234(18):2737–2745

Roberts W, Verplaetse TL, Moore K, Oberleitner L, Picciotto MR, McKee SA (2017b) Effects of varenicline on alcohol self-administration and craving in drinkers with depressive symptoms. J Psychopharmacol 31:906–914

Ryan ML, Falk DE, Fertig JB, Rendenbach-Mueller B, Katz DA, Tracy KA, Strain EC, Dunn KE, Kampman K, Mahoney E, Ciraulo DA, Sickles-Colaneri L, Ait-Daoud N, Johnson BA, Ransom J, Scott C, Koob GF, Litten RZ (2017) A phase2, double-blind, placebo-controlled randomized trial assessing the efficacy of ABT-436, a novel V1b receptor antagonist, for alcohol dependence. Neuropsychopharmacology 42:1012–1023

Sarid-Segal O, Knapp CM, Burch W, Richardson MA, Bahtia S, DeQuattro K, Afshar M, Richambault C, Sickels L, Devine E, Ciraulo D (2009) The anticonvulsant zonisamide reduces ethanol self-administration by risky drinkers. Am J Drug Alcohol Abuse 35:316–319

Schacht JP, Anton RF, Randall PK, Li X, Henderson S, Myrick H (2014) Varenicline effects on drinking, craving and neural reward processing among non-treatment-seeking alcohol-dependent individuals. Psychopharmacology 231:3799–3807

Schacht JP, Voronin KE, Randall PK, Anton RF (2018) Dopaminergic genetic variation influences Aripiprazole effects on alcohol self-administration and the neural response to alcohol cues in a randomized trial. Neuropsychopharmacology 43:1247–1256

Seif T, Simms JA, Lei K, Wegner S, Bonci A, Messing RO, Hopf FW (2015) D-serine and D-cycloserine reduce compulsive alcohol intake in rats. Neuropyschopharmacology 40 (10):2357–2367

Sellers EM, Toneatto T, Romach MK, Somer GR, Sobell LC, Sobell MB (1994) Clinical efficacy of the 5-HT_3 antagonist ondansetron in alcohol abuse and dependence. Alcohol Clin Exp Res 18 (4):879–885

Sills GJ (2006) The mechanisms of action of gabapentin and pregabalin. Curr Opin Pharmacol 6:108–113

Simms JA, Haass-Koffler CL, Bito-Onon J, Li R, Bartlett SE (2012) Mifepristone in the central nucleus of the amygdala reduces yohimbine stress-induced reinstatement of ethanol-seeking. Neuropsychopharmacology 37:906–918

Simpson TL, Saxon AJ, Meredith CW, Malte CA, McBride B, Ferguson LC, Gross CA, Hart KL, Raskind M (2009) A pilot trial of the alpha-1 adrenergic antagonist, prazosin for alcohol dependence. Alcohol Clin Exp Res 33:255–263

Simpson TL, Malte CA, Dietel B, Tell D, Pocock I, Lyons R, Varon D, Raskind M, Saxon AJ (2015) A pilot trial of prazosin, an alpha-1 adrenergic antagonist, for comorbid alcohol dependence and posttraumatic stress disorder. Alcohol Clin Exp Res 39:808–817

Simpson TL, Saxon AJ, Stappenbeck C, Malte CA, Lyons R, Tell D, Millard SP, Raskind M (2018) Double-blind randomized clinical trial of prazosin for alcohol use disorder. Am J Psychiatry 175:1216

Smith RV, Havens JR, Walsh SL (2016) Gabapentin misuse, abuse and diversion: a systematic review. Addiction 111:1160–1174

Swift RM (2003) Topiramate for the treatment of alcohol dependence: initiating abstinence. Lancet 361(9370):1666–1667

Swift RM, Davidson D, Whelihan W, Kuznetsov O (1996) Ondansetron alters human alcohol intoxication. Biol Psychiatry 40:514–521

Vendruscolo LF, Barbier E, Schlosburg JE, Misra KK, Whitfield TW, Logrip ML, Rivier C, Repunte-Canonigo V, Zorrilla EP, Sanna PP, Heilig M, Koob GF (2012) Corticosteroid-dependent plasticity medicates compulsive alcohol drinking in rats. J Neurosci 32:7563–7571

Vendruscolo LF, Estey D, Goodell V, Macshane LG, Logrip ML, Schlosburg JE, McGinn MA, Zamora-Martinez ER, Belanoff JK, Hunt HJ, Sanna PP, George O, Koob GF, Edwards S, Mason BJ (2015) J Clin Invest 125:3193–3197

Voronin K, Randall P, Myrick H, Anton R (2008) Aripiprazole effects on alcohol consumption and subjective reports in a clinical laboratory paradigm–possible influence of self-control. Alcohol Clin Exp Res 32:1954–1961

Watson BJ, Wilson S, Griffin L, Kalk NJ, Taylor LG, Munafo MR, Lingford-Hughes AR, Nutt DJ (2011) A pilot study of the effectiveness of D-cycloserine during cue-exposure therapy in abstinent alcohol-dependent subjects. Psychopharmacology 216:121–129

Wilcox CE, Tonigan JS, Bogenschutz MP, Clifford J, Bigelow R, Simpson T (2018) A randomized, placebo-controlled, clinical trial of prazosin for the treatment of alcohol use disorder. J Addict Med 12(5):339–345

Zallar LJ, Farokhnia M, Tunstall BJ, Vendruscolo LF, Leggio L (2017) The role of the ghrelin system in drug addiction. Int Rev Neurobiol 136:89–119

Zhou Y, Colombo G, Carai MAM, Ho A, Gessa GL, Kreek MJ (2011) Involvement of arginine vasopressin and V1b receptor in alcohol drinking in Sardinian alcohol-preferring rats. Alcohol Clin Exp Res 35:1876–1883

Newly Emerging Drugs of Abuse

Kenichi Tamama and Michael J. Lynch

Contents

1 Introduction 465
2 Opioids 466
2.1 Epidemiology 466
2.2 Chemistry and Chemical Structures 469
2.3 Pharmacology and Physiology Overview 470
2.4 Clinical Effects 473
2.5 Laboratory Detection and Methodology 474
2.6 Treatment 475
3 Cannabinoids 476
3.1 Epidemiology 476
3.2 Chemistry and Chemical Structures 478
3.3 Pharmacology and Physiology Overview 478
3.4 Clinical Effects 479
3.5 Laboratory Detection and Methodology 480
3.6 Treatment 481

Kenichi Tamama and Michael J. Lynch contributed equally to this work.

K. Tamama (✉)
Department of Pathology, University of Pittsburgh School of Medicine, Pittsburgh, PA, USA

Clinical Laboratories, University of Pittsburgh Medical Center Presbyterian Hospital, Pittsburgh, PA, USA

McGowan Institute for Regenerative Medicine, University of Pittsburgh, Pittsburgh, PA, USA

Clinical Laboratory, Children's Hospital of Pittsburgh of UPMC, Pittsburgh, PA, USA
e-mail: tamamakj@upmc.edu

M. J. Lynch (✉)
Division of Medical Toxicology, Department of Emergency Medicine, University of Pittsburgh School of Medicine, Pittsburgh, PA, USA

Pittsburgh Poison Center, Pittsburgh, PA, USA
e-mail: lyncmj@upmc.edu

M. A. Nader, Y. L. Hurd (eds.), *Substance Use Disorders*,
Handbook of Experimental Pharmacology 258, https://doi.org/10.1007/164_2019_260

4 Stimulants/Hallucinogens 482
4.1 Epidemiology 482
4.2 Chemistry and Chemical Structures 484
4.3 Pharmacology and Physiology Overview 484
4.4 Clinical Effects 485
4.5 Laboratory Detection and Methodology 485
4.6 Treatment 486
5 Dissociative Agents 487
5.1 Epidemiology 487
5.2 Chemistry and Chemical Structures 487
5.3 Pharmacology and Physiology Overview 488
5.4 Clinical Effects 488
5.5 Laboratory Detection and Methodology 489
5.6 Treatment 489
6 Sedative-Hypnotics 490
6.1 Epidemiology 490
6.2 Chemistry and Chemical Structures 490
6.3 Pharmacology and Physiology Overview 491
6.4 Clinical Effects 492
6.5 Laboratory Detection and Methodology 492
6.6 Treatment 493
7 Conclusion 493
References 494

Abstract

Drug use and the associated overdose deaths have been a serious public health threat in the United States and the world. While traditional drugs of abuse such as cocaine remain popular, recreational use of newer synthetic drugs has continued to increase, but the prevalence of use is likely underestimated. In this review, epidemiology, chemistry, pharmacophysiology, clinical effects, laboratory detection, and clinical treatment are discussed for newly emerging drugs of abuse in the following classes: (1) opioids (e.g., fentanyl, fentanyl analogues, and mitragynine), (2) cannabinoids [THC and its analogues, alkylindole (e.g., JWH-018, JWH-073), cyclohexylphenol (e.g., CP-47,497), and indazole carboxamide (e.g., FUB-AMB, ADB-FUBINACA)], (3) stimulants and hallucinogens [β-keto amphetamines (e.g., methcathinone, methylone), pyrrolidinophenones (e.g., α-PVP, MDPV), and dimethoxyphenethylamine ("2C" and "NBOMe")], (4) dissociative agents (e.g., 3-MeO-PCP, methoxetamine, 2-oxo-PCE), and (5) sedative-hypnotics (e.g., gabapentin, baclofen, clonazolam, etizolam). It is critically important to coordinate hospital, medical examiner, and law enforcement personnel with laboratory services to respond to these emerging threats.

Keywords

Cannabinoids · Dissociative agent · Drug abuse · Opioids · Sedative-hypnotic · Stimulant

1 Introduction

The world has witnessed a consistent and accelerating rise in overdose deaths for the past 40 years (Jalal et al. 2018). A variety of drug classes have contributed to patterns of recreational use, misuse, addiction, overdose, and death. Over the last two decades, opioids have dominated attention given the unprecedented contribution of this class of drugs to individual and cultural harm in addition to overdose deaths. The overdose death rate tripled from 1999 to 2016 with more than 70,000 overdose deaths reported in 2017, the majority of which were opioid related (Hedegaard et al. 2017; National Institute on Drug Abuse (NIDA) 2018). Nonfatal and fatal overdoses, particularly involving heroin and prescription opioids as well as cocaine, increased worldwide between 1980 and 2013 (Martins et al. 2015). The landscape of drug use has shifted throughout that period within the opioid class of drugs. Beginning in the late 1990s and through the first decade of this century, prescription opioids were the primary cause of overdose mortality with annual overdose deaths exceeding deaths from motor vehicle collisions in 2008. In 2010–2012, opioid prescribing peaked and began to decline in the United States (Guy et al. 2017). At the same time, the cost of high purity heroin was low (Drug Enforcement Administration (DEA) 2017). Overdose death rates from heroin rose precipitously. Then, in 2014, fentanyl and associated analogues began to enter the illicit heroin market, primarily from illicit manufacturers and distributors in China and Mexico (Drug Enforcement Administration (DEA) 2018a). Due to the potency of these drugs and the insidious nature of their introduction to the illicit opioid market, overdose deaths from fentanyl and related synthetic opioids rapidly became the leading cause of unintentional overdose deaths in the years following widespread availability (National Institute on Drug Abuse (NIDA) 2018). Despite the prevalence of fentanyl related compounds and their devastating toll, identification of continuously evolving analogues has proven challenging. Coordination of hospital, medical examiner, and law enforcement personnel with laboratory services has become increasingly important as we continue to respond to this threat (Daniulaityte et al. 2017).

With increasing attention and targeted intervention, prescription opioid and illicit opioid use has declined. However, non-opioid drug use has increased (Substance Abuse and Mental Health Services Administration (SAMHSA) 2018). The classes of illicit drugs available for use have not changed significantly for decades. Classes include stimulants, cannabinoids, sedative-hypnotics, and dissociative agents. However, the specific drugs within these categories have evolved in both receptor specificity and potency leading to an ever-changing landscape of novel psychoactive substances (NPS). Traditional drugs including cocaine, amphetamines, methamphetamines, cannabis, and phencyclidine remain popular. Deaths associated with cocaine and methamphetamine have risen significantly since 2014 (National Institute on Drug Abuse (NIDA) 2018). However, the availability and use of newer synthetic drugs have continued to increase (Drug Enforcement Administration (DEA) 2018a). Due to the influx of newer drugs and variable chemical composition, prevalence of use is likely underestimated given the difficulty in identification and the transient presence of individual drugs within a drug class. Moreover, combinations of drugs such as cocaine adulterated with fentanyl or inclusion of synthetic cannabinoids with fentanyl products have led to unintended and mixed toxicity further complicating clinical management and laboratory identification.

Substance use and associated toxicity have been a continuous phenomena in the United States for decades. The deaths of tens of thousands of Americans per year, primarily from opioid toxicity, have drawn sharp attention to the issues of substance use and addiction. Past experience demonstrates that while the drug of choice will change over time, drug use will continue to be a critical focus of public health and law enforcement policy. Recently, the variety of available drugs has expanded significantly beyond the traditional drugs of just a decade ago. A summary of emerging drugs is presented in Table 1. In order to properly respond to this changing environment, accurate identification of a wide spectrum of drugs will be necessary (Table 2).

2 Opioids

2.1 Epidemiology

Opioid use and misuse have expanded dramatically since the late 1980s–early 1990s. Poorly treated pain as well as a misunderstanding of the potential adverse effects of long-term opioid use combined with pharmaceutical company and regulatory pressures to adequately relieve pain led to marked increases in opioid prescribing from the 1990s through 2010 (Jones et al. 2018). As opioid prescribing began to decline in 2010–2012, illicit use of heroin and then fentanyl rose precipitously (Hedegaard et al. 2017). Starting in 2014, fentanyl and its analogues infiltrated the illicit opioid market. Deaths related to illicitly manufactured fentanyl and associated analogues rose 88% from 2013 to 2016 and rapidly became the most common cause of unintentional overdose death in the United States (Hedegaard et al. 2017). In 2017, 16 fentanyl-related compounds and potent non-fentanyl synthetic opioids like U-47700 were identified in drug seizures by DEA in addition to pure fentanyl (Drug Enforcement Administration (DEA) 2018b). In the first half of 2018, fentanyl accounted for ~75% of opioid identifications by the DEA and was mixed with heroin in 48% of its identifications indicating the significant prevalence of fentanyl in the drug supply as well as the potential for inadvertent use of fentanyl products (Drug Enforcement Administration (DEA) 2018c). Since 2012, 28 new fentanyl analogues have been identified in the European Union, with 18 of them being identified for the first time in 2016–2017. It is important to note that seized products have included pills pressed to look like prescription pharmaceuticals, nasal sprays, and vaping liquids. Seventy percent of European opioid seizures in 2016 were fentanyl and associated analogues (European Monitoring Centre for Drugs and Drug Addiction 2018). The economic burden of the opioid crisis in the United States has been estimated at $78.5 billion/year for prescription opioids alone and at more than $500 billion in 2015 when considering all opioids (Florence et al. 2016). In 2017, the opioid crisis was declared a

Table 1 Examples of emerging drugs of abuse by category. Derived from Drug Enforcement Administration (DEA) (2017)

Opioids	Stimulants	Cannabinoids	Dissociative agents	Sedative-hypnotics
Benzoylbenzyl fentanyl	N-Ethylbuphedrone	FUB-PB-22	3-Methoxy-phencyclidine	Phenazepam
2-Thifuranyl fentanyl	Methylone	5F-EMB-PINACA	Methoxetamine	Diclazepam
U-48800	4-Methylenedioxy-α-pyrrolidinobutiophenone	5F-AB-PINACA	Methoxphenidine	Flubromazolam
Benzylfentanyl	4-Methylethylaminopentiophenone	SDB-005	Deschloroketamine	Flubromazepam
U-49900	α-Pyrrolidinohexanophenone	NM2201	2-Oxo-PCE	Etizolam
Tetrahydrofuran fentanyl	Ethylone	MDMB-CHMICA	Dextromethorphan	Clonazolam
3-Methylfentanyl	Pentylone	5F-AKB48		
Butyryl fentanyl	α-Pyrrolidinovalerophenone	AB-PINACA		
Acryl fentanyl	4-Chloroethcathinone	5F-AMB		
Methoxyacetylfentanyl	Dibutylone	ADB-CHMINACA		
Cyclopropylfentanyl	N-Ethylpentylone	5F-UR-144		
Acetylfentanyl	25I-NBOMe	AB-FUBINACA		
Carfentany78l	25C-NBOMe	MMB-CHMICA		
4-Fluoroisobutyryl fentanyl	4-Bromo-2,5-dimethoxyphenethylamine	ADB-FUBINACA		
U-47700	4-Hydroxy-N-methyl-N-ethyltryptamine	5F-MDMB-PINACA		
Furanyl fentanyl	5-Methoxy-N,N-dimethyltryptamine	FUB-AMB		
Mitragynine	4-Acetoxy-N,N-dimethyltryptamine			
Salvinorin				
Ibogaine				

Table 2 Summary of classes of emerging drugs of abuse including mechanism of action, clinical effects, laboratory testing techniques, and treatment

Drug class	Pharmacology of toxicity	Clinical effects	Laboratory testing	Treatment
Opioids	μ-Opioid receptor agonism (major); δ- and κ-opioid receptor agonism (minor)	Sedation, miosis, respiratory depression	FDA-cleared immunoassays available for opiates, 6-MAM, and fentanyl	Assisted ventilation; titrated naloxone dosing
Synthetic cannabinoids	Potent CB1 receptor agonism; CB2 agonism less clinically relevant for acute toxicity	Paranoia, agitation, tachycardia, hypertension, vomiting	No FDA-cleared immunoassays available	$GABA_A$-agonist sedation (benzodiazepines or barbiturates)
Stimulants and hallucinogens	Norepinephrine, dopamine, and serotonin reuptake inhibition and receptor agonism	Hallucinations, agitation, delirium, seizures, tachycardia, hypertension	Partially cross-reactive with FDA-cleared amphetamine immunoassays	$GABA_A$-agonist sedation (benzodiazepines or barbiturates); dopamine antagonists (antipsychotics)
Dissociative agents	Glutamate NMDA-receptor antagonism	Nystagmus, dissociation, tachycardia, occasionally agitation	Partially cross-reactive with FDA-cleared PCP immunoassays	$GABA_A$-agonist sedation (benzodiazepines or barbiturates)
Sedative-hypnotics	$GABA_A$ and $GABA_B$ receptor agonism	Sedation, hyporeflexia; tachycardia and myoclonus with $GABA_B$ agonists	FDA-cleared immunoassays available for benzodiazepines, but not for GABA derivatives	Supportive care with airway protection if needed; flumazenil in selected scenarios

public health emergency. Given the profound impact opioids have had on medical practice and society in the United States, thorough evaluation and understanding of the effects of these drugs and accurate identification and surveillance are critical (O'Donnell et al. 2017).

2.2 Chemistry and Chemical Structures

Opiates, such as morphine, are opium poppy *Papaver somniferum*-derived psychoactive alkaloids consumed by human beings since the ancient Mesopotamia era circa 3,400 BC (Presley and Lindsley 2018). Opiates have the pentacyclic phenanthrene ring structure (Fig. 1). The major psychoactive alkaloid included in opium poppy is morphine, which is also a direct precursor of heroin. Heroin is 3,6-diacetylmorphine that was pharmaceutically developed by diacetylation of morphine by Bayer in 1898 as a nonaddictive morphine derivative, but it turned out to be strongly addictive. Thebaine, another opiate and biosynthetic precursor to morphine, is chemically modified to develop naloxone (Fig. 1) (Devereaux et al. 2018).

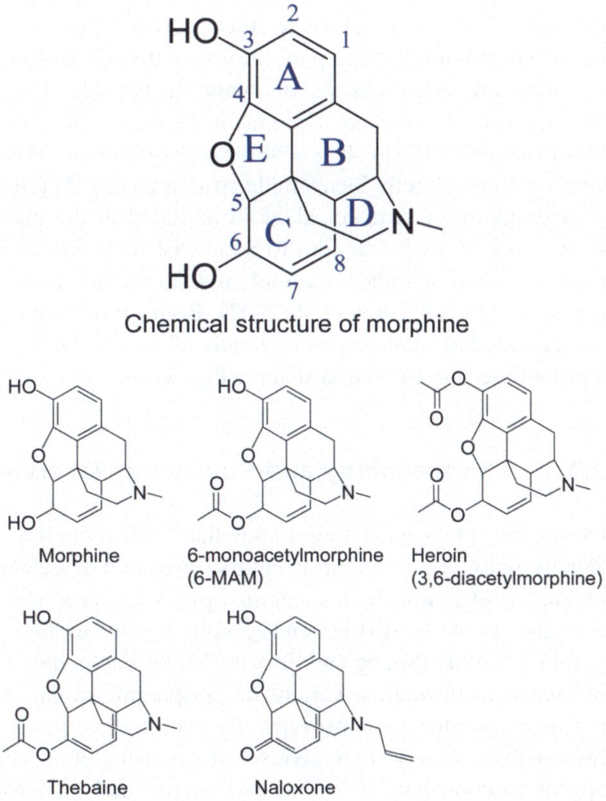

Fig. 1 Chemical structures of morphine and structurally related compounds. The pentacyclic phenanthrene ring structure (ring A–E) and numbering of morphine are also provided in the figure

Fentanyl was first developed by Dr. Paul Janssen, the founder of Janssen Pharmaceuticals and innovative scientist, who developed more than 80 drugs in 1960. He hypothesized that a piperidine ring is the most important chemical structure of morphine and meperidine in their analgesic effect; indeed, fentanyl was synthesized as a piperidine-derivative analgesic and anesthetic agent (Domino 2008; Stanley 1992; Stanley et al. 2008).

Fentanyl and its analogues are synthetic phenylpiperidine or 4-anilidopiperidine opioids (Vuckovic et al. 2009), and its chemical structure substantially differs from that of opiates, even though fentanyl and opiates share the piperidine ring. The fentanyl skeleton consists of N-alkyl chain, piperidine ring, amide group, and aniline ring (Cayman Chemical 2018). Various fentanyl analogues have been developed through substitution of these moieties (Fig. 2).

Nomenclature of these fentanyl analogues is confusing. Typically, the name of the chemical moiety substituting the ethyl or ethoxy moiety in the amide group in fentanyl is added in front of "fentanyl." For example, an ethoxy moiety is replaced with the acetyl moiety in acetylfentanyl, whereas an ethyl moiety is replaced with the butyryl moiety in butyrylfentanyl. Chemical modification can be made in other groups as well. For example, a methyl group is attached to the 3-position in the piperidine ring in 3-methylfentanyl, whereas a carbomethoxy group is attached to the 4-position in the piperidine ring in 4-carbomethoxy fentanyl or carfentanil. A fluorine atom is attached to the *para*-position in the aniline ring in para-fluorobutyrylfentanyl and para-fluoroisobutyrylfentanyl.

There are other classes of synthetic opioids. U-47700 was developed by a pharmaceutical company Upjohn in the 1970s as a more potent opioid analgesic (Szmuszkovicz 1976). It is a structural isomer of AH-7921, a synthetic analgesic with cyclohexylmethylbenzamide structure (Fig. 3) (Brittain et al. 1973).

Mitragynine is a major alkaloid included in the plant *Mitragyna speciosa*, also known as kratom, indigenous to Southeast Asia (Jansen and Prast 1988). 7-Hydroxy mitragynine is a minor alkaloid in kratom, but it is a more potent opioid than mitragynine (Takayama et al. 2002). Both mitragynine and 7-hydroxy mitragynine are classified as monoterpenoid indole alkaloids. These compounds also do not have a piperidine ring in their structure (Fig. 3).

2.3 Pharmacology and Physiology Overview

Opioid receptors exist throughout the CNS including the brain and spinal cord. Traditionally, μ-, δ-, and κ-receptors have been described and studied with subtypes of each and a fourth, nociceptin opioid receptor (NOP), receiving more recent attention due to its distinct endogenous ligand-binding affinity relative to the other opioid receptors (Shang and Filizola 2015). Each type of opioid receptor plays a role in analgesia through a variety of peripheral, spinal, and cerebral activities. The μ-opioid receptor has most typically been targeted as a potent analgesic but is also responsible for undesired adverse effects (Ling et al. 1985). The κ- and δ-receptors appear to contribute to spinal and supraspinal analgesia and represent targets of

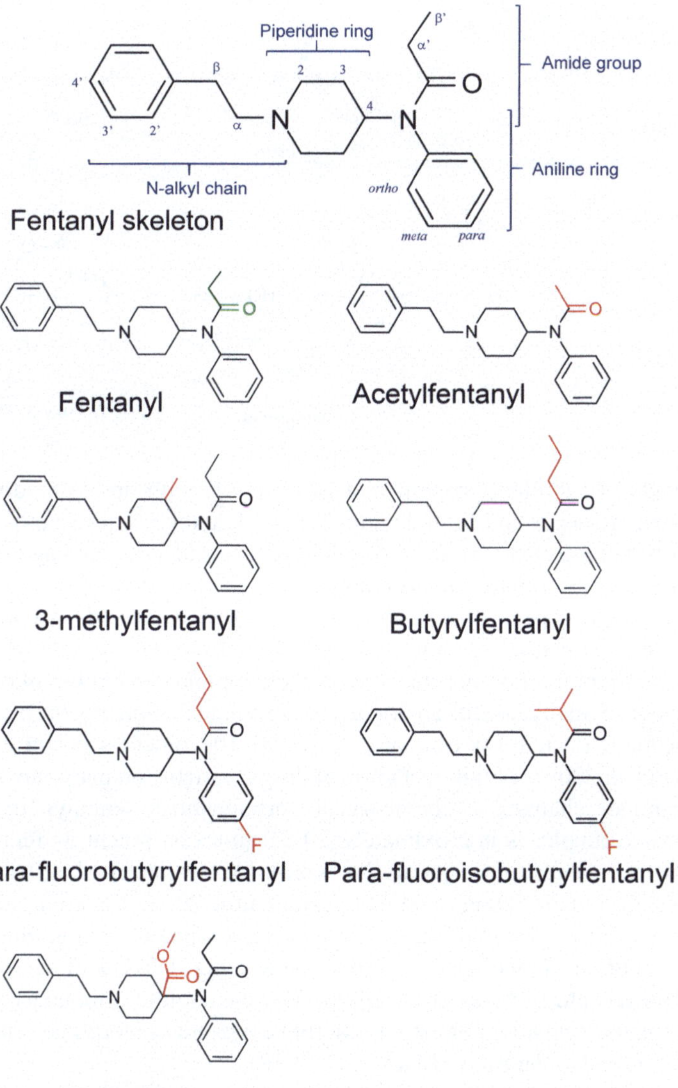

Fig. 2 Chemical structures of fentanyl and fentanyl analogues. The chemical structure of the fentanyl skeleton is also provided. The ethoxy moiety of fentanyl is highlighted in green. The substituting moiety in each fentanyl analogue is highlighted in red

ongoing investigation for therapeutic investigation as well as recreational use, e.g., salvinorin and ibogaine (Gendron et al. 2016; Listos et al. 2011; Litjens and Brunt 2016; Roach and Shenvi 2018). Mitragynine and 7-hydroxy mitragynine, found in kratom, are partial μ-opioid receptor agonists as well as κ- and δ-opioid receptor antagonists. Adrenergic and dopaminergic receptor activation is also described

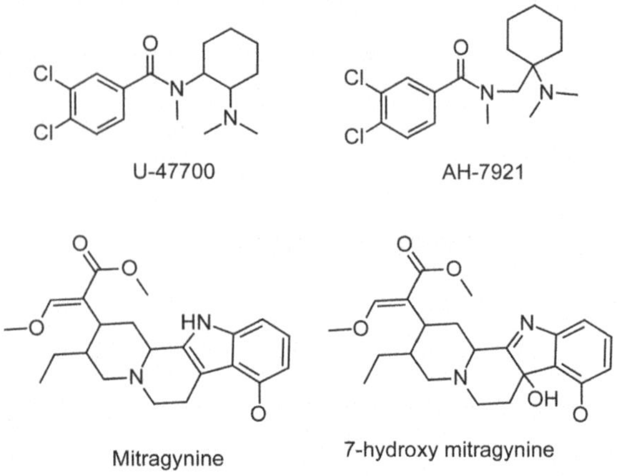

Fig. 3 Chemical structures of U-47700, AH-7921, mitragynine, and 7-hydoxy mitragynine

which results in stimulant properties at lower doses with opioid predominance at higher doses (Kruegel and Grundmann 2018). Naloxone, a μ-receptor antagonist, does not reverse the effects of κ- or δ-opioid receptor activity, and agonists at those sites do not cause respiratory depression.

Time to onset of peak effect and potency of various opioids is conferred by a combination of structural specificity for the opioid receptor as well as capacity to enter the CNS rapidly. For instance, the synthetic opioid class of 4-anilidopiperidine which includes fentanyl and its analogues provides much more potent stimulus of the opioid receptor. Fentanyl is estimated to be 50–100 times as potent as morphine (Vuckovic et al. 2009). Within that class of drugs, variable potency can be seen with relatively minor changes in chemistry. 4-Carbomethoxy fentanyl, or carfentanil (Fig. 2), for example, is approximately 20–30 times as potent as fentanyl and is responsible for deaths throughout the world (Armenian et al. 2018; European Monitoring Centre for Drugs and Drug Addiction 2018; Vuckovic et al. 2009). Heroin results in more rapid onset of euphoria compared to morphine due to its lipophilic addition of two acetyl groups accelerating delivery of morphine to the CNS opioid receptors (Maas et al. 2018). The metabolite, 6-monoacetylmorphine (6-MAM), is nearly pathognomonic for heroin exposure as morphine is not naturally acetylated in the human body (Maas et al. 2018).

Some opioids confer pharmacologic effects other than pure opioid receptor agonism. Serotonin receptor activation secondary to reuptake inhibition has been demonstrated with opioids including tramadol, meperidine, dextromethorphan/dextrorphan, and fentanyl (Baldo 2018). Delayed repolarization of cardiac myocytes with associated QT interval prolongation and risk of polymorphic ventricular tachycardia can be seen with methadone, ibogaine, and loperamide (Behzadi et al. 2018). In addition to serotonin reuptake inhibition, blockade of norepinephrine reuptake by meperidine, tramadol, and their metabolites can result in seizures (Hassamal et al. 2018).

Finally, a variety of adulterating agents have been identified in illicit opioids which may lead to mixed pharmacology and clinical effects. Opioids and other illicit drugs typically are mixed with other compounds which may simply be diluents or bulking agents, e.g., sugars, to deliver a certain weight while minimizing the amount of valuable drug that is included. Adulterants are pharmacologically active constituents that are intentionally included for a variety of reasons that may include enhancing the effect, mitigating associated adverse drug effects, or simply as a lower cost substitute for the primary drug (United Nations Office for Drug Control and Crime Prevention (UNODCCP) 2001). Contaminants, on the other hand, are substances which were not intentionally included and can include bacterial toxins such as botulinum which has been reported worldwide (MacDonald et al. 2013; Palmateer et al. 2013; Yuan et al. 2011). Pharmacologically active adulterants vary significantly by time and geography. However, reported heroin adulterants have included paracetamol/acetaminophen, diphenhydramine, clenbuterol, lidocaine, xylazine, caffeine, diphenhydramine (aka "cheese"), phenobarbital, griseofulvin, diazepam, procaine, quinine/quinidine, chloroquine, methaqualone, and dextromethorphan (Broseus et al. 2016; Phillips et al. 2012; Ruiz-Colon et al. 2014; Solimini et al. 2017). Depending upon the presence and relative concentration of an adulterant, significant clinical effects may manifest that complicate and/or cloud the presentation of a patient with acute opioid intoxication.

2.4 Clinical Effects

Therapeutic use of opioids results in desired effects including potent and rapid reduction in pain as well as cough suppression. However, the distribution and activity of primarily μ-opioid receptors in the medullary respiratory center and gastrointestinal tract result in adverse effects and toxicity at supratherapeutic doses (Minami and Satoh 1995). Additionally, indirect activation of mesolimbic dopamine reward centers and intrinsically rewarding euphoric effects of opioids result in habituation and addiction (Kreek et al. 2012). Opioid use results in constipation with both short- and long-term use (Webster 2015). Acute opioid toxicity includes a typical triad of clinical signs: sedation or coma, hypoventilation, and miosis. Additional toxicity may include seizures, cardiac dysrhythmias, and serotonergic effects depending upon individual drug pharmacology. The onset of respiratory depression and arrest can be rapid, within minutes (Boom et al. 2012). Early signs of respiratory depression are typically hypercapnia followed by hypoxemia meaning that declines in oxygen saturation on pulse oximetry are a later finding. Cyanosis, bluish discoloration of the lips and distal extremities, is a clinical indicator of respiratory failure. Miosis may not be present with some opioids, particularly tramadol and meperidine with concurrent serotonin- and norepinephrine-mediated toxicity. While opioids exert myocardial depressant effects as well as histamine-mediated vasodilation resulting in hypotension, cardiovascular toxicity is primarily the result of hypoxemia and hypoperfusion secondary to respiratory failure. As respiratory failure progresses, secondary cardiac failure and arrest can occur. Pulmonary edema is frequently noted on postmortem examinations as well as in patients who have survived an overdose. There is a reported association of development of pulmonary edema following rapid reversal of acute toxicity with naloxone, but it is unclear if naloxone contributes to this process through catecholamine surge versus unmasking of developing pulmonary edema as part of the natural course of opioid toxicity, sudden inspiration against a closed glottis, or a combination of these factors (Megarbane and Chevillard 2013). Aspiration pneumonitis and pneumonia also frequently complicate opioid toxicity with mental status depression particularly in the presence of vomiting (Table 2).

2.5 Laboratory Detection and Methodology

Laboratory tests used in the clinical laboratories are subject to the law and regulations in each country. In the United States, FDA clearance is required before an immunoassay kit is used in clinical laboratories unless laboratory-developed tests under the Clinical Laboratory Improvement Amendments (CLIA) regulation (Genzen et al. 2017). FDA-cleared opiate immunoassays are included in routine urine drug screening panels. Opiate immunoassays cross-reacts with morphine, 6-MAM, and heroin, but not naloxone, unless its concentration is extremely high (Straseski et al. 2010). As 6-MAM is the immediate metabolite of heroin and morphine is the metabolite of 6-MAM, heroin abuse can be screened by opiate immunoassays, even though the half-life of heroin and 6-MAM is very short in the blood (less than 10 min and 40 min, respectively) (Goldberger et al. 1993). FDA-cleared 6-MAM immunoassays, such as Syva® EMIT® II Plus 6-Acetylmorphine kit (Siemens), are also available, allowing for the rapid screening of previous heroin usage with better specificity to 6-MAM than opiate immunoassays, but the positive results are regarded as "Presumptive" or "Unconfirmed" positive, and MS-based confirmatory testing should be conducted, especially for forensic purposes.

The identification of 6-MAM and/or heroin by mass spectrometry (MS)-based assays is accepted as a proof of previous heroin usage; however, morphine and its glucuronized metabolites are often the only opiates identified in the urine specimens after heroin usage due to the rapid removal of heroin and 6-MAM through metabolism. In this case, it is rather challenging to distinguish heroin usage from opium poppy (e.g., poppy seed) consumption by the laboratory findings. This creates a significant medicolegal issue known as "poppy seed defense" (Chen et al. 2014).

As discussed in the "Chemistry and Chemical Structures" section above, fentanyl and its analogues have a distinct structure to opiates (Figs. 1, 2 and 3); thus, any opiate immunoassays do not cross-react with these compounds (Liu et al. 2018). Instead, various immunoassays have been developed for fentanyl; however, most of them are for forensic or research use. Due to their strong structural similarity, these fentanyl assays should detect various fentanyl analogues with their high cross-reactivity. Currently there is only one FDA-cleared fentanyl immunoassay available on the market (SEFRIA™ Fentanyl Urine Enzyme Immunoassay, Immunalysis, Pomona, CA). The fentanyl immunoassay has not been incorporated in most standard drug screen immunoassay panels yet.

Similarly, any existing opiate immunoassays do not cross-react with U-47700, AH-7921, mitragynine, and 7-hydroxy mitragynine. Even though there are several immunoassay kits commercially available, these are for forensic or research use. There is no FDA-cleared immunoassay kit for these compounds.

Wide availability of FDA-cleared immunoassay kits should enable clinical laboratories to detect more cases of fentanyl (and/or fentanyl analogue) intoxication and misuse in a timely manner, potentially saving more lives.

Besides immunoassays, mass spectrometry (MS) – either gas chromatography-MS (GC-MS) or liquid chromatography-MS (LC-MS) – is used for identification of these synthetic opioids for clinical and forensic cases (summarized in Liu et al. 2018). These compounds can be detected by GC-MS-based untargeted analysis, but LC-MSMS-based targeted analysis is superior in the sensitivity of the assay (Liu et al. 2018).

2.6 Treatment

The primary danger associated with opioid toxicity is respiratory depression with hypercapnia, hypoxemia, and subsequent organ hypoperfusion injury, particularly of the brain and heart. The priority in treatment is to restore ventilation and oxygenation. Assisted ventilation through bag-valve-mask ventilation or endotracheal intubation treats the life-threatening respiratory toxicity associated with opioids. Naloxone, a μ-opioid receptor antagonist, is an effective antidote for acute opioid toxicity. Naloxone was approved for medical use in 1971. More recently, naloxone distribution for bystander use has resulted in reductions in opioid overdose mortality (McDonald and Strang 2016; Walley et al. 2013). Naloxone can be administered via intravenous, intramuscular, intranasal, and endotracheal routes. It is rapidly effective with reversal occurring within minutes of administration (Boyer 2012). Assisted ventilation should not be delayed while preparing or administering naloxone and should continue after administration until the patient is breathing independently. The adverse effects associated with naloxone administration are primarily related to induction of opioid withdrawal in opioid dependent patients (Wermeling 2015). Higher doses of naloxone may be needed depending upon the pharmacologic properties of different agents including receptor-binding affinity (Kd) and potency. However, when delivered promptly and effectively, naloxone is effective for reversal of even the most potent synthetic opioids and fentanyl analogues, though repeated escalating doses may be necessary in some cases (Armenian et al. 2018). If there is no response to even high-dose naloxone, intoxication with a non-opioid agent or advanced irreversible end-organ injury from prolonged hypoperfusion should be suspected. In some cases, the duration of action of the opioid will exceed that of naloxone. In such cases, repeated doses of naloxone and a naloxone infusion may be necessary to maintain ventilation throughout the course of toxicity, while the offending agent is metabolized and eliminated (Boyer 2012).

3 Cannabinoids

3.1 Epidemiology

Cannabis use dates back to ancient China in the fourth century BC and has been part of both social and medical culture since that time (Brand and Zhao 2017). In 1970, the US Controlled Substances Act classified marijuana as a Schedule I drug indicating a high risk of abuse without currently accepted medical use in the United States. However, cannabis-based medications have been approved by the FDA for human medical use including nabilone for chemotherapy-associated nausea and vomiting refractory to other agents; the Δ^9-tetrahydrocannabinol (THC) product, dronabinol, for appetite stimulation in anorexia associated with AIDS and nausea treatment for patients on chemotherapy; and, most recently, the cannabidiol (CBD) product, Epidiolex®, for treatment of specific seizure disorders. While cannabis remains Schedule I at the federal level in the United States, many states have passed legislation permitting the medical use of cannabis products with some states permitting recreational sale of cannabis. Legal status of cannabis is variable throughout the world. CBD, a constituent of marijuana without intoxicating properties, is not scheduled when sold in products that contain <0.3% THC, the primary psychoactive component of marijuana. Overall, marijuana use among Americans has risen significantly since 2003 with approximately 26 million marijuana users over the age of 12 in the United States in 2017 (Substance Abuse and Mental Health Services Administration (SAMHSA) 2018). Approximately 2.5% of the world's population consumes cannabis (World Health Organization Department of Mental Health and Substance Abuse Management of Substance Abuse Team (NMH/MSD/MSB) 2019). In 2008, the use of synthetic cannabinoids began to be recognized, first in Europe and then the United States (Auwarter et al. 2009; European Monitoring Centre for Drugs and Drug Addiction 2009). Their presence was identified in products sold as herbal incense products known colloquially as "K2" or "Spice," terms which have persisted and generally refer to myriad synthetic cannabinoid structures. At that time, the most commonly identified products were JWH-018, JWH-073, JWH-200, and CP-47,497 (Fig. 4) (Brents and Prather 2014). More recently, an even more potent class of synthetic cannabinoids has evolved with marked increases in reported exposures beginning in 2015 (Mowry et al. 2016). This group of cannabinoids including FUB-AMB, ADB-FUBINACA (Fig. 4), and many more are highly potent and result in much more significant toxicity (Table 1). The prevalence of synthetic cannabinoid use is unclear but growing (Law et al. 2015). Synthetic cannabinoids are the largest group of substances monitored by the EU Early Warning System, and cannabinoids were the most frequently seized novel psychoactive substances reported in 2016 (European Monitoring Centre for Drugs and Drug Addiction 2018). A significant barrier to more precise evaluation of prevalence is the difficulty in accurately identifying such a diverse group of continuously evolving chemicals in biological matrices (Castaneto et al. 2014). Synthetic cannabinoids can be identified in blood and urine specimens, but not in routine drug testing in typical healthcare settings highlighting the need for ongoing research and

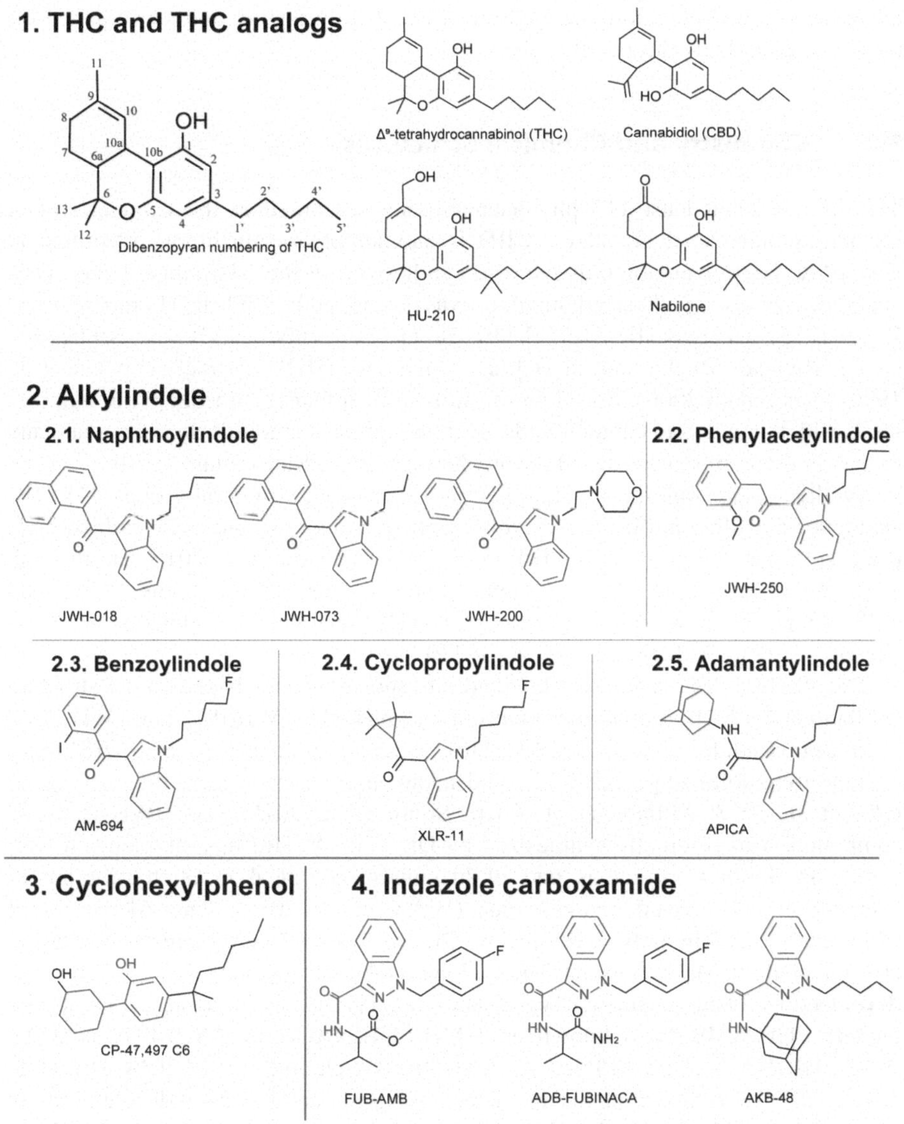

Fig. 4 Chemical structures of phytocannabinoids and synthetic cannabinoids. Based on the structure, these compounds are classified into four major groups: (1) Δ^9-tetrahydrocannabinol (THC) and THC analogues, (2) alkylindoles, (3) cyclohexylphenols, and (4) indazole carboxamide. The alkylindoles are further classified: (2.1) naphthoylindoles, (2.2) phenylacetylindoles, (2.3) benzoylindoles, (2.4) cyclopropylindoles, and (2.5) adamantylindoles. The core chemical structures in each synthetic cannabinoid are highlighted in green in the figure. The dibenzopyran numbering system of THC is also shown (Grotenhermen 2003; Mechoulam 1970)

attention to the application and interpretation of drug testing and surveillance for these compounds (Knittel et al. 2016).

3.2 Chemistry and Chemical Structures

THC is one of at least 113 phytocannabinoids identified in the *Cannabis* plant (Aizpurua-Olaizola et al. 2016). CBD is another phytocannabinoid identified in *Cannabis.* These cannabinoids are also synthesized in the laboratory. Other THC analogues are also synthesized; nabilone was developed by Eli Lilly (Lemberger and Rowe 1975), whereas HU-210 (11-OH-Δ8-THC-dimethylheptyl) was synthesized by Dr. Raphael Mechoulam at Hebrew University (HU) in Israel (Howlett et al. 1990; Mechoulam 2000). Based on the structural similarity, dibenzopyran numbering is widely applied to cannabinoids, even though cannabinoids do not contain any pyrans in their structure (Fig. 4) (Grotenhermen 2003; Mechoulam 1970).

Synthetic cannabinoids are classified into four major structural groups: (1) THC analogue, (2) alkylindole, (3) cyclohexylphenol, and (4) indazole carboxamide (Fig. 4) (Castaneto et al. 2014; Hill et al. 2018; Miliano et al. 2016; Smith et al. 2015; Wiley et al. 2015). Even though synthetic cannabinoids are potent CB1 (and CB2) cannabinoid receptor agonists, non-THC analogue compounds have the chemical structures distinct from that of THC.

The alkylindoles are further classified into several groups based on the structure (Miliano et al. 2016): naphthoylindoles (e.g., JWH-018, JWH-073, and JWH-200), phenylacetylindoles (e.g., JWH-250), benzoylindoles (e.g., AM-694), cyclopropylindoles (e.g., XLR-11), and adamantylindoles (e.g., APICA) (Fig. 4) (Hill et al. 2018; Miliano et al. 2016; Smith et al. 2015). The JWH-series of compounds was originally synthesized by Dr. John W. Huffman at Clemson University in South Carolina as part of his pharmacological research program of synthetic indole-derived cannabinoids (Wiley et al. 2015). The AM-series of compounds was originally developed by Dr. Alexandros Makriyannis at Northeastern University in Massachusetts. The cyclohexylphenols include CP-47.497 that was developed by Pfizer scientists (Weissman et al. 1982). The indazole carboxamides include FUB-AMB (also known as MMB-FUBINACA or AMB-FUBINACA), ADB-FUBINACA, and APINACA (AKB-48) (Gatch and Forster 2018; Hill et al. 2018). APINACA also contains an adamantayl group and has the indazole group in place of the indole ring in APICA, and thus it is structurally similar to APICA, an adamantylindole which can also be classified as an indole carboxamide (Fig. 4).

3.3 Pharmacology and Physiology Overview

Hundreds of cannabinoids, termed phytocannabinoids, and terpenoids have been identified in the *Cannabis* species of plants (Andre et al. 2016). The potential contribution of clinical effects from many of these constituents remains unclear. The primary focus of clinical and pharmacologic evaluation has been with the cannabinoids, THC and CBD. The cannabinoid receptor system is complex with modulatory effects on multiple transmitter-receptor complexes and remains incompletely understood. Endogenous cannabinoids (endocannabinoids), anandamide and 2-arachidonoylglycerol, exert effects upon two identified cannabinoid receptors, CB1 and CB2 (Sugiura and Waku 2002). More recently, activity at the transient receptor potential vanilloid 1 (TRPV1) has been described with implications on both pain and hyperemesis syndromes (Zou and Kumar 2018). The CB1 receptor has been identified throughout the central and peripheral nervous systems with a wide variety of direct effects on neuronal, gastrointestinal, and immune cells as well as pre- and postsynaptic modulation of other neurotransmitters including GABA, acetylcholine, serotonin, glutamate, norepinephrine, and dopamine (Zou and Kumar 2018). Alternatively, CB2 receptors are primarily located in the spleen, testis, and with minimal role in the CNS reward system (Zou and Kumar 2018). Given the wide distribution of cannabinoid receptors and interaction with multiple neurologic pathways, activation results in a complex pattern of activity with many observed and hypothesized effects. THC is a partial agonist at the CB1 and CB2 receptors, while CBD has been described as an allosteric antagonist at cannabinoid receptors with serotonin and TRPV1 agonist activity (Boggs et al. 2018). The relative concentrations of THC and CBD in a cannabis product contribute to the variability in effect and experience with THC typically resulting in more psychoactivating intoxication, while CBD is responsible for the nonintoxicating effects described with cannabis use (Boggs et al. 2018). As opposed to the relatively weak cannabinoid receptor activation by endocannabinoids and the partial agonist and promiscuous activity of phytocannabinoids, synthetic cannabinoids have been developed as full cannabinoid receptor agonists resulting in much more potent activity by orders of magnitude depending upon the specific agent (Castaneto et al. 2014). Synthetic cannabinoids are often available as a liquid formulation which is then applied to vegetative material, e.g., marijuana or tobacco, or used in a vaporizing system. Onset of symptoms after inhalational use is rapid, typically within minutes, and duration can be hours to more than a day depending upon the dose and specific formulation (Castaneto et al. 2014). Marijuana metabolites can persist on urine drug screening for weeks depending upon frequency and magnitude of use (Lowe et al. 2009).

3.4 Clinical Effects

Given the diverse distribution and activity of cannabinoid receptors, there are a wide variety of proven, anecdotal, and theoretical therapeutic opportunities for pharmaceutical modulation. There is growing interest and support, both scientific and social, in the potential of cannabinoids for medical use, but high-level data are generally limited. As of 2017, there was strong evidence to support the benefits of cannabinoid use for nausea, appetite stimulation, modest reductions in chronic pain, and multiple sclerosis related spasticity. Otherwise, available research was unavailable or inadequate to draw definitive conclusions of benefit (National Academies of

Sciences and Medicine 2017). As further research is performed, additional supported indications for medical use may be validated. The diversity of cannabinoid effects also leads to a variety of intended and unintended consequences depending upon the formulation, route of delivery, and specific substance. For nonmedical use, intoxication and/or anxiolysis is typically the goal. Varying relative concentrations of THC and CBD in leaf marijuana as well as edibles, vaping oils, and other formulations of cannabinoids impact the nature and degree of intoxication with higher concentration of THC relative to CBD resulting in greater intoxication, motor impairment, and other adverse effects (Ford et al. 2017). There was a fourfold increase in THC content identified in confiscated marijuana in 2014 compared to 1995 with an increase in THC:CBD concentrations from 14 to 80 times (ElSohly et al. 2016). This rise in potency with availability of high concentration and pure THC alternative products as well as expanded availability has likely contributed to a rise in associated emergency department visits (Zhu and Wu 2016).

Acute phytocannabinoid toxicity is not life-threatening outside of associated trauma or secondary illness but can include impaired motor coordination, altered judgment, impaired short-term memory, nausea, vomiting, tachycardia, vasodilation with hypotension, syncope, paranoia, and psychosis (Volkow et al. 2014). Long-term adverse effects include addiction, impaired cognitive development with associated lower IQ (particularly in adolescent users), worsened educational outcomes, diminished life satisfaction and career achievement, chronic bronchitis, and increased risk of psychosis in individuals with an existing predisposition (Volkow et al. 2014). Cannabinoid hyperemesis syndrome has been described as a cyclical syndrome of vomiting, abdominal cramping, and dehydration in long-term regular users of cannabis with the hallmark feature of patients reporting relief from hot showers or baths (Sorensen et al. 2017).

Synthetic cannabinoids, as full cannabinoid receptor agonists, pose a much more significant immediate threat. In addition to symptoms associated with THC stimulation of cannabinoid receptors, synthetic cannabinoid use has been associated with extreme agitation, delirium, seizures, ventricular dysrhythmias, hemodynamic instability, respiratory failure, rhabdomyolysis, anoxic brain injury, and death (Katz et al. 2016). The degree of agitation and hyperadrenergic toxicity witnessed with use of these drugs is reminiscent of potent stimulant toxicity and may be clinically indistinguishable at the time of initial presentation. Given the relatively recent advent of synthetic cannabinoid availability, difficulty in identification, and limited experience with regular use, data regarding long-term effects are not available (Table 2).

3.5 Laboratory Detection and Methodology

FDA-cleared cannabinoid immunoassays are commonly included in routine urine drug screening panels. These kits are developed to target the inactive Δ9-THC carboxy metabolite, the major urinary excreted form, but they can cross-react with THC due to their structural similarity to the Δ9-THC carboxy metabolite. Some kits can even cross-react weakly with CBD at very high concentrations, as indicated in the published data sheet (e.g., Syva® EMIT-II Plus Cannabinoid immunoassay kit, Siemens) and a published literature (Simpson et al. 1997). Furthermore, CBD products might contain a trace amount of THC (Bonn-Miller et al. 2017). Because of these facts, a urine specimen obtained from a CBD product user might generate a positive result of cannabinoid immunoassays either through its weak cross-reactivity with the immunoassay kit and/or the trace amount of THC included in the CBD products (Kulig 2017), especially if a large amount of CBD products is consumed and a low cutoff is adopted in the immunoassay.

Development of an immunoassay to detect synthetic cannabinoids in urine, the standard type of clinical specimens for analysis, is a challenging task. One major reason is their extensive metabolism. Another confounding factor is the wide structural diversity of these compounds (Fig. 4), which makes the development of a single immunoassay covering the whole class of synthetic cannabinoids unfeasible. Besides THC analogue HU-210, synthetic cannabinoids are structurally dissimilar to Δ9-THC or Δ9-THC carboxy metabolite, as predicted by 2D similarity values to Δ9-THC carboxy metabolite [e.g., JWH-018 (0.382), JWH-073 (0.345)]. That is why synthetic cannabinoids except THC analogues do not cross-react with THC immunoassays targeting Δ9-THC carboxy metabolite (Krasowski and Ekins 2014). Commercially available immunoassays for synthetic cannabinoids (e.g., Randox) can only cover relatively small groups of them with similar chemical structures (Arntson et al. 2013; Namera et al. 2015). None of these kits have received FDA clearance; thus, these kits cannot be used in clinical laboratories.

These limitations in immunoassays make LC-MSMS-based analysis the optimal alternative for the analysis of synthetic cannabinoids (Knittel et al. 2016; Namera et al. 2015; Scheidweiler and Huestis 2014). GC-MS seems not to be suitable for detection of synthetic cannabinoids without proper derivatization pretreatments, presumably because of their polar structures (Liu et al. 2018).

3.6 Treatment

The treatment of cannabinoid toxicity is largely supportive. There is no antidote for cannabinoid toxicity or clinically available CB1 receptor antagonist. Phytocannabinoid toxicity is self-limited, and treatment is aimed at symptom management with antiemetics, IV fluids, safe environment, redirection, and anxiolysis if necessary while intoxicated. Topical capsaicin has been recommended for the treatment of acute exacerbations of cannabinoid hyperemesis syndrome (Sorensen et al. 2017). The primary treatment for acute and chronic toxicity is cessation of use.

Management of synthetic cannabinoid toxicity is also supportive but typically requires much more intensive intervention including escalating doses of parenteral $GABA_A$-agonist medications including benzodiazepines and/or barbiturates to de-escalate agitated delirium associated with risk to both patients and care providers. In cases of severe agitation unresponsive to initial sedation and/or respiratory failure, endotracheal intubation may be necessary to provide adequate ventilation and sedative administration such as propofol or high-dose barbiturates, e.g., phenobarbital. Dosing should be titrated to sedation. Evaluation should include assessment of myocardial ischemia, infarction, or dysrhythmia with electrocardiogram and cardiac enzymes in patients with significant intoxication and cardiovascular vital sign abnormalities. Providers should have a low threshold to evaluate for rhabdomyolysis and associated kidney injury as well as aspiration pneumonitis/pneumonia which are common complications of both stimulant and sedative toxic syndromes. Patients with abnormal movements or encephalopathy out of proportion with intoxication or treatment should be evaluated for nonconvulsive seizure activity in addition to anoxic or traumatic brain injury (Castaneto et al. 2014; Katz et al. 2016).

4 Stimulants/Hallucinogens

4.1 Epidemiology

Cocaine and amphetamine/methamphetamine have been and remain the most commonly used illicit stimulants (Substance Abuse and Mental Health Services Administration (SAMHSA) 2018). Methamphetamine availability and purity are rising, while cost has remained low nationally resulting in increased prevalence of use (Drug Enforcement Administration (DEA) 2018a). Identification of cocaine and methamphetamine in postmortem evaluation of unintentional overdose death victims has risen steadily in recent years (Hedegaard et al. 2017). Additionally, prescription stimulants have been increasingly prescribed and misused (Safer 2016; Substance Abuse and Mental Health Services Administration (SAMHSA) 2018). A diverse group of novel stimulant and hallucinogenic drugs has also grown in popularity. The primary classes of newer stimulant psychoactive substances include β-ketoamphetamines (cathinones), piperazines, tryptamines, and two carbon (2C)-phenylethylamines (Fig. 5) (Graddy et al. 2018). Examples of these can be found in Table 1. Approximately 1.2% of surveyed adults self-reported use of psychoactive substances including cathinones and other novel phenylethylamines, while ~0.7% of high school students reported cathinone use from 2012 to 2014 (Palamar et al. 2015; Patrick et al. 2016). Cathinones are a group of stimulant chemicals derived from the *Catha edulis* (khat) plant. Chewing khat is a common cultural practice in many North African, Eastern Mediterranean, and Middle Eastern countries (Odenwald and al'Absi 2017). Western Europe and US utilization of synthetic stimulants derived from purified cathinone began to be reported in 2009–2010 at which time they were marketed as "bath salts," a name that has persisted and includes a wide variety of distinct cathinone derivatives and other stimulants (Prosser and Nelson 2012). These are often labelled, "Not for human consumption" in order to avoid regulation. While the DEA has classified many of these stimulants as Schedule I, continuous updates and changes to chemical structures make real-time accurate identification and

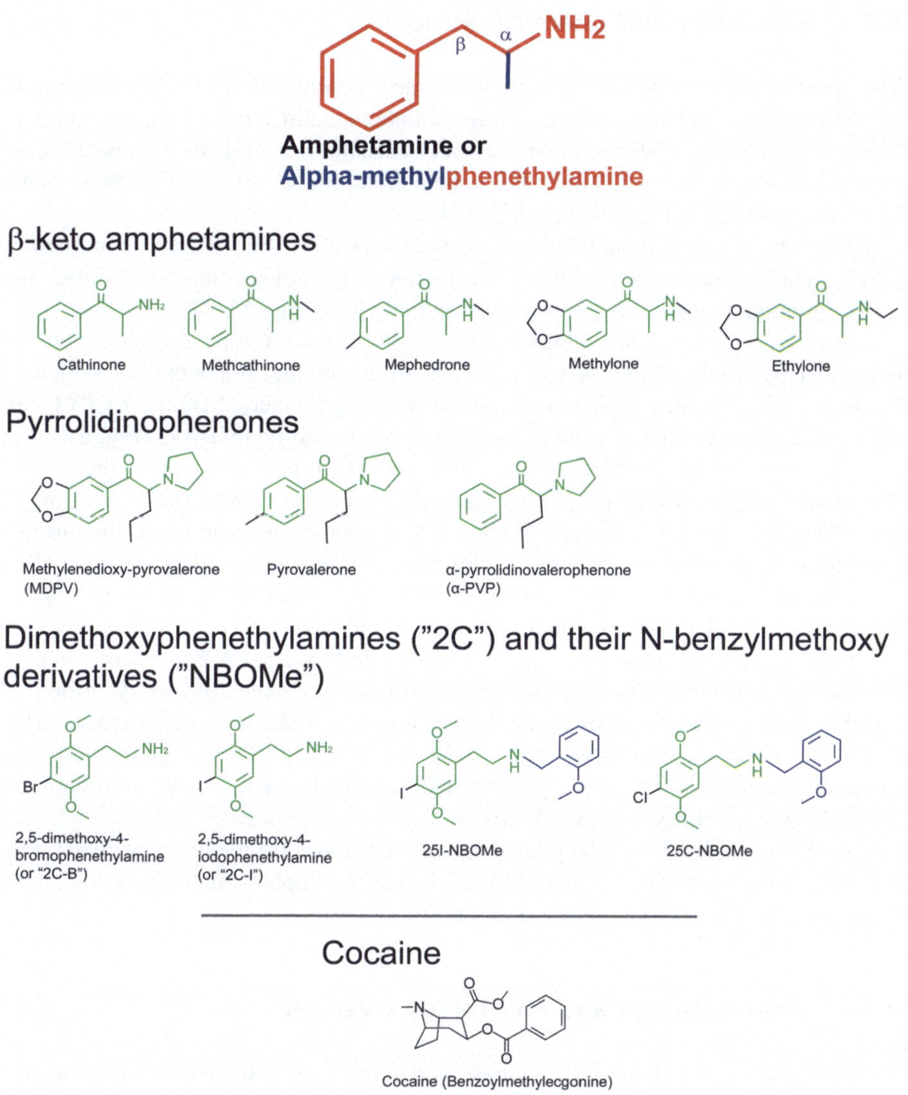

Fig. 5 Chemical structures of amphetamine, amphetamine-derived stimulants/hallucinogens, and cocaine. The chemical structure and nomenclature of amphetamine or alpha-methylphenethylamine are also provided in the figure. The core chemical structure of each class of amphetamine-type stimulants is highlighted in green and blue (for N-benzylmethoxy moiety)

response by regulating agencies difficult (Weinstein et al. 2017). The United Nations estimates that nearly 250 new drug analogues are created each year (Karch 2015). Forensic and clinical laboratories are challenged to keep pace with this fluid market of available stimulants (Glicksberg et al. 2016).

4.2 Chemistry and Chemical Structures

The prototypal compound is amphetamine, contracted from *alpha-m*ethyl-*phe*nethyl*amine*. Besides cocaine, these stimulants/hallucinogens are all amphetamine derivatives. These compounds are classified as β-keto amphetamines, pyrrolidinophenones, and dimethoxyphenethylamines (Fig. 5) (Peters and Martinez-Ramirez 2010; Petrie et al. 2013).

Cathinone is a prototypal β-keto amphetamine (Kalix 1992). There are numerous β-keto amphetamines or cathinone derivatives, including, but not limited to, methcathinone, mephedrone, methylone, and ethylone (Fig. 5).

Pyrrolidinophenones are another class of amphetamine-type stimulants which contain a pyrrolidine ring in place of the amine in the amphetamine skeleton. Examples of pyrrolidinophenones are α-pyrrolidinovalerophenone (α-PVP or "Flakka"), pyrovalerone, and methylenedioxy-pyrovalerone (MDPV) (Fig. 5).

Dimethoxyphenethylamines contain two methoxy groups attached to the 2- and 5-positions of the benzene ring in the phenethylamine backbone. These two carbon phenylethylamines are collectively called "2C." A bromine atom is attached to the 4-position of the benzene ring in 2,5-dimethoxy-4-bromophenethylamine or "2C-B," whereas an iodine atom is attached to the 4-position of the benzene ring in 2,5-dimethoxy-4-iodophenethylamine or "2C-I" (Fig. 5).

Dimethoxyphenethylamines have N-benzylmethoxy or *N-b*enzyl-*o*xy-*me*thyl derivatives called NBOMes. As the name indicates, a 2-methoxybenzyl group is attached to the nitrogen atom of the dimethoxyphenethylamines in NBOMes. The N-benzylmethoxy derivative of 2C-I or 25I-NBOMe [2-(4-Iodo-2,5-dimethoxyphenyl)-N-[(2-methoxyphenyl)methyl]ethanamine] is the prototype of NBOMe (Fig. 5) (Laskowski et al. 2015).

Cocaine or benzoylmethylecgonine is a primary psychoactive tropane alkaloid in *Erythroxylum coca* leaves, structurally distinct from amphetamine-type stimulants/hallucinogens (Fig. 5) (Goldstein et al. 2009).

4.3 Pharmacology and Physiology Overview

Phenylethylamines stimulate the release and inhibit the reuptake of the biogenic amines norepinephrine, dopamine, and serotonin (Graddy et al. 2018). Structural variation imparts distinct patterns of neurotransmitter effects. For instance, methylenedioxymethamphetamine (MDMA) exerts greater serotonin effects leading to a more hallucinogenic experience compared to predominantly adrenergic symptoms with methamphetamine. The constellation of symptoms and clinical effects associated with individual drugs is dictated by the relative intensity of induced neurotransmitter activity. The "2C" compounds and their N-benzylmethoxy derivatives, e.g., 25I-NBOMe ("N-Bombs" or "Smiles"), are primarily potent serotonin receptor agonists with noradrenergic receptor activation, as well (Suzuki et al. 2015). Phenylethylamine drugs can be taken orally, smoked, or injected. 25I-NBOMe has also been sold on paper and referred to as "acid" which can lead to confusion as that colloquial term has been used to describe lysergic diethylamide (LSD). Onset is typically rapid with duration of action of up to 8 h depending upon the specific product (Graddy et al. 2018).

Tryptamines, e.g., 5-Methoxy-N,N-diisopropyltryptamine (5-MeO-DiPT), also known as "Foxy" or "Foxy Methoxy," and piperazines, e.g., 1-benzylpiperazine (BZP) and 1-(3-Trifluoromethylphenyl)piperazine (TFMPP), have primarily serotonergic effects (Arbo et al. 2012; Dinis-Oliveira 2017; Dominguez-Clave et al. 2016).

4.4 Clinical Effects

Stimulants have been used clinically for a variety of purposes, particularly treatment of attention deficit hyperactivity disorder (ADHD) (Safer 2016). However, they also represent a broad and diverse group of illicitly available drugs from cocaine and methamphetamine to a variety of novel psychostimulants and hallucinogens. The toxicity associated with each drug and drug class is conferred by its neurotransmitter-receptor complex activity. Use of phenylethylamine compounds result in a mixture of noradrenergic, dopaminergic, and serotonergic effects including tachycardia, hypertension, diaphoresis, agitation, delirium, seizures, ventricular dysrhythmias, hallucinations, choreiform movements due to dopamine effects, tremor, hyperreflexia, and hyperthermia (Prosser and Nelson 2012). Tryptamines and piperazines, meanwhile, cause primarily serotonergic effects which overlap significantly but with more pronounced tremor and hyperreflexia and without evidence of dopamine-mediated effects such as chorea (Graddy et al. 2018). Dopamine and serotonin activity may both result in "hallucinations" though dopamine is more commonly associated with psychotic and tactile hallucinations, while serotonin is more likely to result in synesthesias (Rolland et al. 2014). Practically, differentiation of the various causative agents is difficult and unlikely to change immediate management. Hyponatremia has been reported with stimulant use, primarily with MDMA but also with the cathinone mephedrone (Prosser and Nelson 2012).

4.5 Laboratory Detection and Methodology

Currently there is no FDA-cleared immunoassay kit specifically targeting β-keto amphetamines, pyrrolidinophenones, and dimethoxyphenethylamine. Due to their moderate structural similarity to amphetamine (Fig. 5) [The 2D similarity value of cathinone, methcathinone, and mephedrone to amphetamine are all 0.45 (Petrie et al. 2013)], β-keto amphetamines appear to cross-react weakly with AxSYM® Amphetamine/Methamphetamine II, CEDIA Amphetamine/Ecstasy kit, and Lin-Zhi Methamphetamine enzyme immunoassays, but not EMIT® II Plus Amphetamines kit (Krasowski and Ekins 2014; Petrie et al. 2013; Regester et al. 2015).

Pyrrolidinophenones, on the other hand, appear not to cross-react with EMIT® II Plus Amphetamines kit, AxSYM® Amphetamine/Methamphetamine II, CEDIA Amphetamine/Ecstasy kit, and Lin-Zhi Methamphetamine enzyme immunoassay due to weak structural similarity to amphetamine [The 2D similarity value of MDPV to amphetamine is 0.22 (Krasowski and Ekins 2014; Petrie et al. 2013; Regester et al. 2015)], but MDPV weakly cross-reacts with Microgenics DRI Phencyclidine enzyme assay, in accord with the moderate 2D similarity value of MDPV to PCP (0.52) (Krasowski and Ekins 2014; Macher and Penders 2013).

Dimethoxyphenethylamines (“2C” compounds) have rather weak structural similarity to amphetamine (Fig. 5) [The 2D similarity values of 2C-I and 2C-B to amphetamine are both 0.33 (Petrie 2013 Excel)]; 2Cs seem not to cross-react with AxSYM® Amphetamine/Methamphetamine II, CEDIA Amphetamine/Ecstasy kit, and Lin-Zhi Methamphetamine enzyme immunoassay; however they weakly cross-react with EMIT® II Plus Amphetamines kit (Petrie et al. 2013; Regester et al. 2015).

These amphetamine-derived stimulants/hallucinogens, at least β-keto amphetamines and pyrrolidinophenones, are detectable by GC-MS-based untargeted analysis without derivatization (Liu et al. 2018). Dimethoxyphenethylamines (“2C” compounds) including NBOMe are also detectable by GC-MS, even without derivatization (Ketha et al. 2017). These compounds are also detectable by LC-MS(MS) (Glicksberg et al. 2016; Laskowski et al. 2015; Namera et al. 2015).

4.6 Treatment

The mainstay of therapy for stimulant and hallucinogen toxicity is sedation to prevent harm associated with agitation. Early recognition and aggressive response to hyperthermia are critical as hyperthermia is an indicator of severe toxicity (Matsumoto et al. 2014). Treatment should include rapid titration of sedative agents including benzodiazepines and barbiturates to both control agitation as well as prevent potential seizures (Prosser and Nelson 2012). While tachycardia and hypertension are key findings, appropriate sedation will often improve both abnormalities. However, if sedation has been achieved, ancillary treatment of persistent severe tachycardia and/or hypertension with agents including α_1-adrenergic antagonists, α_2-adrenergic agonists, and calcium channel blockers is appropriate. Beta blockers are not recommended in the treatment of patients with acute sympathomimetic toxicity (Richards et al. 2017). Many patients will be volume depleted and require isotonic fluid resuscitation. Assessment of sodium concentration should be performed given the association of hyponatremia with some stimulants. Additionally, the psychomotor agitation often associated with stimulant and hallucinogen toxicity can lead to traumatic injuries and rhabdomyolysis with or without compartment syndrome. Careful examination of muscle compartments and for evidence of trauma is important in the management of agitated patients. While CT scan of the head is not absolutely indicated in all patients with agitated toxic encephalopathy, the threshold should be low given both the risks of trauma as well as the potential for intracranial hemorrhage associated with sudden extreme blood pressure elevation (Lappin et al. 2017). Likewise, cardiac evaluation for ischemia, infarction, and dysrhythmia should be performed. Cocaine, in particular, has sodium and potassium channel-blocking properties that can result in QRS and QT prolongation with ventricular dysrhythmia that can be treated with sodium bicarbonate (Stankowski et al. 2015). In addition to GABA agonist sedation, which may require endotracheal intubation to achieve adequate sedation with airway protection, active cooling measures should be employed for hyperthermic patients. Adjunctive therapy with α_2-adrenergic agonists, e.g., dexmedetomidine, is appropriate for sedation as well as sympatholytic effects (Spiller et al. 2013). Patients with predominantly dopaminergic symptoms, including chorea or tactile hallucinations despite appropriate sedation, can be managed with parenteral antipsychotic agents (Wilson et al. 2012) (Table 2).

5 Dissociative Agents

5.1 Epidemiology

Arylcyclohexylamine derivatives of ketamine and phencyclidine have been used illicitly for decades with street names such as "Special K" and "Angel Dust," respectively. Dextromethorphan use, sometimes called "Robotripping" owing to its inclusion in Robitussin® cough suppressants, has also been common, particularly among adolescents (Morris and Wallach 2014). More recently, novel derivatives in this class have gained popularity including 3-methoxy-phencyclidine (3-MeO-PCP), methoxetamine, and 2-oxo-PCE (eticyclidone). Methoxetamine, in particular, emerged through online sales beginning in 2010 (Corazza et al. 2013).

5.2 Chemistry and Chemical Structures

Arylcyclohexylamine derivatives have a phenylcyclohexylamine skeleton (Fig. 6). Phencyclidine or PCP (contracted from "1-(1-*P*henyl*c*yclohexyl)*p*iperidine") is the prototypal compound in this class (Dove 1984). PCP was synthesized as a general anesthetic by Victor Maddox at Parke-Davis in 1956. Even though PCP was quickly abandoned in the clinical scene because of adverse effects in 1963, various arylcyclohexylamine derivatives have been developed at Parke-Davis. A methoxy group is added to the 3-position of the aromatic ring of PCP in 3-MeO-PCP (3-methoxyl-phencyclidine). The piperidine ring of PCP is substituted with the methylamino group in ketamine. Similarly, the piperidine ring of PCP is substituted with the ethylamino group in N-*e*thyl-1-*p*henyl*c*yclohexylamine (PCE) or eticyclidine. An oxo (or "=O") group is attached to the 2-position of the cyclohexyl ring of PCE in eticyclidone or 2-oxo-PCE. A methoxy group is added to the 3-position of the aromatic ring of PCE in 3-methoxyl-eticyclidine (3-MeO-PCE). A methoxy group is further attached to the 3-position of the aromatic ring of eticyclidone in methoxetamine (MXE) (Morris and Wallach 2014).

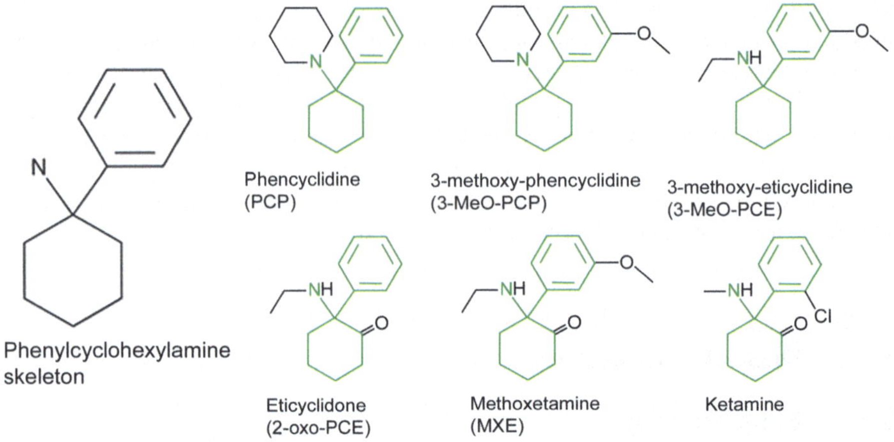

Fig. 6 Chemical structures of arylcyclohexylamines. The phenylcyclohexylamine skeleton is also provided in the figure. The core phenylcyclohexylamine skeleton is also highlighted in each compound in green

5.3 Pharmacology and Physiology Overview

Dissociative agents typically exert their primary pharmacologic effect through blockade of excitatory N-methyl-d-aspartate (NMDA) receptors (Lodge and Mercier 2015). NMDA receptors are stimulated by glutamate and glycine with resulting influx of cations including calcium and sodium (Lakhan et al. 2013). Additional activity as a relatively weak opioid and dopamine receptor agonist has been described as well as effects on serotonergic and noradrenergic pathways (Peltoniemi et al. 2016). The duration of action of phencyclidine and ketamine is relatively brief with a half-life of 2–4 h (Sinner and Graf 2008). However, ketamine and phencyclidine derivative novel psychoactive substances are reported to have longer duration of action than the parent compounds (Corazza et al. 2012). Novel ketamine and phencyclidine derivatives and analogues would be anticipated to share mechanistic function due to class effect, particularly given the reported similarity in clinical syndromes, but dedicated pharmacologic and pharmacokinetic investigation of newly emerging drugs cannot maintain pace with discovery.

5.4 Clinical Effects

Antagonists of the NMDA receptor are promising in the management of a number of acute and chronic conditions. Dissociative agents have been used increasingly for the management of pain, seizures, anesthesia, and alcohol withdrawal (Peltoniemi et al. 2016; Pizon et al. 2018). More recently, there is a growing body of evidence suggesting benefits in the treatment of depression with ketamine and its enantiomer, s-ketamine (Molero et al. 2018). Dextromethorphan, while technically an opioid, is used primarily for its NMDA antagonizing activity (Morris and Wallach 2014). Dissociative symptoms serve as the basis for both desired as well as unintended effects in clinical and recreational use. Despite the common media narrative of severe agitation and superhuman strength associated with use of phencyclidine, the reality is typically much less severe. Clinical effects include a dissociation of thought from the body which can contribute to psychotomimetic effects and the potential for agitation with a detachment of central perception from peripheral pain and action (Morris and Wallach 2014). Additionally, tachycardia, hypertension, catatonia, and nystagmus are hallmark features. A spiritual or "near death" experience is also frequently reported (Corazza et al. 2013).

5.5 Laboratory Detection and Methodology

PCP immunoassays are included as part of routine urine drug screening panels. PCP immunoassays should cross-react with 3-MeO-PCP due to its structural similarity; indeed, the EMIT-II Plus PCP immunoassay exhibits 100% cross-reactivity with 3-Me-PCP (Skaugen et al. 2019). Other arylcyclohexylamine derivatives such as 2-oxo-PCE are not expected to cross-react with PCP immunoassay kits due to the limited structural similarity unless the concentrations of these compounds are very high in the specimen. PCP immunoassays are also known to cross-react various drugs of other classes, such as dextromethorphan, venlafaxine, or tramadol, due to remote structural similarity to PCP (King et al. 2013; Krasowski et al. 2009; Sena et al. 2002).

5.6 Treatment

Toxicity associated with arylcyclohexylamines and related NMDA receptor antagonists is primarily related to the potential for agitation as well as injury associated with dissociative intoxication. Significant cardiovascular toxicity from tachycardia and hypertension as well as seizures have also been reported with the use of newer, more potent analogues (Morris and Wallach 2014). Initial treatment includes providing a safe environment, redirection and reassurance if the patient is demonstrating dysphoric effects, and observation with hydration. However, patients displaying agitation posing a threat to themselves or others should be treated with escalating doses of $GABA_A$ agonists, primarily benzodiazepines (Helander et al. 2015) (Table 2).

6 Sedative-Hypnotics

6.1 Epidemiology

Sedative-hypnotic use and misuse have historically involved prescription pharmaceuticals, e.g., alprazolam, lorazepam, and clonazepam. As opioids have become more tightly regulated and prescribing has declined, prescription alternatives for pain and muscle relaxation have been increasingly utilized with associated rises in misuse and toxicity. Gabapentin and baclofen are commonly used as non-opioid analgesics for neuropathic and musculoskeletal pain. Since 2012, toxicity associated with recreational use of each has accelerated (Shulman et al. 2017). Gabapentin misuse has been estimated as affecting 1% of the population, particularly affecting patients who have an associated opioid use disorder (Smith et al. 2016). At the same time, designer benzodiazepines unavailable for legal prescription or sale in the United States including etizolam and clonazolam, among others, have become increasingly available (Carpenter et al. 2018). Other emerging sedative-hypnotics include phenibut, which is available on the Internet. Phenibut overdose cases have been observed sporadically (Downes et al. 2015; Wong et al. 2015).

6.2 Chemistry and Chemical Structures

γ-aminobutyric acid (GABA) is an inhibitory neurotransmitter in the brain. Most sedative-hypnotics are GABA receptor agonists and/or GABA derivatives. Baclofen, gabapentin, and phenibut (β-phenyl-γ-butyric acid) are all GABA derivatives (Fig. 7). Baclofen was first developed in 1962 by Heinrich Keberle of Ciba in Basel, Switzerland, by adding an aromatic ring to the GABA molecule to increase penetration of the blood-brain barrier (Lapin 2001; Yogeeswari et al. 2006). Similarly, phenibut was developed by Perekalin in Russia in 1964 (Lapin 2001). Gabapentin was developed by adding a cyclohexane ring to GABA molecule at Parke-Davis in 1974 (Satzinger et al. 1975).

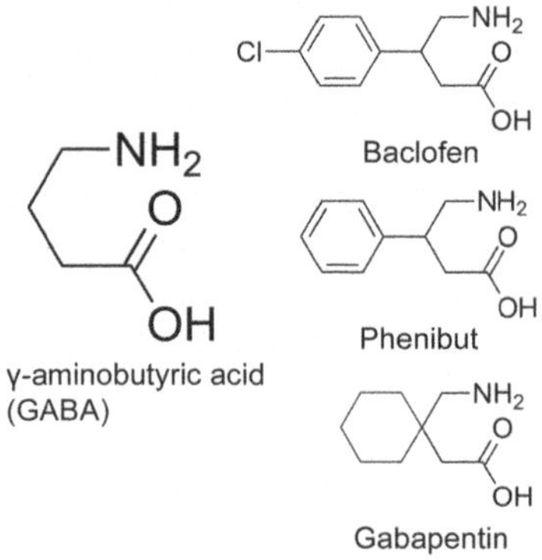

Fig. 7 Chemical structures of γ-aminobutyric acid (GABA) and its derivatives: baclofen, phenibut (β-phenyl-γ-butyric acid), and gabapentin

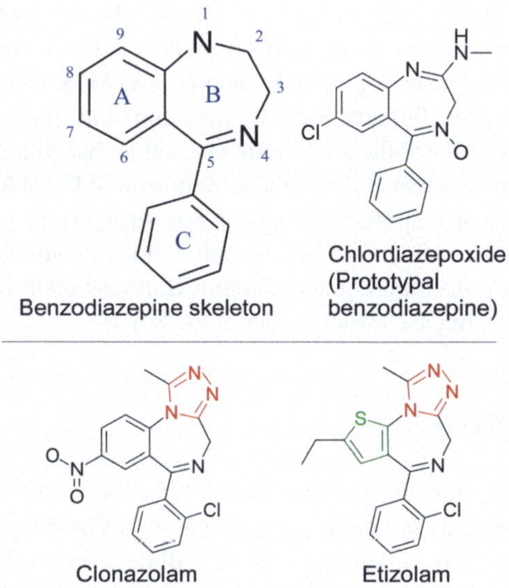

Fig. 8 Chemical structures of benzodiazepines and thienodiazepine. The benzodiazepine skeleton is comprised of the benzene ring (A) fused to a 1,4-diazepine ring (B) and an aryl group (ring C) attached to the 5-position of the diazepine ring (B). A triazole ring (highlighted in red) is fused to the diazepine ring (B) in clonazolam. A thiophene (highlighted in green) substitutes the benzene ring (A), and a triazole ring (highlighted in red) is fused to the diazepine ring (B) in etizolam, one of the thienotriazolodiazepines. The chemical structure of the prototypal benzodiazepine chlordiazepoxide is also shown as a reference in the figure

The prototypal benzodiazepine chlordiazepoxide was first developed in 1960 by Leo Sternbach at Hoffmann-La Roche as a novel synthetic tranquilizer (Sternbach 1979). As the name implies, the benzodiazepine skeleton has a characteristic ring structure with the benzene ring (A) fused to a 1,4-diazepine ring (B). In addition, an aryl group (ring C) is attached to the 5-position of the diazepine ring (B) (Childress and Gluckman 1964) (Fig. 8). Various modifications have been made to develop numerous benzodiazepines. Clonazolam has a triazole ring fused to the 1,4-diazepine ring (B) of the benzodiazepine skeleton. Etizolam also contains a triazole ring fused to the 1,4-diazepine ring (B); however, the diazepine ring is fused to thiophene, not to the benzene ring. That is why it is classified as thienotriazolodiazepine, not benzodiazepine (Tahara et al. 1978).

6.3 Pharmacology and Physiology Overview

Benzodiazepines and other sedative-hypnotics typically act on GABA receptors. From a clinical perspective, the primary GABA receptor subtypes are $GABA_A$ ionotropic and $GABA_B$ metabotropic inhibitory receptors. Each type leads to hyperpolarization, thus causing decreased cellular activity (Jembrek and Vlainic 2015). $GABA_A$ receptor ligands include prescription and designer benzodiazepines, thienotriazolodiazepines, and other sedatives. Both benzodiazepines and thienotriazolodiazepines bind to an allosteric site on the $GABA_A$ receptor; thus, their action depends upon endogenously available GABA (Sanger 2004; Sieghart 2015). $GABA_B$ receptor ligands include baclofen and phenibut among others. $GABA_B$ receptors are distributed on both pre- and postsynaptic membranes and play roles in glutamate release and feedback inhibition of GABA release leading to a heterogeneity of clinical response. Gabapentin is structurally analogous to GABA but does not appear to affect GABA receptors rather inducing sedative effects through the inhibition of voltage-gated calcium channels resulting in reduced excitatory neurotransmitter release (Bockbrader et al. 2010).

6.4 Clinical Effects

As the class name implies, the primary associated clinical effect of sedative use is relaxation, anxiolysis, and sedation, particularly with $GABA_A$ agonists. Typically, individuals suffering $GABA_A$-agonist toxicity will be sedate with relatively minimal effect on heart rate and blood pressure. Airway protective reflexes can be diminished, and reduction in respiratory drive may be observed, especially with concurrent use of another sedative or opioid (Horsfall and Sprague 2017). $GABA_B$-agonist toxicity can be much more diverse. Given the presynaptic distribution of $GABA_B$ receptors with associated inhibition of GABA neurotransmitter release in addition to glutamatergic modulation, $GABA_B$ receptor agonist toxicity may result in sedation, agitation, or an alternating syndrome with both mental states. Additionally, sinus tachycardia, hyperreflexia, and myoclonic jerks may be present unlike with $GABA_A$ toxicity (Schep et al. 2012).

6.5 Laboratory Detection and Methodology

Benzodiazepine immunoassays are included as part of routine urine drug screening panels. Clonazolam and etizolam are moderately detectable by some benzodiazepine immunoassay kits (e.g., CEDIA Benzodiazepine Assay), but these compounds are less detected by other kits (e.g., Syva® EMIT-II Plus Benzodiazepine Assay) (Pettersson Bergstrand et al. 2017; van Wijk et al. 2018). The immunoassays cannot discern designer benzodiazepines/thienodiazepines from prescribed ones because the immunoassays are only capable of screening the presence of multiple compounds within the same class. MS-based assays are required for the identification and confirmation of these compounds, specifically. Indeed, these compounds are successfully identified in serum and urine by LC-high resolution MS (van Wijk et al. 2018).

Regarding the GABA derivatives (baclofen, gabapentin, and phenibut), there are no immunoassays for these compounds commercially available. These compounds are, however, detectable by either GC-MS (Lee et al. 2017; Van Lente and Gatautis 1998) or LC-MS (MS) (Downes et al. 2015; Grinberga et al. 2008; Hou et al. 2014).

Several reference laboratories offer LC-MS(MS)-based quantitative assays for gabapentin and baclofen, but no reference laboratories offer a phenibut assay in the United States (Table 2).

6.6 Treatment

The management of GABA-mediated toxicity is primarily supportive with endotracheal intubation and ventilator therapy for patients who are either unable to protect their airways or who demonstrate evidence of respiratory failure. Flumazenil, a benzodiazepine-specific antagonist on the $GABA_A$ receptor, can be considered in the management of acute sedative-hypnotic toxicity for both therapeutic and diagnostic purposes. Its use is primarily recommended in pediatric populations, patients with isolated benzodiazepine toxicity without known dependence, or those in whom iatrogenic benzodiazepine sedation has resulted in significant adverse effects in order to avoid respiratory complications. However, given the relatively low but real risk of serious adverse events including cardiac dysrhythmias, seizures, agitation associated with abrupt induction of precipitated withdrawal, and/or unmasking of co-occurring stimulant toxicity in contrast to the relatively low risk of toxicity in a medically supervised setting, routine use of flumazenil is not recommended (Penninga et al. 2016).

7 Conclusion

Nonmedical use of medications and illicit drugs represents a critical public health threat worldwide. In the United States, the life expectancy of Americans in 2018 declined due to unintentional overdose and suicide. Overdose deaths have risen substantially in a relatively short period of time and continue to rise each year. In addition to the incredible toll substance use has had on mortality, the overall effect across society is even greater. The nature and prevalence of drugs have evolved over time with a recent acceleration in the variety of chemicals available for use in conjunction with increased ease of access. The result is an incredibly diverse group of novel psychoactive substances derived from traditional categories of drugs which pose significant challenges to healthcare, public health, regulatory, and law enforcement systems. Coordination of these systems built upon accurate identification and surveillance of the rapidly changing environment of drug use is necessary to inform effective and timely therapeutic and policy response to this public health crisis. FDA-cleared immunoassay kits covering these emerging drugs of abuse are required for rapid detection of these drugs in the clinic and hospital (Table 2).

Acknowledgments We are thankful to Jacqueline A. Rymer and Spiros Giannoutsos for their technical assistance in the laboratory.

References

Aizpurua-Olaizola O, Soydaner U, Ozturk E, Schibano D, Simsir Y, Navarro P, Etxebarria N, Usobiaga A (2016) Evolution of the cannabinoid and terpene content during the growth of cannabis sativa plants from different chemotypes. J Nat Prod 79:324–331. https://doi.org/10.1021/acs.jnatprod.5b00949

Andre CM, Hausman JF, Guerriero G (2016) Cannabis sativa: the plant of the thousand and one molecules. Front Plant Sci 7:19. https://doi.org/10.3389/fpls.2016.00019

Arbo MD, Bastos ML, Carmo HF (2012) Piperazine compounds as drugs of abuse. Drug Alcohol Depend 122:174–185. https://doi.org/10.1016/j.drugalcdep.2011.10.007

Armenian P, Vo KT, Barr-Walker J, Lynch KL (2018) Fentanyl, fentanyl analogs and novel synthetic opioids: a comprehensive review. Neuropharmacology 134:121–132. https://doi.org/10.1016/j.neuropharm.2017.10.016

Arntson A, Ofsa B, Lancaster D, Simon JR, McMullin M, Logan B (2013) Validation of a novel immunoassay for the detection of synthetic cannabinoids and metabolites in urine specimens. J Anal Toxicol 37:284–290. https://doi.org/10.1093/jat/bkt024

Auwarter V, Dresen S, Weinmann W, Muller M, Putz M, Ferreiros N (2009) 'Spice' and other herbal blends: harmless incense or cannabinoid designer drugs? J Mass Spectrom 44:832–837. https://doi.org/10.1002/jms.1558

Baldo BA (2018) Opioid analgesic drugs and serotonin toxicity (syndrome): mechanisms, animal models, and links to clinical effects. Arch Toxicol 92:2457–2473. https://doi.org/10.1007/s00204-018-2244-6

Behzadi M, Joukar S, Beik A (2018) Opioids and cardiac arrhythmia: a literature review. Med Princ Pract 27:401–414. https://doi.org/10.1159/000492616

Bockbrader HN, Wesche D, Miller R, Chapel S, Janiczek N, Burger P (2010) A comparison of the pharmacokinetics and pharmacodynamics of pregabalin and gabapentin. Clin Pharmacokinet 49:661–669. https://doi.org/10.2165/11536200-000000000-00000

Boggs DL, Nguyen JD, Morgenson D, Taffe MA, Ranganathan M (2018) Clinical and preclinical evidence for functional interactions of cannabidiol and delta(9)-tetrahydrocannabinol. Neuropsychopharmacology 43:142–154. https://doi.org/10.1038/npp.2017.209

Bonn-Miller MO, Loflin MJE, Thomas BF, Marcu JP, Hyke T, Vandrey R (2017) Labeling accuracy of cannabidiol extracts sold online. JAMA 318:1708–1709. https://doi.org/10.1001/jama.2017.11909

Boom M, Niesters M, Sarton E, Aarts L, Smith TW, Dahan A (2012) Non-analgesic effects of opioids: opioid-induced respiratory depression. Curr Pharm Des 18:5994–6004

Boyer EW (2012) Management of opioid analgesic overdose. N Engl J Med 367:146–155. https://doi.org/10.1056/NEJMra1202561

Brand EJ, Zhao Z (2017) Cannabis in chinese medicine: are some traditional indications referenced in ancient literature related to cannabinoids? Front Pharmacol 8:108. https://doi.org/10.3389/fphar.2017.00108

Brents LK, Prather PL (2014) The K2/spice phenomenon: emergence, identification, legislation and metabolic characterization of synthetic cannabinoids in herbal incense products. Drug Metab Rev 46:72–85. https://doi.org/10.3109/03602532.2013.839700

Brittain RT, Kellett DN, Neat ML, Stables R (1973) Proceedings: anti-nociceptive effects in N-substituted cyclohexylmethylbenzamides. Br J Pharmacol 49:158P–159P

Broseus J, Gentile N, Esseiva P (2016) The cutting of cocaine and heroin: a critical review. Forensic Sci Int 262:73–83. https://doi.org/10.1016/j.forsciint.2016.02.033

Carpenter JE, Murray BP, Dunkley C, Kazzi ZN, Gittinger MH (2018) Designer benzodiazepines: a report of exposures recorded in the National Poison Data System, 2014–2017. Clin Toxicol (Phila) 57(4):282–286. https://doi.org/10.1080/15563650.2018.1510502

Castaneto MS, Gorelick DA, Desrosiers NA, Hartman RL, Pirard S, Huestis MA (2014) Synthetic cannabinoids: epidemiology, pharmacodynamics, and clinical implications. Drug Alcohol Depend 144:12–41. https://doi.org/10.1016/j.drugalcdep.2014.08.005

Cayman Chemical Standardized Naming of Substituted Fentanyls. https://www.caymanchem.com/Literature/standardized-naming-of-substituted-fentanyls. Accessed 4 Dec 2018

Chen P, Braithwaite RA, George C, Hylands PJ, Parkin MC, Smith NW, Kicman AT (2014) The poppy seed defense: a novel solution. Drug Test Anal 6:194–201. https://doi.org/10.1002/dta.1590

Childress SJ, Gluckman MI (1964) 1,4-Benzodiazepines. J Pharm Sci 53:577–590

Corazza O, Schifano F, Simonato P, Fergus S, Assi S, Stair J, Corkery J, Trincas G, Deluca P, Davey Z, Blaszko U, Demetrovics Z, Moskalewicz J, Enea A, di Melchiorre G, Mervo B, di Furia L, Farre M, Flesland L, Pasinetti M, Pezzolesi C, Pisarska A, Shapiro H, Siemann H, Skutle A, Enea A, di Melchiorre G, Sferrazza E, Torrens M, van der Kreeft P, Zummo D, Scherbaum N (2012) Phenomenon of new drugs on the Internet: the case of ketamine derivative methoxetamine. Hum Psychopharmacol 27:145–149. https://doi.org/10.1002/hup.1242

Corazza O, Assi S, Schifano F (2013) From "Special K" to "Special M": the evolution of the recreational use of ketamine and methoxetamine. CNS Neurosci Ther 19:454–460. https://doi.org/10.1111/cns.12063

Daniulaityte R, Juhascik MP, Strayer KE, Sizemore IE, Harshbarger KE, Antonides HM, Carlson RR (2017) Overdose deaths related to fentanyl and its analogs – Ohio, January-February 2017. MMWR Morb Mortal Wkly Rep 66:904–908. https://doi.org/10.15585/mmwr.mm6634a3

Devereaux AL, Mercer SL, Cunningham CW (2018) DARK classics in chemical neuroscience: morphine. ACS Chem Neurosci 9:2395–2407. https://doi.org/10.1021/acschemneuro.8b00150

Dinis-Oliveira RJ (2017) Metabolism of psilocybin and psilocin: clinical and forensic toxicological relevance. Drug Metab Rev 49:84–91. https://doi.org/10.1080/03602532.2016.1278228

Dominguez-Clave E, Soler J, Elices M, Pascual JC, Alvarez E, de la Fuente RM, Friedlander P, Feilding A, Riba J (2016) Ayahuasca: pharmacology, neuroscience and therapeutic potential. Brain Res Bull 126:89–101. https://doi.org/10.1016/j.brainresbull.2016.03.002

Domino EF (2008) Dr. Paul: views through the piperidine ring. Anesth Analg 107:723–724; author reply 724. https://doi.org/10.1213/ane.0b013e31817c737d

Dove HW (1984) Phencyclidine: pharmacologic and clinical review. Psychiatr Med 2:189–209

Downes MA, Berling IL, Mostafa A, Grice J, Roberts MS, Isbister GK (2015) Acute behavioural disturbance associated with phenibut purchased via an internet supplier. Clin Toxicol (Phila) 53:636–638. https://doi.org/10.3109/15563650.2015.1059945

Drug Enforcement Administration (DEA) (2017) 2017 National drug threat assessment. In: U.S. Department of Justice (ed)

Drug Enforcement Administration (DEA) (2018a) 2018 National drug threat assessment. In: U.S. Department of Justice (ed)

Drug Enforcement Administration (DEA) (2018b) Emerging threat report, annual 2017. In: U.S. Department of Justice (ed)

Drug Enforcement Administration (DEA) (2018c) Emerging threat report, mid-year 2018. In: U.S. Department of Justice (ed)

ElSohly MA, Mehmedic Z, Foster S, Gon C, Chandra S, Church JC (2016) Changes in cannabis potency over the last 2 decades (1995-2014): analysis of current data in the United States. Biol Psychiatry 79:613–619. https://doi.org/10.1016/j.biopsych.2016.01.004

European Monitoring Centre for Drugs and Drug Addiction (2009) Understanding the 'Spice' phenomenon. Publications Office of the European Union, Luxembourg

European Monitoring Centre for Drugs and Drug Addiction (2018) Fentanils and synthetic cannabinoids: driving greater complexity into the drug situation. An update from the EU Early Warning System. Publications Office of the European Union, Luxembourg

Florence CS, Zhou C, Luo F, Xu L (2016) The economic burden of prescription opioid overdose, abuse, and dependence in the United States, 2013. Med Care 54:901–906. https://doi.org/10.1097/MLR.0000000000000625

Ford TC, Hayley AC, Downey LA, Parrott AC (2017) Cannabis: an overview of its adverse acute and chronic effects and its implications. Curr Drug Abuse Rev 10:6–18. https://doi.org/10.2174/1874473710666170712113042

Gatch MB, Forster MJ (2018) Cannabinoid-like effects of five novel carboxamide synthetic cannabinoids. Neurotoxicology 70:72–79. https://doi.org/10.1016/j.neuro.2018.11.004

Gendron L, Cahill CM, von Zastrow M, Schiller PW, Pineyro G (2016) Molecular pharmacology of delta-opioid receptors. Pharmacol Rev 68:631–700. https://doi.org/10.1124/pr.114.008979

Genzen JR, Mohlman JS, Lynch JL, Squires MW, Weiss RL (2017) Laboratory-developed tests: a legislative and regulatory review. Clin Chem 63:1575–1584. https://doi.org/10.1373/clinchem.2017.275164

Glicksberg L, Bryand K, Kerrigan S (2016) Identification and quantification of synthetic cathinones in blood and urine using liquid chromatography-quadrupole/time of flight (LC-Q/TOF) mass spectrometry. J Chromatogr B Analyt Technol Biomed Life Sci 1035:91–103. https://doi.org/10.1016/j.jchromb.2016.09.027

Goldberger BA, Darwin WD, Grant TM, Allen AC, Caplan YH, Cone EJ (1993) Measurement of heroin and its metabolites by isotope-dilution electron-impact mass spectrometry. Clin Chem 39:670–675

Goldstein RA, DesLauriers C, Burda AM (2009) Cocaine: history, social implications, and toxicity--a review. Dis Mon 55:6–38. https://doi.org/10.1016/j.disamonth.2008.10.002

Graddy R, Buresh ME, Rastegar DA (2018) New and emerging illicit psychoactive substances. Med Clin North Am 102:697–714. https://doi.org/10.1016/j.mcna.2018.02.010

Grinberga S, Zvejniece L, Liepinsh E, Dambrova M, Pugovics O (2008) Quantitative analysis of phenibut in rat brain tissue extracts by liquid chromatography-tandem mass spectrometry. Biomed Chromatogr 22:1321–1324. https://doi.org/10.1002/bmc.1059

Grotenhermen F (2003) Pharmacokinetics and pharmacodynamics of cannabinoids. Clin Pharmacokinet 42:327–360. https://doi.org/10.2165/00003088-200342040-00003

Guy GP Jr, Zhang K, Bohm MK, Losby J, Lewis B, Young R, Murphy LB, Dowell D (2017) Vital signs: changes in opioid prescribing in the United States, 2006-2015. MMWR Morb Mortal Wkly Rep 66:697–704. https://doi.org/10.15585/mmwr.mm6626a4

Hassamal S, Miotto K, Dale W, Danovitch I (2018) Tramadol: understanding the risk of serotonin syndrome and seizures. Am J Med 131:1382.e1–1382.e6. https://doi.org/10.1016/j.amjmed.2018.04.025

Hedegaard H, Warner M, Minino AM (2017) Drug overdose deaths in the United States, 1999-2016. NCHS Data Brief 294:1–8

Helander A, Beck O, Backberg M (2015) Intoxications by the dissociative new psychoactive substances diphenidine and methoxphenidine. Clin Toxicol (Phila) 53:446–453. https://doi.org/10.3109/15563650.2015.1033630

Hill SL, Dunn M, Cano C, Harnor SJ, Hardcastle IR, Grundlingh J, Dargan PI, Wood DM, Tucker S, Bartram T, Thomas SHL (2018) Human toxicity caused by indole and indazole carboxylate synthetic cannabinoid receptor agonists: from horizon scanning to notification. Clin Chem 64:346–354. https://doi.org/10.1373/clinchem.2017.275867

Horsfall JT, Sprague JE (2017) The pharmacology and toxicology of the 'Holy Trinity'. Basic Clin Pharmacol Toxicol 120:115–119. https://doi.org/10.1111/bcpt.12655

Hou XL, Wu YL, Chen RX, Zhu Y, Lv Y, Xu XQ (2014) Evaluation of two modified quick, easy, cheap, effective, rugged and safe (QuEChERS) sample preparation methods for the analysis of baclofen and gabapentin in feeds by liquid chromatography tandem mass spectrometry. J Pharm Biomed Anal 88:53–59. https://doi.org/10.1016/j.jpba.2013.08.026

Howlett AC, Champion TM, Wilken GH, Mechoulam R (1990) Stereochemical effects of 11-OH-delta 8-tetrahydrocannabinol-dimethylheptyl to inhibit adenylate cyclase and bind to the cannabinoid receptor. Neuropharmacology 29:161–165

Jalal H, Buchanich JM, Roberts MS, Balmert LC, Zhang K, Burke DS (2018) Changing dynamics of the drug overdose epidemic in the United States from 1979 through 2016. Science 361: eaau1184. https://doi.org/10.1126/science.aau1184

Jansen KL, Prast CJ (1988) Ethnopharmacology of kratom and the Mitragyna alkaloids. J Ethnopharmacol 23:115–119

Jembrek MJ, Vlainic J (2015) GABA receptors: pharmacological potential and pitfalls. Curr Pharm Des 21:4943–4959

Jones MR, Viswanath O, Peck J, Kaye AD, Gill JS, Simopoulos TT (2018) A brief history of the opioid epidemic and strategies for pain medicine. Pain Ther 7:13–21. https://doi.org/10.1007/s40122-018-0097-6

Kalix P (1992) Cathinone, a natural amphetamine. Pharmacol Toxicol 70:77–86

Karch SB (2015) Cathinone neurotoxicity ("The 3Ms"). Curr Neuropharmacol 13:21–25. https://doi.org/10.2174/1570159X13666141210225009

Katz KD, Leonetti AL, Bailey BC, Surmaitis RM, Eustice ER, Kacinko S, Wheatley SM (2016) Case series of synthetic cannabinoid intoxication from one toxicology center. West J Emerg Med 17:290–294. https://doi.org/10.5811/westjem.2016.2.29519

Ketha H, Webb M, Clayton L, Li S (2017) Gas chromatography mass spectrometry (GC-MS) for identification of designer stimulants including 2C amines, NBOMe compounds, and cathinones in urine. Curr Protoc Toxicol 74:4.43.1–4.43.10. https://doi.org/10.1002/cptx.33

King AM, Pugh JL, Menke NB, Krasowski MD, Lynch MJ, Pizon AF (2013) Nonfatal tramadol overdose may cause false-positive phencyclidine on Emit-II assay. Am J Emerg Med 31(444): e5–e9. https://doi.org/10.1016/j.ajem.2012.05.028

Knittel JL, Holler JM, Chmiel JD, Vorce SP, Magluilo J Jr, Levine B, Ramos G, Bosy TZ (2016) Analysis of parent synthetic cannabinoids in blood and urinary metabolites by liquid chromatography tandem mass spectrometry. J Anal Toxicol 40:173–186. https://doi.org/10.1093/jat/bkv137

Krasowski MD, Ekins S (2014) Using cheminformatics to predict cross reactivity of "designer drugs" to their currently available immunoassays. J Cheminform 6:22. https://doi.org/10.1186/1758-2946-6-22

Krasowski MD, Pizon AF, Siam MG, Giannoutsos S, Iyer M, Ekins S (2009) Using molecular similarity to highlight the challenges of routine immunoassay-based drug of abuse/toxicology screening in emergency medicine. BMC Emerg Med 9:5. https://doi.org/10.1186/1471-227X-9-5

Kreek MJ, Levran O, Reed B, Schlussman SD, Zhou Y, Butelman ER (2012) Opiate addiction and cocaine addiction: underlying molecular neurobiology and genetics. J Clin Invest 122:3387–3393. https://doi.org/10.1172/JCI60390

Kruegel AC, Grundmann O (2018) The medicinal chemistry and neuropharmacology of kratom: a preliminary discussion of a promising medicinal plant and analysis of its potential for abuse. Neuropharmacology 134:108–120. https://doi.org/10.1016/j.neuropharm.2017.08.026

Kulig K (2017) Interpretation of workplace tests for cannabinoids. J Med Toxicol 13:106–110. https://doi.org/10.1007/s13181-016-0587-z

Lakhan SE, Caro M, Hadzimichalis N (2013) NMDA receptor activity in neuropsychiatric disorders. Front Psychiatry 4:52. https://doi.org/10.3389/fpsyt.2013.00052

Lapin I (2001) Phenibut (beta-phenyl-GABA): a tranquilizer and nootropic drug. CNS Drug Rev 7:471–481

Lappin JM, Darke S, Farrell M (2017) Stroke and methamphetamine use in young adults: a review. J Neurol Neurosurg Psychiatry 88:1079–1091. https://doi.org/10.1136/jnnp-2017-316071

Laskowski LK, Elbakoush F, Calvo J, Exantus-Bernard G, Fong J, Poklis JL, Poklis A, Nelson LS (2015) Evolution of the NBOMes: 25C- and 25B- sold as 25I-NBOMe. J Med Toxicol 11:237–241. https://doi.org/10.1007/s13181-014-0445-9

Law R, Schier J, Martin C, Chang A, Wolkin A, Centers for Disease C (2015) Notes from the field: increase in reported adverse health effects related to synthetic cannabinoid use – United States, January–May 2015. MMWR Morb Mortal Wkly Rep 64:618–619

Lee HZS, Ong MC, Lim JLW, Yap TWA (2017) Challenges in GC-MS analysis: case studies on phenibut and ethylphenidate. Forensic Sci Int 277:166–178. https://doi.org/10.1016/j.forsciint.2017.06.002

Lemberger L, Rowe H (1975) Clinical pharmacology of nabilone, a cannabinol derivative. Clin Pharmacol Ther 18:720–726

Ling GS, Spiegel K, Lockhart SH, Pasternak GW (1985) Separation of opioid analgesia from respiratory depression: evidence for different receptor mechanisms. J Pharmacol Exp Ther 232:149–155

Listos J, Merska A, Fidecka S (2011) Pharmacological activity of salvinorin A, the major component of Salvia divinorum. Pharmacol Rep 63:1305–1309

Litjens RP, Brunt TM (2016) How toxic is ibogaine? Clin Toxicol (Phila) 54:297–302. https://doi.org/10.3109/15563650.2016.1138226

Liu L, Wheeler SE, Venkataramanan R, Rymer JA, Pizon AF, Lynch MJ, Tamama K (2018) Newly emerging drugs of abuse and their detection methods: an ACLPS critical review. Am J Clin Pathol 149:105–116. https://doi.org/10.1093/ajcp/aqx138

Lodge D, Mercier MS (2015) Ketamine and phencyclidine: the good, the bad and the unexpected. Br J Pharmacol 172:4254–4276. https://doi.org/10.1111/bph.13222

Lowe RH, Abraham TT, Darwin WD, Herning R, Cadet JL, Huestis MA (2009) Extended urinary Delta9-tetrahydrocannabinol excretion in chronic cannabis users precludes use as a biomarker of new drug exposure. Drug Alcohol Depend 105:24–32. https://doi.org/10.1016/j.drugalcdep.2009.05.027

Maas A, Madea B, Hess C (2018) Confirmation of recent heroin abuse: accepting the challenge. Drug Test Anal 10:54–71. https://doi.org/10.1002/dta.2244

MacDonald E, Arnesen TM, Brantsaeter AB, Gerlyng P, Grepp M, Hansen BA, Jonsrud K, Lundgren B, Mellegard H, Moller-Stray J, Ronning K, Vestrheim DF, Vold L (2013) Outbreak of wound botulism in people who inject drugs, Norway, October to November 2013. Euro Surveill 18:20630

Macher AM, Penders TM (2013) False-positive phencyclidine immunoassay results caused by 3,4-methylenedioxypyrovalerone (MDPV). Drug Test Anal 5:130–132. https://doi.org/10.1002/dta.1371

Martins SS, Sampson L, Cerda M, Galea S (2015) Worldwide prevalence and trends in unintentional drug overdose: a systematic review of the literature. Am J Public Health 105:e29–e49. https://doi.org/10.2105/AJPH.2015.302843

Matsumoto RR, Seminerio MJ, Turner RC, Robson MJ, Nguyen L, Miller DB, O'Callaghan JP (2014) Methamphetamine-induced toxicity: an updated review on issues related to hyperthermia. Pharmacol Ther 144:28–40. https://doi.org/10.1016/j.pharmthera.2014.05.001

McDonald R, Strang J (2016) Are take-home naloxone programmes effective? Systematic review utilizing application of the Bradford Hill criteria. Addiction 111:1177–1187. https://doi.org/10.1111/add.13326

Mechoulam R (1970) Marihuana chemistry. Science 168:1159–1166

Mechoulam R (2000) Looking back at Cannabis research. Curr Pharm Des 6:1313–1322

Megarbane B, Chevillard L (2013) The large spectrum of pulmonary complications following illicit drug use: features and mechanisms. Chem Biol Interact 206:444–451. https://doi.org/10.1016/j.cbi.2013.10.011

Miliano C, Serpelloni G, Rimondo C, Mereu M, Marti M, De Luca MA (2016) Neuropharmacology of new psychoactive substances (NPS): focus on the rewarding and reinforcing properties of cannabimimetics and amphetamine-like stimulants. Front Neurosci 10:153. https://doi.org/10.3389/fnins.2016.00153

Minami M, Satoh M (1995) Molecular biology of the opioid receptors: structures, functions and distributions. Neurosci Res 23:121–145

Molero P, Ramos-Quiroga JA, Martin-Santos R, Calvo-Sanchez E, Gutierrez-Rojas L, Meana JJ (2018) Antidepressant efficacy and tolerability of ketamine and esketamine: a critical review. CNS Drugs 32:411–420. https://doi.org/10.1007/s40263-018-0519-3

Morris H, Wallach J (2014) From PCP to MXE: a comprehensive review of the non-medical use of dissociative drugs. Drug Test Anal 6:614–632. https://doi.org/10.1002/dta.1620

Mowry JB, Spyker DA, Brooks DE, Zimmerman A, Schauben JL (2016) 2015 annual report of the American Association of Poison Control Centers' national poison data system (NPDS): 33rd annual report. Clin Toxicol (Phila) 54:924–1109. https://doi.org/10.1080/15563650.2016.1245421

Namera A, Kawamura M, Nakamoto A, Saito T, Nagao M (2015) Comprehensive review of the detection methods for synthetic cannabinoids and cathinones. Forensic Toxicol 33:175–194. https://doi.org/10.1007/s11419-015-0270-0

National Academies of Sciences E and Medicine (2017) The health effects of cannabis and cannabinoids: the current state of evidence and recommendations for research. The National Academies Press, Washington

National Institute on Drug Abuse (NIDA) (2018) Overdose death rates. https://www.drugabuse.gov/related-topics/trends-statistics/overdose-death-rates. Accessed 15 Nov 2018

O'Donnell JK, Halpin J, Mattson CL, Goldberger BA, Gladden RM (2017) Deaths involving fentanyl, fentanyl analogs, and U-47700 – 10 states, July-December 2016. MMWR Morb Mortal Wkly Rep 66:1197–1202. https://doi.org/10.15585/mmwr.mm6643e1

Odenwald M, al'Absi M (2017) Khat use and related addiction, mental health and physical disorders: the need to address a growing risk. East Mediterr Health J 23:236–244

Palamar JJ, Martins SS, Su MK, Ompad DC (2015) Self-reported use of novel psychoactive substances in a US nationally representative survey: prevalence, correlates, and a call for new survey methods to prevent underreporting. Drug Alcohol Depend 156:112–119. https://doi.org/10.1016/j.drugalcdep.2015.08.028

Palmateer NE, Hope VD, Roy K, Marongiu A, White JM, Grant KA, Ramsay CN, Goldberg DJ, Ncube F (2013) Infections with spore-forming bacteria in persons who inject drugs, 2000-2009. Emerg Infect Dis 19:29–34. https://doi.org/10.3201/eid1901.120044

Patrick ME, O'Malley PM, Kloska DD, Schulenberg JE, Johnston LD, Miech RA, Bachman JG (2016) Novel psychoactive substance use by US adolescents: characteristics associated with use of synthetic cannabinoids and synthetic cathinones. Drug Alcohol Rev 35:586–590. https://doi.org/10.1111/dar.12372

Peltoniemi MA, Hagelberg NM, Olkkola KT, Saari TI (2016) Ketamine: a review of clinical pharmacokinetics and pharmacodynamics in anesthesia and pain therapy. Clin Pharmacokinet 55:1059–1077. https://doi.org/10.1007/s40262-016-0383-6

Penninga EI, Graudal N, Ladekarl MB, Jurgens G (2016) Adverse events associated with flumazenil treatment for the management of suspected benzodiazepine intoxication – a systematic review with meta-analyses of randomised trials. Basic Clin Pharmacol Toxicol 118:37–44. https://doi.org/10.1111/bcpt.12434

Peters FT, Martinez-Ramirez JA (2010) Analytical toxicology of emerging drugs of abuse. Ther Drug Monit 32:532–539. https://doi.org/10.1097/FTD.0b013e3181f33411

Petrie M, Lynch KL, Ekins S, Chang JS, Goetz RJ, Wu AH, Krasowski MD (2013) Cross-reactivity studies and predictive modeling of "Bath salts" and other amphetamine-type stimulants with amphetamine screening immunoassays. Clin Toxicol (Phila) 51:83–91. https://doi.org/10.3109/15563650.2013.768344

Pettersson Bergstrand M, Helander A, Hansson T, Beck O (2017) Detectability of designer benzodiazepines in CEDIA, EMIT II Plus, HEIA, and KIMS II immunochemical screening assays. Drug Test Anal 9:640–645. https://doi.org/10.1002/dta.2003

Phillips KA, Hirsch GA, Epstein DH, Preston KL (2012) Cardiac complications of unwitting co-injection of quinine/quinidine with heroin in an intravenous drug user. J Gen Intern Med 27:1722–1725. https://doi.org/10.1007/s11606-012-2089-2

Pizon AF, Lynch MJ, Benedict NJ, Yanta JH, Frisch A, Menke NB, Swartzentruber GS, King AM, Abesamis MG, Kane-Gill SL (2018) Adjunct ketamine use in the management of severe ethanol withdrawal. Crit Care Med 46:e768–e771. https://doi.org/10.1097/CCM.0000000000003204

Presley CC, Lindsley CW (2018) DARK classics in chemical neuroscience: opium, a historical perspective. ACS Chem Neurosci 9:2503–2518. https://doi.org/10.1021/acschemneuro.8b00459

Prosser JM, Nelson LS (2012) The toxicology of bath salts: a review of synthetic cathinones. J Med Toxicol 8:33–42. https://doi.org/10.1007/s13181-011-0193-z

Regester LE, Chmiel JD, Holler JM, Vorce SP, Levine B, Bosy TZ (2015) Determination of designer drug cross-reactivity on five commercial immunoassay screening kits. J Anal Toxicol 39:144–151. https://doi.org/10.1093/jat/bku133

Richards JR, Hollander JE, Ramoska EA, Fareed FN, Sand IC, Izquierdo Gomez MM, Lange RA (2017) Beta-blockers, cocaine, and the unopposed alpha-stimulation phenomenon. J Cardiovasc Pharmacol Ther 22:239–249. https://doi.org/10.1177/1074248416681644

Roach JJ, Shenvi RA (2018) A review of salvinorin analogs and their kappa-opioid receptor activity. Bioorg Med Chem Lett 28:1436–1445. https://doi.org/10.1016/j.bmcl.2018.03.029

Rolland B, Jardri R, Amad A, Thomas P, Cottencin O, Bordet R (2014) Pharmacology of hallucinations: several mechanisms for one single symptom? Biomed Res Int 2014:307106. https://doi.org/10.1155/2014/307106

Ruiz-Colon K, Chavez-Arias C, Diaz-Alcala JE, Martinez MA (2014) Xylazine intoxication in humans and its importance as an emerging adulterant in abused drugs: a comprehensive review of the literature. Forensic Sci Int 240:1–8. https://doi.org/10.1016/j.forsciint.2014.03.015

Safer DJ (2016) Recent trends in stimulant usage. J Atten Disord 20:471–477. https://doi.org/10.1177/1087054715605915

Sanger DJ (2004) The pharmacology and mechanisms of action of new generation, non-benzodiazepine hypnotic agents. CNS Drugs 18(Suppl 1):9–15; discussion 41, 43–45. https://doi.org/10.2165/00023210-200418001-00004

Satzinger G, Hartenstein J, Herrmann M, Heldt W (1975) Cyclic amino acids. US4024175A

Scheidweiler KB, Huestis MA (2014) Simultaneous quantification of 20 synthetic cannabinoids and 21 metabolites, and semi-quantification of 12 alkyl hydroxy metabolites in human urine by liquid chromatography-tandem mass spectrometry. J Chromatogr A 1327:105–117. https://doi.org/10.1016/j.chroma.2013.12.067

Schep LJ, Knudsen K, Slaughter RJ, Vale JA, Megarbane B (2012) The clinical toxicology of gamma-hydroxybutyrate, gamma-butyrolactone and 1,4-butanediol. Clin Toxicol (Phila) 50:458–470. https://doi.org/10.3109/15563650.2012.702218

Sena SF, Kazimi S, Wu AH (2002) False-positive phencyclidine immunoassay results caused by venlafaxine and O-desmethylvenlafaxine. Clin Chem 48:676–677

Shang Y, Filizola M (2015) Opioid receptors: structural and mechanistic insights into pharmacology and signaling. Eur J Pharmacol 763:206–213. https://doi.org/10.1016/j.ejphar.2015.05.012

Shulman J, Pizon A, Lynch M (2017) Trends in gabapentin abuse reported to poison centers, 2012-2015 (abstract). Clin Toxicol (Phila) 55:689–868. https://doi.org/10.1080/15563650.2017.1348043

Sieghart W (2015) Allosteric modulation of GABAA receptors via multiple drug-binding sites. Adv Pharmacol 72:53–96. https://doi.org/10.1016/bs.apha.2014.10.002

Simpson D, Braithwaite RA, Jarvie DR, Stewart MJ, Walker S, Watson IW, Widdop B (1997) Screening for drugs of abuse (II): cannabinoids, lysergic acid diethylamide, buprenorphine, methadone, barbiturates, benzodiazepines and other drugs. Ann Clin Biochem 34 (Pt 5):460–510. https://doi.org/10.1177/000456329703400502

Sinner B, Graf BM (2008) Ketamine. Handb Exp Pharmacol 182:313–333. https://doi.org/10.1007/978-3-540-74806-9_15

Skaugen JM, Scoccimarro A, Pizon AF, Rymer JA, Giannoutsos S, Ekins S, Krasowski MD, Tamama K (2019) Novel ketamine analogs cause a false positive phencyclidine immunoassay. Ann Clin Biochem 56:598–607. https://doi.org/10.1177/0004563219858125

Smith JP, Sutcliffe OB, Banks CE (2015) An overview of recent developments in the analytical detection of new psychoactive substances (NPSs). Analyst 140:4932–4948. https://doi.org/10.1039/c5an00797f

Smith RV, Havens JR, Walsh SL (2016) Gabapentin misuse, abuse and diversion: a systematic review. Addiction 111:1160–1174. https://doi.org/10.1111/add.13324

Solimini R, Rotolo MC, Pellegrini M, Minutillo A, Pacifici R, Busardo FP, Zaami S (2017) Adulteration practices of psychoactive illicit drugs: an updated review. Curr Pharm Biotechnol 18:524–530. https://doi.org/10.2174/1389201018666170710184531

Sorensen CJ, DeSanto K, Borgelt L, Phillips KT, Monte AA (2017) Cannabinoid hyperemesis syndrome: diagnosis, pathophysiology, and treatment-a systematic review. J Med Toxicol 13:71–87. https://doi.org/10.1007/s13181-016-0595-z

Spiller HA, Hays HL, Aleguas A Jr (2013) Overdose of drugs for attention-deficit hyperactivity disorder: clinical presentation, mechanisms of toxicity, and management. CNS Drugs 27:531–543. https://doi.org/10.1007/s40263-013-0084-8

Stankowski RV, Kloner RA, Rezkalla SH (2015) Cardiovascular consequences of cocaine use. Trends Cardiovasc Med 25:517–526. https://doi.org/10.1016/j.tcm.2014.12.013

Stanley TH (1992) The history and development of the fentanyl series. J Pain Symptom Manag 7: S3–S7

Stanley TH, Egan TD, Van Aken H (2008) A tribute to Dr. Paul A. J. Janssen: entrepreneur extraordinaire, innovative scientist, and significant contributor to anesthesiology. Anesth Analg 106:451–462, table of contents. https://doi.org/10.1213/ane.0b013e3181605add

Sternbach LH (1979) The benzodiazepine story. J Med Chem 22:1–7

Straseski JA, Stolbach A, Clarke W (2010) Opiate-positive immunoassay screen in a pediatric patient. Clin Chem 56:1220–1223. https://doi.org/10.1373/clinchem.2009.137596

Substance Abuse and Mental Health Services Administration (SAMHSA) (2018) Key substance use and mental health indicators in the United States: results from the 2017 National Survey on Drug Use and Health. In: US Department of Health and Human Services (ed)

Sugiura T, Waku K (2002) Cannabinoid receptors and their endogenous ligands. J Biochem 132:7–12

Suzuki J, Dekker MA, Valenti ES, Arbelo Cruz FA, Correa AM, Poklis JL, Poklis A (2015) Toxicities associated with NBOMe ingestion-a novel class of potent hallucinogens: a review of the literature. Psychosomatics 56:129–139. https://doi.org/10.1016/j.psym.2014.11.002

Szmuszkovicz J (1976) Analgesic n-(2-aminocycloaliphatic)benzamides. US4098904A

Tahara T, Araki K, Shiroki M, Matsuo H, Munakata T (1978) Syntheses and structure-activity relationships of 6-aryl-4H-s-triazolo[3,4-c]thieno[2,3-e] [1,4]diazepines. Arzneimittelforschung 28:1153–1158

Takayama H, Ishikawa H, Kurihara M, Kitajima M, Aimi N, Ponglux D, Koyama F, Matsumoto K, Moriyama T, Yamamoto LT, Watanabe K, Murayama T, Horie S (2002) Studies on the synthesis and opioid agonistic activities of mitragynine-related indole alkaloids: discovery of opioid agonists structurally different from other opioid ligands. J Med Chem 45:1949–1956

United Nations Office for Drug Control and Crime Prevention (UNODCCP) (2001) Drug characterization and impurity profiling – background and concepts. United Nations Publication, New York

Van Lente F, Gatautis V (1998) Cost-efficient use of gas chromatography-mass spectrometry: a "piggyback" method for analysis of gabapentin. Clin Chem 44:2044–2045

van Wijk XMR, Yun C, Hooshfar S, Arens AM, Lung D, Wu AHB, Lynch KL (2018) A liquid-chromatography high-resolution mass spectrometry method for non-FDA approved benzodiazepines. J Anal Toxicol 43:316–320. https://doi.org/10.1093/jat/bky092

Volkow ND, Baler RD, Compton WM, Weiss SR (2014) Adverse health effects of marijuana use. N Engl J Med 370:2219–2227. https://doi.org/10.1056/NEJMra1402309

Vuckovic S, Prostran M, Ivanovic M, Dosen-Micovic L, Todorovic Z, Nesic Z, Stojanovic R, Divac N, Mikovic Z (2009) Fentanyl analogs: structure-activity-relationship study. Curr Med Chem 16:2468–2474

Walley AY, Xuan Z, Hackman HH, Quinn E, Doe-Simkins M, Sorensen-Alawad A, Ruiz S, Ozonoff A (2013) Opioid overdose rates and implementation of overdose education and nasal naloxone distribution in Massachusetts: interrupted time series analysis. BMJ 346:f174. https://doi.org/10.1136/bmj.f174

Webster LR (2015) Opioid-induced constipation. Pain Med 16(Suppl 1):S16–S21. https://doi.org/10.1111/pme.12911

Weinstein AM, Rosca P, Fattore L, London ED (2017) Synthetic cathinone and cannabinoid designer drugs pose a major risk for public health. Front Psych 8:156. https://doi.org/10.3389/fpsyt.2017.00156

Weissman A, Milne GM, Melvin LS Jr (1982) Cannabimimetic activity from CP-47,497, a derivative of 3-phenylcyclohexanol. J Pharmacol Exp Ther 223:516–523

Wermeling DP (2015) Review of naloxone safety for opioid overdose: practical considerations for new technology and expanded public access. Ther Adv Drug Saf 6:20–31. https://doi.org/10.1177/2042098614564776

Wiley JL, Marusich JA, Lefever TW, Antonazzo KR, Wallgren MT, Cortes RA, Patel PR, Grabenauer M, Moore KN, Thomas BF (2015) AB-CHMINACA, AB-PINACA, and FUBIMINA: affinity and potency of novel synthetic cannabinoids in producing delta9-tetrahydrocannabinol-like effects in mice. J Pharmacol Exp Ther 354:328–339. https://doi.org/10.1124/jpet.115.225326

Wilson MP, Pepper D, Currier GW, Holloman GH Jr, Feifel D (2012) The psychopharmacology of agitation: consensus statement of the american association for emergency psychiatry project Beta psychopharmacology workgroup. West J Emerg Med 13:26–34. https://doi.org/10.5811/westjem.2011.9.6866

Wong A, Little M, Caldicott D, Easton C, Andres D, Greene SL (2015) Analytically confirmed recreational use of Phenibut (beta-phenyl-gamma-aminobutyric acid) bought over the internet. Clin Toxicol (Phila) 53:783–784. https://doi.org/10.3109/15563650.2015.1059944

World Health Organization Department of Mental Health and Substance Abuse Management of Substance Abuse Team (NMH/MSD/MSB) Cannabis. https://www.who.int/substance_abuse/facts/cannabis/en/. Accessed 6 June 2019

Yogeeswari P, Ragavendran JV, Sriram D (2006) An update on GABA analogs for CNS drug discovery. Recent Pat CNS Drug Discov 1:113–118

Yuan J, Inami G, Mohle-Boetani J, Vugia DJ (2011) Recurrent wound botulism among injection drug users in California. Clin Infect Dis 52:862–866. https://doi.org/10.1093/cid/cir005

Zhu H, Wu LT (2016) Trends and correlates of cannabis-involved emergency department visits: 2004 to 2011. J Addict Med 10:429–436. https://doi.org/10.1097/ADM.0000000000000256

Zou S, Kumar U (2018) Cannabinoid receptors and the endocannabinoid system: signaling and function in the central nervous system. Int J Mol Sci 19:833. https://doi.org/10.3390/ijms19030833

The manufacturer's authorised representative in the EU is Springer Nature Customer Service Centre GmbH, Europaplatz 3, 69115 Heidelberg, Germany. If you have any concerns regarding our products, please contact ProductSafety@springernature.com

Printed and bound by CPI Group (UK) Ltd, Croydon, CR0 4YY
05/10/2026
02228422-0005